Differential Diagnosis
in Otorhinolaryngology

Differential Diagnosis in Otorhinolaryngology

Symptoms, Syndromes and Interdisciplinary Issues

Hans Heinz Naumann

With contributions by
Frank Martin, Hans Scherer and Karin Schorn

63 illustrations, 193 tables

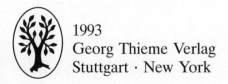

1993
Georg Thieme Verlag
Stuttgart · New York

Thieme Medical Publishers, Inc.
New York

Library of Congress Cataloging-in-Publication Data
Die Deutsche Bibliothek − CIP-Einheitsaufnahme

Naumann, Hans Heinz:
[Differentialdiagnostik in der Hals-Nasen-Ohrenheil-kunde, English]
Differential diagnosis in otorhinolaryngology : symptoms, syndromes, and interdisciplinary issues / Hans Heinz Naumann, with contributions by Frank Martin, Hans Scherer, and Karin Schorn.
Includes bibliographical references and index.
ISBN 3-13-113501-8 (G. Thieme Verlag). −
ISBN 0-86577-507-9 (Thieme Medical Publishers)
1. Otolaryngology−Diagnosis. 2. Diagnosis, Differential.
I. Martin, Frank, Prof. Dr. II. Scherer, Hans.
III. Schorn, Karin. IV. Title.
[DNLM: 1. Otorhinolaryngologic Diseases−diagnosis.
2. Diagnosis, Differential. WV 150 N311d 1993]
RF48.N3813 1993
617.5'1075−dc20
DNLM/DLC
for Library of Congress   93-26903
                                                            CIP

Prof. Dr. Hans Heinz Naumann
Emerit. Direktor der Klinik und Poliklinik für Hals-Nasen-Ohrenkranke (ENT Department) der Universität München
Klinikum Großhadern
Marchioninistraße 15
D-81377 München

Prof. Dr. Frank Martin
Klinik und Poliklinik für Hals-Nasen-Ohrenkranke der Universität München
Klinikum Großhadern
Marchioninistraße 15
D-81377 München

Prof. Dr. Hans Scherer
Direktor der Hals-Nasen-Ohren-Klinik
mit Poliklinik
Klinikum Steglitz der Freien Universität Berlin
Hindenburgdamm 30
D-12203 Berlin

Prof. Dr. Karin Schorn
Klinik und Poliklinik für Hals-Nasen-Ohrenkranke der Universität München
Klinikum Großhadern
Marchioninistraße 15
D-81377 München

This book is an authorized, and updated translation of the German edition published and copyrighted 1990 by Georg Thieme Verlag, Stuttgart, Germany. Title of the German edition:
Differentialdiagnostik in der
Hals-Nasen-Ohren-Heilkunde

Translated by: Terry C. Telger
Illustrated by: Günther Bosch

© 1993 Georg Thieme Verlag, Rüdigerstraße 14,
D-70469 Stuttgart, Germany
Thieme Medical Publishers, Inc.,
381 Park Avenue South, New York, NY 10016
Typesetting by Primustype Hurler,
D-73274 Notzingen
Printed in Germany by K. Grammlich,
D-72124 Pliezhausen

ISBN 3-13-113501-8 (GTV, Stuttgart)
ISBN 0-86577-507-9 (TMP, New York)   1 2 3 4 5 6

Important Note: Medicine is an ever-changing science undergoing continual development. Research and clinical experience are continually expanding our knowledge, in particular our knowledge of proper treatment and drug therapy. Insofar as this book mentions any dosage or application, readers may rest assured that the authors, editors and publishers have made every effort to ensure that such references are in accordance with the state of knowledge at the time of production of the book.
Nevertheless this does not involve, imply, or express any guarantee or responsibility on the part of the publishers in respect of any dosage instructions and forms of application stated in the book. Every user is requested to examine carefully the manufacturers' leaflets accompanying each drug and to check, if necessary in consultation with a physician or specialist, whether the dosage schedules mentioned therein or the contraindications stated by the manufacturers differ from the statements made in the present book. Such examination is particularly important with drugs that are either rarely used or have been newly released on the market. Every dosage schedule or every form of application used is entirely at the user's own risk and responsibility. The authors and publishers request every user to report to the publishers any discrepancies or inaccuracies noticed.

Preface

This reference book is intended primarily to aid the otorhinolaryngologist in making a differential diagnosis. It can also provide a useful source of up-to-date information for colleages in other specialties who deal with symptoms and clinical issues that relate to otorhinolaryngology and allied fields.

The *concept* of the book: The chapters are organized according to symptoms and dieseases occuring in ten different regions of the head and neck. Each of the ten chapters is divided into sections devoted to a particular *main symptom*. Each "symptom" section contains a *synopsis* — a table-like chart in which the disorders associated with the symptom are listed and grouped according to various criteria. The reader who is already an expert in ENT diagnosis can use the synopsis as a „checklist" for relevant disorders to be considered in the evaluation of a particular case. For the less experienced user, the principal disorders are discussed in *brief commentaries*, which either follow the synopsis or appear elsewhere in the book. Generally these commentaries include a description of *main and associated symptoms*, notes on *pathogenesis*, a review of necessary *diagnostic steps*, and a list of *alternatives* to be considered in the differential diagnosis.

Numerous *tables*, easily distinguished visually from the synopses, are included to provide additional useful information.

The schematic *illustrations* further aid differential-diagnostic decision making by providing a quick recapitulation of anatomic and functional relationships.

Many diseases have *more than one* main symptom and so must be considered in the differential diagnosis of various symptoms. To minimize repetitions of text, we generally present *only one* brief commentary for each disorder. To make it easier to *locate the brief commentaries*, the disease names listed in the synoptic tables are followed by a page reference in cases where the associated commentary does not immediately follow the synopsis but is presented elsewhere in the book.

An asterisk (*) after a disease name in the tables indicates that a brief commentary is *not* provided for that disorder. These diseases were listed for the sake of completeness but were not given special commentary because they were considered too banal or too irrelevant for the otorhinolaryngologist.

The reader has *two ways to find detailed information on a particular disease when a symptom is known:*

1. The logical sequence is as follows: region or organ → symptom → synopsis of relevant disorders → brief commentary
2. Information on a particular disorder can be found quickly by referring to the extensive index at the back of the book

Consistent with the purpose of the book, very few authors and references are cited within the actual text. A comprehensive list of cited references and other suggested reading is presented at the end of the book.

I wish to thank Prof. Dr. K. Schorn of Munich, Prof. Dr. F. Martin of Munich, and Prof. Dr. H. Scherer of Berlin for their contributions to the text, which are credited as such and deal with the specialized fields of audiology, phoniatrics, and neurotology. I am grateful to them as well for their ongoing support in the planning and realization of this project.

I thank Prof. Dr. E. Kastenbauer and Prof. Dr. T. P. U. Wustrow, both of Munich, for critically reviewing the manuscript and offering valuable suggestions.

I am grateful to Prof. Dr. O. Braun-Falco, Head of the Dermatology Department at the University of Munich, Dr. T. Ruzicka of Munich, senior staff member of the Dermatology Department, and Prof. Dr. W. Forth, Head of the Walther Straub Institute for Pharmacology and Toxicology of the University of Munich, who checked the timeliness and technical accuracy of text passages relating to their fields of expertise. I also thank Prof. Dr. M. Eder, Head of the Department of Pathology of the University of Munich, for his valuable advice on selected topics in pathologic anatomy.

The idea for this book was suggested some years ago by the publisher, Georg Thieme Verlag. Dr. med. h. c. G. Hauff, Dr. D. Bremkamp, and Mr. A. Menge were constantly available with advice on the publishing aspects of the book and vigorously supported its completion. I gratefully acknowledge their help and that of all those at Thieme Verlag who assisted in the project, including Mr. G. Bosch, who furnished the artwork.

This book is designed to meet the requirements of the practitioner in otorhinolaryngology. Consequently, greater emphasis was placed on a comprehensive scope and a user-friendly format than on completeness of detail. I hope nonetheless that this book will prove to be a valuable resource in the daily practice of many colleagues. I would welcome any suggestions for improvements that may arise from the practical utilization of this book.

Munich, fall, 1993   *H. H. Naumann*

Contents

1. Ear

Differential Diagnosis in General Clinical Otology

The Symptoms

- Otalgia, p. 3
- Dysesthesia, p. 18
- Otorrhea, p. 27
- Tinnitus, p. 92
- Morphologic change (swelling, tumor), p. 27
- Malformation and congenital functional disturbance of the inner ear, p. 32
- Change in the tympanic membrane, p. 34
- Otogenic facial paralysis, p. 36
- Intracranial otogenic complications, p. 40
- Hearing loss, p. 58
- Vertigo, p. 101

Clinical syndromes relating to multiple cranial nerve lesions (Table 1.**18**), p. 48

Common malformation syndromes involving the ear (Table 1.**19**), p. 52

Principal Diagnostic Methods

- *Inspection, palpation* (auricle and surrounding tissues, regional lymph nodes).

- *Otoscopy* (after cleaning of the external auditory canal, surgical cavity, etc.). Some cases warrant use of the *pneumatic otoscope* (of Siegle) with straight or angled *rod or fiber optics* and/or the *otomicroscope*.

- *Audiologic tests,* see p. 55.
- *Vestibular function tests,* see p. 97.
- *Radiographic evaluation* using the *standard projections* of Schüller, Stenvers, E. G. Mayer and the *Tomography* is still in use in some places, but today the *computed tomography* (CT) using various projections and special techniques is the method of choice. *Angiography* (conventional and DSA, superselective angiography, retrograde venography) is particularly useful for evaluating otologic tumors. *Radionuclide studies* are occasionally employed (e.g., for neoplasms and questionable osteomyelitis).

- *Magnetic resonance imaging* (MRI). The indications for this relatively new modality have not yet been fully elucidated for otologic investigations. It definitely improves the diagnosis of acoustic neuroma and other mass lesions involving the petrous pyramid and the rest of the skull base, and it contributes significantly to the detection of inflammatory processes involving the brain and CSF spaces.[*]

---

[*] The rapid evolution of CT and MRI and the resultant advances in diagnostic capabilities are reshaping the indications for the various imaging procedures. Their practical value, however, is partly a matter of availability. Most otorhinolaryngologic disorders can be correctly diagnosed without "high-tech" apparatus. Economy is another concern. This book devotes much space; therefore, to older, proven imaging procedures that are universally available. Where several procedures are mentioned for certain diagnostic inquiries, this is done to acknowledge available alternatives and does not imply that *all* the procedures should be used.

○ *Eustachian tube function* can be tested *qualitatively* by the Valsalva maneuver, politzerization, or eustachian catheterization and *quantitatively* by tympanometry (see p. 57) or measurements of *intratympanic pressure* and *eustachian tube resistance*, which are more technically complex and less often used in the clinical setting.

Symptom   **Otalgia**

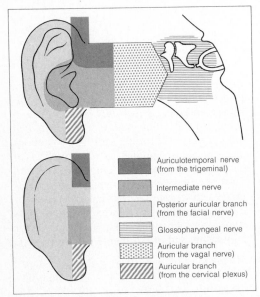

Auriculotemporal nerve (from the trigeminal)

Intermediate nerve

Posterior auricular branch (from the facial nerve)

Glossopharyngeal nerve

Auricular branch (from the vagal nerve)

Auricular branch (from the cervical plexus)

Fig. 1.**1**   Sensory nerve supply of the external ear and tympanic cavity

Although "otalgia" in the strict sense means pain referred to the ear from a distant or regional source (e.g., neuralgia) while "otodynia" denotes pain originating within the ear, this distinction is not consistently followed, and "otalgia" is customarily used to denote all forms of ear pain.

The *character* of otalgia is as variable as its *location* owing to the complex sensory innervation of the ear (Fig. 1.1). This does not apply to the inner ear, which lacks a sensory nerve supply.

External Ear (Auricle and External Auditory Canal)

Injuries of the External Ear

In general, the differential diagnosis of trauma to the external ear is not a problem since the history and findings tend to be obvious. The greatest difficulty is excluding concomitant involvement of the middle or inner ear. If the history is vague or equivocal, one should consider the possibility of deception due to psychosis or criminal intent.

Main symptoms: Typical findings are noted on inspection, palpation, and otoscopy (lacerations, contusions, stab wounds, bites, cuts, or abrasions of the auricle and/or injuries of the meatal soft tissues, the latter usually accompanied by a bloody discharge in the ear canal). Tragal tenderness, painful mastication (proximity of temporomandibular joint [TMJ]) may be present.

Other symptoms and special features: Mechanical obstruction of the external auditory canal (by blood, soft tissues, etc.) may cause hearing loss even if the middle and inner ear are not involved.

Diagnosis:
● Detailed history and documentation of findings (also important for forensic reasons!). Otoscopy (or otomicroscopy) is used to determine the extent of involvement of meatal soft tissues and exclude trauma to the tympanic membrane and middle ear.
● If involvement (fracture) of the temporal bone is suspected: radiographic evaluation

Table 1.**1** *Symptom* Otalgia

Synopsis

External ear (auricle and external auditory canal)

Injuries

Burns and chemical injury

Frostbite

Chondrodermatitis nodularis chronica helicis

Auricular skin diseases, see p. 145

(Herpes) zoster oticus

Perichondritis

Erysipelas

Foreign bodies in the external auditory canal and cerumen impaction, see p. 19

Circumscribed otitis externa (furuncular otitis)

Diffuse otitis externa

Malignant (necrotizing) otitis externa

Bullous (hemorrhagic) otitis externa, see p. 10

Myringitis, see Tab. 1.**10**

Exostoses of the external auditory, canal, see p. 20

Tumors

Middle ear

Injuries

– Traumatic tympanic membrane perforation

– Barotrauma (aerotitis)

Disturbances of eustachian tube ventilation, see p. 21

Acute purulent otitis media

Special forms:

– Otitis media in infants and small children

– Influenzal otitis (acute hemorrhagic otitis media)

– Mucosus otitis

– Hyperacute otitis media

– Swimmer's otitis

– Otitis media in measles and scarlet fever

Mastoiditis

Otogenic facial nerve paralysis, see Table 1.**11**

Petrositis (suppuration of the petrous apex)

Chronic otitis media, see p. 24

Previous middle ear surgery

Tumors

Inner ear and internal auditory canal

Inflammatory processes

Tumors

Neuralgias

Neuralgia of the geniculate ganglion (Hunt syndrome)

– of the auriculotemporal nerve

– of the glossopharyngeal nerve (and the Jacobson nerve), see p. 162

– of the vagus nerve, see p. 163

– of the pterygopalatine ganglion (Sluder syndrome), see p. 162

Vascular anomalies, see Table 2.**10**

Vasomotor headache, see p. 165

Miscellaneous causes of otalgia

Psychogenic otalgia

Pain referred to the ear from surrounding structures

Congenital aural fistula, see p. 32

Periauricular lymphadenitis, see pp. 31 and Table 10.**7**

Temporal arteritis, see p. 167

Temporomandibular joint disease

Myoarthropathies

Dentogenic causes, see p. 158

Diseases of the large salivery glands, see pp. 298 ff.

Pathologic processes in the mouth, nose, paranasal sinuses, pharynx, larynx, or neck

Facial nerve paralysis (nonotogenic), see p. 150

Otogenic intracranial complications, see p. 40

Vertebragenic causes (C0–C3), see p. 393

(Schüller view, possibly Stenvers view; temporal bone, CT scans) to demonstrate fracture lines and clouding or shadowing of the middle ear space, ossicular discontinuity, TMJ fracture, etc. See Table 1.**12.**
● If hearing impairment is present: audiologic status (see p. 55). If vertigo is present: test for nystagmus and vestibular nerve status (see p. 97). Check TMJ function (impaired mastication).

Differential diagnosis must exclude involvement of the middle ear (tympanic membrane rupture, temporal bone fracture), inner ear (windows, longitudinal and transverse pyramidal fractures), and adjacent structures (parotid gland, TMJ).

Burns and Chemical Injuries of the External Ear

Main symptoms: *First degree* burns: erythema of the skin: *second degree* burns: erythema and blistering; *third degree* burns: charring and necrosis. Electrical burns produce "current marks." Pain is initially constant, severe, and burning, later becoming intermittent. Perichondritic irritation is further marked by severe tenderness to pressure and in some cases by the full-blown symptoms of auricular perichondritis (see p. 5).

Causes: Accident or occupational injury (by dry or moist heat, chemical agents, hot metal, electric current, etc.).

Diagnosis does not require detailed description owing to the typical history and local findings. Note, however, that damage apparently confined to the external ear may additionally involve the middle ear (e.g., burns from welding spatter). See p. 8.

Frostbite of the Auricle

Main symptoms: *Acute* frostbite injury: pallor and numbness mainly localized to the auricular margin. Thawing of the affected area is followed by hyperemia and swelling (first degree frostbite), vesiculation (second degree frostbite), or necrotic demarcation (third degree frostbite). The initial numbness is replaced by constant pain, depending on the severity of the frostbite. After acute manifestations subside,

auricular pain may persist, especially in response to temperature changes, and may be accompanied by chronic itching.

Other symptoms and special features: *Chronic state, see p. 18.*

The **diagnosis** is made from the history and local findings.

Chondrodermatitis Nodularis Chronica Helicis

Main symptoms: A solitary, firm, pale livid nodule the size of a rice grain or peppercorn, usually occurring on the superior rim of the auricle in males over 40 years of age and frequently bilateral. The lesion is very tender to pressure and is painful when the patient lies on the ear. Though the nodule itself is harmless, the pain is usually severe enough to necessitate removal.

Diagnosis: Excisional biopsy encompassing the whole lesion (also curative).

Differentiation is required from gouty tophus (biopsy, metabolic tests) and nodulus cutaneus (rare; biopsy shows fascicular fibroma; generally **painless**). Also: pressure sores on the auricle (e.g., in persons who wear headphones or ear plugs at work). Biopsy differentiates the lesion from basal cell carcinoma, early spindle-cell carcinoma, and its occasional precursor, cutaneous horn.

(Herpes) Zoster Oticus

Main symptoms: Onset is marked by intense neuralgiform ear pain involving areas supplied by specific nerves. Rapid formation of clustered vesicles on an erythematous base, present for only a few days and involving the auricle and/or the external ear canal (rarely the tympanic membrane). Severe general malaise with fever.

Other symptoms and special features: Partial or complete facial paralysis in approximately 60% of cases. Possible sensorineural hearing loss ranging to deafness, and/or vestibular dysfunction (approximately 40%) ranging to labyrinthine failure, presenting various combinations and degrees of severity. All age groups are affected, with a definite peak between 40 and 60 years of age.

Cause: Neurotropic reactivation of varicella zoster virus.

Diagnosis:
● The causative organism can sometimes be recovered from the contents of the vesicles. Currently available virologic (serologic) test methods are not yet reliable enough.
● Function testing, especially of cranial nerves VII, VIII, IX, and X when zoster oticus is suspected (may require serial testing at frequent intervals).
● In patients with meningitic or premeningitic symptoms: CSF examination (pressure elevation, increased protein, and cellularity) (see Table 1.**15**).

Differentiation is required from diffuse otitis externa and "idiopathic" facial nerve paralysis (absence of vesicles and malaise, generally little or no pain). Also from statoacoustic nerve disorders of other cause (see p. 103 ff.) and from influenzal otitis.

Auricular Perichondritis

Main symptoms: Extreme tenderness on pressure of affected cartilage areas; circumscribed redness and doughy thickening of the overlying skin, later affecting a larger area and progressing to a pad-like swelling chiefly affecting the *anterior side* of the auricle. With onset of cartilage necrosis, balloon-like deformity of the auricle with subcutaneous fluctuation. Eventual breakthrough of pus with a draining fistula. Usually the tragus is tender to pressure!

Other symptoms and special features: Severe malaise, at least in the acute stage. Temperature elevation, left shift in WBC, elevated ESR.

Cause: Bacterial infection of the nutrient perichondrium.

Diagnosis:
● Locate the portal of entry for the infection (microtrauma, gross trauma, mechanical damage to the auricle, prior ear surgery, etc.). Bacteriologic examination of drainage or aspirate (usually demonstrates staphylococci, sometimes *Pseudomonas* or other "problem organisms"); antibiotic sensitivity testing.
● Otoscopy and radiographs (Schüller view: mastoid, zygomatic process) to exclude middle ear disease.

Differentiation is required from erysipelas of the external ear, which also affects the earlobe (rarely involved by perichondritis).

Recurring bouts of perichondritis can produce "cauliflower ear" deformity with gross thickening and coarsening of the cartilage skeleton giving the ear a hard rubbery consistency. The loss of elasticity predisposes the auricle(s) to mechanical irritation and pain.

Auricular Erysipelas

Main symptoms: Swelling, tension, and redness of the auricular skin. The erythematous area is sharply demarcated, and the skin appears glossy. The area of involvement generally includes the earlobe. There is moderate pain or only a sensation of fullness and heat, possibly with itching. Rapid spread of cutaneous manifestations.

Other symptoms and special features: Fever, often commencing with chills. Involvement or regional lymph nodes.

Cause: Streptococcal organisms, which mainly attack the cutaneous lymphatics through small epidermal defects.

Diagnosis: The clinical picture is very characteristic. Identification of the causative organism is problematic, and in doubtful cases a presumptive diagnosis must be made empirically based on rapid response to antibiotic therapy. See also p. 173.

Differentiation is required from perichondritis, erysipeloid (slower progression, vesiculation, no fever), and (herpes) zoster oticus.

Foreign Bodies in the External Auditory Canal
See p. 19.

Cerumen Impaction
See p. 19.

Circumscribed Otitis Externa (Furunculosis of the External Auditory Canal)

Main symptoms: Traction on the auricle and pressure on the tragus are painful, as is mastication. Pain may be throbbing and often radiates through the entire side of the head. Occasional fever and severe malaise.

Other symptoms and special features. Hearing loss occurs when there is luminal obstruction of the external auditory canal. A furuncle on the posterior or superior canal wall can produce swelling in the retroauricular crease; an anterior wall lesion can cause preauricular swelling extending to the eye. Other features: swollen and painful regional lymph nodes (anterior to the tragus, behind the ear ["pseudomastoiditis"], below the auricular base), occasionally with liquefying lymphadenitis. Left shift in differential blood count and elevated ESR.

Cause: Staphylococcal infection secondary to microtrauma ("cleaning") of the external ear canal.

Diagnosis:
• Inspection, palpation (tragal tenderness).
• Otoscopy shows variable ear canal obstruction by red and swollen soft tissues. Furuncles form only at sites where the skin of the external canal bears hairs or hair appendages. Central necrosis is often apparent. Opening the furuncle releases a purulent discharge into the ear canal. Lesions may be multifocal!
• Bacteriologic smear and sensitivity testing. Exclusion of individual disposition (proneness to general furunculosis; diabetes; occupational situation, e.g., a dusty work environment).
• Auditory tests in patients with hearing loss.
• In doubtful cases, Schüller radiograph or CT (to evaluate the mastoid air cells).

Conditions requiring **differentiation:** See Table 1.2.

Diffuse Otitis Externa

Main symptoms: Tragal tenderness; diffuse swelling of the skin of the external auditory canal, occasionally with complete luminal obstruction (hearing loss).

Other symptoms and special features: Depending on the cause: purulent discharge or scaling and/or crusting of the skin ("wet" or "dry" otitis externa). Symptoms are highly diverse. Typical course is chronic and relapsing and is often bilateral with involvement transcending the ear canal. Stages may be characterized as "quiescent," "dry," "exacerbated," or "wet." Diffuse ear pain, if present, is generally confined to the wet stages. "Dry" stages are often associated with intense pruritus.

Causes: A basic distinction is drawn between otitis externa having an *eczematous* cause (microbial eczema, contact eczema, seborrheic eczema, atopic eczema) and noneczematous forms. External otitis also may be classified by etioliogic agent as *bacterial* (due to staphylococci, *Proteus, Pseudomonas,* or other "problem organisms"), *virogenic, mycogenic* (see. p. 20), or mixed. Exogenous skin damage (chlorinated pool water, dusty work environment, chemical agents, medications, purulent middle ear discharge, etc.), endogenous factors (metabolic disorders, especially diabetes), and local conditions (exostoses) may have causal significance.

Diagnosis:
• A detailed recent and long-term history are essential. A protracted, relapsing course suggests an eczematous base, fungal infection, or an occupational or "endogenous" disposition. Differential diagnosis can be extremely difficult and may ultimately prove unsuccessful!
• Otoscopy may show a swollen, red, moist, macerated ear canal with a fetid, sticky discharge, or it may show a dry and perhaps scaly canal whose skin may be thin and "atrophic" or thick and puffy. Stenosis of the ear canal is a common finding. Generally the tympanic membrane is intact in episodic otitis externa. Diffuse external otitis may develop as a sequel to acute or chronic suppurative otitis media; corresponding tympanic membrane changes are evident on otoscopy. Slight redness of the tympanic membrane does not necessarily signify middle ear involvement (audiologic tests!).
• Bacteriologic and mycologic smears from the external auditory canal.
• A prolonged, recurrent, refractory course warrants dermatologic consultation to evaluate for eczema and/or examination by an inter-

Table 1.2   Differentiating features of diffuse otitis externa, acute otitis media, and chronic otitis media

Symptom	Diffuse otitis externa	Acute otitis media	Chronic otitis media with mucosal suppuration	Chronic otitis media with bony suppuration
Otalgia	Tragel tenderness; possible persistent earache or intense itching	Severe pain that may throb with the pulse; subsides with the onset of otorrhea	Generally no pain (except with acute exacerbation)	Generally no pain, but there my be a sensation of pressure. Pain heralds incipient complication
Discharge	Greasy or watery, usually scant with little odor	Profuse, creamy, purulent discharge follows tympanic membrane perforation, odorless, gradually increasing in consistency and viscocity	Stretchy, mucopurulent discharge with little odor, alternating moist and dry phases	Greasy, gritty, very fetid discharge of variable quantity; dry phases may occur
Tympanic membrane findings	Pale, normal	Thickened, reddened, sometimes bulging; with spontaneous perforation; very small rent with pulsating purulent discharge	Central perforation or total defect	Marginal perforation
Hearing	Unaffected except with total obstruction of the auditory canal	Severe (conductive) hearing loss	(Conductive) hearing loss depending on tympanic membrane perforation and middle ear status	Conductive or combined hearing loss, depending on damage to middle ear
Radiograph of mastoid process (Schüller)	Normally aerated air cell system in the mastoid process	Clouding or shadowing of the mastoid air cells	Pneumatization usually absent or deficient	Pneumatization usually absent or deficient; visible bone defect may be present

nist to exclude diabetes and other predisposing factors.

Differentiation is required from a general eczematous disposition, early furuncular otitis, otomycosis (wet and dry!), otitis media, and possibly erysipelas. See Table 1.2.

Malignant (Necrotizing) Otitis Externa

Main symptoms: Lancinating ear pain of increasing severity. Aural discharge usually emanates from a granulating area on the floor of the external auditory canal. Characteristic fistula formation at the junction of the cartilaginous and bony external canal or closer to the tympanic membrane.

Other symptoms and special features: Diabetics are predisposed. *Pseudomonas aeruginosa* is recovered in virtually all cases. Infection spreads to produce cranial nerve deficits, first affecting the facial nerve then the nerves of the posterior group. Males over 50 years of age are chiefly affected.

Causes: Slowly progressive inflammation of soft tissues and bone in the region of the petrous pyramid and neighboring structures with abscess formation, osteonecrosis, and involvement of vital structures (venous sinuses, nerves, bone). Middle and inner ear involvement is possible in the late stage! Abscess formation may penetrate toward the pharynx (retropharyngeal abscess, see p. 266).

Diagnosis:
● Otoscopy (granulating inflammation in the external ear canal).
● Histologic examination of the granulation tissue (to exclude malignancy).
● Bacteriologic smear (multiple smears may be needed for identification of *Pseudomonas*), antibiotic sensitivity tests. Metabolic status (diabetes).
● Complete cranial nerve status (repeated tests may be required).
● Temporal bone radiographs especially high-resolution CT scans (to detect osteomyelitic foci). MRI (to evaluate soft tissues at the inferior surface of the skull base). Additionally radionuclide bone scans of the petrous pyramid and the rest of the middle skull base (serial, to detect areas of bone resorptive activity).

Differentiation is required from a malignant tumor of the external auditory canal, petrous pyramid, or skull base (biopsy), extension of an atypical chronic otitis media, tertiary syphilis, and extension of suppurative parotitis to the external auditory canal.

Bullous (Hemorrhagic) Otitis Externa
See p. 10.

Myringitis
See Table 1.**10.**

Exostoses of the External Auditory Canal
See p. 20.

Tumors of the External Ear

Malignant and even ulcerating tumors of the *auricle* (basal cell carcinoma, squamous cell carcinoma, melanoma, etc.) rarely cause ear pain in their initial stage. This also applies to a small percentage of malignant tumors arising within the *external auditory canal*. Most tumors of the external canal are associated with potentially severe pain, especially in the advanced stage. (See p. 31 for further details.)

Middle Ear

Injuries

Acute trauma to the middle ear causes an immediate, severe otalgia whose intensity diminishes rapidly with time, even if the effects of the trauma have not been corrected or resolved.

Traumatic Perforations of the Tympanic Membrane

This is the most common type of middle ear injury.

Main symptoms (with a previously intact tympanic membrane): Very severe pain at the moment of injury, gradually diminishing thereafter. Tinnitus (rushing, ringing, or pure tone) is a frequent accompaniment beginning immediately with the trauma and continuing. Fresh tympanic membrane perforations are visible on otoscopy.

Other symptoms and special features: Rarely there is (slight) bleeding from the external auditory canal. Conductive hearing loss. Some membrane ruptures are accompanied by ossicular disarticulation, rupture of an inner ear window, and/or a laterobasal fracture (see pp. 39, 40, 63).

Causes: Occupational, athletic, or traffic injuries, which may involve trauma to the ear canal, tympanic membrane, and/or tympanic cavity with or without foreign bodies (e.g., wood splinters, grain fibers, straw, welding spatter, etc.). Many perforations are self-inflicted (cleaning instrument, knitting needle, etc.) or iatrogenic (by instruments). Others are caused by the action of high pressure (explosion, blow to the ear, platform diving, underwater diving, etc.) (see p. 58ff.) or by barotrauma (see below and p. 64).

Diagnosis:
● Recent history. Otoscopy reveals tympanic membrane perforation with jagged edges and fresh blood on and in the drumhead. Bleeding is seldom profuse. Foreign bodies or foreign material may be found near the perforation in the external canal or tympanic cavity. Optical magnification (magnifying otoscope or otomicroscope) is advised! Precise documentation of local findings (also necessary on forensic grounds).
● If injury by welding spatter is suspected, obtain a Schüller radiograph and/or CT to locate the metallic foreign body in the middle ear.
● Audiologic testing (conductive hearing loss is typical but depends on the severity of the trauma!), see p. 58ff. Exclude vestibular irritation or dysfunction (nystagmus), see p. 107.
● When tympanic membrane rupture is part of a severe head injury, perform a thorough otologic–traumatologic workup (and documentation!) including CT and a neurologic and/or neurosurgical evaluation.

Differentiation is required from an isolated injury of the external auditory canal. Exclude concomitant trauma to the inner ear, TMJ, facial nerve, ossicular chain (discontinuity), and temporal bone (fracture).

Barotrauma of the Middle (Aerotitis, Barotitis)

Main symptoms: Acute, severe pain in the ear, sudden hearing loss, pulsatile tinnitus.

Other symptoms and special features: Balance disturbances, possible bleeding into the tympanic membrane, hemotympanum. Rupture of the tympanic membrane is *not* generally present!

Causes: Eustachian tube dysfunction due to a sudden, large pressure difference between the environment and the middle ear space. Most common during rapid descent (flying, diving).

Diagnosis:
● Typical history. Otoscopy: thickened and possibly hemorrhagic tympanic membrane and/or hematotympanum.
● Audiologic tests (findings depend on severity of trauma, see p. 58ff.).
● Endoscopic examination of the nose and nasopharynx to exclude mechanical obstruction of eustachian tube ventilation.
● With a suspected *rupture of the round window membrane* (see p. 63): exploratory paracentaris.

Differentiation is required from sudden deafness (see p. 72), acute suppurative otitis media, and "swimmer's ear" (see p. 11).

Disturbances of Eustachian Tube Ventilation

See pp. 21 and 73.

Acute Suppurative Otitis Media

Main symptoms: Onset (1–2 days) marked by increasingly severe lancinating or throbbing otalgia; hearing loss; (pulsatile) tinnitus (hissing, rushing); typical changes in the tympanic membrane (see below).

Other symptoms and special features: (Severe) malaise and fever, which may be high in children (who may have initial chills). Purulent otorrhea, usually profuse, follows in 3–8 days (due to spontaneous tympanic membrane perforation or tympanocentesis), with lessening of pain. Most cases undergo full recovery in 3–4 weeks. Prompt initiation of antibiotics significantly improves symptoms and shortens the course while preventing tympanic membrane perforation and otorrhea. See also p. 24.

Causes: Usually tubogenic, less commonly hematogenous or posttraumatic infection of the middle ear space (90% rate of monomicrobial infection by streptococci, pneumococci, *Haemophilus influenzae*, staphylococci, etc.). Some cases result from viral infection, usually followed by a bacterial superinfection.

Diagnosis:
● Otoscopic findings vary with the stage of disease: "injected drum"; hyperemia involving part and then all of the tympanic membrane;

progressive bulging and effacement of membrane landmarks; congested ear drum; possible nipple formation; drumhead opacity with scaly deposits or vesicles. Later: bulging regresses due to spontaneous perforation (usually very small and emitting a pulsatile discharge) or paracentesis. As discharge subsides the membrane becomes less opaque, "cleaning of drum heads" and the perforation heals by scarring.
● When discharge is present: bacteriologic smear and sensitivity studies.
● Serial audiologic tests.
● With a suspected atypical course (incipient complications, presence of a "special form" [see below]): Schüller radiographs, or CT.

Differentiation is required from otitis externa, see Table 1.**2.**

Special Forms of Acute Suppurative Otitis Media:

Otitis Media in Infants and Small Children

Main symptoms: *Severe* systemic illness. High fever (sometimes with an undulant pattern), often accompanied by dyspepsia, irritability, and crying. "Ear tugging" and burrowing the head in the pillow are helpful local signs. Spontaneous tympanic membrane perforation is rare. Spread of inflammation to adjacent tissues is relatively common and leads rapidly to swelling and discharge behind, in front of, or above the auricular base. In cases treated with antibiotics or in infections of low virulence, the disease may take a protracted, relapsing, or "undulating" course lasting 6−8 weeks or longer!

Diagnosis:
● Otoscopy: The tympanic membrane can be *very* difficult to evaluate in small children due the oblique, slit-like lumen of the external auditory canal. Also, marked redness may be absent or equivocal because of hyperemia due to crying. Use a *small* ear speculum even if it is inconvenient for optical magnification (otoscope or otomicroscope). Watch for periauricular lymph node swelling.
● Exploratory tympanocentesis.
● With otorrhea: bacteriologic smear and sensitivity testing (*H. influenzae* and *E. coli* are more common in infantile than adult cases). Incidence of complications is particularly high in small children!
● Pediatric consultation may be advised.

Differentiation is required from otitis externa and systemic infections (early-stage acute exanthema, infectious nutritional deficit, etc.).

Influenzal Otitis (Acute Hemorrhagic Otitis Media)

Main symptoms: Severe to excruciating otalgia. Formation of blood blisters in the external auditory canal, on the tympanic membrane, and/or in the middle ear mucosa (not visible otoscopically but responsible for the occasionally severe middle ear symptoms). Inner ear symptoms (cochlear and/or vestibular nerve involvement) may occur. Severe systemic signs. Paracentesis releases a pink, serous discharge, later (within days) becoming thicker and purulent. Frequent otogenic complications! See p. 105.

Causes: Infection with influenza virus A, B, or C. Increased capillary fragility.

Diagnosis:
● Otoscopy: Blood blisters in the external canal and/or on the tympanic membrane.
● With statoacoustic nerve symptoms: Audiologic and neuro-otologic status.
● Notation of other symptoms of true viral influenza (see p. 183).
● Immunologic and serologic detection of influenza viruses.

Mucosus Otitis (Subacute Otitis Media)

Main symptoms: Otitis media with mild symptoms and a protracted course.

Other symptoms and special features: Mild local complaints (fullness, slight earache). Otoscopy shows a pale, thickened, doughy, and/or flaky tympanic membrane. Children predominate. Frequent complications.

Causes: Infection with type III *Pneumococcus mucosus* or occasionally with streptococci, other pneumococci, etc. Proliferating mucosal inflammation in the tympanic cavity; gradual bone resorption with complications supervening. An insidious "masked" course can follow inadequate antibiotic treatment or chemotherapy.

Diagnosis:
● Long history of vague middle ear symptoms. Otoscopic findings (see above). After weeks or months of low-grade symptoms, very severe complications (mastoiditis, labyrinthitis, meningitis, etc.) can arise in a setting of apparent good health.
● If mucosus otitis is suspected, an attempt should be made to identify the causal organism, and serial radiographs (Schüller or CT) should be taken at frequent intervals.

Hyperacute Otitis Media

Generally rare but fulminating form that mainly affects children. Symptoms are *extremely severe:* initial chills followed by high fever; very severe otalgia, sometimes accompanied by signs of meningeal irritation and cerebral signs such as vomiting, convulsions, and somnolence. Otoscopic features are typical of acute otitis media (see above). After spontaneous perforation or tympanocentesis, the dramatic symptoms subside and the disease takes a "normal" course.

Swimmer's Otitis ("Swimmer's Ear")

Main symptoms: Severe, unilateral or bilateral earache occurring a few hours after swimming, with typical otoscopic features of acute otitis media.

Cause: Probably a tubogenic infection by virulent organisms present in the water.

Differentiation is required from otitis externa developing within a short time after swimming (see Table 1.2).

Otitis Media in Measles and Scarlet Fever

These infectious diseases may be associated with an otitis media whose symptoms are indistinguishable from simple acute otitis media, but rarely there are differentiating features: *Measles* is occasionally associated with multiple persistent tympanic membrane perfora-

tions. In *scarlet fever* (which has become very rare), there may be a necrotizing otitis media with a subtotal or total defect in the tympanic membrane and expulsion of bony sequestra from the petrous pyramid (sequestrating osteomyelitis).

In both types of infection there may be a high rate of otogenic complications arising from middle ear disease.

Mastoiditis

Main symptoms: Tender, doughy swelling and redness over the mastoid plane, prominence of the auricle, purulent otorrhea, progressive hearing loss. Mastoiditis is the most common otogenic complication.

Other symptoms and special features: Onset usually occurs in the "resolution stage" of acute otitis media (3rd–4th week) with a resurgence of fever (in some cases), throbbing earache, increasing (purulent, nonfetid) otorrhea, and possibly increased malaise. Laboratory tests show leukocytosis with a left shift and a markedly elevated ESR. The main symptoms progress, culminating in discharge of pus to the outside and the formation of a subperiosteal abscess on the mastoid plane (other typical routes for extension of infection are noted below).

"Initial tenderness" over the mastoid on the 1st–4th day of acute otitis media is not clinically important (irritative symptom) and should not be confused with *tenderness after 3–4 weeks' illness signifying the liquefaction of bone!* On the other hand, a "masked" mastoiditis, mostly due to insufficient antibiotic treatment, may not become clinically apparent for several months.

Causes: Increasing osteitic destruction of the petrous air cell system (most common site is the mastoid; other sites of liquefaction and extension are noted below). Mastoiditis is generally secondary to an acute otitis media; chronic cases may rarely develop as a complication of chronic otitis media.

Diagnosis:
● Very thorough otologic history, typical local findings (see above). Otoscopy: Tympanic membrane thickened and hyperemic, usually

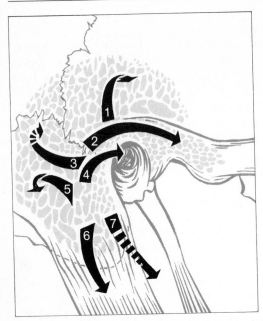

Fig. 1.**2** Potential routes for spread of infection in mastoiditis

1 Toward the temporal squama and middle cranial fossa
2 Toward the zygomatic arch (zygomaticitis)
3 Toward the sigmoid sinus and posterior cranial fossa
4 Toward the external auditory canal (sagging of the posterosuperior canal wall)
5 Toward the mastoid plane (subperiosteal abscess)
6 Toward the tip of the mastoid and the attachment of the sternocleidomastoid muscle (Bezold mastoiditis)
7 Toward the medial surface of the mastoid (Mouret mastoiditis, parapharyngeal abscess)
(See also Fig. 1.**5**)

with a copious, creamy, purulent, *nonfetid* discharge. Audiologic evaluation (conductive hearing loss).
● Radiographs (Schüller or CT): After initial clouding, films show progressive shadowing of the air cell system of the mastoid process and increasing destruction of intracellular partitions. Suspected early mastoiditis warrants serial radiographs at 4- to 8-day intervals, depending on symptoms.

Differentiation (Table 1.**3**) is required from furuncular otitis externa, pseudomastoiditis

(periauricular lymphadenitis, as in pediculosis capitis [result of scratching]). Parotid disease. Gouty tophi.

Other Common Routes for the Extension of Infection in Mastoiditis

(Fig. 1.**2**)

Breakthrough into the External Auditory Canal

Sagging of the posterior (superior) canal wall (otoscopy). Differentiation is required from furunculosis of the external auditory canal (see Table 1.**3**).

Zygomaticitis

Osteitic liquefaction in the air cells and root of the zygomatic arch. May lead to collateral involvement of the TMJ ("otogenic arthritis"). The swelling anterior to the ear may extend to the lateral orbital region.

Extension to the Temporal Squama

With a heavily pneumatized petrous squama, infection can spread above the auricular attachment causing *downward displacement* of the prominent auricle.

Extension to the Occiput (Citelli Abscess)

Swelling with abscess formation between the mastoid and occiput or back of the neck (gravitation abscess!) Very rare.

Extension to the Tip or Medial Wall of the Mastoid: Bezold Mastoiditis

Gravitational settling of the mastoid abscess to the attachment of the sternocleidomastoid muscle leads to a typical guarded head posture in which the head is tilted toward the affected side ("otogenic" wryneck, see Table 10.**11**). Pus tracking downward from the medial surface of the sternocleidomastoid muscle produces Mouret mastoiditis with deep cervical cellulitis or extension into the parapharyngeal space (see p. 265, 266 and Fig. 4.**2a**).

Table 1.3 Differential diagnosis of retroauricular swelling

Clinical symptoms	Furuncle of the external auditory canal	Mastoiditis	"Pseudomastoiditis" (periauricular lymphadenitis)	Erysipelas
History	Very short	3 weeks or longer	Very short	Very short
Fever	Possible	Usually high fever	–	Precipitously high fever
Pain	Very severe and continuous, intensified by chewing. Tragal tenderness	Gradually increasing, throbbing pain. Tenderness over the mastoid plane	Retroauricular tenderness	Feeling of tension. No pain
Redness and swelling	Ear canal red and swollen; possible circumscribed, conical swelling. Swelling behind the retroauricular crease	Broad area of redness and swelling over the mastoid plane	Redness and swelling in the area of the retroauricular crease	Diffuse but sharply demarcated redness and firm swelling affecting the entire auricle and possibly the external auditory canal
Involvement of the external auditory canal	Inevitable; significant narrowing	Relatively uncommon	–	Occasional
Discharge from the ear canal	Sparse, brief, late	Copious, watery, persistent, often pulsatile	–	–
Tympanic membrane	Normal	Reddened, thickened, very often perforated	Normal	Normal
Hearing	Not affected (except with auditory canal occlusion)	Severely impaired	Not affected	Not affected
Regional lymph nodes	Usually involved	Not involved	Involved	Involved

Extension to the Posterior or Middle Cranial Fossa

Marked by typical symptoms of an otogenic intracranialcomplication (see p. 40 and Fig. 1.5).

"Recurrent" Mastoiditis

A tender, erythematous swelling develops rapidly in the area of the retroauricular scar left by a previous mastoidectomy (may occur years after surgery). Usually there is rapid fluctuation, often commencing in the lower half of the scar. The diagnosis is easily made from the history (prior surgery), the presence of a retroauricular scar, and local findings.

The **diagnostic workup** is essentially the same as for "classic" mastoiditis but is adapted to the modified local symptoms.

Mastoiditis in Infants

Main symptoms:
a) *Overt form:* redness, retroauricular swelling, and abscess formation occur *very rapidly* (usually with 1 week) after the onset of otologic symptoms. Otorrhea and tympanic membrane perforation may be absent due to the nonpneumatized mastoid in infants. Syndesmoses about the petrous pyramid create pathways for very rapid spread of infection from the eardrum to the mastoid plane.
b) *Occult form:* The otologic symptoms are subtle (infiltration or possibly congestion of the tympanic membrane, usually no discharge) while systemic signs are alarming and predominant: Severe systemic toxicity with rapidly progressive dyspepsia.

Diagnosis: These small children (usually < 1 year of age) are generally referred by a pediatrician. Even with mild otoscopic findings, CT, or even exploratory antrotomy is indicated for differential diagnosis when corresponding systemic signs are present.

Petrositis (Suppurative Petrous Apicitis)

Main symptoms: The Gradenigo triad (otorrhea, ipsilateral trigeminal neuralgia, abducens nerve palsy).

Other symptoms and special features: Throbbing pain "deep in the ear," inside the skull, or diffuse pain at the "center of the head"; may radiate to the temporoparietal area or perhaps the TMJ. Increasing malaise; occasionally vertigo, vomiting, and/or hearing loss (even deafness). Progresses to involvement of additional cranial nerves (facial, glossopharyngeal, vagus, less commonly the accessory and hypoglossal) and symptoms of intracranial spread (see p. 40ff.). Generally occurs in *acute* otitis media. See also Table 1.**18**.

Causes: Spread of a destructive inflammatory process (osteitis) via the paralabyrinthine cells to the petrous apex in a patient with a well-pneumatized petrous pyramid (Fig. 1.**5**). From there the infection spreads to neighboring structures (gasserian ganglion, oculomotor nerves, especially the abducens nerve) and involves the labyrinth, dura, subarachnoid space, and the base of the brain (see p. 42ff.). Spread occurs more readily to the posterior cranial fossa than to the middle fossa; also to the internal auditory canal and down through the skull base to produce retropharyngeal abscess, "peritonsillar" abscess, or nasopharyngeal abscess (fistula) (see p. 265, 266 and Fig. 1.**5**). Collateral meningeal irritation is common.

Diagnosis:
• History of ipsilateral otitis media. Otoscopy generally shows residual signs of otitis media.
• Diagnostic imaging. Plain radiographs (Stenvers: both petrous pyramids for comparison of the apices; Schüller view); CT of the pyramids and/or MRI.
• Audiologic and neuro-otologic evaluation, all with follow-ups, are indicated whenever petrositis is suspected!
• Leukocytosis with a left shift, increased ESR.

Differentiation is required from sinus phlebitis (petrous sinus, cavernous sinus, or jugular bulb), osteomyelitis secondary to malignant otitis externa, otogenic sepsis, brain abscess, and noninflammatory mass lesion near the skull base.

Chronic Otitis Media

See pp. 22 and 24 and Table 1.**2**.

Otalgia Following Ablative and Reconstructive Middle Ear Surgery
(Tympanoplasty)

This type of pain is very rare except in the immediate postoperative period. Even with recurrent inflammation of the tympanic region, otalgia almost never occurs, though otorrhea is common. Significant pain can result, however, from postoperative perichondritis, missed (concealed) osteitic or osteomyelitic foci, incipient otogenic complications, and occasionally from neuralgias caused by unfavorable wound healing or scar formation. "Radical cavities" can also lead to pain resulting from acute dermatitis, a weeping cavity wall, or insufficient cleansing.

Diagnosis:
- History (including operation report!); inspection and palpation of the ear, operative area, and cavity.
- Radiographs, especially CT.
- Location of pain is helpful for excluding perichondritis and an incipient otogenic complication (mastoiditis, sinus phlebitis, petrositis, intracranial involvement [see p. 40]).

Tumors of the Middle Ear

Pain is not among the cardinal symptoms of the rare histologically *benign* tumors that arise in the middle ear region (such as osteomas, osteofibromas, angiomas, neuromas, etc.). Rarely, nonchromaffin paragangliomas and chemodectomas (glomus tympanicum and glomus jugulare tumors) cause neuralgiform pain due to the irritation of adjacent nerves, but only in the advanced stage. Generally by that time the tumor has already been diagnosed from characteristic symptoms (see p. 31).

Carcinomas (squamous cell carcinoma and adenocarcinoma) are the most common *malignant* tumors of the middle ear. Advanced malignancies cause increasing, deep ear pain that may become intolerable once the tumor has reached the dura ("dural pain"), the gasserian ganglion (fifth nerve), or the perichondrium of the external ear.

Main symptoms: Pain may be mild to moderate initially but invariably becomes severe in later stages. The tympanic cavity and/or external auditory canal contain granulating tissue that bleeds easily ("polyps"); often this tissue is first discovered and examined during surgical exploration for a symptomatic otitis media. Progressive hearing impairment. Sanguinous, usually fetid aural discharge. More common in males over 50 years of age than in women.

Diagnosis:
- If malignancy is suspected: detailed long-term history and meticulous examination using the otoscope and otomicroscope.
- Radiographic evaluation (CT scans) to identify sites of bone destruction in the petrous pyramid. MRI eventually for the differentiation toward the adjacent soft tissues.

- Audiologic and neuro-otologic evaluation.
- Biopsy, repeated as needed until the tentative diagnosis is confirmed or refuted. Given the relative scarcity of middle ear malignancies, their very consideration is the most important step in making a correct diagnosis!

Differentiation is mainly required from malignant (necrotizing) otitis externa (see p. 7) and a middle ear complication spreading to the external auditory canal (see p. 11).

Inner Ear and Internal Auditory Canal

Pain is not a characteristic symptom of inner ear disorders except when the disease spreads beyond the inner ear to involve adjacent structures (dura, cranial nerves, etc.); the resultant pain signifies that a complication has already developed. The increasing headache that accompanies the development of acoustic neuroma (especially in stage III) is a symptom of rising intracranial pressure and is not tumor-specific (see pp. 31, 78).

Neuralgias Involving the Ear

Common symptoms: Lancinating otalgia of sudden onset and brief duration, usually localized within the ear or in the otobase. May be very severe or "intolerable" and is sometimes triggered by external stimuli. The pain is often perceived beyond the confines of the ear and may radiate to several regions at once.

Neuralgia of the Geniculate Ganglion (Hunt Syndrome)

Main symptoms: Sharp, stabbing pain, continuous or paroxysmal, in the external ear canal and periauricular region, occasionally radiating to the roof of the palate and deep into the ear and face.

Other symptoms and special features: Abnormal taste sensations in the anterior two-thirds of the tongue as well as increased salivation. Rarely combined with facial paralysis (e.g., with concomitant zoster oticus).

Causes: Unclear; possibly infection with a neurotropic virus (zoster).

Diagnosis: First exclude ear disease and zoster oticus (history!). Zoster infection is marked by moderate pleocytosis with a slight elevation of CSF protein (see Table 1.**15**). (Presumptive) diagnosis is usually one of exclusion. The external auditory canal may be a trigger zone.

Differentiation is required from trigeminal neuralgia, glossopharyngeal neuralgia, auriculotemporal neuralgia, the Costen syndrome, and otitis media.

Neuralgia of the Auriculotemporal Nerve
(Branch of the Mandibular Division of the Trigeminal Nerve)

Main symptoms: Paroxysmal, burning pain anterior to the ear and deep in the ear, radiating to the cheek and temple. Principally affects the tragus and the root of the helix. Triggered or intensified by gustatory sensation and mastication.

Other symptoms and special features: Cutaneous erythema and hyperesthesia in the distribution of the nerve; occasional (gustatory) sweating, mydriasis, widening of the palpebral fissure. An attack lasts for several minutes.

Causes: Not fully understood; high association with disease and surgery of the parotid gland.

Diagnosis:
● History (with special attention to the parotid!), typical symptomatology during an attack.
● With local hyperhidrosis: starch test (see Table 5.**8**, "gustatory sweating").

Differentiation is required from trigeminal neuralgia, Costen syndrome, and Hunt syndrome.

Glossopharyngeal Neuralgia
See p. 162.

Vagus Neuralgia
See p. 163.

Sluder Neuralgia
(Irritation of the pterygopalatine ganglion)
See p. 162.

Vasomotor Headache
See p. 165.

Vascular Anomalies
See Table 2.**10.**

Miscellaneous Causes of Otalgia

Otalgia can occur in association with *poisonings* (e.g., mercury, lead, phosphorus, arsenic) and *systemic diseases* such as gout, diabetes, arteriosclerosis, tabes, etc. In these cases, however, otalgia is not the main symptom leading to a diagnosis but is only a possible feature of the underlying disorder.

Psychogenic Otalgia

Ear pain, like disturbances of hearing and balance, may have a psychogenic cause. The symptoms do not correlate with any somatic or organic findings, nor do they correspond to typical nerve distributions. Complaints on the quality and nature of the pain are strikingly variable and disjointed.

Diagnosis of Neuralgias Involving the Ear:
● Thorough history that includes the characteristics of the pain; identification of possible trigger zone(s); exclusion of inflammatory or neoplastic disease in the painful area and all the nerves supplying the area.
● Palpation, inspection, otoscopy.
● Screening test for hearing loss.
● Radiographic views may be helpful (Schüller, Stenvers, paranasal sinuses, tomograms and/or CT scans).
● Anesthesia of the presumptive trigger zone(s) may temporarily relieve the neuralgia. Neurologic consultation may be required.

Otalgia Referred from Surrounding Structures

Pain can be referred to the ear from regional or distant inflammatory processes, tumors, or functional disturbances, simulating a primary ear disease. The main conditions to be considered are the following, very heterogeneous disturbances:

Congenital Aural Fistula
See p. 32.

Periauricular Lymphadenitis
See p. 31 and Table 10.8.

Temporal Arteritis
See p. 167.

Temporomandibular Joint Disorders

Main symptoms: Pain radiating to the ear, exacerbated by biting, chewing, and movement of the joint. Tenderness to pressure over the joint, with possible redness and swelling. Grinding or clicking sound in the joint during jaw movements. Possible trismus or mechanical obstruction of joint excursions. Costen syndrome: see pp. 158–159. Pain on movement of the TMJ is characteristic!

Causes: Temporomandibular arthritis; prior malreduction of condylar fracture; malocclusion, faulty bite (e.g., poorly fitting denture).

Diagnosis:
● History, exclusion of an otogenic cause.
● Radiography of the TMJ (possibly by CT and/or pantomography); dental or oral surgical consultation.

Myoarthropathies

Caused by unphysiologic use of the muscles of mastication (pterygoid muscles, masseter muscle, temporal muscle, digastric muscle) and faulty loading of the TMJs. Otalgia and tinnitus may occur in addition to headache, neck pain, TMJ pain, and dental pain. Myoarthropathies chiefly affect women over 50 years of age. Emotional disturbances (aggressiveness, anxiety reactions) may have causal significance.

Diagnosis: Consultation with a dentist or oral surgeon may be indicated after the exclusion of otolaryngologic disease. Psychiatric evaluation also may be advised.

Dentogenic Causes
See p. 236.

Diseases of the Major Salivary Glands

Acute or recurrent inflammation, stones, and malignant tumors of the major salivary glands may be associated with otalgia, but never without symptoms typical of the salivary gland disease (see p. 299 ff.).

A true, otalgia-associated combined disease involving the salivary gland and ear is present when a parotid abscess breaks through into the external auditory canal (see p. 23) or a malignant tumor of the parotid gland spreads to involve the external auditory canal (or vice versa).

Otalgia Due to Diseases of the Oral Cavity, Paranasal Sinuses, Pharynx, or Cervical Organs

This category includes inflammatory processes such as abscesses and ulcers of the tongue base; peritonsillar or intratonsillar infiltration, ulcers, abscesses, or cellulitis; and retropharyngeal abscesses. Sphenoidal sinusitis and/or maxillary sinusitis can occasionally cause ear pain.

Otalgia on swallowing is an important potential early warning sign of a malignant tumor of the tongue, tonsils, nasopharynx, oropharynx, hypopharynx, esophagus, or thyroid gland! Inflammatory endopharyngeal diseases such as epiglottitis, epiglottic abscess, and pharyngeal perichondritis of diverse causes (see p. 317) as well as laryngeal carcinoma often cause severe pain radiating to the ear, especially when perichondritis is also present.

Causes: Neurosensory connections linking the oropharynx and hypopharynx, upper esophagus, and larynx with the ear (external canal and middle ear) (auricular branch of the vagus nerve, also connections with the glossopharyngeal nerve).

Diagnosis:
● Exclusion of an otogenic cause.
● Otalgia on swallowing in a patient with a normal otologic examination always requires a thorough evaluation of the nasopharynx, oro-

pharynx, hypopharynx, larynx, upper esophagus, and thyroid by palpation and endoscopy. Suspect findings are an indication for biopsy and perhaps diagnostic imaging.

Otalgia in Nonotogenic Facial Paralysis
See p. 150.

Pain Due to Otogenic Intracranial Complications
See p. 40 ff.

Dysplasias at the Craniocervical Junction

Like basilar impression (impression of the foramen magnum, occipital hypoplasia, high dens, shortened clivus), these deformities can cause otalgia in addition to disturbances of the medulla, long spinal tract, and inner ear.

Vertebragenic Otalgia
See p. 393.

Symptom   **Dysesthesia (Fullness, Pressure, Itching) in the Ear**

A feeling of fullness, pressure, or itching about the ear are pathologic sensations (dysesthesias), which are often produced by innocuous conditions but may also result from serious disorders and sometimes occur as precursors or residua of painful ear diseases. Compared with the symptom of otalgia, patients tend to be less precise in describing the *character*, *location*, and *time course* of the dysesthesia. Especially in patients who lack objective symptoms, the differential diagnosis relies critically on a careful history that gives specific attention to these details.

External Ear (Auricle and External Auditory Canal)

Inflammatory Skin Diseases of the Auricle

Main symptoms: Itching; typical eruptions that may spread from the auricle to the external auditory canal (or vice versa).

Relatively common conditions are *impetigo, eczema* (contact, microbial, seborrheic, atopic), *comedo acne, chloracne, scratch dermatitis* (e.g., in pediculosis), *erysipelas, erysipeloid,* and *psoriasis.* See also p. 145.

Diagnosis:
● Detailed history, taking note of analogous eruptions elsewhere on the body.
● Otoscopic delineation of skin changes with respect to the middle ear and exclusion of otitis media.
● Bacteriologic and mycologic smear. Dermatologic consultation may be required.

Previous Frostbite

Main symptoms: Chronic itching of the auricle, exacerbated by temperature changes. "Nibbled" auricular margin, sometimes with marked losses of auricular substance in cases with previous cartilage necrosis. There may be firm, bluish-red, nodular thickenings on the auricular margin with an ulcerative tendency (perniones or chilblains).

Differentiation is required from basal cell carcinoma or incipient carcinoma (biopsy!). Carcinoma is believed to occur more frequently in an auricle damaged by frostbite or burn.

Othematoma

Main symptoms: Puffy swelling, initially noninflammatory, involving the *anterior side* of the auricle (and occasionally the posterior side following loss of cartilage substance). Feeling of tension, occasional mild itching.

Other symptoms and special features: Fluctuation; pale white, yellowish, or violet discoloration of the skin, depending on the contents (serum or blood). Fluid contents become organized in long-standing cases. The end result is a coarse, rigid, grossly thickened auricle (see p. 4).

Causes: Effusion between the perichondrium and cartilage caused by a blunt shearing trauma or occurring "spontaneously," i.e., with no recollection of trauma.

Diagnosis: History is often diagnostic; some cases require needle aspiration (useful for diagnosis *and* treatment).

Differentiation is required from incipient perichondritis (always associated with pain and other signs of inflammation!).

Foreign Bodies in the External Auditory Canal

Main symptoms: Feeling of pressure. Severe pain may occur in certain circumstances (incarceration, skin irritation, cerumen impaction, etc.) and is accentuated by chewing (proximity of TMJ).

Other symptoms and special features: Conductive hearing loss occurs when the object totally occludes the ear canal (see p. 58). Incrustation and foreign-body dermatitis or decubitus leads to a purulent, possibly foul-smelling otorrhea. Living foreign bodies (maggots, insects, etc.) cause itching of varying intensity.

Diagnosis:
- Barring diffuse accompanying inflammation and swelling of the ear canal, otoscopy generally establishes the presence of a foreign body (or impacted cerumen) without difficulty.
- Radiograph(s) are rarely necessary as an adjunct.
- Some cases may require surgical opening of the ear canal with diagnostic and therapeutic intent.

Table 1.**4** *Symptom* Dysesthesias (fullness, pressure, itching) in the ear

Synopsis
External ear (auricle and external auditory canal)
Inflammatory skin diseases
Previous frostbite
Othematoma
Foreign bodies
Cerumen impaction and epidermal plug
Idiopathic (symptomatic) pruritus
Diffuse otitis externa (noneczematous, eczematous), see p. 6
Fungal infection
Exostoses of the external auditory canal
Stenoses and posttraumatic scars of the external auditory canal
Tumors, see p. 8
Middle ear
Disturbances of eustachian tube ventilation
Chronic otitis media (nonspecific and specific)
Tumors
Inner ear and internal auditory canal
Labyrinthitis
Inner ear (sensorineural) hearing loss, see p. 58ff.
Ménière disease, see p. 82, 112
Sudden deafness, see p. 72
Acoustic trauma, see p. 58ff.
Noise-induced hearing loss, see p. 61, 77
Tumors in the internal auditory canal, see p. 31, 78, 108
Regional causes
Lymphadenopathies
Salivary gland tumors
Metabolic disorders
TMJ disorders, malocclusion

Cerumen Impaction

Main symptom: Abrupt unilateral or bilateral hearing loss, sometimes with associated tinnitus. Pain occurs only if the plug is very large and hard and is then often exacerbated by chewing.

Diagnosis:
- Otoscopy (yellow to dark brown obstruction plug). Auditory testing may be indicated to evaluate conductive hearing loss.
- Irrigation confirms the presumptive diagnosis (irrigate only after excluding a tympanic membrane perforation!).

Differentiation is required from foreign bodies (e.g., a cotton wad) and from the (very rare) *"epidermal plug"* (keratosis obturans or "cholesteatoma of the external ear canal"), which consists of a hard, firm, yellowish-white mass of epidermal debris that is generally located within, and completely fills, the bony ear canal. The hard, scaly material must be repeatedly softened (e.g., with salicylic alcohol or resorcinol) to allow piecemeal removal by irrigation. Do not confuse an epidermal plug with a middle ear cholesteatoma!

Idiopathic (Symptomatic) Pruritus of the Ear

Main symptoms: Itching of variable intensity, generally bilateral and often very severe, in the external auditory canal. Alternates with quiescent periods. Typically there are no remarkable local otologic findings aside from a thin, atrophic canal skin and insufficient cerumen.

Other symptoms and special features: Predominantly affects women over 60 years of age.

Causes: Unknown. Hormonal (menopause), diatetic, metabolic (diabetes), and autonomic dysfunctions have been postulated.

Diagnosis: Exclusion of organic ear or skin disease. Evaluation by an internist (see above).

Diffuse Otitis Externa
See p. 6.

Fungal Infections of the Ear

Main symptoms: Severe itching or burning sensation in the external ear canal. Feeling of fullness; pain is uncommon (may reflect superinfected otitis externa). Fungal mycelia may be visible in the ear canal (forming a coating like "dust," "cotton," or "powder"). Alternation between *"dry"* and *"wet"* *phases.* The coating material may appear whitish, gray, greenish, yellow, or black, depending on the infecting organism.

Other symptoms and special features: Inclination to granuloma formation in the external ear canal or on the tympanic membrane (fungal myringitis). Variable inflammatory reaction of affected areas of the canal skin (and in radical surgical cavities!) with scratch trauma at the meatal inlet and within the canal. Involvement of the tympanic cavity is rare but can occur via a large tympanic membrane perforation.

Causes: Primary or secondary infection with various species of *Aspergillus, Candida (albicans), Penicillium, Mucor,* dermatophytes, yeasts, etc. Fungal involvement is said to be present in some 20% of ear canal inflammatory conditions. Common (but not exclusive!) in tropical and subtropical zones and damp environments. May predispose to bacterial superinfection or may develop secondarily to a bacterial infection.

Diagnosis:
- History (travel in warm countries, work in a damp environment, recurrent bouts of itching, etc.).
- Otoscopy often shows a discolored material coating the external ear canal (see above), possibly with plug formation or a colored discharge within the canal. Otomicroscopy is indicated. *However:* Fungal infection may be present even in a dry, apparently "clean" external auditory canal!
- Mycologic and bacteriologic smear (if infection is suspected, study may have to be repeated several times until fungi are identified).

Exostoses of the External Auditory Canal

Main symptoms: Feeling of pressure or fullness, itching in the ear canal. Intermittent hearing impairment (e.g., ear remains "plugged up" for some time after swimming). Otoscopy usually shows multiple, circumscribed, bony hard, conical, or rounded protrusions of the ear canal wall that may occlude most of the canal lumen.

Table 1.**6**   Methods of dedecting CSF in aural or nasal discharge

Method	Principle and capabilities	Remarks
Qualitative test for CSF in bloody discharge	Hemorrhagic discharge on gauze or filter paper: appearance of a light halo around a bloody center (pure blood has sharp margins)	Very crude screening test
Glucose test	*Nasal discharge:* glucose elevated with cerebrospinal rhinorrhea (dipstick test, then laboratory glucose determination	*Cannot* be used when blood is present
Protein determination	*Nasal discharge:* protein elevated when CSF is present	*Cannot* be used when blood is present
β_2-transferrin determination	Gel electrophoresis assay. Biochemical detection of the CSF-specific constituent β_2-transferrin. Method of Oberascher and Arrer* or of Reisinger, Lempart, and Hochstrasser**	Currently the most reliable method of detection. * Laryng. Rhinol. Otol. 65 (1986) 158 ** Laryng. Rhinol. Otol. 66 (1987) 255
Prealbumin/albumin ratio	Screening test to determine the concentrations of prealbumin and albumin in the discharge. CSF contains more prealbumin than serum. Compared against albumin level in serum and CSF	If test is inconclusive, β_2-transferrin determination is required (see**)
Na fluorescein test	After intrathecal administration of 0.5 cm³ Na fluorescein 0.5%, CSF fluoresces under u. v. or blue light. Used to detect CSF leakage from the subarachnoid space and pinpoint the location of the fistula. Caution: Excessive intrathecal dye concentration can induce generalized seizures	Useful for localization of CSF fistula
Radionuclide detection	Intrathecal administration of isotope-labeled albumin (analogous to Na fluorescein test). Radionuclide can be detected, for example, by placing cotton over the suspected leak and testing it with a pulse counter.	Useful for localization of CSF fistula
Endoscopic detection	Even without labeling, a "CSF track" or profuse CSF discharge can sometimes be detected using optical magnification	Relatively crude screening study

All the detection methods listed above are useful only when the history and other clinical findings are known

- Biopsy.
- General examination to exclude tuberculosis in another organ.

Differentiation is required from syphilis, fungal infection, and HIV infection.

Tumors of the External Auditory Canal and Middle Ear
See p. 28 ff.

Other symptoms and special features: As occlusion of the ear canal progresses, marked signs of inflammation appear (due to deficient self-cleansing). The exostoses may arise from the bone on a pedicle (usually on the lateral canal wall) or on a broad base (usually on the medial wall near the tympanic membrane). They grow very slowly and remain asymptomatic for a long time.

Causes: Formation of small cortical osteomas, probably triggered by frequent cooling of the bone of the external auditory canal by cold water (swimming, water sports).

Diagnosis: Otoscopic findings are diagnostic.

Differentiation is required from furunculosis of the external ear canal or a solitary polyp extending from the tympanic cavity into the external canal.

Stenoses and Scars
of the External Auditory Canal

Main symptoms: Feeling of pressure and fullness in the ear canal; also itching and/or pain when retention is present.

Other symptoms: Deficient self-cleansing leads to retention of debris and recurrent external otitis with discharge.

Causes: Previous trauma to the external auditory canal, also ear surgery; rudimentary or mild anomalies. Secondary stenoses (even atresia!) may follow cutaneous diseases of the ear canal. Mechanical irritation or intolerance (plastics in earpieces, etc.) can also incite stenosis formation in the ear canal.

Diagnosis:
● History provides clues to the cause; otoscopic findings are diagnostic. It is important to differentiate a pure connective-tissue (cicatricial) stenosis from a bony stenosis (e.g., following a fracture of the auditory canal).
● In doubtful cases: CT scans of the affected region of the ear canal.
● Audiologic evaluation (e.g., exclusion of concomitant middle ear involvement).

Differentiation is required from exostoses, malformations, and manifestations of other bony or connective-tissue outgrowths or neoplasms.

Tumors of the External Auditory Canal
See p. 28 ff.

Middle Ear

Disturbances of Eustachian Tube Ventilation (Tubotympanic Catarrh, Catarrhal Otitis Media, Otitis Media Simplex, Sero[muco]tympanon)

Main symptoms: Acute feeling of pressure and fullness in the ear (often accompanied by catarrh): "water in the ear" with a perceptible fluid shift during head movements. Occasional autophony and/or a gurgling or deep rushing sound in the ear. Occasional bouts of lancinating ear pain. Crackling sound in the ear on swallowing, yawning, and noseblowing. More or less pronounced hearing impairment, which can vary markedly in severity (conductive hearing loss, see p. 59). *Chronic* cases do not have sharp pain but a constant "plugged up" feeling in the ear with hearing impairment and a ringing or rushing tinnitus.

Other symptoms and special features: Otoscopy shows a pale, usually retracted tympanic membrane with radial injection in acute cases. Transudate in the middle ear produces an amber-yellow discoloration or oily opacity of the tympanic membrane. Occasionally a fluid level is visible behind the membrane and may shift with head movements. Bubbles may appear behind the membrane following air insufflation.

Long-standing eustachian tube dysfunction leads to pallor and marked retraction of the tympanic membrane. Organized residua and adhesions may already be present in some cases, along with a "scarred" membrane showing dark, blue-violet discoloration ("blue drum"). Eustachian tube catheterization no longer improves hearing due to progressive luminal obliteration of the tympanic cavity. Severe, stable conductive hearing loss is present (see p. 73).

Causes: Impaired transtubal ventilation and drainage of the middle ear due to eustachian tube dysfunction. This may be transient due to mucosal swelling (e.g., catarrh) or irreversible due to intratubal stenosis, scars, or obturating lesions adjacent to the tube (nasopharynx, middle ear, skull base).

Diagnosis:

● Otoscopic findings, besides those listed above, include shortening of the malleus handle, a projecting short process of the malleus, an altered tympanic membrane reflex, and abnormal membrane folds. Often there is a highly viscous, "mucogelatinous" discharge in the tympanic cavity ("glue ear"). Drumhead mobility is decreased. Fluid level is visibly affected by use of the pneumatic (Siegle) otoscope.
● Valsalva maneuver, politzerization, or tubal catheterization with concurrent otomicroscopic observation of the tympanic membrane or auscultation of the insufflation sound via a listening tube passed into the ear canal.
● Audiologic testing and tympanography (impedance testing) (see p. 57).
● Schüller radiograph usually shows good pneumatization in cases taking a short, acute course and decreased pneumatization in chronic cases.
● Search for the cause of the eustachian tube obstruction or irritation: nasopharynx, adenoids, nasopharyngeal neoplasms, inflammatory lesions of the nose and paranasal sinuses, middle ear, (submucous) cleft palate, endocrine causes (e.g., pregnancy), disturbances or oropharyngeal innervation).

Differentiation is required from incipient acute otitis media (little or no pain with a nonpurulent effusion), chronic otitis media (tympanic membrane findings), adhesive process (partial or complete fixation of the tympanic membrane in a retracted position, opaque "scarred" drumhead). Also otosclerosis: freely mobile, usually very delicate membrane in a normal position. Radiographs show a well-pneumatized mastoid process; tomographic evaluation of the ossicular chain may be helpful.

Special Situation: Patulous (Abnormally Patent) Eustachian Tube

Main symptoms: Feeling of pressure and/or fullness in the ear; autophony (or "tympanophony"), i.e., a harsh, jarring perception of one's own voice. Otoscopy generally shows a thin, bulging, distended tympanic membrane.

Other symptoms and special features: Respiratory-associated sounds within the head. Audiologic findings, see p. 57 ff.

Cause: Believed to result from an incompetent tubal closure mechanism of varying etiology.

Chronic Otitis Media

Aural pressure and fullness, though *not* among the *main symptoms* of chronic otitis media, are still common features of this condition and are reported in patients with chronic mucosal suppuration (especially with acute recurrence and in wet stages) as well as in cholesteatomatous or bony suppuration and chronic cases of specific causation. Patients rarely experience these complaints as severe, however. Pressure or fullness of acute onset may be an early sign of incipient dermatitis in a previously dry radical surgical cavity. Pressure or fullness following tympanoplasty may signify impaired middle ear ventilation or a recurrence of middle ear disease. Progression to *otalgia* heralds an acute exacerbation or incipient complication. See p. 24 for further details.

Otologic Tumors

Early-stage neoplasms, both benign and malignant, can cause a diffuse feeling of pressure or fullness in the ear, which initially may be the only subjective symptom of disease. The diagnosis is made from clinical (and histologic) local findings. See also pp. 15 and 28 ff.

Diseases of the Inner Ear

Aural pressure or fullness is a feature of certain inner ear diseases including *labyrinthitis, Ménière disease* (ear pressure of varying intensity), *sudden hearing loss, acoustic trauma,* and *noise-induced hearing loss* — although each of these disorders is associated with other predominant subjective and objective signs (see pp. 61, 72, 81, 112).

Labyrinthitis

Main symptoms: Vertigo, nausea, nystagmus (*irritative* toward the affected ear, *paralytic* away from the affected ear). Auditory function in the affected ear diminishes to the point of deafness. Tinnitus may be present. There is no otalgia, but aural pressure my be experienced. Symptoms of vestibular and cochlear nerve dysfunction are predominant, accompanied by a partial or complete loss of inner ear function. See pp. 64 and 106 for further details (causes, diagnosis, differential diagnosis).

Causes of Pressure and Fullness not Located in the Ear

These occasional causes include:
● Inflammatory or neoplastic diseases of regional lymph nodes (see p. 399).
● Salivary gland diseases (functional disturbances, early inflammatory diseases, sialadenoses, neoplasms) (see p. 298).
● TMJ disorders (malocclusion, abortive Costen syndrome, osteoarthritis, previous trauma, etc.) (see pp. 17, 31, 144, 158).

Symptom   Otorrhea (Aural Discharge)

Otorrhea refers to discharge from the external auditory canal of a material that is produced in the auditory canal, middle ear, or (rarely) elsewhere in the petrous pyramid or endocranium. The discharge may be characterized as serous, mucous, purulent, flaky, bloody (or blood-tinged), watery (CSF), stretchy, gelatinous, etc. The discharge may be odorless, or the odor can range from taint to fetid. The otorrhea may be intermittent or continuous, scant to profuse, and may be combined with other aural symptoms (pain, itching, burning, etc.). The consistency, color, and odor of the discharge are generally very useful for differential diagnosis. Stained microscopic slides rarely contribute to diagnosis, but useful information can be gained from bacteriologic and mycologic smears and, when CSF otorrhea is suspected, biochemical examination of the fluid (see Table 1.6).

Table 1.5 *Symptom*   Otorrhea (aural discharge)

Synopsis
Causes in the external ear (and immediate surroundings)
Circumscribed otitis externa (furuncle of the ear canal), see p. 6
Diffuse otitis externa (eczematous/noneczematous), see p. 6
Fungal infections of the ear, see p. 20
Malignant otitis externa, see p. 7
Parotid fistula
Causes in the middle ear
Acute purulent otitis media
– With special forms
Chronic otitis media
– Mucosal suppuration
– Bony (cholesteatomatous) suppuration
– Previous ear surgery
– Tuberculous otitis media
Tumors, see p 28 ff.
Causes at the skull base and/or in the cranial cavity
CSF otorrhea
Petrositis, see p. 14
Otogenic intracranial complications, see p. 40

External Ear

Circumscribed Otitis Externa (Furuncle of the External Auditory Canal)
See p. 6.

Diffuse Otitis Externa
See p. 6.

Fungal Infections of the Ear
See p. 20.

Malignant Otitis Externa

See p. 7.

Parotid Fistula

A pseudo-otorrhea can result from trauma or breakthrough of a parotid abscess into the external ear canal, establishing a communication between the ear canal and the duct system of the parotid gland. Usually the discharge from the ear canal is initially purulent (abscess contents or wound exudate) and becomes more watery as the fistula consolidates. The quantity varies with the activity of the gland (greater before and after meals). The fistulous opening is always located on the floor or anterior wall of the cartilaginous ear canal (Santorini fissures). A rare disorder.

Diagnosis:

● History of parotid disease or injury. Quantity of aural discharge may vary around mealtimes.
● Identification of the discharge as saliva (salivary chemistry, see Table 5.5).

Middle Ear

Acute Suppurative Otitis Media

Otorrhea is not invariably a feature of acute middle ear inflammatory lesions and is not considered an early sign. It is more common in children with acute otitis media than in adults. The discharge in simple otitis media is initially thin, occasionally blood-tinged, serous, odorless (and perhaps pulsatile). In subsequent days the discharge becomes increasingly viscous and purulent before assuming a mucoid consistency in the resolution stage (1st to 2nd week). Discharge subsides during the 3rd or 4th week. See p. 9 for further details.

In *otitis in infants and small children* (*not* to be confused with *infantile mastoiditis*, p. 14), spontaneous perforation of the tympanic membrane releases a discharge that is generally mucopurulent, stretchy, odorless, and pulsatile (see also p. 9).

In *hemorrhagic (influenzal) otitis*, the discharge is initially blood-tinged (pink to red). This is a *cardinal symptom* for the diagnosis of influenzal otitis! As the disease progresses, the discharge becomes more viscous and gradually becomes creamy and purulent. See p. 10 for further details.

Chronic Otitis Media

Otorrhea is the leading symptom of chronic otitis media. The character of the discharge is an important criterion for differentiating between the two main forms of this disease group, which are discussed separately below.

Chronic Mucosal Suppuration

The aural discharge in the wet stage of the disease is an odorless, stretchy, mucous to muropurulent fluid, depending on the state of middle ear inflammation. Discharge in the uncleaned ear may become foul-smelling due to decomposition. The discharge may be constant or interrupted by dry phases over a period of weeks, months, or years. The quantity varies greatly, ranging from a slight moisture of the ear canal to a profuse, very troublesome discharge, which drips from the ear canal and stains pillows and clothing. Irritation of the canal skin is common (weeping dermatitis or diffuse external otitis).

Generally there is a central tympanic membrane perforation of variable size (from a pinhole to complete loss of the tympanic membrane).

Other symptoms and special features: Pain is very rare in this form of chronic otitis media and, if present, is very mild and tends to occur briefly during an acute exacerbation. Hearing loss varies with the size of the tympanic membrane perforation and other middle ear defects (see p. 73 ff). Balance disturbances also may occur (see p. 104 ff).

Chronic Bony Suppuration
(With and Without Cholesteatoma)

Again, the otorrheic manifestations are diverse. Rarely there is a dry or almost dry tympanic membrane perforation, but profuse discharge is also uncommon. Usually the tympanic membrane and portions of the ear canal are coated with a discolored, oily, purulent, foul-smelling discharge. The odor remains fetid despite cleansing of the ear. The discharge has a "gritty," crumbly consistency, which is *not* mucoid or stretchy. It may contain whitish scales (from cholesteatoma), especially during or after irrigation of the ear. In other cases the discharge may be so slight that it produces only a brownish, lacquer-like crust about the marginal perforation. When the crust has been softened, cholesteatoma constituents can usually be mobilized and flushed from the ear.

The tympanic membrane perforation is marginal, often occurring in the pars flaccida or at the posterior (superior) margin of the membrane. But it can occur anywhere on the bony annulus, especially after temporal bone fractures. Usually the perforation is easily identified, but it may be hidden behind encrusted discharge or may be so small and concealed that optical magnification is required for its detection.

Other symptoms and special features: Typically there is a vague feeling of aural pressure. Pain is unusual and signifies retention or a complication. Hearing loss may occur depending on the type and location of the pathologic change (see p. 58). Balance disturbances are relatively common (with and without fistula formation, see p. 105).

Diagnosis:
● Otoscopy permits detection and classification of a tympanic membrane perforation. Smear is taken for microbiologic evaluation and sensitivity testing.
● Audiologic and neuro-otologic evaluation (vestibular nerve) including the "fistula test" (with a labyrinthine fistula, compression of air in the external meatus generally provokes nystagmus toward the affected side, while aspiration provokes nystagmus toward the opposite or untested side). *But:* A negative test does not prove that a fistula-like erosion of bone has not already occurred!
● Radiographs (standard projections of Schüller and Stenvers, possibly the E. G. Mayer view) for detecting and delineating areas of bone destruction. High-resolution CT scans may be needed, say, to detect a fistula in

the labyrinthine system, ossicular caries, or an area of destruction threatening or involving the middle or posterior cranial fossa, facial nerve, or labyrinth.

Differentiation is required from diffuse otitis externa, tuberculous otitis media, malignant tumors of the external auditory canal or middle ear, and syphilis.

Special Situation:

Previous Surgery on the Middle Ear

Otorrhea following middle ear surgery may arise from dermatitis involving the lining of a radical surgical cavity (inadequate and/or improper care) or may signify a recurrence of middle ear disease (graft perforation, suppuration of residual air cells, recurrent cholesteatoma, rejection of implant material, etc.).

Tuberculous Otitis Media

Main symptoms: Like those of a nonspecific chronic or subacute otitis media. Painless onset, usually followed by a painless course with scant purulent otorrhea. The tympanic membrane is thickened and usually shows multiple perforations, which may enlarge rapidly and coalesce to a total defect. Granulation (= tubercle) formation on the drum, in the tympanic cavity, and/or in the external auditory canal. Severe (conductive) hearing loss.

Other symptoms and special features: Chronic mastoiditis or petrositis may develop, especially in children; also labyrinthine involvement. Regional lymph node involvement, occasionally with the formation of a cold abscess and/or cervical fistula. Productive or exudative (usually mixed) course of the disease.

Causes: Primary infection is most common in children. Other age groups: generally a post-primary infection with tubercle bacilli.

Diagnosis:
● Otoscopy shows typical tympanic membrane findings.
● Smear and bacteriologic study. Organism may be detected using laboratory animal tests.
● Radiography: Schüller, Stenvers views; possibly CT scans of the petrous pyramid.

Table 1.6 Methods of dedecting CSF in aural or nasal discharge

Method	Principle and capabilities	Remarks
Qualitative test for CSF in bloody discharge	Hemorrhagic discharge on gauze or filter paper: appearance of a light halo around a bloody center (pure blood has sharp margins)	Very crude screening test
Glucose test	*Nasal discharge:* glucose elevated with cerebrospinal rhinorrhea (dipstick test, then laboratory glucose determination	*Cannot* be used when blood is present
Protein determination	*Nasal discharge:* protein elevated when CSF is present	*Cannot* be used when blood is present
β_2-transferrin determination	Gel electrophoresis assay. Biochemical detection of the CSF-specific constituent β_2-transferrin. Method of Oberascher and Arrer* or of Reisinger, Lempart, and Hochstrasser**	Currently the most reliable method of detection. * Laryng. Rhinol. Otol. 65 (1986) 158 ** Laryng. Rhinol. Otol. 66 (1987) 255
Prealbumin/albumin ratio	Screening test to determine the concentrations of prealbumin and albumin in the discharge. CSF contains more prealbumin than serum. Compared against albumin level in serum and CSF	If test is inconclusive, β_2-transferrin determination is required (see**)
Na fluorescein test	After intrathecal administration of 0.5 cm³ Na fluorescein 0.5%, CSF fluoresces under u. v. or blue light. Used to detect CSF leakage from the subarachnoid space and pinpoint the location of the fistula. Caution: Excessive intrathecal dye concentration can induce generalized seizures	Useful for localization of CSF fistula
Radionuclide detection	Intrathecal administration of isotope-labeled albumin (analogous to Na fluorescein test). Radionuclide can be detected, for example, by placing cotton over the suspected leak and testing it with a pulse counter.	Useful for localization of CSF fistula
Endoscopic detection	Even without labeling, a "CSF track" or profuse CSF discharge can sometimes be detected using optical magnification	Relatively crude screening study

All the detection methods listed above are useful only when the history and other clinical findings are known

● Biopsy.
● General examination to exclude tuberculosis in another organ.

Differentiation is required from syphilis, fungal infection, and HIV infection.

Tumors of the External Auditory Canal and Middle Ear
See p. 28 ff.

Causes of Otorrhea
Located at the Otobase

Basal skull fractures, especially longitudinal fractures of the pyramid, create dural defects and fracture lines that may allow CSF drainage into the middle ear and external auditory canal. The resulting discharge, especially if not profuse, can be difficult to distinguish from a middle ear effusion. Sometimes there is concomitant CSF drainage to the pharynx via the ipsilateral eustachian tube!

Symptom   **Tinnitus**

See p. 92.

Symptom   **Morphologic Change (Swelling, Tumor)**

This group of symptoms includes visible changes in the shape and contour of the ear and its immediate surroundings caused by a transient or permanent volume increase (edema, inflammation, growth) as well as typical otologic tumors, such as acoustic neuromas and glomus tumors, which are either invisible externally or become visible only at a very late stage.

Diseases Arising from the Ear

Othematoma
See p. 18.

Auricular Perichondritis
See p. 5.

Congenital Aural Fistula
See p. 32.

Cysts and Celes

Main symptoms: Very slowly increasing, painless swelling located on or more commonly adjacent to the auricle. Doughy or tense consistency. Aspiration may yield a yellowish fluid or solid material.

Causes: Retention cysts (atheromas, etc.) or branchial cleft anomalies (see p. 32).

Otogenic Inflammatory Complications

Mastoiditis (see p. 11), zygomaticitis, Bezold mastoiditis (see p. 12ff.), sinus thrombosis (see p. 41), intracranial abscess (see p. 43).

Tuberculous Otitis Externa

Main symptoms: Formation of a firm, painless, hazelnut- to walnut-size lesion, usually on the lobule of the ear, with red to livid discoloration of the overlying skin. Very protracted course.

Cause: Tuberculoma formation by bacilli "inoculated" through small skin defects (e.g., caused by earrings).

Diagnosis:
- Typical location and local findings. Biopsy.
- Complete otologic status and general examination (lung!).

Table 1.**7** *Symptom* Morphologic change,
(swelling, tumors)

Synopsis
Arising from the ear
Othematoma, see p. 18
Perichondritis, see p. 5
Congenital aural fistula, see p. 32
Cysts and celes
Otogenic inflammatory complications
– Mastoiditis, see 11
– Sinus thrombosis, see p. 41
– Intracranial abscess formation, see p. 43 ff.
Tuberculous otitis externa
Benign tumors
– Atheroma
– Hemangioma, lymphangioma
– Lipoma
– Osteoma
– Glomus tumor (chemodectoma)
– Acoustic neuroma
– Rare benign neoplasms
– Adenoma
– Pleomorphic adenoma
– Osteofibroma
– Ossifying fibroma
– Giant-cell tumor
– Histiocytosis X
Malignant tumors
– Squamous cell carcinoma
– Adenocarcinoma
– Sarcomas of varying composition
– Malignant melanoma
Arising from surrounding structures
Parotid origin, see p. 302 ff.
– TMJ
– Regional lymph nodes

Differentiation is required from a Boeck sarcoid, fibroma, sarcoma, lipoma, and leukemic infiltration. Tuberculoma of the auricle has become rare. *Tuberculous otitis media,* see p. 25.

Benign Tumors

Only a few benign tumors that cause visible swelling are reasonably common in the ear region. They include *fibromas, atheromas, epidermoids, dermoids, angiomas, lipomas,* and *osteomas.* If local findings are equivocal, the diagnosis is established by biopsy.

Several *guidelines for differential diagnosis* are presented below:

Atheroma (Sebaceous Cyst), Epidermoid, Dermoid

Main symptoms: Well-circumscribed, rounded, subcutaneous mass of variable size, which moves with the skin. Mass is painless (unless inflamed). Common on the earlobe, mastoid, and posterior auricular surface.

Causes: Diverse. Some lesions represent true heterotopic ectoderm, others are retention cysts caused by obliteration of gland excretory ducts.

Diagnosis: Excisional biopsy.

Differentiation is required from fibroma, lipoma, and Besnier–Boeck–Schaumann disease. "Artificial" atheromas, pseudocholesteatomas, and keloid formation can occur in the area of old surgical scars. *True* cholesteatomas arising in the temporal bone due to epithelial heterotopia and having no connection with the middle ear spaces are very rare.

Hemangioma and Lymphangioma

Main symptoms: Diffuse, pad-like tumor of variable size embedded in the skin and subcutaneous tissue. Overlying skin color may be normal or show reddish-purple discoloration (nevus flammeus). Lymphangiomas are far less common than hemangiomas. Displaceability varies, but very few of these tumors move independently of the skin. Most are present at birth.

Other symptoms and special features: Hemangiomas may present as a nevus on the auricle, possibly accompanied by facial nevi. In small children the tumor volume expands during crying (especially with cavernous hemangioma). Preauricular occurrence is most common (parotid region). Spontaneous regression is possible during the first years of life. See also pp. 146, 308, and 405.

Cause: True congenital neoplasm with a capillary or cavernous structure.

Diagnosis:
● Typical "pad" findings on inspection and palpation.
● Lesions of suitable location and extent may be visualized by the selective injection of radiographic contrast medium through a feeding artery (superselective angiography). CT and MRI or both can be helpful in some cases.
● Some cases may require biopsy.

Differentiation is required from arteriovenous aneurysm (congenital or posttraumatic, predilection for the auricle; occasional pulsatile tinnitus, typical angiographic findings), hemangiopericytoma (may undergo malignant change!), and malignant vascular tumors (hemangiosarcoma, hemangioendothelioma).

Lipoma

Main symptoms: Easily displaceable, smooth-walled, subcutaneous neoplasm.

Diagnosis: Excisional biopsy.

Osteoma

Main symptoms: Circumscribed or diffuse, nondisplaceable, nontender mass located beneath the soft tissue covering the cranial bone (mastoid, temporal squama).

Diagnosis:
● Radiographic evaluation (may include CT); biopsy may be required.
● Osteomas at certain sites can be diagnosed by examination of the middle and inner ear.

Special Clinical Forms:

Glomus Tumor (Jugulotympanic Paraganglioma, Chemodectoma)

Main symptoms: Pulsatile tinnitus (unilateral), feeling of pressure "deep in the ear," progressive hearing loss (may progress to deafness). Balance disturbances. In later stages: facial paralysis and possible posterior cranial nerve involvement: foramen jugulare syndrome (see Table 1.**18**). Involvement of the trigeminal, abducens, and oculomotor nerves is also possible in the late stage.

Other symptoms and special features: Peak occurrence is in the 4th–6th decades with about a 3:1 preponderance of females over males. Glomus tumors grow in the skull base, showing both extracranial (middle/inner ear) and intracranial extension. Otoscopy may initially show a reddish area visible through the lower half of the tympanic membrane or, with a tympanic membrane perforation, a red *"polyp" that bleeds easily and briskly when touched.* There is gradual destruction of the middle and inner ear with labyrinthine failure. Advanced tumors may cause life-threatening compression of the pons, cerebellum, medulla oblongata, and internal carotid artery. Penetration to the auditory canal and/or mastoid is common.

Cause: Nonchromaffin chemodectoma growing by infiltration and expansion. Potential sites of origin: a) *Glomus tympanicum* (tumor initially confined to the tympanic cavity), b) *glomus jugulare* (confined to the tympanic cavity and jugular bulb), c) *further spread from b)* to the bony skull base and/or cranial cavity.

Diagnosis:
● Otoscopy.
● Audiologic and neuro-otologic evaluation (see pp. 75 and 108).
● Diagnostic imaging: Schüller and Stenvers radiographs and special views (e.g., Mifka) of the jugular foramen. More efficient are high-resolution CT scans. MRI is also rewarding; both modalities may be combined. Common carotid and vertebral angiograms (DSA). Superselective angiography (feeding vessels, embolization) is also an option. Suspected occlusion of the sigmoid sinus is evaluated by retrograde jugulography.

Differentiation is required from cholesterol granuloma of the middle ear, a high-riding jugular bulb, and a laterally displaced internal carotid artery. Also differentiate from neuromas of cranial nerves IX, X, XI, or XII (radiographs generally show *sharply* marginated bone defects, contrasting with the blurred, indistinct margins associated with glomus tumors).

Acoustic Neuroma

Main symptoms: Initial tinnitus and slight hearing loss, followed by mild balance disturbances. Three stages (tumor size) with focal,

Table 1.**8** Symptoms of acoustic neuroma

Three stages:	I:	Small intrameatal tumors, maximum diameter less than 8 mm (focal symptoms see below)
	II:	Intrameatal–intracranial tumors, maximum diameter less than 2.5 cm (focal and regional symptoms, see below)
	III:	Intracranial tumors; maximum diameter greater than 2.5 cm (focal, regional, and cerebral compression symptoms, see below)
Focal symptoms:		– Tinnitus and increasing (retrocochlear) sensorineural hearing loss. Negative recruitment. Audiologic details, see p. 78 – Vertigo and balance disturbances (initially subtle, often the first symptom). Neuro-otologic details, see p. 108
Regional symptoms:		– Trigeminal nerve: facial hypoesthesia, diminished corneal reflex, positive Hitzelberger sign (hypoesthesia of the posterosuperior external auditory canal) – Facial nerve: facial twitches or facial paralysis (unilateral) – Abducens nerve: diplopia – Glossopharyngeal nerve and/or vagus nerve: dysphagia, sometimes combined with hoarseness (recurrent nerve) – Cerebellum: ataxia, uncoordinated limb movements, dysdiadochokinesis
Cerebral compression symptoms:		– Headache (often most pronounced occipitally) – Projectile vomiting – Decreased visual acuity (papilledema) – Personality change
CSF:		Elevated protein (> 100 mg/100 cm^3, but no pleocytosis); with an advanced mass lesion: increased CSF pressure (see p. 43)

regional, and possible cerebral compression symptoms (see Table 1.**8**). Peak occurrence is in the 3rd–6th decades. Incidence of bilaterality is approximately 2%. Acoustic neuroma is the most common neoplasm of the cerebellopontine angle (70–90%).

Cause: Histologically benign schwannoma that can cause extensive damage by expansive growth.

Diagnosis:
● Audiologic evaluation (see p. 78).
● Neuro-otologic evaluation (see p. 108).
● Diagnostic imaging: CT with or without air contrast. Meatal cisternography (contrast medium in the subarachnoid space) has declined in importance, while MRI has become the modality of choice.
● CSF examination: protein elevated >100 mg/100 mL, but no increase in cellularity!

Differentiation is required from Ménière disease, sudden hearing loss, primary ("true") cholesteatoma of the petrous pyramid or cerebellopontine angle, and middle ear cholesteatoma invading the internal auditory canal. Meningioma is the second most common cerebellopontine angle tumor (5–10%) (roentgenograms usually show a defect clearly outlined by a sclerotic bony "shell"; demonstrable by CT or also MRI): Facial or trigeminal nerve neuroma. Epidermoid (3–6%), glomus jugulare tumor, chondroma, cerebellar tumor, vascular anomaly, aneurysm. Lymphoma. Syphilis (especially congenital).

Rare Causes

Rare causes of swelling about the ear include benign neoplasms such as *adenomas* ("ceruminoma," hidradenoma), *pleomorphic adenomas* (parotid gland!), *chondromas, osteofibromas, ossifying fibromas, giant cell tumors,* "pseudo-tumors" (bone cysts), also *Paget disease of bone* and *osteitis fibrosa cystica generalisata* (Recklinghausen disease), which may be combined with "brown tumors" (giant cell tumors). Bony "swellings" about the ear may also be a feature of the *histiocytosis X* group, which includes *eosinophilic granuloma, Hand–Schüller–Christian disease,* and *Letterer–Siwe disease.*

Diagnosis: Radiology, biopsy, general examination!

Malignant Tumors

Epithelial malignancies of the ear (squamous cell carcinomas and adenocarcinomas) are generally manifested initially by ulceration, bleeding, fetid otorrhea, and sometimes otalgia, rather than by a visible swelling (see pp. 8 and 15). Peak occurrence is 60–70 years with a 7:1 preponderance of males. Massive swelling (of soft tissues covering the lateral skull) may occur as a *late* finding. The same applies to "secondary" malignancies of the ear arising from the parotid gland or skull base. *Early* swelling, rather, is characteristic of *metastatic malignancies* from the digestive tract, breast, and hypernephroma as a result of tumor seeding to periauricular lymph nodes.

The very rare *mesenchymal malignancies* of the ear (spindle cell sarcoma, fibrosarcoma, rhabdomyosarcoma, etc.) are often manifested initially by a marked, rapidly enlarging, painless soft-tissue swelling in the periauricular region. Sarcomas are more common than carcinomas in adolescents! *Malignant melanomas* of the external ear can likewise produce marked, early swelling due to rapid metastasis to the periauricular nodes, depending on the grade of tumor malignancy (see p. 150).

Diagnosis:
- History, palpation, general ENT status.
- Diagnostic imaging; may include CT and/or MRI depending on local findings.
- Biopsy.

Other Swellings Not Arising Primarily from the Ear

Parotid Gland
See p. 298 ff.

Temporomandibular Joint (Trauma, Arthritis, Osteoarthritis)

Main symptoms: Swelling *anterior* to the tragus, occasional tenderness over the TMJ, painful mastication.

Diagnosis: History of trauma, dental extraction, or articular rheumatism. Dental consultation.

Regional Lymph Nodes

Main symptoms: Swelling, occasionally with tenderness in the preauricular area (parotid region) or retroauricular area (mastoid plane), about the mastoid tip, and at or below the sternocleidomastoid insertion. Enlarged regional lymph nodes are palpable and displaceable.

Causes: Inflammation in the area drained by these groups of nodes (mainly the ear and its surroundings, also the scalp; also "pseudomastoiditis" secondary to scratching for head lice). Diseases of the lymphatic system (see Tables 10.**6**, 10.**8**, 10.**12**). Lymphogenous metastasis from the ear, face, or scalp. See p. 397 ff. for further details.

Diagnosis:
- Detailed history, palpation.
- Otoscopy (exclusion of otogenic inflammatory cause).
- Exclusion of a primary head and neck tumor, including a "concealed" primary behind the hairline (e.g., melanoma).
- ESR and differential blood count.
- Biopsy (or at least cytodiagnostic aspiration) especially of lesions that do not regress or are unresponsive to treatment.
- Internal medical consultation may be required (to exclude a generalized lymphatic disease, see p. 406 ff.).

Symptom   **Malformation of the Ear**

The mandibular and hyoid arches, and thus the first and second branchial arches and the first pharyngeal pouch, play a crucial role in the ontogenesis of the middle ear region. The inner ear, meanwhile, develops from the ectodermal otocyst. Complex formative stages during embryonic development account for the exceptionally broad spectrum of potential isolated anomalies of the ear region and the diverse combinations of deformities that can affect the ear, face, and neck.

Not all ear malformations present as *morphologic changes* that are visible externally or detectable by otoscopy. Malformations that affect only the tympanic cavity and/or labyrinthine system are manifested by *other cardinal symptoms*, which include various forms of *hearing loss, vestibular dysfunction* and, less commonly, *facial nerve dysfunction*. These symptoms may be associated with visible dysmorphias of the ear, face, or neck that arouse specific clinical interest at an early stage (see Table 1.19). The principal ear malformations are listed in Table 1.9 according to differential diagnostic criteria. Audiologic differential diagnosis is discussed on p. 55 ff.

Since visible malformations cause parents to seek medical attention for their child at a very early age, but diagnostic options are still limited in small children, it is useful to stage the diagnostic workup according to the patient's age, physical and mental development, and therapeutic requirements so that the evaluation can be expanded and completed at the appropriate time (see p. 83).

Diagnosis:
● Inspection (whole body), otoscopy, and general ENT findings. Start with a gross classification of the deformity and identify the involved portions of the ear.
● Radiography (depending on the patient's age). Standard Schüller and Stenvers projections; CT scans of the petrous pyramids.
● The most accurate and complete audiologic workup possible for age (see p. 55).
● Age-appropriate neuro-otologic status (see p. 97) including testing of facial nerve function (see p. 152 ff.).
● Exclusion of additional, generalized malformations. Pediatric and/or genetic consultation.

Congenital Aural Fistula

Main symptoms: Preauricular (usually anterior to the ascending helix), circumscribed, extremely tender area of recurrent swelling and redness. During noninflamed periods the lesion appears as a dimple in the skin (fistulous opening), which occasionally emits a cloudy

Table 1.**9** *Symptom* Malformation of the ear

Synopsis		
Location and type of malformation	Type of hearing impairment	Clinical remarks
External ear		
Congenital auricular tags	None	Cosmetically conspicuous
Auricular anomalies such as Darwin ear, macacus ear, cat's ear, lop ear, Wildemuth ear, Stahl ear, macrotia, apostasis	None	Cosmetically conspicuous
Split earlobe	None	Cosmetically conspicuous
Congenital aural fistula	None	Cosmetically conspicuous at times; recurrent inflammation and retention of secretions

Table 1.**9**   (cont.)

Synopsis		
Congenital otocervical fistula	None	Malformation of the 1st and/or 2nd branchial cleft creating cysts, ducts, or fistulae of variable extent between the auricle, auricular base, parotid gland, external auditory canal, tympanic cavity, mandibular angle, submental and cervical region. See also p. 402
Microtia		Usually combined with atresia of the external ear canal and middle ear anomalies
– Without ear canal atresia	None	
– With ear canal atresia	Conductive hearing loss	
Stenosis of the ear canal (connective-tissue or bony)	Possible conductive hearing loss	Proneness to otitis externa
Atresia of the ear canal	Conductive hearing loss	
Duplicated ear canal	Possible conductive hearing loss	Retention, recurrent suppuration, etc.
Middle ear		
Aplasia or dysplasia of the tympanic membrane	Conductive hearing loss	
Dysplasia of the tympanic cavity	Conductive hearing loss, possible inner ear involvement	Depends on type and severity of the malformation
Ossicular dysplasia and/or dysmorphia	Conductive hearing loss	Variable degree of hearing impairment
Persistent stapedial artery	Conductive hearing loss	Possible pulsatile tinnitus
Atypical course and/or branching of the facial nerve	Possible conductive hearing loss	Facial nerve dysfunction may be present or absent
Dysplasia of the petrous pyramid	Variable auditory findings	Variable findings
Inner ear		
Classic types of deformity (Michel, Bing–Siebenmann, Mondini, Scheibe)	See Table 1.**42**	
Various genetic hearing impairments or deafness	See Table 1.**42**	
Without other dysplastic manifestations	See Table 1.**42**	
With dysplasias in conjunction with malformation syndromes	See Table 1.**43**	
Internal auditory canal		
Narrowing of the internal acoustic meatus	Sensorineural hearing loss or deafness	

Malformations in the area of the *craniocervical junction* can also cause otalgia and hearing loss (see p. 18)

fluid. The fistulous tract may open near the tympanic membrane in the external auditory canal or even within the tympanic cavity (type I). A type II fistula, the most common, consists of a relatively shallow, superficial cavity system terminating near the ear canal in the anterior cervical triangle below the mandibular angle or at the junction of the cartilaginous and bony ear canal. Some type II fistulas pass with the facial nerve through the parotid gland! Both types may be associated with cysts and/or sinuses anterior to the tragus.

Causes: Anomalous development of ducts or duct systems based on the first or occasionally the second branchial cleft system. Some cases may also reflect abnormalities in the fusion of second and third auricular hillocks. Retained secretions in the fistulous tract lead to marked inflammatory signs or even abscess formation.

Diagnosis:
● History (recurrent bouts of inflammation at the same, typical location). Generally a small dimple is visible in the area of redness and swelling. In the noninflamed state, milky fluid can usually be expressed from the fistulous opening, and a probe can be passed into the fistulous tract.
● The extent of the noninflamed fistula can be established radiographically by the injection of contrast medium.

Differentiation is required from auricular perichondritis, furunculosis, and abscess formation (e.g., due to insect bite).

Combined Malformations of the External and Middle Ear

Main symptoms; Auricular dysplasia (e.g., microtia, anotia) may coexist with atresia (or stenosis) of the external auditory canal (bony or, rarely, connective-tissue form) in various combinations. Associated facial dysplasias are common (see Tables 1.**19** and 2.**13**). There are varying degrees of hearing impairment, mostly conductive hearing loss. Inner ear malformations may coexist. For further details see p. 83 and Tables 1.**19** and 1.**43**.

Causes: Genetic and/or exogenous factors.

Diagnosis:
● Inspection and palpation.
● Radiography: CT scans.
● Complete audiologic and neuro-otologic status.

Malformations and Congenital Dysfunctions of the Inner Ear
See p. 83 ff.

Symptom   **Cutaneous Change around the Ear**

See Table 2.**4**.

Symptom   **Change in the Tympanic Membrane**

Table 1.**10**   Typical tympanic membrane changes

Changes	Causes
Position	
Irregular, partial, or complete displacement of the plane of the tympanic membrane	Previous middle ear surgery or trauma
Lateralization of the tympanic membrane	Congenital bony or connective-tissue atresia of the ear canal
	Acquired (secondary) connective-tissue atresia following surgery, trauma, or chronic dermatosis
Funnel-shaped tympanic membrane	Partial atresia of the ear canal
Retracted tympanic membrane, prominent short process of malleus, with or without middle ear effusion	Subacute or chronic eustachian tube dysfunction Adhesive process Previous middle ear surgery

Table 1.**10**   (cont.)

Changes	Causes
Bulging tympanic membrane (grayish-brown)	Cholesterol granuloma
Bulging tympanic membrane (chalky white)	Middle ear cholesteatoma
Bulging tympanic membrane (red color visible behind membrane)	Glomus tympanicum and other middle ear tumors
Tympanic membrane bulging, transparent, very thin	Patulous eustachian tube
Structure	
Thickened and opaque tympanic membrane	Previous middle ear surgery (tympanic membrane graft) Mucosus otitis Resolving acute otitis media Fungal infection
Scarred, relatively immobile tympanic membrane of nonuniform structure	Previous trauma Previous middle ear surgery Chronic eustachian tube dysfunction with scars and adhesions
Color	
Red to purple	Hematotympanum
Blue ("blue drum")	Chronic seromucous otitis media
Pink, translucent	Middle ear effusion due to acute disturbance of eustachian tube ventilation Otosclerosis
Yellow (amber)	Older middle ear effusion due to impaired eustachian tube ventilation
Blackish-gray (can be wiped off)	Coated with *Aspergillus niger*
White (can be wiped off)	Coated with *Candida albicans*
Grayish-white to brownish (may be slightly glossy)	Cholesterol granuloma
White (chalky or glossy-translucent)	Middle ear cholesteatoma
Reddened with dark brown bullae	Hemorrhagic (influenzal) otitis
Membrane surface	
Scaly or flaky coating	Incipient or resolving acute suppurative otitis media Involvement by otitis externa
Granulating	Simple myringitis, often caused by: − Fungal infection of the drumhead − Tuberculosis
Common tympanic perforations	
Single central perforation, usually very small and draining	Acute otitis media
Single central perforation with smooth edges; size ranges from pinhole to oval- or kidney-shaped perforation to a total defect	Chronic otitis media, mucosal suppuration type Rarely, suppurating cholesteatoma ("tensacholesteatoma type") Tuberculous otitis media (rare)
Single central perforation with jagged edges that may show bloody inhibition; variable size	Recent trauma
Single marginal perforation of variable size and location	Chronic otitis media, suppurating cholesteatoma type Previous severe trauma separating the tympanic membrane from the annulus (e. g., longitudinal temporal fracture)
Multiple (central) perforations	Tuberculous otitis media, otitis in measles

Symptom   Otogenic Facial Nerve Paralysis

Facial nerve paralysis can have numerous causes (see p. 154). An *otogenic cause* is relatively common, and *otogenic facial paralysis* represents a special category in differential diagnosis owing to its close relationship with various ear diseases. Hence a separate section is devoted to the differential diagnosis of *otogenic facial paralysis*.

To avoid repetition, we also refer the reader to the section on *Facial Paralysis* (see p. 150 ff.), which lists the *most important diagnostic options* and reviews the differentiation of *nonotogenic facial paralysis*.

Otogenic facial paralysis is *always* a *peripheral* paralysis that may be partial or complete, transient or permanent. Further details are given on p. 150 and in Figures 1.**3**, 1.**4**, and 1.**5**.

Inflammatory Causes

Facial Paralysis in Acute Otitis Media

Main symptoms: *Early facial nerve paralysis,* marked by onset of (often partial and/or transient) paralysis during the initial days of otitis media, is not uncommon, especially in children. Produces typical flaccid paralysis of the mimetic muscles with inability to whistle, frown, or inflate the cheek on the affected

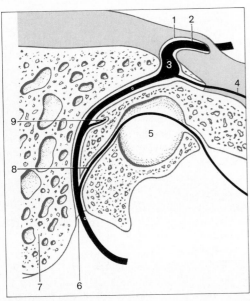

Fig. 1.**3**   Course of the facial nerve in the petrous part of the temporal bone

1 Bony wall of the internal acoustic meatus
2 Facial nerve
3 Geniculate ganglion of the facial nerve
4 Greater petrosal nerve
5 Tympanic cavity
6 Stylomastoid foramen
7 Mastoid with air cells
8 Chorda tympani
9 Stapedius nerve

Table 1.**11**   *Symptom*   Otogenic facial nerve paralysis

Synopsis
Inflammatory causes
Acute otitis media
Chronic otitis media
Malignant otitis externa, see p. 7
(Herpes) zoster oticus, see p. 4
Traumatic causes
Longitudinal temporal bone fracture
Transverse temporal bone fracture
Iatrogenic
Obstetric trauma
Neoplastic causes
Arising from the facial nerve
– Neuroma
With secondary involvement of the facial nerve
– Acoustic neuroma, see pp. 29, 78, 108
– Cerebellopontine angle tumor
– Primary (true) cholesteatoma
– Histiocytosis X, see p. 218
– Leukemic deposits, see p. 406
– Angioma, see pp. 146, 308, 405
– Glomus tumor (chemodectoma), see p. 29
– Carcinoma, see p. 31
– Sarcoma, see p. 31
Congenital

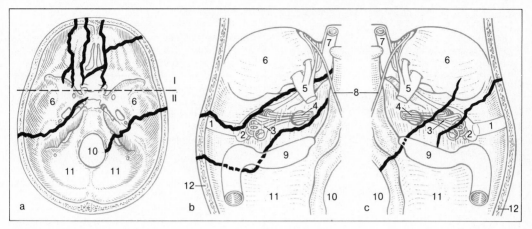

Fig. 1.**4a−c**   Types of basal skull fracture (**b** and **c** modified from Patten)

a Overall skull base, showing frontobasal (I) and laterobasal (II) fractures
b Typical longitudinal temporal bone fractures
c Typical transverse temporal bone fractures
  1 External auditory canal
  2 Tympanic cavity
  3 Labyrinth with cochlea and semicircular canals
  4 Internal acoustic meatus with facial nerve and statoacoustic nerve
  5 Semilunar (gasserian) ganglion of trigeminal nerve
  6 Middle cranial fossa
  7 Internal carotid artery
  8 Abducens nerve
  9 Sigmoid sinus
  10 Foramen magnum
  11 Posterior cranial fossa
  12 Cranial bone (in section)
(See also Table 1.**12**)

side. Facial distortion and asymmetry during speaking and laughing. Eating and drinking difficulties. The Bell phenomenon (upward and medial eye movement on attempt to close the eye). The paralysis may also have a later onset, especially with incipient or advanced bone destruction (mastoiditis), occurring at *any* time during acute middle ear inflammation. Pain, if present, is caused less by the nerve lesion than by otitis media.

Other symptoms and special features: Possible disturbance of taste sensation (ipsilateral). Abortive paralytic symptoms can occur when disease is limited to isolated nerve fiber bundles (see Fig. 4.**4**).

Causes: Collateral transmission (especially in early paralysis) or direct involvement of nerve tissue by an inflammatory or destructive process in the middle ear region. Transmission is facilitated by sites of bone dehiscence in the fallopian canal.

Diagnosis:
● Detection of middle ear inflammation is crucial. This can be difficult in infants (obliquity of the tympanic membrane relative to the ear canal axis, very firm membrane, absence of tympanic perforation, absence of pneumatization, etc.; see p. 10).
● After infancy, otoscopic findings are supplemented by radiographs (Schüller; CT).
● Audiologic status.
● Bacteriologic examination of aural discharge and sensitivity tests.
● Possible exploratory (and decompressive) paracentesis.
● Additional age-appropriate nerve function tests (see p. 152).

Differentiation is required from other possible causes of the paralysis (see Table 1.**11**).

Facial Paralysis in Chronic Otitis Media

Main symptoms: Like those in acute otitis media (see above), but usually there is a long his-

Table 1.**12**   Symptoms associated with temporal bone fractures (see Fig. 1.**4**)

Longitudinal fractures (approximately 70–80%, caused chiefly by violence from the side)	Transverse fractures (approximately 20%, caused chiefly by violence from the front or back)
Middle ear symptoms predominate	*Inner ear symptoms predominate*
Bleeding from the ear canal	Ear canal and tympanic membrane intact
Hematotympanum	Possible hematotympanum
Rupture of the tympanic membrane	
Discontinuity in the bony annulus and/or external ear canal	
Ossicular discontinuity	
Impression of the mandibular head in the ear canal	
Conductive hearing loss (may be combined with sensorineural hearing loss)	Deafness Vertigo and spontaneous nystagmus toward the unaffected side (due to labyrinthine damage)
Facial nerve paralysis (in about 20%) (typical site of injury: geniculate ganglion or 2nd genu of facial nerve)	Facial nerve paralysis (in about 50%) (typical site of injury: labyrinth or internal auditory canal)
CSF otorrhea (through middle ear and external auditory canal)	Otogenic CSF leak (rhinorrhea), frequently through the eustachian tube to the nasopharynx
Standard radiographs (Schüller): Fracture line through the squama, middle ear, posterior canal wall, mastoid	Standard radiographs (Stenvers): Fracture line through the labyrinth or internal auditory canal
Other structures at risk: middle meningeal artery (epidural hematoma), sigmoid sinus, cavernous sinus, petrosal sinus	Other structures at risk: internal carotid artery, trigeminal nerve, abducens nerve

Mixed and *bilateral fractures* also occur

tory of otitic symptoms. A cholesteatoma or granulating process is generally present.

Diagnosis:
● Otoscopy (tympanic membrane perforation typical of chronic otitis media; detection or exclusion of cholesteatoma).
● Schüller and Stenvers radiographs (to detect bone destruction about the facial nerve). Preferable, tomograms or CT scans to detect erosion of the facial canal.

● Complete inner ear evaluation (auditory and vestibular testing). Nerve function tests (see p. 152).

Differentiation is required from the other causes listed in Table. 1.**11**.

Facial Paralysis in Malignant Otitis Externa
See p. 7.

Facial Paralysis in Zoster Oticus

See p. 4.

Traumatic Causes

Main symptoms: Temporal correlation between onset of facial paralysis and an adequate traumatic event (injury, accident, surgery).

Other symptoms and special features: Degree (temporary, permanent) and extent (partial, complete) of the paralysis depend on the mechanism of the injury, the violence of the trauma, etc.

Diagnosis:
- Otoscopy and complete audiologic and neuro-otologic evaluation.
- Radiography: CT scans.
- Nerve function tests (see p. 152).

Special Situation:

Temporal Bone Fracture (Fig. 1.4a–c)

With a *longitudinal fracture of the petrous pyramid* (the most common temporal bone fracture), complete or partial facial paralysis may be concomitant with the injury or may ensue after a period of hours or days ("late paralysis"). The latter type is caused by reactive edema in tissues surrounding the nerve or by a hematoma. Late facial paralysis has a favorable prognosis. *Middle ear symptoms* are predominant with a longitudinal fracture (hematotympanon, tympanic perforation, conductive hearing loss, typical fracture signs in the ear canal and/or mastoid) (Table 1.**12** and Fig. 1.**4b**).

A *transverse temporal bone fracture* almost always causes (complete) facial paralysis at the time of the injury. *Inner ear symptoms* are predominant with this injury (deafness, vestibular dysfunction) (Table 1.**12** and Fig. 1.**4c**). The location and course of any temporal bone fracture are radiographically (CT) analyzed and documented.

Other Injuries

Self-inflicted injuries (knitting needle, twig, ear spoon, etc.), also facial nerve paralysis during or after *ear operations.* Paralysis developing hours or days after the injury, surgical procedure, packing, or removal of packing have a significantly better prognosis than paralysis occurring simultaneously with the surgery or manipulation.

Obstetric injury and *intrauterine pressure injury* are rare causes of facial nerve paralysis. The resulting paralysis is usually incomplete. Facial asymmetries or at least symptoms of a pressure insult are generally apparent immediately after birth.

Facial Nerve Paralysis Due to Tumor Growth

Main symptoms: Paralysis is typically painless, persistent, and slowly progressive; may be partial initially.

Other symptoms and special features: Warning signs are often absent initially and later depend on the type and location of the tumor. Progressive hearing loss is not uncommon (see p. 72). Besides the facial nerve, middle ear tumors may also involve the glossopharyngeal, vagus, and/or accessory nerves (jugular foramen syndrome, see Table 1.**18**).

Causes: It is relatively rare for tumors causing facial nerve paralysis to *arise from the nerve itself* (facial neuroma, see p. 156). Peak occurrence in middle age. Facial neuromas affect the mastoid segment of the nerve more frequently than the tympanic segment.

Facial nerve paralysis is caused far more commonly by benign or malignant tumors developing *in proximity to the nerve:* acoustic neuromas and other histologically benign tumors of the petrous pyramid or cerebellopontine angle; also primary cholesteatomas, histiocytosis X, leukemic deposits, angiomas, glomus jugulare tumors (chemodectomas), and carcinomas of the ear and other rare malignancies (e.g., rhabdomyosarcomas).

Diagnosis:
- Otoscopy usually reveals normal findings (at least initially). Tumor-related facial paralysis is often dismissed initially as "idiopathic." Facial paralysis that does not improve in 2–3 months (electrophysiologic tests) *must* be thoroughly evaluated to rule out neoplastic disease.

- Complete inner ear evaluation (audiologic and neuro-otologic).
- Diagnostic imaging: CT. Increasingly, MRI is also used depending on the inquiry.
- Neurologic consultation. Follow-ups at 2-month intervals.

Differentiation is required from (herpes) zoster oticus and other neurotropic viral dis-

eases that present few symptoms. Severe "idiopathic" paralysis with neurotmesis. Tumors involving the extratemporal part of the nerve (parotid gland, face). See p. 156.

Even a *congenital* facial paralysis can be called *"otogenic"* with some justification if it is combined with a *malformation of the middle ear.* See Tables 1.**9**, 1.**19**, and 2.**13**.

Symptom   **Intracranial Otogenic Complications**

Seee Table 1.**13** and Figure, 1.**5** and 1.**6**.

Table 1.**13**   Major symptoms of otogenic complications

Disease	Fever	Chills	Head-ache	Abnor-mal neu-rologic findings	Abnor-mal CSF findings	Typical radio-graphic findings	Details
Mastoiditis	+++	–	Mastoid pain	–	–	+++	see p. 11
Petrositis	++	–	++	++	(+)	+++	see p. 14
Sigmoid sinus thrombosis	+++	+++ (not in children)	Affected side	–	–	(+)	see p. 41
Otitic hydrocepha-lus	–	–	++	(+)	++ (pres-sure)	(+)	see p. 46
Epidural abscess	(+)	–	+ to ++	–	–	(+)	see p. 42
Subdural abscess	+	–	+	Possible	+	(+) to ++	see p. 42
Bacterial menin-gitis	+++	–	+++	+++	+++	–	see p. 42
Brain abscess	(+) to ++	–	+++	+++	++	+++	see p. 43

(+) = Occasionally present
+   = Present but not always with clear diagnostic significance
++   = Pronounced
+++ = Always present and very pronounced

Otogenic Sinus Thrombosis (Generally Affecting the Sigmoid Sinus)

Main symptoms: Chills, intermittent ("septic") temperatures spikes above 40 °C or continuous pyemic fever. Rapid pulse. Frequent chills with corresponding septic temperatures are an ominous sign!

Other symptoms and special features: Nausea and vomiting, lethargy ranging to somnolence, possible papilledema. The Griesinger sign: tenderness to pressure at the posterior border of the mastoid (site of emergence of mastoid emissary vein). Later, tenderness and palpable firmness may be found along the internal jugular vein at the anterior border of the sternocleidomastoid muscle. Stiff neck (with accompanying meningitis), dyspnea (with pulmonary metastases). Splenomegaly. Jaundice (with septic hepatic metastases). Muscle and joint complaints (septic joint metastases) and petechial hemorrhages in the skin. Chills are generally absent in children, who have only a high sustained or intermittent fever. Chills and septic temperatures also may be absent in patients receiving antibiotics. Inadequate antibiotic treatment can prolong prodromal symptoms and obscure warning signs (masking effect).

Causes: Spread of infection from the ear (mastoid) with periphlebitis, phlebitis, thrombosis, and increasing obliteration of the sinus lumen. This complication has become rare. See also Figures 1.**5** and 1.**6**.

Diagnosis:
- Otoscopy shows unresolved otitis media.
- Schüller radiograph, CT. Additional MRI may be indicated. Carotid angiography may show an obstruction in the (sigmoid) sinus during the runoff phase.
- Internal medical consultation (septic metastases?).
- Bacteriologic examination of the blood (serum cultures, preferably on blood drawn during episode of chills). Urinanalysis (e.g., hematuria, albuminuria, and cylindruria with interstitial focal nephritis). Differential blood count shows leukocytosis and a left shift with markedly increased ESR.
- CSF often shows mild pleocytosis and increased protein.

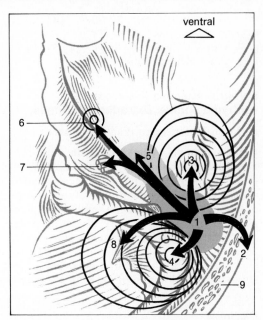

Fig. 1.**5**   Potential routes of spread for purulent otogenic complications (schematic diagram)

1 Middle ear region
2 Extension to the outside
3 Spread to middle cranial fossa and temporal lobe
4 Spread to sigmoid sinus
5 Involvement of inner ear and labyrinth
6 Spread to petrous apex (the Gradenigo syndrome)
7 Spread to the subarachnoid space via the internal auditory canal
8 Spread to the posterior cranial fossa and cerebellum
9 Lateral cranial bone (in section)
(See also Fig. 1.**2**)

Differentiation is required from influenza, typhus, malaria, Bang disease, viral pneumonia, miliary tuberculosis. Postanginal sepsis, septic endocarditis. Thrombosis of other dural sinuses, e.g.:
- *Transverse sinus thrombosis:* The Griesinger sign very often positive.
- *Extension through the superior petrosal sinus to the cavernous sinus:* Swelling of the upper lid, chemosis, possible proptosis, papilledema, oculomotor paralysis. See p. 214, Figure 1.**6**, and Table 1.**18**.

• *Thrombosis of the jugular bulb:* Sometimes associated with paralysis of the glossopharyngeal, vagus, or accessory nerve—jugular foramen syndrome (see Table 1.**18**).

Epidural Abscess (External Pachymeningitis, Extradural Abscess)

Lacks characteristic cardinal symptoms.

Other symptoms and special features: Headache (dull and boring, sometimes throbbing). Fever may be present, but often there is vague malaise with subfebrile temperatures. Cerebral symptoms (vomiting, somnolence, slow pulse) are unusual. Primary disease is often acute otitis media, less commonly chronic otitis media. Given its nonspecific symptoms, epidural abscess is often first discovered during surgical exploration of the middle ear (cf. Fig. 3.**6**).

Diagnosis:
• Detection of otitis media, which may already appear resolved!
• Suspected epidural abscess should be confirmed or excluded by imaging studies (CT, MRT, possibly angiography). Site of predilection is the posterior cranial fossa (often near the sinus); less common site is the middle cranial fossa near the mastoid air cell system.

Differentiation is required from epidural hematoma (different history; trauma), headache of other etiology (see p. 157 ff.), and other otogenic complications in the developing stage.

Subdural Abscess (Internal Pachymeningitis)

Subdural abscess, like epidural abscess, usually does not cause characteristic symptoms. There may be headache and somnolence. Aphasia, seizures, and hemiplegia are rare. Especially in patients receiving inadequate antibiotic treatment, subdural abscess is a precursor of meningitis or brain abscess (see analogous situation in Fig. 3.**6**). Suspicion of one or more subdural abscesses can be confirmed by CT or MRI and possibly by other neuroradiologic studies such as EEG, echoencephalography, and radionuclide imaging. Subdural abscess and otogenic meningitis may coexist!

Otogenic Meningitis (Leptomeningitis)

Main symptoms: Otitis media (may be largely asymptomatic or "resolved"). Severe headache, stiff neck; high sustained fever. Photophobia, agitation. Nausea and vomiting. Positive Kernig sign.

Other symptoms and special features: Increasing daze. Scaphoid abdomen (opisthotonos). Motor irritation signs (tonic—clonic spasms). Cranial nerve paralysis (abducens, oculomotor, facial) may occur. Highly variable pulse. Disturbance of mentation. Possible eyeground changes (papilledema). Positive pyramidal tract signs (Babinski, Gordon, Oppenheim). Blood count shows pleocytosis with a left shift. Possible sudden onset of symptoms with rapid deterioration, sometimes within a few hours!

Causes: Spread of bacterial infection from the middle ear and labyrinth to the leptomeninx through preexisting pathways or by osteomyelitic destruction and dural penetration.

Diagnosis:
• Assessment of current otologic and rhinologic findings.
• Radiography: Schüller and Stenvers projections, possibly paranasal sinus views (exclusion of hidden foci). CT, MRI, and radionuclide scans are options for exclusion of brain abscess.
• Lumbar or suboccipital puncture (Tables 1.**14** and 1.**15**): pressure elevation (>200 mmH$_2$O), pleocytosis, CSF protein content markedly increased (positive Pandy), glucose reduced, chlorides increased.
• Bacteria (predominantly pneumococci, also streptococci, staphylococci, Haemophilus influenzae, etc.) can be identified if antibiotics have not yet been administered.

Differentiation is required from epidemic meningitis, others, especially nonpurulent meningitides, tuberculous meningitis (glucose markedly reduced!). Incipient brain abscess. Especially when "stiff neck" is present, consider: cerebral concussion or contusion, polyradiculitis, intracranial hemorrhage, brain tumor, cervical spine pathology, and tetanus. See also Table 10.**2**.

Table 1.**14** Typical cerebrospinal fluid findings

CSF finding	Disorder
Increased pressure (normal = 70–120 mmH$_2$O)	Brain tumor; subdural hematoma; brain abscess; meningitis; sinus thrombosis
Increased total protein (normal = 25–40 mg/100 mL)	Meningitis; chronic subdural hematoma; encephalitis; multiple sclerosis (in some cases); poliomyelitis, etc.
Discoloration Blood-tinged	Acute subarachnoid hemorrhage; intracerebral hematoma; possible after lumbar puncture; cranial trauma
Xanthochromic	Older intracranial hemorrhage; internal hemorrhagic pachymeningosis; brain tumor; chronic icterus
Pleocytosis Predominantly granulocytes	Bacterial meningitis in acute stage; brain tumor; previous trauma, hemorrhage, abscess; encephalitis; subarachnoid hemorrhage
Predominantly lymphocytes	Serous meningitis; syphilis; multiple sclerosis; poliomyelitis; resolution stage of bacterial meningitis
Increased glucose	Diabetes; encephalitis; stroke; (brain tumor); (hypertension)
Decreased glucose	Bacterial meningitis; subacute meningitis; brain abscess; hypoglycemia
Increased chlorides	Brain tumor; encephalitis; myelitis
Decreased chlorides	Meningitis; cerebellar tumor; cerebral syphilis; acute infectious diseases

Otogenic Brain Abscess

Otogenic brain abscesses, though much less frequent since the advent of antibiotic therapy, can still occur. Their relative scarcity makes a given abscess all the more dangerous, because the classic symptoms are often masked (especially with antibiotic treatment) and are apt to be overlooked or misinterpreted on initial examination. Otogenic brain abscesses develop by direct extension, i.e., they are always located near the primary focus in the temporal lobe of the cerebrum (approximately two-thirds) or in the cerebellum (approximately one-third) (see Fig. 1.**5**).

Both sites are associated with similar, nonspecific *general symptoms*. They differ, however, with regard to *cerebral compression symptoms* and *focal symptoms*.

General symptoms: Malaise, anorexia, "endocranial facies." Fever (in some cases). Severe, dull headache (see p. 157 ff.); possible tenderness to cranial percussion. Pulse rate initially increased and/or irregular, becoming slower as the disease progresses (<60/min, "pressure pulse"). Personality change, slowed mental responses, occasional disorientation; psychic lability; daze and drowsiness ranging to somnolence or even coma; "organic brain

Table 1.15 CSF findings that are useful for differential diagnosis

	Pressure	Appearance	Cell count and type	Total protein	Glucose	Chlorides	Pandy reaction
Normal findings	70–120 mmH$_2$O	clear like water	< 12/3 cells	25–40 mg/100 mL	40–90 mg/100 mL	680–760 mg/100 mL	
Disease:							
Bacterial meningitis	Moderately increased	Yellowish-white, turbid	> 500 (–20 000)/3; initially granulo-cytes, increasing lympho-cytes in the resolu-tion stage	50–1500 mg/100 mL	< 35 mg/100 mL	Decreased	+ to +++
Viral meningitis	Normal (to slightly increased)	Clear (rarely slightly opales-cent)	Slightly increased (< 500/3)	Gradually increasing (to approx. 120 mg/100 mL	Normal	Normal	Gradually more posi-tive
Tuberculous menin-gitis	Increased	Clear, "web-like clots"	Moderate lymphocy-tosis	Increased	Decreased	Decreased	+
Zoster oticus	Normal	Clear, colorless	> 800/3; predomi-nantly lym-phocytes	Often increased	Normal	Normal	+
Spontaneous sub-arachnoid hemor-rhage (pachy-meningitis, tumor)	Usually increased	Xantho-chromic	In some cases old erythro-cytes, granu-locytes	Markedly increased	Increased	Normal	+++
Intracranial trauma	Usually increased	With bledding: red, flesh-colored, or xantho-chromic; otherwise clear	In some cases old erythro-cytes, granu-locytes	Increased	Normal or increased	Normal	++ to +++
Brain abscess	Normal to increased	Clear to opalescent	Mild pleo-cytosis	Normal to slightly increased	Normal to (+)	Normal	(+) to +++
Brain tumor	Increased	Clear (some-times yellowish)	Mild pleo-cytosis	Increased	Normal, occasion-ally +	Normal, occasion-ally –	+

Table 1.**15**   (cont.)

	Pressure	Appearance	Cell count and type	Total protein	Glucose	Chlorides	Pandy reaction
Normal findings	70–120 mmH₂O	clear like water	<12/3 cells	25–40 mg/100 mL	40–90 mg/100 mL	680–760 mg/100 mL	
ENT tumors that have secondarily invaded the skull base	Normal to (+)	Opalescent	Mild pleocytosis, also tumor cells	Greatly increased	Normal	Normal	+++
Acoustic neuroma	(+) to +++	Clear	Not increased	+ to ++	Normal	Normal	

Note: Grade of finding increases from (+) to +++

Table 1.**16**   Features differentiating brain abscess from purulent bacterial meningitis

Symptom	Purulent meningitis	Brain abscess
Puls rate	Increased	(Markedly) decreased
Fever	High	Low or absent
Headache	Sharp and intermittent	Dull and constant
Proneness to convulsions	High	Low
Root irritation	Very common	Uncommon
CSF	Pleocytosis (intitially leuko-cytosis, later lymphocytosis)	Little or no increase in cellu-larity
Optic fundus	Normal	Frequent papilledema

syndrome." Profuse or projectile vomiting (sometimes *without* nausea!). Irregular (Cheyne–Stokes) respiration may occur in the late (terminal) stage. ESR greatly increased. Differential blood count: leukocytosis with a left shift. CSF: pleocytosis, initially with leukocyte predominance; proteins greatly increased with a shift toward the globulins in the electrophoretogram.

Several features are useful for *differential diagnosis* (Table 1.**16**). *Headache due to brain abscess* generally is dull, initially unilateral, and shows an undulating intensity with mild or marked obtundation. Often the patient does not report the headache until specifically questioned. *Meningitis headache,* on the other hand, tends to be sharp and accompanied by motor unrest. The head is moved about, and there is increasing agitation with quiet intervals of lessening duration.

Local Cerebral Symptoms (Focal and Pressure-related Symptoms)

Temporal Lobe Abscess

Papilledema (sometimes subtle!). Amnestic aphasia (word-finding difficulty) or sensory aphasia (word deafness) (in *right-handed* patients with a *left* temporal lobe abscess; may be no analogous pattern in *left-handed* patients!). Tonic perseveration. Occasional alexia and agraphia. Visual disturbances in the form of quadrant hemianopia and/or gaze paralysis of other ocular movements. (Subtle) olfactory dysfunction is also possible. Usually there is marked involvement of motor pathways with impairment of gross strength, crossed partial or complete hemiparesis (leg, arm, facial expression), and marked pyramidal signs (Babinski, Oppenheim, Mendel−Bechterev). Also motor irritation signs: (tonic−)clonic spasms, convulsions. Cranial nerves I−VIII may be affected, especially III (oculomotor), VI (abducens), and VII (facial); facial nerve paralysis may be ipsilateral or contralateral! Subtle central auditory disturbances and acoustic hallucinations.

Cerebellar Abscess

Papilledema is generally pronounced! Intention tremor. Cerebellar ataxia (wide-based, unsteady stance and/or gait, "sailor's gait"). Incoordination of the extremities (adiadochokinesia), upper limb tonus discrepancy (pointing test). Vertigo. Tilted head position and/or abnormal posture in recumbency. Nuchal stiffness can also occur (accompanying meningitis). Cranial nerves III−VII may be involved (especially VI). Gaze-induced nystagmus and/or conjugate deviation "away from the focus." Nondirectional provocative vestibular nystagmus. On walking with eyes closed, gait deviates toward the affected side.

The *four classic stages* of otogenic brain abscess (initial, latent, manifest, terminal) are not always apparent since the condition may take an acute, peracute, or even a chronic "intermittent" course whose symptoms may be further obscured by antibiotics. Multifocality is not uncommon and generally affects a single region (i.e., the temporal lobe *or* the cerebellum). See also Table 1.**17**.

Diagnosis:
● Otoscopic confirmation of a "resolved" or florid otitis media (or sinusitis).
● Complete audiologic and neuro-otologic workup (see pp. 55, 97, and 110).
● Electroencephalogram, echoencephalogram.

● Radiography: Schüller, Stenvers, standard skull films, depending on clinical picture. Paranasal sinus views may be indicated. CT. Radionuclide brain scan. Cerebral angiography (subtraction technique; carotid angiography usually more rewarding than vertebral angiography). Ventriculography (pneumoencephalography, cisternography).
● MRI has assumed major importance in the assessment of these lesions.
● CSF examination (see Tables 1.**14**, 1.**15**, 1.**16**).
● Neurologic and perhaps ophthalmologic consultation may be required.

Depending on the site of the abscess, **differentiation** is required from stroke, brain trauma, brain tumor (slow, protracted course; marked papilledema; CSF findings; more "stable" symptoms), tuberculous meningitis. Diabetic or uremic coma. Infectious diseases (influenza, typhus, etc.). Labyrinthitis, acute labyrinthine failure. Subarachnoid hemorrhage. Nonotogenic and nonrhinogenic (viral) encephalitis, diffuse encephalitis, multiple sclerosis. Cerebellar tumor, cerebellopontine angle syndrome. See also p. 107 ff.

Otitic Hydrocephalus

Main symptoms: Headache, possibly accompanied by ipsilateral facial paralysis or abducens paralysis, occurring several weeks after resolution of an acute otitis media or after sigmoid sinus thrombosis. Nausea and vomiting are the only systemic signs. Chiefly affects children and adolescents. A *very rare* condition.

Cause: Increased intracranial pressure, presumably due to venous congestion.

Diagnosis:
● History of "resolved" acute otitis media or sinus thrombosis. Corresponding local otoscopic findings.
● Optic fundus: Papilledema.
● CSF findings: Markedly increased pressure (>300 mmH$_2$O); fluid clear with no increase in protein or cellularity.
● Neurologic findings: No focal signs.

Differentiation is required from localized meningitis, brain abscess, and brain tumor.

Table 1.**17** Differentiation of temporal lobe abscess, cerebellar abscess, and frontal lobe abscess

Temporal lobe abscess (usually otogenic)	Cerebellar abscess (usually otogenic)	Frontal lobe abscess (usually rhinogenic)
Balance disturbances rare, no nystagmus, no dysdiadocho-kinesia	Nystagmus (central), balance disturbances, adiadochokinesia, past pointing	Possible contralateral ataxia. Paroxysmal gaze deviations with head rotation to the opposite side
Paralysis on the opposite side (but complete hemiplegia is rare!)	Paralysis on the same side, ataxia	Cortical epileptic seizures can occur. Large lesions can produce hemiplegic symptoms
Speech disturbance (word-finding difficulty = amnestic aphasia if the dominant hemisphere is involved	No speech disturbance except possible dysarthria	Mental changes (talkativeness, inappropriate joking, lack of critical thinking). Somnolence, memory loss, apathy
Visual field defects	No visual field defects	
Papilledema rare	Papilledema common and pronounced	Papilledema may occur
Oculomotor dysfunction common	Oculomotor dysfunction less common	Possible (unilateral) anosmia
Abducens paralysis common	Abducens paralysis common	Possible paralysis of ocular muscles
Conjugate deviation ("looks toward the affected side")	Conjugate deviation ("looks away from the affected side")	
Contra- or ipsilateral facial paralysis	Only ipsilateral facial paralysis (central type predominant)	
	Tendency to fall toward the affected side	

Clinical Syndromes Involving Multiple Cranial Nerve Lesions

These conditions may be caused by numerous intracranial and extracranial disorders. Otogenic, rhinogenic, and pharyngogenic causes are not uncommon. For anatomic reasons, *ear diseases* tend preferentially to involve cranial nerves V−XII in various combinations. Since overlapping etiologies are possible in the skull base region (Fig. 1.**6**), the listing in Table 1.**18** includes *all* of the more common clinical skull base syndromes, even though many are non-otogenic, in order to make the connections more clear.

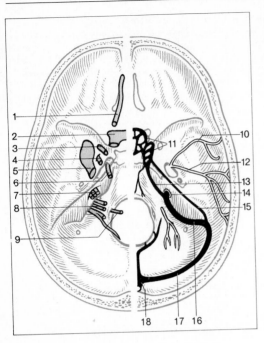

Fig. 1.6 Structures of the skull base (left side of figure: cranial nerves; right side: major blood vessels)

1 Olfactory nerve (I)
2 Chiasm of optic nerve (II)
3 Oculomotor nerve (III)
4 Trochlear nerve (IV)
5 Trigeminal nerve (V) with semilunar (gasserian) ganglion
6 Abducens nerve (VI)
7 Facial nerve (VII) and statoacoustic nerve (VIII) in the internal auditory canal
8 Glossopharyngeal nerve (IX), vagus nerve (X), and accessory nerve (XI) in the jugular foramen
9 Hypoglossal nerve (XII)
10 Frontal and parietal branches of the middle meningeal artery
11 Cavernous sinus
12 Meningeal branch of the middle meningeal artery
13 Inferior petrosal sinus
14 Jugular foramen with jugular vein
15 Superior petrosal sinus
16 Sigmoid sinus
17 Transverse sinus
18 Confluence of sinuses

Table 1.18 Clinical syndromes involving multiple cranial nerve lesions (see also Fig. 1.6)

Name (and synonyms)	Main clinical symptoms	Anatomic substrate	Causes	Clinical remarks
Olfactory syndrome	Unilateral, then bilateral anosmia; vision loss (optic nerve atrophy); possible frontal lobe syndrome	Cranial nerves I, II	Frontobasal fractures, nasopharyngeal tumors, frontobasal meningiomas	DD: Foster–Kennedy syndrome
Foster–Kennedy syndrome	Unilateral optic nerve atrophy and contralateral papilledema	Cranial nerve II, possible involvement of rhinencephalon	Frontal lobe tumors, frontobasal trauma, olfactory meningioma	Also possible: cerebral compression signs, status epilepticus
Orbital fissure syndrome	Unilateral paresis of oculomotor nerve and lesion of trochlear nerve, trigeminal nerve (1st division = ophthalmic nerve), abducens nerve. End result: ophthalmoplegia with ptosis and mydriasis. Intra- and periocular pain	Cranial nerves III, IV, V_1, VI	Sphenoid and/or ethmoid sinusitis, frontobasal trauma, intracerebral aneurysm, orbital tumors. Also tumors and/or granulomatous inflammatory conditions of the middle cranial fossa. Sphenoid tumors, internal carotid aneurysm	Precursor of orbital apex syndrome; DD: cavernous sinus syndrome, Jacod syndrome

Table 1.**18**   (cont.)

Name (and synonyms)	Main clinical symptoms	Anatomic substrate	Causes	Clinical remarks
Orbital apex syndrome	Vision loss, ptosis, diplopia, exophthalmos, severe temporoparietal pain	Cranial nerves II, III, IV, V, VI	Craniocerebral trauma, intraorbital tumors, epipharyngeal tumors, retro-orbital tumors, Paget diseases. Also ethmoid and/or sphenoid sinusitis	Possible hypoesthesia of the forehead (1st trigeminal nerve division)
Cavernous sinus syndrome (Jefferson syndrome, Foix syndrome, foramen lacerum syndrome, parasellar syndrome)	Ophthalmoplegia and exophthalmos (possibly pulsatile), trigeminal hypoesthesia (diminished corneal reflex), fixed pupil, frontal and ocular pain. With cavernous sinus thrombosis: very severe septic signs (see p. 213)	"Anterior" syndrome: cranial nerve III, possible involvement of cranial nerve VI (not II) and V_1. "Middle" syndrome: cranial nerves III + V_1 + V_2. "Posterior" syndrome: cranial nerves III + V_1 + V_2 + V_3 (and possibly VI)	Tumors (pituitary), craniopharyngioma, neuromas, nasopharyngeal tumors. Tumors of middle cranial fossa, internal carotid aneurysms. Wegener granulomatosis. Sinus cavernous thrombosis. Sella tumors. Also sinusitis!	Similar to orbital fissure syndrome. Cause of cavernous sinus thrombosis may be otogenic or tonsillogenic as well as rhinogenic. Furuncle of the upper lip also possible
(Posttraumatic) carotid–cavernous sinus syndrome, "carotid–cavernous fistula"	Severe retro-ocular headache, pulsatile bruit over the nasal root or temple. Pulsatile exophthalmos. Congestion of fundal veins, conjunctiva, and nasal mucosa	Aneurysms between the internal carotid artery and cavernous sinus	Posttraumatic or spontaneous	Bruit disappears on compression of the ipsilateral carotid artery. The a-v shunt can lead to deficient perfusion of the ipsilateral cerebral hemisphere
Sphenoid wing syndrome	Unilateral temporal bone tenderness to percussion. Gradual exophthalmos on the affected side. Function deficits of cranial nerves III, IV, V_1, VI	Mass effect or pressure atrophy in the sphenoid wing area with involvement of cranial nerves III, IV, V_1, and VI	Diverse tumors such as sphenoid meningioma	Medially situated meningiomas can produce Foster–Kennedy syndrome
Gradenigo syndrome	Otorrhea, abducens palsy, severe concomitant attacks of facial pain. Cranial nerves VII and VIII may also be involved. Diminished corneal reflex	Suppurative petrous apicitis with involvement of gasserian ganglion	Purulent otogenic complication with petrositis; malignant tumors of the petrous apex; also nasopharyngeal tumors	

Table 1.**18**   (cont.)

Name (and synonyms)	Main clinical symptoms	Anatomic substrate	Causes	Clinical remarks
Cerebello-pontine an-gle syn-drome	Hearing loss, bal-ance disturbances, facial paralysis	Cranial nerves V, VII, VIII, and pos-sibly IX	Acoustic neuroma, meningioma, der-moid	Relatively com-mon in the ENT region
Retrolaby-rinthine symptom complex (Zange syn-drome)	Like Gradenigo + ipsilateral hearing loss + rotatory nys-tagmus	Petrous apex de-struction involving the cochlea, ves-tibular apparatus, and internal audi-tory canal	Inflammatory or neoplastic destruc-tion in the medial part of the petrous pyramid, also basal skull fractures	Progression may lead to Garcin syndrome. DD: Raeder syndrome
Jacod syn-drome (pe-trosphenoi-dal syn-drome), syndrome of middle cranial nerve group	Unilateral ophthal-moplegia, ptosis, vi-sion loss ranging to blindness, trigeminal paresthesia, de-creased corneal re-flex, possible mas-seter paralysis	Partial or com-plete cranial nerve II–VI deficit with destruction of adjacent skull base	Nasopharyngeal tu-mors, eustachian tube tumors; neo-plasms traversing the cavernous sinus and/or foramen lace-rum	Possible hearing disturbance if the middle ear is in-volved!
Raeder syn-drome	Incomplete Horner syndrome, periorbi-tal pain (without tri-geminal nerve invol-vement), possible in-volvement of cranial nerves III, IV, V, VI. Accompanying au-tonomic syndrome (always on the same side)	Involvement of in-ternal carotid ar-tery by parasellar mass lesion or in-fection	Bing–Horton (clus-ter) headache; chronic paroxysmal hemicrania, vascular headache (see p. 165). Tumors, trauma, or inflamma-tory complications	True Bing–Horton headache (see p. 166) must be excluded, also hypertension and organic disease of the internal ca-rotid artery. DD: otitis media and-its complications, Horner syndrome of other etiology

Syndromes involving the lower cranial nerves:

Jugular fo-ramen syn-drome (Ver-net syn-drome)	Glossopharyngeal neuralgia with sen-sory disturbances in the distribution of cranial nerve IX. Hy-poglossal paralysis, motor disturbances of cranial nerve X (soft palate, pharynx, recurrent nerve). Al-so taste disturbance in the posterior third of the tongue	Cranial nerves IX, X, and XII in the area of the jugular foramen	Inflammatory pro-cesses about the jugular foramen. Ba-sal skull fracture. Ex-tra- or intracranial tumors, nasopharyn-geal tumors. Throm-bophlebitis of the jugular bulb. Menin-gitis. Aneurysms	Inflammatory oto-genic cause rela-tively common, al-so nasopharyn-geal tumors. Ba-sal skull fracture with jugular fora-men symptoms and possible dis-placement of bone fragments = Siebenmann syn-drome

Table 1.**18**   (cont.)

Name (and synonyms)	Main clinical symptoms	Anatomic substrate	Causes	Clinical remarks
Avellis syndrome	Ipsilateral paralysis of the recurrent nerve and soft palate ("palatolaryngeal hemiplegia"). Partial anesthesia of pharyngeal mucosa	Cranial nerves IX and X	Lesions of brain stem nuclei, trauma, benign and malignant mass lesions. Brain stem infarction	
Schmidt syndrome	Like Avellis syndrome + ipsilateral paralysis of trapezius and sternocleidomastoid muscles ("scapulopalatopharyngeal hemoplegia")	Cranial nerves IX, X, XI	Nuclear, intramedullary, and/or peripheral root lesions. Basal skull fracture. Brain stem infarction	
Tapia syndrome	Paralysis of the recurrent nerve and tongue ("glossolaryngeal hemiplegia")	Cranial nerves X and XII	Injury just below the bony skull base, also iatrogenic trauma (intubation, operation). Benign and malignant tumors	
Jackson syndrome	Recurrent nerve paralysis, lingual paralysis, paralytic dysphagia ("glossopalatolaryngeal hemiplegia")	Cranial nerves X, XI, and XII	Tumor extension involving the jugular foramen *and* hypoglossal canal. Cervical trauma. Damage is mostly peripheral, but intramedullary damage can also occur	Relatively common in ENT region (tumors)
Collet–Sicard syndrome	Hoarseness, lingual paralysis, taste disturbance in the posterior third of the tongue, nuchal pain, accessory nerve paralysis, dysphagia	Cranial nerves IX, X, XI, and XII	Affected: jugular foramen, hypoglossal canal, anterior occipital condyles. Trauma, abscess formation (pharynx), thrombophlebitis of transverse sinus: glomus jugulare tumor	Not uncommon with "ENT" tumors
Villaret syndrome	Like Collet–Sicard syndrome + ipsilateral Horner syndrome (usually *not* complete)	Cranial nerves IX, X, XI, XII, and sympathetic (cervical) trunk	Trauma (including parapharyngeal space). Benign and malignant tumors (parotid gland, pharynx, glomus, lymphoma), parapharyngeal abscess	ENT etiology relatively common

Table 1.**18**   (cont.)

Name (and synonyms)	Main clinical symptoms	Anatomic substrate	Causes	Clinical remarks
Garcin syndrome	Symptoms depend on location and type of damage. Often the complete picture develops gradually	Various combinations of cranial nerve I–XII neuropathies	Osteomyelitis of the skull base, basal meningitis, basal aneurysms, cavernous sinus thrombophlebitis, cranial nerve polyneuritis. Carcinomas. Basal skull trauma also a potential cause	*No* signs of increased intracranial pressure; usually *no* headache, *no* vomiting; no peripheral motor hemiparesis. Often due to locally invasive tumors of the nasopharynx, oropharynx, or salivary glands

Congenital Syndromes that Involve the Ear

Table 1.**19** lists the more *common syndromes* in which anomalies affecting various body regions are associated with congenital otologic disease. Facial paralysis is also a feature of some of these syndromes. For congenital inner ear disorders, see also Table 1.**19**.

Table 1.**19**   Common congenital syndrome involving the ear (selection)

Syndrome	Features	Typical ENT deficits	Other typical symptoms
Albers-Schönberg syndrome (marble bone disease)	Generalized diffuse osteosclerosis	Sensorineural hearing loss (rarely deafness); conductive hearing loss also possible. Involvement of additional cranial nerves (II, VI, VIII)	Growth retardation, bone fragility, anemia; may commence with long asymptomatic period
Alport syndrome	See Table 1.**43**		
Alström syndrome	See Table 1.**43**		
Apert syndrome	See Table 1.**43**		
van Buchem syndrome	See Table 1.**43**		
Cockayne syndrome	Combination of dwarfism, hearing loss, and retinitis pigmentosa	Conductive hearing loss, dysplasia, and dystopia of the external ear. Malformation of the middle ear	Microcephaly, oligophrenia
Crouzon syndrome	See Tables 1.**43** and 2.**13**		

Table 1.19   (cont.)

Syndrome	Features	Typical ENT deficits	Other typical symptoms
Down syndrome (trisomy 21)	See Table 2.13		
Franceschetti–Zwahlen syndrome	See Tables 1.43 and 2.13		
Goldenhar syndrome	See Table 2.13		
Gregg syndrome	Rubella embryopathy (maternal infection during the first weeks of pregnancy)	Varying degrees of sensorineural hearing loss ranging to deafness	Congenital cataract, anomalies of the heart and other internal organs. Microcephaly
Halgren–von Graefe syndrome	See Table 1.43		
Hunter syndrome	See Table 1.43		
Klippel–Feil syndrome	Synostosis (synostoses) of the cervical vertebrae	Short neck. Possible dysplasia of external auditory canal and/or middle ear. Possible cleft palate, sensorineural hearing loss	High scapula. Barrel chest. Various vertebral deformities
Marfan syndrome	See Table 1.43		
Moebius syndrome	Congenital paralysis of one or more cranial nerves	Vestibular dysfunction. Moderate to severe sensorineural hearing loss. Conductive hearing loss also possible with malformations of the external and/or middle ear	Ocular muscle palsy. Paralytic dysphagia. Mimetic rigidity
Nager–de Reynier syndrome	See Table 2.13		
Osteogenesis imperfecta (van der Hoeve–de Kleyn syndrome)	See Table 1.43		
Paget disease (osteitis deformans syndrome)	Localized fibrotic osteodystrophy	Possible inner ear involvement with sensorineural hearing loss; conductive or mixed hearing loss also possible	Increase in head circumference. Visual defects (optic nerve atrophy). Neurologic deficits are possible. Deformity of long bones
Pendred syndrome	See Table 1.43		

Table 1.**19**   (cont.)

Syndrome	Features	Typical ENT deficits	Other typical symptoms
von Pfaundler–Hurler syndrome (Hunter–Hurler syndrome)	See Table 2.**13**		
Refsum syndrome	See Table 1.**43**		
Robin syndrome	See Table 2.**13**		
Thalidomide syndrome	Embryopathy due to maternal thalidomide use during pregnancy	Aplasia or dysplasia of the external and/or middle ear with conductive or mixed hearing loss. Possible paralysis of cranial nerves VI and VII	Hypoplastic or aplastic dysmelias (multiple). Malformations of internal organs also possible
Trisomy 13–15, 18, 21 (Trisomy 18 = Edward syndrome, Trisomy 21 = Down syndrome)	See Tables 2.**13** and 4.**26**		
Turner syndrome (Ullrich–Turner syndrome)	See Table 1.**43**		
Usher syndrome	See Table 1.**43**		
Vourmann–Vourmann syndrome	See Table 1.**43**		
Waardenburg syndrome	See Table 2.**13**		
Wildervanck syndrome	See Tables 1.**43** and 2.**13**		

Differential Diagnosis of Hearing Disorders

K. Schorn

The diseases reviewed in this section are associated with hearing loss or can be diagnosed with the aid of special auditory tests.

Principal Diagnostic Methods

○ *History:* Attention is given to: hereditary disorders in the family, especially familial hearing loss, mental disorders or syndromes; childhood illnesses, especially ototoxic infectious diseases; late diseases such as autoimmune disorders, use of ototoxic drugs; exposure to noise, injuries involving the head or cervical spine; and current complaints including the development, severity, and type of hearing loss and characteristics of tinnitus; (vertigo history, see p. 97).

○ *Inspection,* palpation, otoscopy, radiography, and eustachian tube function tests (see p. 1).

○ *Tuning fork tests* for qualitative differentiation of conductive and sensorineural hearing loss.
Weber test: Binaural comparison of bone conduction with the tuning fork placed on the midline of the skull.
Rinne test: Monaural comparison of air and bone conduction.
Gellé test: Tuning fork is placed on the cranial midline, and air is insufflated into the ear canal with a Politzer bag. In a positive (normal) test the sound is diminished by increasing the pressure, due to stiffening of the ossicular chain (ossicular fixation). In a negative test, the loudness of the sound does not change.

○ *Pure-tone audiometry:* For quantitative assessment of conductive or sensorineural hearing loss in the frequency range of 125 Hz to 10,000 Hz.

○ *Whispered and spoken voice test:* Measurement of the distance at which a whispered and spoken voice can be heard. The discrepancy between the ability to hear whispered and spoken speech is minimal with conductive hearing loss but substantial with sensorineural hearing loss.

○ *Speech audiometry*
Freiburg speech test: Tests the subject's ability to comprehend spoken numbers and monosyllabic words for the quantitative investigation of hearing loss.
− Conductive hearing loss: Shift of the number curve and the monosyllable curve toward greater loudness levels.
− Pancochlear hearing loss with recruitment: Distance between number and monosyllable curves is only minimally increased. Loss of speech discrimination is common.
− High-tone hearing loss with recruitment: Marked separation of the number and monosyllable curves. Loss of discrimination is possible depending on the degree of the hearing impairment.
− Low-tone hearing loss with recruitment: Marked hearing loss for numbers, possible loss of monosyllable discrimination.
− Sloping loss with recruitment: Marked discrepancy between numbers and monosyllabic words, usually with loss of discrimination.
− Retrocochlear hearing loss: Marked deviation of the monosyllable curve, usually with discrimination loss, from an essentially normal number curve.

Dichotic speech tests such as the *Feldmann test* for diagnosing central hearing loss:
− Normal hearing, conductive impairment, or cochlear impairment: 100% comprehension of multisyllabic words in both ears.
− Retrocochlear or central hearing loss: unilateral or bilateral disturbance of word comprehension.

○ *Testing of recruitment:* Patients with cochlear dysfunction are hearing-impaired for faint sounds, but can hear loud sounds normally.

The Fowler test: Subjective loudness balance between an impaired ear and an unimpaired opposite ear. Positive test = loudness bal-

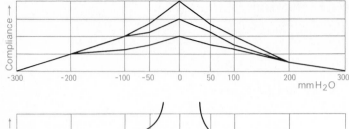

Fig. 1.**7**   Normal tympanometric patterns

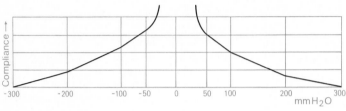

Fig. 1.**8**   Tympanogram of an abnormally mobile tympanic membrane

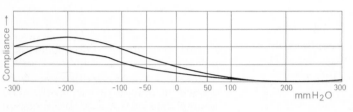

Fig. 1.**9**   Tympanograms indicating negative pressure in the middle ear

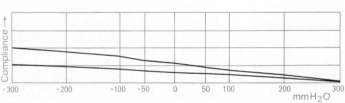

Fig. 1.**10**   Tympanograms indicating massive negative pressure in the middle ear or atresia

ance = cochlear impairment. Negative test = loudness imbalance = retrocochlear impairment.

SISI (short increment sensitivity index) test: Periodically superimposed 1-dB increments of 0.2-s duration on a continuous pure tone. The test is presented at 20 dB above threshold. Only patients with recruitment hear the increments.

SISI 1 dB = 70−100%   = positive recruitment
SISI 1 dB = 0−30%   = no recruitment
SISI 1 dB = 40−60%   = borderline

The Lüscher test: Amplitude-modulated tones are differentiated from unmodulated tones. The amplitude of the tone is changed every 0.3−0.5 s by an adjustable dB or percentage value.

Cochlear   impairment   =   differentiation threshold diminished.
Retrocochlear impairment = differentiation threshold normal or increased.

○ *Hearing fatigue tests:* Threshold shift is evidence of retrocochlear impairment.

The Carhart test or TTDT (threshold tone decay test): If the tone becomes inaudible (= tone decay, threshold shift), its intensity is increased at once by 5 dB.
Negative test = subject hears tone for 1 min at 10 to a maximum of 20 dB above his threshold level = no tone decay. Positive test = increase of 30 dB is required before the tone is heard for 1 min = evidence of retrocochlear lesion.

Langenbeck noise audiometry: Threshold determination during simultaneous presen-

Table 1.**20**   Gross differential diagnosis of acute hearing loss

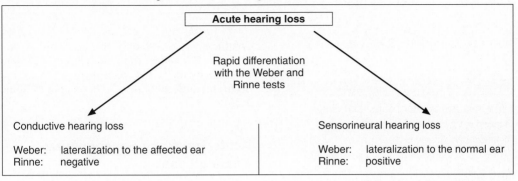

tation of Langenbeck noise. Suitable for downsloping or rising patterns.
Cochlear impairment: Shifted threshold in noise is continuous with the threshold out of noise.
Retrocochlear impairment: Shifted threshold in noise parallels the theshold out of noise.

o *Impedance measurement:*
Tympanometry: Indirect measurement of middle ear pressure with an intact tympanic membrane in response to pressure changes in the external auditory canal.
Type I: Centered peak = normal pattern (Fig. 1.**7**).
Type II: Peak is centered but truncated at the top = tympanic membrane is abnormally mobile due to ossicular discontinuity, atrophic areas in the ear drum, etc. (Fig. 1.**8**).
Type III: Peak in the negative pressure range = negative pressure in the middle ear (Fig. 1.**9**).
Type IV: Flat tympanogram with no peak = severe negative pressure or atresia (Fig. 1.**10**).
Stapedius reflex: The acoustic stapedius reflex is elicited to assess recruitment. The reflex is also used indirectly for objective threshold measurement and for topodiagnostic testing of the facial nerve.
– Conductive impairment: Stapedius reflex is absent in the test ear on ipsilateral and contralateral sound stimulation.

– Cochlear impairment: Distance between auditory and reflex threshold ≤70 dB.
– Retrocochlear impairment: Absence of reflex in the stimulated ear, or distance between auditory and reflex threshold ≥90 dB.
– Facial nerve paralysis: Reflex absent in the test ear implies paralyses central to the origin of the stapedius nerve.

o *Electric-response audiometry (ERA)*
– Brain stem electric response audiometry (BERA) = Auditory brain stem response (ABR): Auditory evoked acoustic-nerve and brain stem potentials can be measured to confirm or exclude retrocochlear hearing loss. ABR also provides objective threshold measurements in children and malingerers.

o *Audiometric testing in infants and small children:* Reflex audiometry (cochleopalpebral reflex positive in 96% of normal-hearing newborns), behavioral observation audiometry, and delayed otoacoustic emissions (DEOAE), are useful only for auditory screening. The BERA test is the most reliable (see above).

Symptom   **Acute Hearing Loss**

Table 1.**21**   *Symptom*   Acute conductive hearing loss

Synopsis
With external auditory canal pathology
Ceruminal plug, see p. 19
Foreign bodies, see p. 19
Furuncle of the external auditory canal, see p. 6
Diffuse otitis externa, see p. 6
With tympanic membrane pathology
Injuries, see p. 8
Myringitis, see Table 1.**10**
Influenzal otitis, see p. 10
With middle ear pathology
Acute otitis media, see p. 9
Mastoiditis, see p. 11
Traumatic ossicular discontinuity, see p. 8
Longitudinal temporal bone fracture, see p. 39
Barotrauma, see p. 9
Acute eustachian tube dysfunction, see p. 21

The hearing loss may be unilateral or bilateral and may develop within seconds, hours, or overnight. It may be maximal at once or may progress in stages over a period of days. All degrees of hearing loss can occur from mild impairment to total deafness (Table 1.**20**).

Acute Conductive Hearing Loss

Because diseases associated with acute conductive hearing loss usually have a clinical picture dominated by otalgia, dysesthesia, otorrhea, or otogenic facial paralysis, the individual disease entities are discussed elsewhere (see page references in Table 1.**21**).The audiologic findings associated with middle ear diseases are summarized in Table 1.**22**.

Acute Sensorineural Hearing Loss

Many forms of acute sensorineural hearing loss are grouped under the heading of Sudden Deafness, in which only the symptom is described. But since true "idiopathic" sudden deafness by no means accounts for all cases, an accurate differentiation is essential (Table 1.**23**).

Acute Traumatic Sensorineural Hearing Loss

All forms in this group are preceded by a traumatic event, so the history is the basis for differential diagnosis (Table 1.**24**).

Gunshot Trauma

Main symptoms: Bilateral hearing loss accompanied by tinnitus and often by stabbing pain. The ear directed toward the noise source sustains greater damage than the opposite ear.

Other symptoms and special features: High-pitched tinnitus is common. Tympanic membrane is intact. Vestibular involvement is rare.

Hearing loss is often pronounced initially and tends to improve in days or weeks. Progression occurs only if the primary hearing loss is greater than 70–80 dB.

Causes: Single or repeated exposure to "impulse noise," i.e., a powerful pressure wave of *very brief duration* (1–3 ms) with a peak amplitude between 160 and 190 dB.

Diagnosis: Hearing loss is generally asymmetric with a notch of variable width, which is maximal between 3 and 6 kHz (Fig. 1.**11**). More severe damage produces a sloping loss that converts to a high-tone notch during recovery. Severe hearing loss rarely develops. Tinnitus is generally in the 4–6 kHz range and can be masked at the auditory threshold.

Vertigo is very rare and signifies a circumscribed lesion of the vestibular apparatus (otoliths).

Differential diagnosis in the acute stage is not difficult. Otherwise differentiation is required from noise-induced hearing loss or head trauma.

Table 1.**22**   Acute conductive hearing loss with middle ear pathology

Disorder	Main symptoms	Tympanic membrane	Pure-tone audiogram	Tympanogram
Acute otitis media	Severe otalgia, possible pulsatile tinnitus	Reddened, bulging, or retracted	Conductive impairment uncharacteristic	Fig. 1.**9**
Mastoiditis	Throbbing otalgia, auricular prominence, mastoid tenderness, otorrhea	Reddened, thickened, usually perforation with purulent discharge	Moderate to severe pancochlear conductive hearing loss	Faulty seal
Traumatic ossicular discontinuity or fracture	Pain, hearing loss	Normal appearance	Severe pancochlear conductive hearing loss	Fig. 1.**8**
Longitudinal temporal bone fracture	Bleeding, hearing loss, possible facial paralysis or CSF otorrhea	Hematotympanon, visible step in ear canal, possible tympanic membrane perforation	Severe pancochlear conductive hearing loss	Uncharacteristic trace or faulty seal
Barotrauma	Severe otalgia, pulsatile tinnitus	Hematotympanon, hemorrhagic tympanic membrane	Conductive hearing loss uncharacteristic	Figs. 1.**9** or 1.**10**
Acute eustachian tube dysfunction	Paroxysmal dysesthesia with feeling of pressure and fullness, clicking, lancinating pain	Retracted, possible radial congestion or effusion	Moderate to severe pancochlear conductive hearing loss	Figs. 1.**9** or 1.**10**

Fig. 1.**11**   Audiograms of gunshot trauma

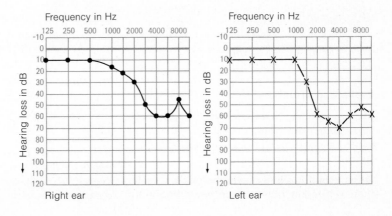

Right ear

Left ear

Table 1.**23** *Symptom*   Acute sensorineural sensorineural hearing loss

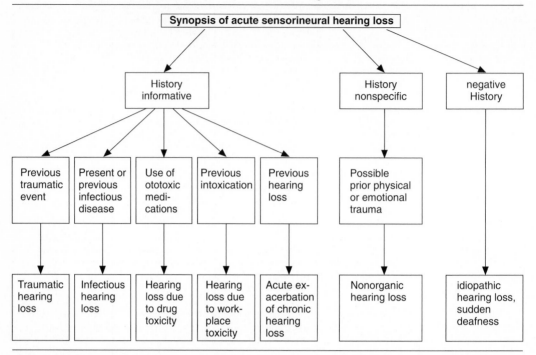

Table 1.**24** *Symptom*   Acute traumatic sensorineural hearing loss

Synopsis
Gunshot trauma
Explosion trauma
Acute noise trauma
Acoustic accident
Blunt head trauma with no fracture in the ear region
Transverse temporal bone fracture
Window rupture
Barotrauma
Electric shock and lightning strike

Explosion Trauma

Main symptoms: Stabbing pain, often in both ears. Immediate bilateral hearing loss accompanied by tinnitus. The ear toward the blast sustains greater damage.

Other symptoms and special features: Usually there is bleeding from one and sometimes both ears by a rupture of the tympanic membrane. Possible vestibular damage.

The conductive component of the hearing loss improves with spontaneous healing of the tympanic membrane lesion. Progression to chronic otitis media may occur. Inner ear damage and tinnitus are usually irreversible. Progression of sensoneural hearing loss is rare but is more common than with gunshot trauma.

Causes: Powerful acoustic wave with pressure peak at 160−190 dB *lasting longer than 3 ms.* Generally a single event, e.g., explosion, bomb or cannon shell blast, exploding pressure vessel or boiler, or blowout of a large truck tire.

Diagnosis: Otoscopy reveals a central tympanic membrane perforation with jagged edges, at least on the side toward the blast and sometimes bilaterally. There may be accompanying ossicular fracture or discontinuity with resulting conductive hearing loss whose severity depends on the size of the drum perforation and degree of ossicular involvement. Inner ear damage is variable (Fig. 1.**12**). The c^5 notch

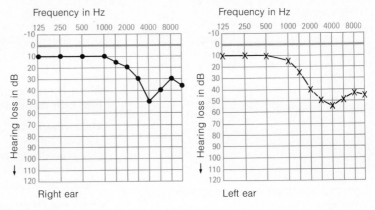

Fig. 1.12 Audiograms of bilateral explosion trauma rupturing the left tympanic membrane

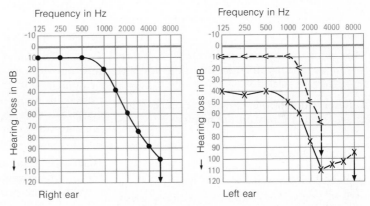

Fig. 1.13 Audiograms of acute noise trauma

characteristic of gunshot trauma is usually absent or may be present only in the less damaged ear. The puretone audiogram shows a sharpy downsloping or flat pattern. Recruitment is positive but may be masked by conductive hearing loss. One-fourth of cases have profound unilateral hearing loss or deafness; bilateral deafness is very rare. Tinnitus is usually high-pitched.

Vertigo is more common than with gunshot trauma. Tullio phenomenon or vestibular hyporeactivity with paretic nystagmus (see pp. 107, 113).

Differential diagnosis is obvious in acute cases. In compensation cases, Schüller radiographs should be obtained to assess the pneumatization of the mastoid process and to exclude pediatric otitis with preexisting damage to the tympanic membrane.

Acute Noise Trauma

Main symptoms: Hearing loss noticed immediately after occupational noise exposure; tends to improve markedly in hours or days. Hearing loss is usually symmetric but may be milder on the side away from the noise source.

Other symptoms and special features: Main associated symptom is tinnitus, usually bilateral and high-pitched. Ear pressure and vertigo are rare.

Causes: Exposure to sound levels at 130–160 dB of several minutes' duration caused by gaseous or steam discharge from boilers, jet engines, firing ranges, etc.

Diagnosis: Audiogram shows high-tone loss with a c^5 notch, similar to advanced noise-induced hearing loss; usually symmetric; recruitment always present (Fig. 1.13). Tinnitus is in

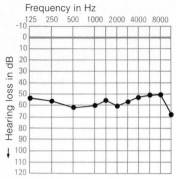

Frequency in Hz

Fig. 1.**14**   Audiogram of acoustic accident

the 4−6 kHz range with a masking level at the auditory threshold.

Mild, nonspecific vestibular symptoms are rare and imply circumscribed lesion of the vestibular apparatus (otoliths).

Differentiation from noise-induced hearing loss is based entirely on the history.

Acoustic Accident

Main symptoms: Acute hearing loss in one ear noticed immediately after occupational noise exposure, usually accompanied by tinnitus.

Other symptoms and special features: *Acute* vestibular symptoms are absent. Careful history may elicit vertigo, which lasts only seconds, or unsteadiness on rapid head and body movements.

Causes: Moderate-level noise exposure at 90−120 dB coinciding with unphysiologic loading of the cervical spine with decreased blood flow to one ear caused by a strained head position. Preexisting cervical spine pathology is often demonstrated.

Diagnosis: Unilateral sensorineural hearing loss with a flat, pancochlear, or trough-shaped audiometric curve (Fig. 1.**14**). Positive recruitment. Tinnitus of variable frequency is usually present.

Direction-changing nystagmus may be provoked by head movements, with an abnormal neck rotation test in the ENG. Radiographs may show cervical spine pathology.

Differentiation from idiopathic sudden deafness must rely on a description of the patient's work situation with strained head position.

Blunt Head Trauma with No Apparent Fracture about the Ear

Main symptoms: Unilateral or bilateral hearing loss, tinnitus, vertigo, headache, and general postconcussional symptoms with unconsciousness or daze dominate the clinical picture in various combinations and degrees.

Other symptoms and special features: Hearing loss tends to improve in days or weeks, but secondary deterioration of various degrees up to total deafness can occur, especially if the primary injury was severe.

Causes: The site of the trauma is more critical than the absolute force of the impact in terms of otologic insult. Inner ear damage may be caused by temporal, parietal, and especially occipital violence, the trauma-producing pressure wave being transmitted by bone conduction to the inner ear.

Diagnosis: Pure-tone audiogram typically shows circumscribed high-tone notches and possibly a sharp downslope in the high-tone range. A flatter pattern is seen with severe injury (Fig. 1.**15**).

A temporal or temporoparietal blow causes significantly greater damage to the ipsilateral ear, while an occipital blow commonly produces a symmetrical hearing loss. Recruitment is usually positive but may be absent if the patient was unconscious, especially following occipital trauma, in which case threshold decay can be demonstrated. The stapedius reflex may be absent, and prolonged latencies are found in auditory evoked brain stem and auditory nerve potentials. Tinnitus is often high-pitched but may occur in the middle and lower frequencies.

The nonspecific vertigo that often dominates subjective complaints generally represents a central vestibular disturbance; rarely it may signify lesions of the peripheral labyrinths (see p. 107).

Differentiation from preinjury sensorineural hearing loss is difficult. Cerebral deficits and

Fig. 1.**15** Audiogram patterns of head trauma of varying degree (right ear affected)

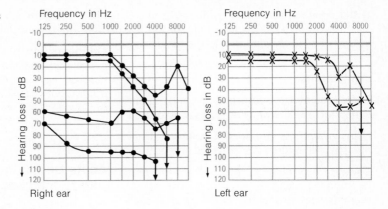

Right ear   Left ear

concentration difficulties resulting from the head trauma can markedly accentuate a preexisting hearing loss, which then may be attributed to the trauma itself.

Transverse Temporal Bone Fracture

Main symptoms: Unilateral deafness and severe vertigo based on unilateral vestibular dysfunction.

Other symptoms and special features: Unilateral tinnitus and frequently unilateral facial nerve paralysis. Hearing loss in the opposite ear is common. Anosmia is rare (see p. 225).

Causes: Burst fracture due to violence from the back and less commonly from the front; the fracture line running transversely through the labyrinth and/or the internal ear canal. Double transverse temporal bone fractures are very rare.

Diagnosis: Clinical hallmark is complete unilateral deafness. Bone conduction transmits a disruptive pressure wave to the opposite ear, which shows a typical c^5 notch with positive recruitment. The tinnitus is usually unilateral and high-pitched, and may occur through all frequencies. If contralateral tinnitus is present, it is high-pitched (see Table 1.**12**).

Vestibular symptoms are pronounced (see p. 107).

Differentiation from preexisting hearing loss is difficult.

Rupture of the Round or Oval Window

Main symptoms: Unilateral hearing loss of acute onset, which may fluctuate, progress until to deafness, or remain constant. Over 70% of patients have vertigo, and over 50% have tinnitus that is often pulsatile, as well as ear pressure or a feeling of fullness perceived throughout the head.

Causes: Operative or traumatic ruptures more commonly affect the oval window. Spontaneous ruptures of the round window may result from inner ear implosion due to accoustic trauma, head trauma, impedance audiometry, etc., or from explosive inner ear pressures caused by a rise in CSF pressure or physical exertion, possibly combined with a negative pressure in the middle ear (as in barotrauma). Congenital or inflammatory weakness of the round window membrane or vascular insufficiency should be considered in children.

Diagnosis: Very few patients have middle ear effusion with a negative shift in the tympanogram. The pure-tone threshold test does not show a consistent pattern, although the low frequencies are commonly more affected than the high frequencies. All patients show markedly positive recruitment. Hearing loss may be exacerbated by straining and by infusion therapy. Tinnitus is variable in pitch and loudness and is not always present.

Vertigo is generally paroxysmal, of variable intensity, and occurs at varying intervals. The Valsalva maneuver, straining, and air insufflation often evoke a positive fistula sign (see pp. 113, 117).

Differentiation from Ménière disease and cervical hearing disorder is based on an accurate history of acute symptoms and the fistula test.

Barotrauma

Main symptoms: Acute hearing impairment, unilateral or bilateral, with vertigo and otalgia.

Other symptoms and special features: Tinnitus, possible middle ear effusion (see p. 9).

Causes: Barotrauma of the inner ear is caused by a sudden change in ambient pressure (e.g., rapid descent during diving, fall of cabin pressure in an aircraft, or descending flight with an occluded eustachian tube).

Diagnosis: Conductive hearing loss due to serotympanon and/or sensorineural hearing loss of variable degree ranging to deafness. Recruitment is usually positive; tinnitus is high-, low-, or medium-pitched and rarely pulsatile.

The vestibular damage is like the cochlear injury, i.e., hyporeactivity or failure with corresponding symptoms.

Differentiation is required from decompression sickness (caisson disease), which is distinguished by neurologic symptoms such as paresthesias ("diver's fleas"), pulmonary complaints with coughing fits, burning pain, respiratory distress ("chokes"), joint pain, as well as focal and generalized seizures.

Electric Shock and Lightning Strike

Main symptoms: Inconsistent. Acute unilateral or bilateral hearing loss often goes unnoticed initially due to the prominent neurologic symptoms.

Causes: The effects of the trauma depend critically on the current strength (low voltage <1 mV and high voltage >1 mV) and the path taken by the current. The typical, massive disruption of electrical conductivity throughout the body leads to a very diverse clinical picture.

Diagnosis: Pure-tone audiometry shows a variable pattern and degree of hearing loss. The site of the lesion may be labyrinthine, retrolabyrinthine, or central. Accordingly, the vestibular symptoms may be peripheral or central. Neurologic consultation is indicated.

Differentiation is required from psychogenic hearing loss, since psychogenic overlay and neurosis appear to be more common than in other modes of injury.

Acute Sensorineural Hearing Loss Due to Infectious Toxic Disease

While sensorineural hearing loss due to bacterial infection has become uncommon, hearing loss secondary to viral infection presents a broad spectrum (Table 1.25). Differential diagnosis of the various infectious diseases is based on otologic findings in conjunction with the results of internal medical or neurologic consultation.

Meningoencephalitis

Otogenic and rhinogenic meningoencephalitis are described elsewhere (see pp. 42), so the present discussion is limited to *viral meningitis*.

Main symptoms: Very severe headache, sudden fever, neurologic deficits, and cerebral impairment. Otologic consultation is generally sought to evaluate hearing loss which is generally bilateral and exclude cranial neuropathies. Vertigo, facial weakness, and speech impediment may also be present.

Diagnosis: A "typical" pure-tone audiogram is not recorded during or after meningitis. Possible features are high-tone hearing loss, pancochlear hearing loss of variable degree, and deafness with or without residual hearing. The hearing loss is almost always symmetrical. It may occur during the disease or after a disease-free interval and may be progressive. Suprathreshold tests, if applicable, are nonspecific. Recruitment may be positive or absent. Threshold decay is frequently present, and the stapedial reflex is usually absent. Hearing loss after a disease-free interval usually signifies retrocochlear disease. Tinnitus may be present or absent and is nonspecific. Vertigo is also nonspecific; paretic nystagmus is common (see p. 106).

Zoster Oticus

Main symptoms: Fifty percent of cases show profound unilateral hearing loss or even total deafness of acute onset, combined with vertigo and/or facial paralysis. Other symptoms are noted on p. 4.

Diagnosis: Severe, typically unilateral sensorineural hearing loss with a slight downslope along the 70- to 90-dB line or a high-tone loss (Fig. 1.**16**). Complete deafness and tinnitus are rare. Suprathreshold tests yield mixed positive and negative results.

Vestibular involvement, which may occur later, causes a paretic nystagmus with a corresponding spontaneous and provoked nystagmus toward the opposite ear (see p. 105).

Differentiation is required from idiopathic sudden hearing loss and other agents that can cause virogenic cochlear neuritis such as parainfluenza virus, influenza virus, Coxsackie virus, enterovirus, and adenovirus. Serum tests are required for identification, especially if vesicular eruptions are absent.

Mumps

Main symptoms: Disease is generally confined to the parotid glands (see p. 300). Rare cases cause complete, usually unilateral permanent deafness, which is more common in adults than in children.

Diagnosis: Hearing loss occurs as complete sensironeural deafness with no residual hearing (cochlear neuritis).

Concomitant involvement of the vestibular apparatus, manifested by vestibular hyporeactivity or failure, is rare. An almost asymptomatic meningoencephalitis develops in some cases.

Serologic tests are needed to **differentiate** mumps-associated hearing loss from other forms of unilateral deafness in nonacute states when parotid swelling is absent.

Syphilis

Note: General ENT symptoms are discussed on p. 247ff. The present section deals exclusively with auditory symptoms.

Table 1.**25** *Symptom* Acute sensorineural hearing loss due to infectious disease

Synopsis
During or following:
Meningoencephalitis
Zoster oticus
Mumps
Syphilis
Toxoplasmosis
Lyme disease
Typhus
Measles and scarlet fever
Spotted fever
Brucellosis
AIDS
Infectious diseases with occasional ototoxic effect

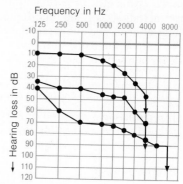

Fig. 1.**16** Audiogram patterns in zoster oticus

Main symptoms: Hearing loss is usually bilateral; it may come on acutely or take an indolent or intermittent course with exacerbations that may culminate in deafness. Common accompanying symptoms are episodic vertigo and, less commonly, tinnitus. The symptoms usually appear in stages II and III.

Diagnosis: Pure-tone threshold findings are nonspecific, showing pancochlear patterns or low-tone hearing losses between 250 and 1000 Hz with sharp high-tone losses beyond 4000 Hz. Recruitment may be positive or absent. Tinnitus can occupy various frequency ranges and generally cannot be masked at the auditory threshold.

Vertigo tests yield nonspecific findings consistent with a central vestibular disorder (see p. 108). Dermatologic and/or neurologic consultation is indicated.

Differentiation is required from Ménière disease and acoustic neuroma. Congenital syphilis, see Table. 1.**44**.

Toxoplasmosis

Main symptoms: Hearing loss is nonspecific and often associated with ataxia and attacks of vertigo. Other symptoms are listed in Table 4.**28**.

The audiometric findings of toxoplasmosis are variable and inconsistent. Besides complete bilateral deafness, audiometry may show moderate pancochlear hearing losses, high-tone losses (symmetric or asymmetric), and trough configurations in the mid-frequency range. Recruitment may be present or absent depending on the mode of infection.

Vestibular testing shows a nonspecific pattern with unilateral or bilateral peripheral vestibular dysfunction and central vestibular signs.

Differentiation is required from other forms of toxic sensorineural hearing loss.

Lyme Dysease

Main symptoms: Hearing loss of acute onset, sometimes episodic, of varying degree affecting one or both ears and usually accompanied by tinnitus.

Other symptoms and special features: Suspicion is raised by isolated macular or papular lesions with annular erythema mainly affecting the extremities and associated with fever, headache, and limb pain mimicking a flu-like infection. Stage II is marked by neurologic and cardiac manifestations with hyper-, hypo-, and paresthesias at various body sites and cranial nerve involvement with unilateral or bilateral facial paralysis and, less commonly, abducens or oculomotor neuropathy. The neurologic symptoms of stage III can mimic the features of multiple sclerosis.

Causes: Infection, usually tick-borne, with the bacterium *Borrelia burgdorferi* (100 times more prevalent than the spring–summer meningitis virus, also transmitted by ticks).

Diagnosis: Unilateral or bilateral sensorineural hearing loss, usually occurring in stage II. High-tone hearing loss is most common, but hearing losses with a pancochlear pattern ranging to deafness can also occur. Recruitment is usually positive but may be absent in some cases. Tinnitus is usually high-pitched, may be unilateral or bilateral, but is absent in many cases.

Vestibular testing may show unilateral or bilateral reduced response or even complete failure (see p. 105).

The diagnosis is established by identifying antibodies against *Borrelia burgdorferi*.

Differentiation is required from other forms of toxic sensorineural hearing loss.

Typhus

Main symptoms: Bilateral hearing loss develops in 90% of cases, generally regresses when fever subsides. Balance disturbances are rare. Major symptoms such as headache, fever, as well as abdominal complaints and diarrhea are internal.

Diagnosis: Pure-tone audiogram shows unequal sensorineural high-tone hearing loss without recruitment, which generally is reversible.

Bilateral vestibular hyporeactivity is uncommon.

Measles and Scarlet Fever

Irreversible sensorineural hearing loss, mostly unilateral, develops rarely in the setting of a measles or scarlet fever infection. It is generally associated with otitis media (see p. 11).

Spotted Fever

Main symptoms: Bilateral hearing loss with pronounced tinnitus is present in 80% of cases, however, this disease has nearly vanished from this part of the world.

Other symptoms: High fever of rapid onset, severe headache, conjunctivitis with photophobia, and maculous exanthema on the trunk and extremities.

Causes: The causative organism is *Rickettsia prowazeki,* transmitted by the contaminated feces of infected body lice percutaneously or by direct interpersonal contact.

Diagnosis: Established by an internist or infectious disease specialist.

Pure-tone audiogram shows bilateral, asymmetric, nonspecific sensorineural hearing loss without recruitment, usually with a high-tone loss. Tinnitus can be masked only at the suprathreshold level. Prognosis is good for hearing loss of early onset but poor for hearing loss commencing in the 9th week of the disease. Balance disturbances are only occasionally observed.

Differentiation is required from influenza, abdominal typhus, infectious hepatitis, malaria, leptospirosis, chickenpox, measles, smallpox, and tularemia.

Brucellosis

Main symptoms: Acute hearing loss may be a feature of chronic brucellosis, which has become a rare disease. Balance disturbances have also been observed. Systemic symptoms consist chiefly of recurrent febrile episodes and joint and muscle pain. See Table 4.28 for further details.

Diagnosis: Pure-tone audiogram usually shows bilateral sensorineural hearing loss without recruitment. Patients with chronic brucellosis may develop mastoiditic−meningitic complications with profound cochlear−retrocochlear hearing loss or total deafness.

Occasional vestibular neuritis with corresponding vestibular hyporeactivity or failure.

Differentiation is required from typhus, tularemia, malaria, influenza, tuberculosis, and other febrile diseases.

AIDS

Main symptoms: It is currently thought that cerebral symptoms initiate the clinical presen-

Table 1.**26**   *Symptom*   Acute sensorineural hearing loss due to drug toxicity

Synopsis
Aminoglycoside antibiotics
Loop diuretics
Salicylates
Local anesthetics
Cytostatic drugs
Tuberculostatic drugs
Drugs with infrequent ototoxic effect (quinidine, practolol, tricyclic antidepressants, aryl acetate derivatives, tetanus antitoxin, smallpox antitoxin, marihuana, alcohol and nicotine abuse

tation of AIDS in more than half of the HIV-infected population. Among these symptoms are fluctuating hearing loss and nonspecific vertigo. Other symptoms are discussed on pp. 108 and 245.

Infectious Diseases with Occasional Ototoxic Effect

Anthrax and *smallpox* have little epidemiologic significance today. These infections may be associated with sensorineural hearing loss, usually with nonspecific pure-tone audiometric curves. Recruitment may be negative in rare cases. Hearing loss is usually reversible.

Sensorineural hearing loss has been reported in isolated cases of *malaria, tetanus,* and *trichinosis.* There is no precise information on audiometric findings or recruitment.

Sensorineural Hearing Loss Due to Drug Toxicity

Because this type of hearing loss is a sequela of medical treatment, an accurate diagnosis can have substantial medicolegal or compensational significance. Common drugs with known ototoxicity are listed in Table 1.**26**.

Aminoglycoside Antibiotics

Main symptoms: Sensorineural hearing loss of acute onset, generally bilateral and, due to

Table 1.**27**   Commonly used aminoglycoside antibiotics (after Federspil and Mees)

International nonproprietary name	Product names	Ototoxic dose
Gentamicin	Gentamicin Beecham Gentamicin POS Gentamicin Ratiopharm Duragentamicin Gentamix Gentamytrex Michogencin Refobacin Septopal Sulmycin	50 mg/kg b.w.
Tobramycin	Gernebcin	75 mg/kg b.w.
Sisomicin	Extramycin	75 mg/kg b.w.
Netilmicin	Certomycin	200 mg/kg b.w.
Amikacin	Biklin	120 mg/kg b.w.

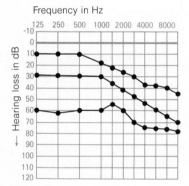

Fig. 1.**17** Audiogram patterns in aminoglycoside ototoxicity

high-tone loss, manifested initially by difficulties speech comprehension in conversations with several persons or when background noise is present. Hearing loss progresses in days or weeks to involve lower tones. Occasional acute onset of profound bilateral hearing loss or deafness.

Other symptoms and special features: Markedly abnormal pain threshold for loud stimuli. Tinnitus is usually bilateral but may be unilateral. Bilateral ear pressure, cranial fullness; vertigo and unsteadiness.

Follow-ups are necessary because the hearing loss may progress to deafness even after the antibiotic is discontinued. Improvement of hearing or vestibular reactivity is very rare.

Causes: Commonly used aminoglycoside antibiotics are listed in Table 1.**27**. The toxic effect is dose-dependent, with an increased sensitivity in infants and small children. The critical predisposing factor is renal dysfunction. Contributory factors are noise, otitis media, hypoxia, diabetes, and the concomitant use of diuretics or other antibiotics. Local use in the presence of gastrointestinal infection or chronic otitis media can cause severe ototoxic side effects.

Diagnosis: Bilateral sensorineural hearing loss with very strong recruitment and initial high-tone hearing loss progressing to a pancochlear configuration (Fig. 1.**17**). The tinnitus, usually bilateral, is high-pitched and easily masked. There is variable peripheral vestibular hyporeactivity or failure depending on the particular drug used. With gentamicin, vestibular symptoms are predominant (see pp. 107, 121).

Differentiation from other ototoxic drug effects is based only on the history and audiologic monitoring.

Loop Diuretics

Main symptoms: Bilateral high-tone hearing loss, generally with tinnitus, develops within hours or days after use. Hearing loss and tinnitus are reversible with immediate withdrawal of the drug.

Causes: High doses of loop diuretics (Table 1.28) causes an inhibition of enzyme activity, which interferes with electrolyte transport in the cochlea. Virtually all cases reported to date have had coexisting renal function impairment.

Diagnosis: Demonstration of high-tone sensorineural hearing loss with markedly positive recruitment, often with a shallow notch at 2000–4000 Hz in the pure-tone audiogram (Fig. 1.18). Speech discrimination is good. Tinnitus is usually bilateral, medium-pitched, and easily masked.

Differentiation is required from other ototoxic drug effects.

Salicylates

Main symptoms: Acute hearing loss of variable degree, usually bilateral.

Other symptoms and special features: Tinnitus and vertigo. Sensitivity is believed to be particularly high in children. The symptoms are reversible and disappear rapidly after salicylate withdrawal.

Causes: Higher doses (2–6 g/day) of salicylates (aspirin, Aspro, ASS Woelm, Acetylin, Colfarit, Solpyron, Trineral).

Diagnosis: Sensorineural hearing loss of variable degree with a pancochlear curve (Fig. 1.19). Preexisting inner ear damage produces a parallel shift. Recruitment is markedly positive with no threshold decay. Speech audiogram shows good discrimination with a helmet curve. Tinnitus is high-pitched and easily masked.

Vestibular dysfunction with bilateral hypoexcitability is possible (see pp. 107, 121).

Table 1.**28**   Commonly used ototoxic diuretics

International non-proprietary name	Product names
Ethacrynic acid	Hydromedin
Furosemide	Lasix Furo–Puren Furosemide Ratiopharm Furosemide Stada Hydro Rapid Fusid
Bumetanide	Fordiuran
Piretanide	Arelix

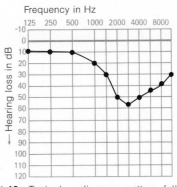

Fig. 1.**18**   Typical audiogram pattern following the use of loop diuretics

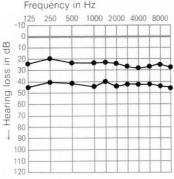

Fig. 1.**19**   Audiogram patterns in salicylate ototoxicity

Table 1.**29** Commonly used cytostatic drugs with ototoxic properties

International non-proprietary name	Product names
Cyclophospha-mide	Cyclostin Endoxan
Cisplatin	Cisplatin Solution Medag Cisplatin Solution Behring Cisplatin R.P. Solution Platiblastin Platinex
Ototoxic risk increased when dosage exceeds 200 mg/cm² body surface area	

Table 1.**30** Commonly used tuberculostatic drugs with ototoxic properties

International non-proprietary name	Product names
Streptomycin	Solvo-Strept Streptomycin Sarbach Streptomycin Heyl Streptothenate
Rifampicin (rifampin)	Rifa Rimactan
Capreomycin	Ogostal

Differentiation is required from aminoglycoside antibiotics and other ototoxic drugs.

Local Anesthetics

Main symptoms: Mild hearing loss, usually unilateral. Nonspecific vertigo.

Causes: Use of local anesthetics in the middle ear, e.g., added to otic drops or administered during ear surgery. Also spinal anesthesia.

Diagnosis: Audiometry shows sensorineural hearing loss with a flat curve and recruitment. Reduced peripheral vestibular response. Hearing loss and vertigo are generally transient, but late reactions including deafness have been demonstrated experimentally.

Differential diagnosis includes aminoglycoside antibiotics and loop diuretics.

Cytostatic Drugs

Main symptoms: Acute bilateral exacerbation of preexisting hearing loss. Impairment in a previously normal-hearing ear is extremely rare.

Other symptoms and special features: Tinnitus and vertigo are rare. Some cases develop irreversible hearing loss, some show spontaneous improvement.

Causes: Use, especially long-term, of cytostatic drugs (Table 1.**29**).

Diagnosis: Preexisting cochlear hearing loss is exacerbated parallel to the baseline curve. Recruitment is always positive with no threshold decay. Speech discrimination is good. Tinnitus of new onset is rare, but preexisting tinnitus is often increased. Peripheral vestibular hypoactivity is occasionally observed.

Tuberculostatic Drugs

Main symptoms: Acute hearing loss of variable degree, usually bilateral. Tinnitus may be present or absent. Vertigo is usually present.

Cause: Treatment with tuberculostatic drugs (Table 1.**30**).

Diagnosis: Bilateral high-tone sensorineural hearing loss or bilateral low-tone sensorineural hearing loss with recruitment. Tinnitus is usually high-pitched.

Vestibular testing shows bilateral hyperactivity, which often precedes cochlear damage, especially after streptomycin use (see pp. 107, 121).

Drugs and Vaccines with Occasional Ototoxic Effect

Main symptoms: Acute hearing loss of variable degree, generally bilateral. Tinnitus and vertigo are very rare. Hearing loss is generally reversible.

Causes: Instances of transient hearing loss have been associated with use of the following drugs: quinidine, practolol (beta-adrenergic blocking agent), tricyclic antidepressants, aryl acetate derivatives such as indomethacin and diclofenac, tetanus and smallpox antitoxin, marijuana, alcohol and nicotine abuse. There are no reliable reports of hearing problems associated with other drugs such as heroin or cocaine.

Diagnosis: Pure-tone audiogram usually shows high-tone sensorineural hearing loss with recruitment, occasional vestibular hyporeactivity (e.g., with tofranil).

Hearing Loss Due to Occupational Toxicity

Acute and chronic intoxication from exposure to substances like those in Table 1.**31** have become uncommon as a result of strict workplace safety regulations.

Main symptoms: Nausea with vomiting and headache.

Other symptoms and special features: A common accompanying symptom is hearing loss, which is more frequent than involvement of the vestibular apparatus. There may be other neurologic symptoms as well as toxic effects on the liver, kidney, and bone marrow.

Diagnosis: The hearing loss generally affects both ears with a high-tone loss or pancochlear configuration. Recruitment is often negative as a result of damage to the spinal ganglion.

Differentiation from preexisting hearing loss is frequently difficult.

Acute Exacerbations of Chronic Hearing Loss

Diseases that lead to a *chronically* progressive sensorineural hearing loss are listed in Table 1.**32**. Because these diseases often take an episodic course, they sometimes present an acute sensorineural hearing impairment.

Nonorganic Acute Hearing Loss

Nonorganic hearing disorders may be *psychogenic* in origin or may represent a *feigning* or *exaggeration* of hearing impairment.

Table 1.**31** *Symptom* Acute sensorineural hearing loss due to workplace toxicity

Synopsis
Aminobenzol
Lead
Fluorine
Carbon monoxide
Nitrobenzol
Mercury
Carbon disulfide

Table 1.**32** Acute exacerbations of chronic hearing loss

Disorders	Frequency of episodes
Cochlear hearing loss	
In renal dysfunction	Common
In thyroid dysfunction	Rare
In diabetes mellitus	Very rare
In vascular disorders	Very common
In immune diseases	Possible
In cervical syndrome	Common
Retrocochlear hearing loss	
Acoustic neuroma	Possible
Vascular damage in the brain stem region	Common
Brain stem tumors	Possible
Multiple sclerosis	Common
Hearing loss in children	
Monosymptomatic progressive recessive hearing loss	Common
Pendred syndrome	Common
van Buchem syndrome	Rare
Congenital syphilis	Common

Psychogenic Hearing Loss

Main symptoms: Sudden, usually bilateral hearing loss or deafness following a stressful event.

Other symptoms and special features: Common associated symptoms include speech difficulties, gait disturbances, and persistent trembling or shaking ("war psychosis"). Young persons are commonly affected.

Causes: Acute or chronic abnormal response to a stressful incident, e.g., self-blame for an automobile accident causing the death of a family member, or a failed suicide attempt.

Diagnosis: Except with complete bilateral deafness, hearing for speech is generally better than hearing for pure tones. Audiogram shows a pancochlear pattern, usually along the 40- to 50-dB line. Otoacoustic emissions (OAEs) are positive. Recruitment and fatigue tests are unrewarding. Except with severe hysteria, the stapedius reflex is intact. The classic tests for feigned hearing loss (Lombard test, Stenger test, Lee delay test) are unremarkable. A discrepancy may be noted between the results of brain stem and cortical audiometry. Measurement of auditory evoked brain stem and auditory nerve potentials shows stimulus responses like those of normal hearers, while auditory evoked cortical potentials are difficult to record and interpret.

Differentiation from exaggerated hearing impairment and organic hearing loss may require repeated auditory testing.

Feigned or Exaggerated Hearing Impairment (Pseudohypacusis)

Main symptoms: Unilateral or bilateral, asymmetric hearing loss that develops some time after a traumatic event. Patient's behavior is often demonstrative (e.g., cupping the hand behind the auricle, exaggerated lip reading by a patient who speaks with normal loudness and timbre).

Other symptoms and special features: Pretended headache, general physical weakness, nonspecific vertigo. Direct questioning always elicits additional problems such as impairment of short-term and long-term memory, concentration difficulties, and contradictory statements of difficulty or discomfort.

Causes: The most common stated cause is antecedent trauma (cranial injury, acoustic trauma, etc.).

Diagnosis: Auditory tests show lack of test–retest reliability. Pure-tone hearing is usually better than speech hearing, with Békésy audiometry showing a type V configuration (continuous tone heard better than intermittent tone). The SISI test is always negative, and the standard tests for feigned hearing loss (Lombard test, Stenger test, Dörfler–Stuart test, Lee delay test) indicate exaggeration of hearing impairment. The stapedius reflex is intact and OAEs, positive. Cortical audiometry generally elicits remarkably good stimulus responses that are even better than in normal hearing subjects. A patient familiar with the test, however, could suppress responses to alter the test outcome.

Differentiation from organic and psychogenic hearing loss is often difficult, because all three can occur as mixed forms.

Idiopathic Acute Hearing Loss

If we regard acute hearing loss not as a symptom but more correctly as an idiopathic condition ("idiopathic acute hearing loss"), we can diagnose this disease only if the previously described disorders have been excluded. That is why the commentary on this clinically important disorder has been placed last in this section. Two forms are recognized:

Sudden Deafness

Main symptom: Acute, usually unilateral hearing loss developing within seconds, minutes, or hours in a patient with no history of ear disease. Often accompanied by tinnitus.

Other symptoms and special features: None!

Causes: Vascular and/or viral etiologies have been postulated.

Diagnosis: No consistent audiometric findings. Patients may have a complete deafness with residual hearing, low-tone hearing loss, high-tone hearing loss with a sharp downsloping or flat pattern, or mid-frequency hearing loss. Recruitment is obligatory. Tinnitus pitch is variable and is easily masked at the auditory threshold.

Differentiation is required from acute sensorineural hearing loss of other etiology (see Table 1.**23**).

Labyrinthine Apoplexy

Main symptoms: Acute, unilateral profund hearing loss, mostly total deafness with severe vertigo. High-pitched tinnitus is generally present.

Causes: Presumably caused by an acutely disturbed blood supply in the inner ear.

Diagnosis: Pure-tone audiogram usually shows deafness (with possible residual hearing) or severe pancochlear sensorineural hearing loss, often without loudness balance. Paretic nystagmus with corresponding spontaneous and provoked nystagmus (see p. 107).

Differentiation especially from acoustic neuroma is accomplished by CT and MRI.

Symptom   Chronic Hearing Loss

The hearing impairment is generally bilateral and develops gradually over a period of months or years. The degree of impairment ranges from mild to profound. Complete deafness is extremely rare. There is virtually no propensity for spontaneous improvement (Table 1.**33**).

Chronic Conductive Hearing Loss

There are many diseases associated with chronic conductive hearing loss (Table 1.**34**). However, otologic referral is usually prompted by a different predominant symptom, such as otalgia, dysesthesia or otorrhea. Chronic conductive hearing loss caused by disease of the external auditory canal is nonspecific and is diagnosed from otoscopic findings. The clinical audiology of chronic middle ear diseases is summarized in Table 1.**35**.

Diseases whose cardinal symptom is chronic

hearing loss include *otosclerosis, adhesive process*, and *tympanosclerosis*.

Table 1.**34**   *Symptom*   Chronic conductive hearing loss

Synopsis
With external auditory canal pathology
Ceruminal plug, see p. 19
Exostoses, see p. 20
Stenoses, see p. 21
Tumors, see p. 28
With middle ear pathology (see Table 1.**35**)
Chronic otitis media, see p. 22
Middle ear tumors, see p. 28 ff.
Chronic disturbances of eustachian tube ventilation, see p. 21
Otosclerosis
Adhesive process
Tympanosclerosis

Table 1.**33** Gross differential diagnosis of chronic hearing loss

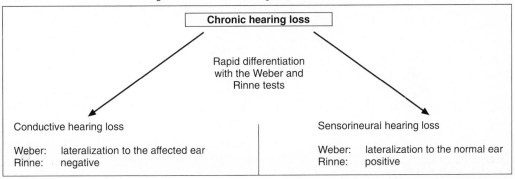

Chronic hearing loss

Rapid differentiation with the Weber and Rinne tests

Conductive hearing loss

Weber: lateralization to the affected ear
Rinne: negative

Sensorineural hearing loss

Weber: lateralization to the normal ear
Rinne: positive

Table 1.**35**   Chronic hearing loss with middle ear pathology

Disorder	Main symptoms	Tympanic membrane findings	Pure-tone audiogram	Tympanogram	Further details
Chronic mucosal suppuration	Aural discharge usually mucoid and odorless; little if any pain	Central perforation of variable size	Pancochlear conductive hearing loss of variable degree	Faulty seal	see p. 24
Chronic bone suppuration	Aural discharge fetid, usually purulent or crumbly, may contain whitish flakes; vague feeling of pressure, possible balance disturbances	Marginal perforation usually in area of Schrappnell membrane or posterosuperiorly	Mild to moderate conductive hearing loss, rarely severe	Faulty seal or pattern as in Fig. 1.**9**	see p. 24
Otosclerosis	Slowly progressive unilateral hearing loss, later becomes bilateral; tinnitus usually unilateral	Normal appearance, possible Schwartze sign	Initial low-frequency conductive hear loss, later pancochlear pattern with Carhart notch	Fig. 1.**7**	see p. 75
Adhesive process	Slowly progressive hearing loss in patients with prior history of otitis (usually in childhood)	Thickened, scarred membrane with atrophic areas, often retracted	Usually severe pancochlear conductive hearing loss	Fig. 1.**9** or Fig. 1.**10**	see p. 76
Tympanosclerosis	Progressive bilateral hearing loss, usually commencing in childhood	Membrane scarred and thickened with calcium deposits, atrophic areas, and possible visible sclerotic foci	Severe pancochlear conductive hearing loss	Fig. 1.**10**	see p. 76
Benign tumors	Feeling of fullness, pressure, later progressive hearing loss	Membrane retracted or bulging, depending on type and location of tumor (which may be visible through the membrane)	Nonspecific	Negative pressure or positive pressure	see p. 28

Table 1.**35**   (cont.)

Disorder	Main symptoms	Tympanic membrane findings	Pure-tone audiogram	Tympanogram	Further details
Glomus tumors	Pulsatile tinnitus, aural fullness, pressure, rarely pain, later progressive hearing loss	Livid tumor visible through the membrane	Pancochlear conductive haering loss of variable degree	Negative pressure or positive pressure	see p. 29
Malignant tumors	Otorrhea, increasing pain, progressive hearing loss	Granulating tissue that bleeds easily	Severe pancochlear conductive hearing loss	Faulty seal or pattern as in Fig. 1.**9**	see p. 31
Chronic disturbances of eustachian tube ventilation	Constant sensation of hearing obstruction with fluctuating hearing loss; clicking sound may be heard on noseblowing and swallowing	Retracted, possibly with visible fluid level	Nonspecific conductive hearing loss	Fig. 1.**9** or Fig. 1.**10**	see p. 21

Otosclerosis

Main symptom: Slowly, sometimes episodically progressive hearing loss, initially affecting one ear and later becoming bilateral in most cases.

Other symptoms and special features: Increasing tinnitus, generally unilateral, which is commonly frequently low-pitched but may be high-pitched. Most common in the white race. Familial occurrence is described in 50−60% of cases (3:1 females to males). Often coincides with pregnancy.

Causes: Poorly understood. Besides congenital disposition, endocrine and metabolic disturbances are thought to have causal significance.

Diagnosis: Conductive hearing loss begins in the low frequencies; high frequencies are not affected until the advanced stage. Carhart notch is present. High-tone loss is increasingly apparent in the bone conduction curve (Fig. 1.**20**). Normal tympanometric curve with absent stapedius reflex. Gellé test is pathologic. Radiographs generally show good pneumatization of the petrous pyramid.

Fig. 1.**20** Audiogram in severe bilateral otosclerosis

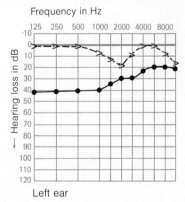

Left ear

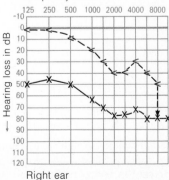

Right ear

Table 1.**36** *Symptom* Chronic sensorineural hearing loss

Synopsis
Noise-induced hearing loss
Presbycusis
Hearing loss due to metabolic and circulatory diseases
– In renal dysfunction
– In thyroid dysfunction
– In diabetes mellitus
– In vascular disorders
– In immune disorders
Acoustic neuroma
Central auditory dysfunction
– Bulbopontine hearing disorders
– Mesencephalic hearing disorders
– Multiple sclerosis
– Cortical–subcortical hearing disorders

Causes: Sequel to chronic otitis media with a poorly ventilated tympanic cavity. Cholesterol granuloma formation and fibrosis involving the entire tympanic cavity. Partial destruction of the auditory ossicles and cicatric fixation of the ossicular chain with occlusion of the windows.

Diagnosis: The tympanic membrane is scarred, thickened, retracted, and contains atrophic areas. Radiographs generally show deficient pneumatization of the petrous pyramids. Pure-tone audiogram usually shows severe pancochlear conductive hearing loss, rarely accompanied by high-tone sensorineural impairment. The tympanogram is flat and shifted toward the negative pressure range. The stapedius reflex is absent.

Differentiation is required from other causes of conductive hearing loss such as otosclerosis, tympanosclerosis, and tumors.

Differentiation from middle ear deformities, ossicular discontinuity, and adhesive processes is based on impedance audiometry and temporal bone radiographs:

○ *Ossicular or tympanic deformity:* Completely flat tympanogram.

○ *Ossicular discontinuity:* No measurable deflections in tympanogram, absent stapedius reflex.

○ *Fracture of stapes crura:* No measurable deflections in tympanogram, but a demonstrable stapedius reflex.

○ *Adhesive process:* Flattened tympanogram shifted into negative pressure range, deficient pneumatization of the petrous pyramids.

○ *Fixation of the malleus head:* Requires surgical diagnosis.

Adhesive Processes

Main symptom: Hearing loss, often bilateral and usually present for some years.

Other symptoms and special features: Tinnitus is rarely present, and otorrhea is sometimes present in connection with an infection.

Tympanosclerosis

Main symptom: Increasing conductive hearing loss, usually commencing in childhood and frequently bilateral.

Causes: Tympanosclerotic transformation of the middle ear mucosa mainly in the stapes area and later in the epitympanum or entire tympanic cavity. Morphologic changes include swelling of the collagen fibers and hyaline degeneration with subsequent calcium deposition.

Diagnosis: Tympanic membrane is scarred and thickened and contains calcium deposits and possibly atrophic areas. A whitish material may be visible through the membrane. Pneumatization of the petrous pyramids is usually deficient.

Pure-tone audiogram generally demonstrates severe pancochlear conductive hearing loss. The tympanogram is flat and shifted toward negative pressures.

Chronic Sensorineural Hearing Loss

See Table 1.**36**.

Noise-Induced Hearing Loss (Chronic Acoustic Trauma)

Main symptoms: The hearing loss is often first noticed by family members. With passage of time, patient has difficulty comprehending speech when more than one person is talking, in a noisy environment, in echo-filled rooms, and while watching TV. This can lead to problems of social isolation. In advanced stages, the patient has difficulty discriminating speech with a single person.

Other symptoms and special features: Unilateral or bilateral high-pitched tinnitus and marked noise sensitivity are common. When questioned, the patient reports having experienced a deafening effect from occupational noise exposure, sometimes combined with headache, ear pressure or tinnitus, before the hearing loss became established. Increasingly, the complaints tended to persist for several hours after leaving work. Hearing and tinnitus may improve after discontinuation of occupational noise exposure, but progression indicates that another disease process is involved.

Causes: 1) Noise intensity. Normal ears are not damaged by levels below 85 dB(A). 2) Noise frequency spectrum. High frequencies are more damaging than low frequencies. 3) Duration of noise exposure. 4) Individual noise sensitivity.

Diagnosis: Initially there is a characteristic c^5 notch, which widens and deepens as hearing loss progresses. This is followed by a sloping pattern, sometimes steep, starting above 1000 Hz. The middle and lower frequencies are involved later (Fig. 1.**21**).

Recruitment is always markedly positive. Even slight asymmetries are uncommon and are based on the specific occupational situation (e.g., right-handed metal forging work). Whispered and spoken voice testing shows a marked discrepancy between the ability to comprehend whispered and conversational speech. Speech audiometry shows remarkably good monosyllabic discrimination. Tinnitus is easily masked and is usually matched to a 4- to 6-kHz tone, but with a sharply sloping loss the tinnitus is localized to the descending flank.

Vestibular tests are normal.

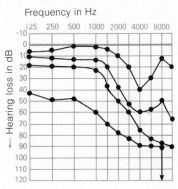

Fig. 1.**21** Audiogram patterns in noise-induced hearing loss

Differentiation is required from progressive degenerative sensorineural hearing loss, presbycusis, cervicogenic hearing loss, and hearing loss due to ototoxicity.

Presbycusis

Main symptoms: Marked initially by poor speech discrimination when more than one person is talking or when background noise is present ("cocktail party effect") and in rooms with poor acoustics (e.g., old churches). High frequencies (e.g., cricket chirps) are no longer perceived. In advanced stage even conversation with one person becomes difficult, and speech becomes distorted.

Other symptoms and special features: Noise sensitivity is common, and tinnitus is often present but causes little annoyance. Though vertigo is not among the true associated symptoms, direct questioning often elicits unsteadiness and transient dizziness during particular head and body movements.

Causes: The term "presbycusis" is not precisely defined. It refers not only to the physiologic sensorineural hearing loss and the neural and central deterioration that accompany aging but also to the sensorineural hearing loss, which is caused solely by old age, cardiovascular and metabolic disorders, and long-term environmental influences.

Table 1.**37** Chronic sensorineural hearing loss due to metabolic or circulatory diseases

Disorder	Pure-tone audiogram	Recruitment	Tinnitus	Change in findings	Vestibular findings
Renal dysfunction	Bilateral high-tone hearing loss; rarely moderate to severe pancochlear pattern	+	Rare	Progression of variable degree, frequent flareups	Asymmetric hyporeactivity
Thyroid dysfunction	Bilateral high-tone hearing loss, rarely pancochlear pattern	+/−	Rare	Slow progression, flareups, may respond to therapy	Hyporeactivity possible
Diabetes mellitus	Bilateral high-tone hearing loss, usually with sloping pattern	+/−	Rare	Slow progression, adolescents may show positive therapeutic response	Usually normal
Vascular disorder	Strictly symmetrical high-tone hearing loss with sloping or diagonal pattern	+	Common, high- or medium-pitched	Episodic and/or continuous progression of variable degree	Bilateral hyporeactivity
Immune disorders	Unilateral of bilateral hearing loss, sloping or pancochlear pattern	+/−	Nonspecific	Continuous and/or episodic progression, may respond to therapy	Unilateral or rarely bilateral hyporeactivity

Diagnosis: Pure-tone audiogram may show a symmetrical, gradually sloping high-tone loss, a sharply sloping high-tone loss, or a more pancochlear configuration. Recruitment is often slight or only partially manifested. Frequency resolution is impaired in the high-tone range, with a markedly pathologic temporal resolution when background noise is present. Hearing is often quite good in the absence of background noise and even shows a good result on dichotic testing, while monosyllabic discrimination, on the other hand, is too poor compared with pure-tone testing. Speech discrimination in noise is generally poor, especially when sentences are tested. Tinnitus is usually high-pitched and often must be masked 10−20 dB above the auditory threshold.

Central vestibular dysfunction is not uncommon.

Differentiation is required from noise-induced hearing loss, ototoxicity, or cervicogenic hearing loss.

Chronic Sensorineural Hearing Loss Due to Metabolic or Circulatory Disorders

See Table 1.**37**.

Acoustic Neuroma

Main symptoms: Unilateral hearing loss and tinnitus.

Other symptoms and special features: Although the tumor develops from the vestibular part of cranial nerve VIII, vertigo is an infrequent complaint due to the slow rate of progression. Balance disturbances are not usually

Table 1.**38** Central auditory dysfunction

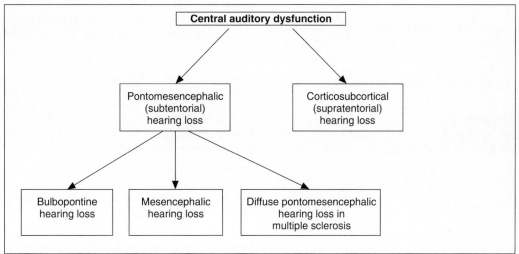

experienced until the brain stem and cerebellum become involved (see p. 110). Other symptoms are facial paresthesias, headache (usually occipital), vomiting, decreased and blurred vision, and facial twitching and paralysis. Progressive brain stem compression may incite ipsilateral or contralateral spastic signs. Finally the obstruction of CSF drainage produces the symptoms of increased intracranial pressure with severe headache, bilateral papilledema, and increasing daze (see Table 1.**8**).

Diagnosis: Slowly progressive, unilateral hearing loss that starts in the high frequencies. Signs of retrocochlear impairment include pathologic threshold fatigue. Initially, there is absence of recruitment with an absent stapedius reflex in more than 80% of cases and also a relatively large loss of discrimination. Brain stem audiometry in 95% of patients shows prolonged latencies consistent with retrocochlear dysfunction. As the tumor enlarges, it can cause acute exacerbation of hearing loss, in the course of which recruitment becomes positive.

More than 95% of patients show a reduced caloric response on the side of the lesion (see p. 108). Trigeminal nerve involvement is marked by a diminished corneal reflex. Positive Hitselberger sign (hypoesthesia of the posterosuperior wall of the external auditory canal). Conventional Stenvers radiographs

may not always demonstrate slight asymmetry of the internal auditory canal (at least 2 mm), but cranial CT scans are positive in over 95% of cases. Cranial MRI is rewarding in virtually all cases, especially when a contrast medium is used. Typically there is a marked rise in CSF protein content.

Differentiation is required from Ménière disease, cervicogenic sensorineural hearing loss, and retrocochlear hearing loss of diverse etiology. Special case: Recklinghausen neurofibromatosis (see p. 138) and Gardner−Turner syndrome (see Table 4.**26**).

Central Auditory Dysfunction

There are two potential sites for central nerve damage causing auditory dysfunction (Table 1.**38**).

Bulbopontine Hearing Disorders

Main symptoms: Neurologic symptoms with central vestibular dysfunction are predominant.

Other symptoms: Auditory symptoms are variable and can range from mild unilateral or bilateral hearing deficits causing little subjective distress to unilateral progressive hearing loss as well as acute deterioration of hearing. Tinnitus may be present or absent.

Causes: Mass effect from basal gangliomas, meningiomas, cranial nerve VIII or V neuromas, or tumors of the fourth ventricle. Vascular disorders such as hemorrhage or malacia with crossed symptoms. Infectious and degenerative lesions are less common.

Diagnosis: Pure-tone threshold audiometry is not informative, but generally there is a marked threshold decay and often an absence of recruitment with a contralateral and ipsilateral absent or fatigued stapedius reflex. Auditory localization is impaired. Speech audiometry shows relatively poor discrimination, especially on dichotic testing. Temporal resolution is impaired, and level difference thresholds are increased. An essential diagnostic procedure is ABR with measurement of the middle potentials, which are often poorer than the subjective auditory threshold. Analysis of the early potentials shows changes in latency and amplitude.

There are pronounced vestibular symptoms with ataxia, disinhibition, direction-changing nystagmus, and optokinetic impairment (see p. 109). Certain tumor locations and bleeding sites produce typical neurologic brain stem symptoms, which may involve cranial nerves II−XI, with tonic spasms, hemiparesis, or even decerebrate rigidity. Neurodiagnostic procedures include EEG, lumbar puncture, cranial CT, and MRI.

Mesencephalic Hearing Disorders

Main symptoms are neurologic with damage to individual cranial nerves of the pyramidal tracts and of the sensory, cerebellar, and extrapyramidal systems, leading to contralateral central pareses or sensory disturbances involving the trunk and extremities.

Other symptoms: Hearing impairment is never reported spontaneously, but careful questioning elicits paracusis, diplacusis, or paramusia.

Causes: Damage to the peduncle or quadrigeminal bodies by mass lesions (gliomas, tuberculomas, pinealomas), intracranial hypertension, or the much rarer alternating syndromes of vascular origin.

Diagnosis: Hearing loss in the pure-tone audiogram is subtle and nonspecific, but changes are apparent in binaural tone localization and integration and in sensitized speech tests. Binaural speech tests may show changes that are often bilateral and sometimes contralateral to a lesion located above the crossing of the auditory pathways. Accelerated speech tests indicate damage to the reticular substance. Despite the minimal subjective hearing impairment, early brain stem potentials exhibit marked changes.

ENG shows evidence of central vestibular dysfunction. The diagnosis is based on a neurologic workup consisting of clinical examination, EEG, CT, MRI, and CSF analysis.

Diffuse Pontomesencephalic Hearing Disorders in Multiple Sclerosis

Main symptoms: Cranial nerve deficits, motor and sensory system manifestations, and disturbances of the cerebellar and the autonomic nervous system contribute to the diverse symptomatology of these disorders. The optic nerve is most commonly affected, and unilateral or bilateral amaurosis may develop in a matter of days. Often the initial symptoms are mild hearing deficits, which may increase steadily or episodically with passage of time and often fluctuate sharply. Another early symptom is vestibular dysfunction with attacks of rotating vertigo induced by any change of position.

Other symptoms and special features: Paralysis of ocular movement (abducens nerve), facial paresthesias or trigeminal neuralgias, speech disturbances, and rarely disturbances of taste and smell.

Causes: Poorly understood. A persistent viral infection evoking an individually varied immune response has been suggested.

Diagnosis: Repeated, systematic audiometric examinations are necessary due to the variability of auditory function and suprathreshold test results. Pure-tone audiometry shows nonspecific, often bilateral sensorineural hearing loss with mild threshold decay and variable recruitment. The contralateral and/or ipsilateral stapedius reflex is absent but may return in rare cases. Speech audiometry shows relatively poor discrimination, especially in the sensitized and dichotic tests. Recordings of early auditory evoked potentials show amplitude changes and prolonged latencies as well as desynchronization and discrepancies between the subjective and objective thresholds.

Vestibular testing reveals a dissociated gaze nystagmus with changing peripheral reactivity. Cerebellar ataxia is often predominant (see p. 110). The diagnosis is established by neurologic studies.

Differentiation is required from tumors and hemorrhage. In the event of an organic brain seizure with unconsciousness, the diagnosis should be reconsidered since this symptom is not characteristic of multiple sclerosis (MS).

Corticosubcortical Hearing Disorders

Main symptoms: Organic brain deficits of varying degree with associated sensory, psychic, and vegetative aura phenomena.

Other symptoms and special features: Auditory hallucinations and illusions that may be expressed in words or music. There may be accompanying gnostic disturbances of hearing, manifested as global auditory agnosia or dissociated agnosia. The latter is confined to noises, music, or the spoken word. Speech disturbances are also present in most cases. Rare cases experience a vestibular or vertiginous aura with nonspecific rotating vertigo or even an olfactory aura (see p. 227).

Causes: Hemispheric, temporal, or juxtatemporal lesions. Causes in younger patients include vascular disorders such as rupture of an aneurysm or angioma. Older patients may have postthrombotic or postembolic malacia, tumors, temporal epilepsy, or injuries due to temporal contusion.

Diagnosis: Standard hearing tests are usually normal, but tests for acoustic localization, binaural integration, and acoustic reaction time are frequently pathologic, either bilaterally or on the side opposite the lesion. Sensitized speech tests are most reliable but are difficult to perform in aphasic or confused patients. Early brain stem potentials show normal latencies and amplitudes, while the middle and late potentials show altered stimulus responses with lengthened amplitudes or with deficits. The diagnosis is established by EEG recording during an attack and by CT or MRI.

Differentiation from brain stem lesions can be accomplished by CT and MRI.

Symptom   **Fluctuating Hearing**

Complaints other than hearing loss tend to dominate the symptomatology of fluctuating hearing. With fluctuating *conductive hearing loss*, the principal complaints are otorrhea, pain, or dysesthesias such as itching and aural fullness (see p. 18). With fluctuating *sensorineural hearing loss*, vertigo is generally predominant. The disorders are described fully in the section on Vertigo (see p. 97ff.); here they are summarized in Tables 1.**39** and 1.**40** only.

Table 1.**39** *Symptom* Fluctuating sensorineural hearing loss

Synopsis
Ménière disease, see Table 1.**40** and p. 112
Lermoyez disease, see Table 1.**40** and p. 113
Labyrinthine fistula, see Table 1.**40** and p. 113
Cervicogenic sensorineural hearing loss, see Table 1.**40** and pp. 106, 113
Metabolic sensorineural hearing loss, see Table 1.**40**
Cogan syndrome, see Table 1.**40**

Table 1.**40** Fluctuating sensorineural hearing loss

Disorder	Pure-tone audiogram	Recruitment	Tinnitus	Vertigo	Special features
Ménière disease	Unilateral fluctuating low-tone hearing loss below 1 kHz, later assuming a pancochlear pattern, usually along the 70 dB line	Strongly positive	Unilateral, usually low-pitched, rarely high-pitched	Attacks initially last seconds to minutes, later persist for hours or days; increasing unilateral hyporeactivity; alternation of paretic nystagmus and recovery nystagmus	Attacks increasingly preceded by ear pressure, with gradual deterioration of hearing
Lermoyez disease	Unilateral fluctuating low-tone hearing loss	Strongly positive	Unilateral, usually low-pitched	Attacks from seconds to minutes in duration; alternation of paretic and recovery nystagmus	Hearing and tinnitus improve during vertiginous attacks
Labyrinthine fistula	Unilateral fluctuating low-tone hearing loss, later involving middle and high frequencies and progressing to total deafness	Strongly positive	Unilateral, nonspecific	Positive fistula sign, paroxysmal vertigo during straining, increasing unilateral hyporeactivity	None
Cervicogenic sensorineural hearing loss	Unilateral or bilateral fluctuating low-tone hearing loss with a notch at 500 Hz	Positive	Unilateral or bilateral, usually in 500-Hz range	Paroxysmal vertigo with direction-alternating provoked nystagmus	Cervical spine complaints
Metabolic sensorineural hearing loss	Bilateral asymmetric fluctuating sensorineural hearing loss in low-frequency range, rarely pancochlear or involving high frequencies	Usually positive	Unilateral or bilateral, nonspecific	Usually absent	Hyperlipoproteinemia or hypoglycemia or hypothyroidism
Cogan syndrome	Bilateral asymmetric sensorineural hearing loss, predominantly in the high-frequency range or pancochlear	Positive	May be unilateral or bilateral, nonspecific	Increasing asymmetric hyporeactivity on both sides; episodic vertigo need not be present	Interstitial keratitis

Symptom   **Hearing Loss in Children**

The diagnosis of hearing impairment in the pediatric age groups is of major importance owing to its critical influence on both, the speech development and the overall personal and social development of the affected child. Even in very early infancy, ABR testing can establish the presence, nature, and degree of hearing impairment. Common malformations of the external and middle ear that are associated with conductive hearing loss are listed in Tables 1.**9** and 1.**19**. The present section deals exclusively with *sensorineural* hearing losses

and mixed hearing losses in the pediatric population. The major types of pediatric sensorineural hearing loss are summarized in Table 1.**41**. The clinical audiology of *congenital monosymptomatic* and *progressive monosymptomatic* sensorineural hearing losses is reviewed in Table. 1.**42** and that of *hereditary polysymptomatic* sensorineural hearing losses (syndromes) in Table 1.**43**. The clinical audiology of *acquired* pediatric sensorineural hearing losses is summarized in Table 1.**44**.

Table 1.**41**   *Symptom*   Sensorineural hearing loss in children

Synopsis	

Congenital, hereditary monosymptomatic hearing losses
  – Dominant
  – Recessive
  – Sex-linked
 	
Progressive monosymptomatic hearing losses
  – Dominant hereditary high-frequency hearing loss
  – Dominant hereditary mid-frequency hearing loss
  – Dominant hereditary low-frequency hearing loss
  – Recessive hereditary hearing loss
  – Sex-linked hereditary hearing loss
 	
Polysymptomatic hearing losses (syndromes)
 	
o Hearing loss with external ear deformity
  – Vourmann–Vourmann syndrome
 	
o Hearing loss with ophthalmic diseases
  – Usher syndrome
  – Refsum syndrome
  – Hallgren syndrome or von Graefe–Hallgren syndrome
  – Alström syndrome
  – Laurence–Moon–Biedl syndrome
 	
o Hearing loss with renal disease
  – Alport syndrome
 	
o Hearing loss with thyroid disease
  – Pendred syndrome
	o Hearing loss with integumentary anomalies
	  – Crouzon syndrome
	  – Mandibulofacial dysostosis (Franceschetti syndrome)
	  – Wildervanck syndrome
	  – Marfan syndrome
	  – Albers-Schönberg disease
	  – van Buchem syndrome
	  – Craniometaphyseal dysplasia (Pyle syndrome)
	  – Paget disease
	  – van der Hoeve–de Kleyn disease
	
	o Hearing loss with mucopolysaccharidoses
	  – Hunter syndrome
	  – Scheie syndrome
	  – Morquio syndrome
	
	o Hearing loss with chromosomal abnormalities
	  – 5p syndrome (cri du chat)
	  – Turner syndrome
	
	o Hearing losses acquired in utero
	  – Rubella
	  – Cytomegaly
	  – Toxoplasmosis
	  – Congenital syphilis
	  – Toxic insult
	
	o Hearing losses acquired perinatally
	  – Neonatal asphyxia
	  – Prematurity
	  – Kernicterus
	
	o Postnatal hearing losses

Table 1.**42**   Congenital and progressive monosymptomatic sensorineural hearing loss

Disorder	Audiologic symptoms	Recruitment	Vestibular symptoms	Change in findings	Special features
Congenital hearing loss					
Dominant hereditary hearing loss	Unilateral or bilateral complete deafness or profound hearing loss	If measurable, positive	Possible unilateral or bilateral hyporeactivity or failure	Progression may occur in the first years of life	Bone *aplasia* of the cochlea (Michel type) when onset is before week 4 of embryonic development, bone *dysplasia* (Mondini type) when onset is in week 7 or after
Recessive hereditary hearing loss	Strictly bilateral hearing loss Type I: steep downslope past 1.5 kHz Type II: sloping pattern Type III: residual hearing up to 2 kHz	If measurable, positive	Bilateral vestibular hyporeactivity or failure	None	Membranous aplasia or dysplasia of the cochlear duct and often of the saccule (Scheibe's type); most common form of congenital hearing loss
Sex-linked hereditary hearing loss	Very severe or profound hearing loss, usually bilateral, with a pancochlear pattern	Positive	None	None	Overt disease occurs only in males; females can transmit the disorder as a recessive trait
Progressive hearing loss					
Dominant high-frequency hearing loss	High-frequency hearing loss above 1 kHz up to 80 dB; progresses much later to involve other frequencies	Markedly positive	None	Onset at school age with very slow progression	Partial damage to membranous labyrinth (Alexander type), most common progressive hereditary hearing loss

Table 1.**42**   (cont.)

Disorder	Audiologic symptoms	Recruitment	Vestibular symptoms	Change in findings	Special features
Dominant mid-frequency hearing loss	Bilateral shallow notch at 1–2 kHz; loss progresses even later to involve high and then low frequencies	Positive	None	Onset at school age, slow progression, hearing aid needed by 3rd–4th decade	Alexander type
Dominant low-frequency hearing loss	Symmetric hearing loss below 2 kHz, later progressing in the high-frequency range, even pancochlear loss at 50–60 dB	Positive	None	Onset at school age, very slow progression to pancochlear pattern at the 50–60 dB level by the 5th–6th decade	Alexander type
Recessive hearing loss	Bilateral hearing loss with pancochlear pattern ranging to deafness with residual hearing	If measurable, generally positive	None	Early onset, rapid progression, often episodic	Speech defects are common
Sex-linked hearing loss	Always bilateral pancochlear pattern, increasing to profound impairment	Nonspecific	Unknown	Onset at school age, very slow progression; hearing loss does not become profound until 5th to 6th decade	Affects either males or females exclusively within a family

Table 1.**43**   Hereditary polysymptomatic sensorineural hearing loss (syndromes)

Disorder	Audiologic symptoms	Vestibular symptoms	General symptoms	Change in findings
With malformations of the external ear				
Vourmann–Vourmann syndrome	Mild to moderate bilateral high-frequency hearing loss	Rarely, bilateral hyporeactivity	Bilateral aural and cervical fistula	Hearing: slow progression

Table 1.**43**   (cont.)

Disorder	Audiologic symptoms	Vestibular symptoms	General symptoms	Change in findings
With ophthalmic disease				
Usher syndrome	Bilateral hearing loss Type I: sloping pattern at 40–70 dB Type II: deafness with or without residual hearing Type III (rare): low-frequency hearing loss at 20–40 dB	Bilateral hypo-reactivity	Retinitis pigmentosa with bilateral night blindness and visual field defects, possible migraine	Hearing: no change Vision: onset in 1st decade, progression to blindness
Refsum syndrome	Asymmetric high-frequency hearing loss with sloping pattern, later progressing to involve mid-frequency ranges	Later spinocerebellar ataxia	Retinitis pigmentosa with night blindness, narrowing of visual fields, and pale pupils; later: cataract, polyneuritis in arms and legs, ichthyosis, anosmia, and A-V block	Hearing: onset in 2nd–3rd decade, slow progression to profound (but not total) deafness Vision: onset in 1st–2nd decade, slow progression Polyneuritis: starts in advanced age, often takes episodic course
Hallgren syndrome (von Graefe–Hallgren syndrome)	Severe bilateral congenital hearing loss	Direction alternating provoked, nystagmus, vestibulo-cerebellar ataxia	Retinitis pigmentosa with visual field narrowing and cataract; possible oligophrenia, clubfoot, kyphosis, growth retardation	Hearing: unchanged Vision: onset in first years of life with marked progression Ataxia: marked progression
Alström syndrome	Progressive bilateral hearing loss, usually pancochlear or with sloping pattern	Direction alternating provoked nystagmus	Pigmentary degeneration of the retina and optic nerve atrophy with visual deterioration, divergent strabismus, obesity, hypogenitalism, hyperuricemia, eventual renal failure	Hearing: onset at school age, slow progression Vision: onset in early childhood, gradual progression to blindness Diabetes mellitus: onset in 2nd decade Renal failure: onset in 3rd decade

Table 1.**43**   (cont.)

Disorder	Audiologic symptoms	Vestibular symptoms	General symptoms	Change in findings
Laurence–Moon–Biedl syndrome	Usually bilateral, nonspecific sensorineural hearing loss of variable degree	None	Retinitis pigmentosa with ptosis, iris coloboma, epicanthus, strabismus, possible cataract; hypogenitalism; possible mental retardation, polydactyly, or cardiac defects	Hearing: possible slow progression Vision: slow progression to blindness
With renal disease				
Alport syndrome	Progressive, bilateral, roughly pancochlear hearing loss slightly more pronounced in the middle frequencies; pronounced recruitment; later sloping pattern progressing to deafness	Bilateral hyporeactivity	Nephritis with progressive renal failure and hematuria, frequently cataract and fundus albipunctatus	Hearing and vision: onset late in 1st decade, progression more pronounced in males than females
With thyroid disease				
Pendred syndrome	Severe bilateral congenital hearing loss progressing to deafness	Frequent bilateral hyporeactivity	Euthyroid struma, enzymopathy (impaired iodine utilization)	Hearing: onset at birth with gradual, sometimes episodic progression Struma: onset in early childhood
With integumentary disease				
Waardenburg syndrome	Congenital bilateral hearing loss of variable degree, usually moderate impairment with a pancochlear pattern	Bilateral hyporeactivity corresponding to the hearing loss	Pigmentation changes in the iris, skin, and hair; large, white forelock; lateral displacement of medial canthus; wide, flat nasal dorsum; brachydactyly, syndactyly, dental anomalies, possible cardiac anomaly and genital dysplasia	None

Table 1.**43**   (cont.)

Disorder	Audiologic symptoms	Vestibular symptoms	General symptoms	Change in findings
With skeletal disease				
Crouzon syndrome (see Table 2.**13**)	Usually bilateral, severe, pan-cochlear conductive hearing loss, unilateral or bilateral sensori-neural hearing loss of variable degree	Possible unilateral or bilateral hyporeactivity	Cranial anomalies, ocular anomalies with hypertelorism, exophthalmos, and strabismus; optic nerve atrophy; parrot beak nose, maxillary dysplasia, ossicular anomalies	Hearing: onset of sensorineural hearing loss in early childhood, gradual progression Vision: onset at preschool age, gradual progression to blindness
Franceschetti–Zwahlen syndrome (see also Table 2.**13**)	Severe unilateral or bilateral conductive hearing loss, possible unilateral sensorineural haering loss of variable degree	Possible unilateral hyporeactivity	Lateral coloboma of eyelid, antimongoloid position of palpebral fissures, bird face, microtia and atresia of external auditory canal, hypoplastic zygoma, macrostomia	None
Wildervanck syndrome	Severe conductive hearing loss, frequent sensorineural hearing loss of variable degree	Usually bilateral hyporeactivity	Cervical vertebral fusion, abducens paralysis, exophthalmos, atresia of external auditory canal or middle ear deformities, cleft palate rare	None
Marfan syndrome	Unilateral or bilateral conductive hearing loss, mixed hearing loss, or pure sensorineural hearing loss	Possible unilateral or bilateral hyporeactivity	Arachnodactyly, ectopia lentis, cardiac and pulmonary anomalies, ocular motor palsies, paralytic dysphagia, possible mimetic rigidity	None

Table 1.**43**   (cont.)

Disorder	Audiologic symptoms	Vestibular symptoms	General symptoms	Change in findings
Albers-Schön-berg syndrome	Typically bilateral, pro-gressive, mixed hearing loss; conductive loss starts in the low frequencies, sen-sorineural loss in the high fre-quencies	None	Increasing facial paralysis and vi-sion loss, pro-gressive osteo-sclerosis of all bones	Hearing and vision: onset in childhood, gradual progression to deafness and blindness
van Buchem syndrome	Severe bilateral conductive hear-ing loss, pro-gressive retro-cochlear sensori-neural hearing loss with pan-cochlear pattern	Increasing bi-lateral hypo-reactivity	Hyperostosis of cranium, man-dible, clavicle, and ribs; in-creasing facial paralysis and progressive visu-al loss	Hearing and vision: onset during puber-ty, steady progres-sion to deafness and blindness
Pyle syndrome	Severe conduc-tive hearing loss, increasing retro-cochlear impair-ment	Eventual hypo-reactivity	Hyperostosis of the facial skele-ton, splaying of the metaphyses of the long bones	Hearing: conductive hearing loss is con-genital, sensorineu-ral loss starts at pre-school age and steadily progresses to deafness Cranial deformities: onset in very early childhood, continual progression
Paget syndrome (see also Table 1.**19**)	Unilateral or bilateral conduc-tive hearing loss with pancochlear pattern, mixed hearing loss, or pure sensorineu-ral hearing loss, starting with the high frequencies	Unilateral or bilateral hypo-reactivity	Deforming oste-itis of the cra-nium and lower extremities	Hearing and osteitis: onset in middle age, gradual progression
van der Hoeve–de Kleyn syndrome	Slowly progres-sive, often mixed hearing loss; stapes fixation	None	Blue sclerae, bone fragility, dental anomalies	Hearing: onset vari-able, slow progres-sion to deafness

Table 1.**43**   (cont.)

Disorder	Audiologic symptoms	Vestibular symptoms	General symptoms	Change in findings
With mucopolysaccharidosis				
Hunter syndrom type B	Usually bilateral, nonspecific, progressive sensorineural hearing loss; conductive component also may be present	Unknown	General developmental retardation, mucopolysacchariduria, possible chronic recurring rhinitis	Hearing: onset in infancy, slow progression
Scheie syndrome	Usually bilateral, progressive mixed hearing loss	Possible hyporeactivity	Mental retardation, facial dysmorphia, hand and foot deformities, possible corneal opacity	Hearing: onset at school age, slow progression
Morquio syndrome	Bilateral, slowly progressive mixed hearing loss	Possible bilateral hyporeactivity	Dwarfism with short neck and deformed trunk, changes in dental enamel	Hearing: onset in teens, very slow progression Growth disturbance: onset in 1st or 2nd year of life
Chromosome abnormalities				
Cri-du-chat syndrome	Severe mixed hearing loss; bilateral deafness is common	None	Severe disturbance of mental and motor development, microencephaly, severe ocular malformation, short neck, simian palm crease	None
Turner syndrome	Bilateral sensorineural hearing loss with a notch in the midfrequency range	None	Short stature, shield-shaped thorax, low-set ears, myopathic facies, short neck, intellectual impairment, sexual infantilism	None

Table 1.**44**   Acquired sensorineural hearing loss in children

Disorder	Audiologic symptoms	Vestibular symptoms	General symptoms	Change in findings
Acquired in utero				
Rubella	Complete bilateral deafness with no residual hearing; less commonly severe sensorineural hearing loss, usually of cochlear type, with nonspecific audiometric curve	Usually bilateral vestibular failure	Amaurosis or severe visual impairment, cardiac defects, frequently cleft palate, dental anomalies, microcephali, motor retardation, possible thrombocytopenia	Hearing and vision: losses may progress during the first years of life
Cytomegaly	Bilateral cochlear impairment of variable degree	Unilateral or bilateral hyporeactivity of varying degree	None	Progression may occur during the first years of life
Toxoplasmosis	Usually bilateral high-frequency hearing loss of mild degree; severe pancochlear hearing loss is possible	Usually bilateral hyporeactivity of variable degree	None	None
Congenital syphilis	Highly variable ranging from mild hearing loss to deafness, unilateral or bilateral, cochlear or retrocochlear	Asymmetric hyporeactivity of variable degree; often positive fistula sign with Tullio phenomenon	Hutchinson teeth, interstitial keratitis, periostitis of cranium and tibia	Progression is variable and usually episodic, but remissions can occur
Drug toxicity, see Table 1.**26**				
Acquired perinatally				
Neonatal asphyxia	Hearing loss of variable degree, unilateral or bilateral; usually high-frequency sensorineural hearing loss with recruitment	None	Central damage with debilitation is possible	None

Table 1.**44**   (cont.)

Disorder	Audiologic symptoms	Vestibular symptoms	General symptoms	Change in findings
Prematurity	Cochlear and retrocochlear impairment of variable degree showing various audiometric patterns, unilateral or bilateral	Possible ataxia and central vestibular dysfunction	Frequent central damage with debilitation	None
Kernicterus	Moderate to severe bilateral cochlear impairment with sloping pattern; central damage with agnosia also possible	Possible central vestibular dysfunction	Muscle spasms, seizures, mental retardation, choreoathetosis	Possible progression after seizures
Acquired postnatally, see Table 1.**25**				

Symptom   **Tinnitus**

The gross differential diagnosis of tinnitus is based on the site of tinnitus generation (Table 1.**45**). The relevant disorders are not discussed again in this section; page references in Tables 1.**46**–1.**48** will direct the reader to the appropriate brief commentaries.

Table 1.**45**   Gross differential diagnosis of tinnitus

Site of generation	Main features
Middle ear tinnitus	Constant or pulsatile, usually low-pitched, can be masked at auditory threshold
Cochlear tinnitus	Usually high-pitched, can be masked at auditory threshold
Cervical tinnitus	Fluctuating, usually low-pitched, masking level is 10–20 dB above threshold
Mixed cochlear–neural tinnitus	Tone is variable, masking level is 10–20 dB above threshold
Neural tinnitus	Strictly unilateral, masking level is well above threshold
Central tinnitus	Diffuse "head tinnitus," resistant to masking

Middle Ear Tinnitus

Characteristic features: This subjectively very troublesome tinnitus is usually combined with conductive hearing loss and pathologic findings on impedance audiometry.

Relevant disorders are listed in Table 1.46.

Table 1.46   Middle ear tinnitus

Disorder	Quality	Sidedness	Pitch	Tympanic membrane findings	Pure-tone audiogram	Tympanogram	Stapedius reflex	Details
Traumatic tympanic membrane injury	Constant	Unilateral	Variable, usually high-pitched	Perforation with jagged edges in acute cases	Slight conductive hearing loss, rarely with associated high-frequency sensorineural loss	Faulty seal	Faulty seal	See p. 8
Acute otitis media	Pulsatile	Unilateral	Variable	Congested or with draining perforation	Nonspecific conductive hearing loss	Negative pressure or faulty seal	Absent	See p. 9
Otosclerosis	Constant	Usually unilateral	Variable, usually low-pitched	Normal appearance, possible Schwartze sign	Conductive hearing loss with Carhart notch	Fig. 1.7	Absent	See p. 75
Barotrauma	Pulsatile	Unilateral	Variable, usually low-pitched	Hemorrhagic, hematotympanon, rarely perforation	Conductive or mixed hearing loss	Usually negative pressure	Absent	See p. 64
Glomus tumor	Synchronus with the pulse	Unilateral	Low-pitched	Livid mass occasionally visible through membrane	Conductive hearing loss	Variable	Absent	See p. 29
Patulous eustachian tube	Respiration-dependent	Unilateral or bilateral	Variable	Normal	Normal	Fig. 1.7	Normal	See p. 22
Myoclonic soft palate	Pulsatile but synchronous with the pulse	Unilateral or bilateral	Variable	Normal	Normal	Fig. 1.7	Normal	

Cochlear Tinnitus

Characteristic features: The tinnitus has a tonal character and is localized in the ear. It is associated with sensorineural hearing loss that usually involves the high frequencies. Recruitment is demonstrated.

Relevant disorders are listed in Table 1.**47**.

Table 1.**47**   Cochlear tinnitus

Disorder	Sidedness	Pitch	Pure-tone audiogram	Vestibular testing	Details
Traumatic etiology					
Gunshot trauma	Unilateral or bilateral	High-pitched, usually 4–6 kHz	Asymmetric high-frequency loss with c^5 notch	Usually normal	See p. 58
Explosion trauma	Bilateral	High-pitched, usually 3–4 kHz	Asymmetric high-frequency sensorineural loss with a sharp downslope in one ear, usually accompanied by a conductive component of variable degree	Paralytic nystagmus uncommon	See p. 59, 60
Acute noise trauma	Usually bilateral	High-pitched in 4–6 kHz range	High-frequency sensorineural loss with a c^5 notch	Normal	See p. 61
Acoustic accident	Unilateral	Variable	Pancochlear configuration	Normal or direction-changing provoked nystagmus	See p. 62
Blunt head trauma	Usually unilateral	Variable, usually high-pitched	c^5 notch or steep downslope	Nonspecific	See p. 62
Transverse temporal bone fracture	Unilateral	Variable, usually high-pitched	Deafness	Paretic nystagmus	See p. 63
Noise-induced hearing loss	Bilateral or unilateral	High-pitched, usually 3–6 kHz	c^5 notch	Normal	See p. 77

Table 1.**47** (cont.)

Disorder	Sidedness	Pitch	Pure-tone audiogram	Vestibular testing	Details
Toxic etiology					
Aminoglycoside antibiotics	Bilateral	High-pitched, usually 6–12 kHz	High-frequency loss, later converting to pan-cochlear pattern	Bilateral hypo-reactivity	See p. 67
Loop diuretics	Usually bi-lateral	Medium-pitched, 2–4 kHz	Sensorineural notch between 2 and 4 kHz	Possible hypo-reactivity	See p. 68
Salicylates	Bilateral	High-pitched	Pancochlear con-figuration is most common	Bilateral hypo-reactivity	See p. 68
Vascular etiology					
Sudden deafness	Unilateral	Usually high-pitched	Variable		See p. 72
Labyrinthine apoplexy	Unilateral	Variable	Severe hearing loss or total deaf-ness	Paretic nystag-mus	See p. 73
Ménière disease	Unilateral	Usually low-pitched, rarely high-pitched	Low-frequency notch, changing later to pan-cochlear pattern	Hyporeactivity with episodic vertigo	See p. 81, 112
Lermoyez disease	Unilateral	Variable, usually low-pitched	Fluctuating low-frequency notch	Hyporeactivity with episodic vertigo	See p. 81, 113

Cervical Tinnitus

Characteristic features: Cervical tinnitus is usually unilateral and seldom bilateral. It is constant and very rarely pulsatile. The sound tends to be more noticeable early in the morning than in the evening. The tinnitus changes pitch and loudness frequently with changes in head position, is usually low-pitched, and often can be masked only at a slightly supra-threshold level; sometimes it may be accentuated by masking. The tinnitus is combined with a fluctuating, usually low-frequency sensorineural hearing loss with marked recruitment and a direction-changing provoked nystagmus.

Mixed Cochlear–Neural Tinnitus

Characteristic features: The tinnitus may be unilateral or bilateral and can be masked at the auditory threshold or 10–20 dB above threshold. The masking level and frequency are variable and the tinnitus may occur in all frequencies and can be combined with a sensorineural hearing loss of variable degree, with or without recruitment. Vestibular findings are non-specific.

Relevant disorders are listed in Table 1.**48**.

Table 1.**48** Mixed cochlear–neural tinnitus

Disorder	Sidedness	Pitch	Pure-tone audiogram	Vestibular testing	Details
Presbycusis	Usually bilateral	Usually high-pitched, not very bothersome	High-frequency downslope or diagonal downslope, weak recruitment	Nonspecific	See p. 77
Spotted fever	Bilateral	Variable, usually high-pitched	Nonspecific, no recruitment	Nonspecific	See p. 66
Syphilis	Unilateral or bilateral	Nonspecific	Nonspecific	Nonspecific; peripheral or central vestibular dysfunction	See p. 65

Neural Tinnitus

Characteristic features: The tinnitus is strictly unilateral and perceived deep within the ear. It is constant and usually high-pitched. The characteristic symptom is a masking level well above the auditory threshold, combined with sensorineural hearing loss that shows the features of retrocochlear impairment on suprathreshold testing. Vestibular testing generally shows hyporeactivity.

Relevant disorders: Acoustic neuroma and other neoplastic or vascular disorders of the cerebellopontine angle.

Central Tinnitus

Characteristic features: Diffuse "head tinnitus" without laterality. The masking level is well above threshold and equal in both ears, combined with sensorineural hearing loss without recruitment and with marked threshold decay. Central vestibular dysfunction is common.

Specific disorders are listed in Table 1.**38**.

Rare Forms of Tinnitus

Tinnitus with a completely *normal auditory threshold* is most likely psychogenic.

"Allergic tinnitus" varies in occurrence, pitch, and loudness. It is caused chiefly by the consumption of milk products and pork and less commonly by cereals, coffee, and other foods. It is combined with a fluctuating low-frequency or high-frequency hearing loss and variable vertiginous symptoms.

Differential Diagnosis of Vestibular Disorders

H. Scherer

The Sense of Equilibrium and its Evaluation

The diagnosis of balance disorders is based on a knowledge of the peripheral sensory receptors and their afferent information, and of the neuronal mechanisms in the vestibular and their efferent connections. A thorough history and examination tailored specifically to the system of interest will furnish a diagnosis. A brief overview of available diagnostic methods is presented below.

Essential Diagnostic Procedures

History

Obtaining an accurate vestibular history, though time-consuming, can bring the examiner very close to a diagnosis when properly conducted.

Seven critical questions should be directed to the vertiginous patient:

1. What is the *nature of the complaint?* The patient should describe the complaints in his or her own words; the examiner may classify these as a sensation of rotation, a sensation of swaying, a feeling of dysequilibrium, or a disturbance of consciousness.
2. What are the *temporal characteristics* of the vertiginous episodes including onset, time prior to onset, and course?
3. Are there any factors that *precipitate, exacerbate, or alleviate* complaints?
4. Are there *associated symptoms* including audiologic, neurologic, or cervical phenomena?

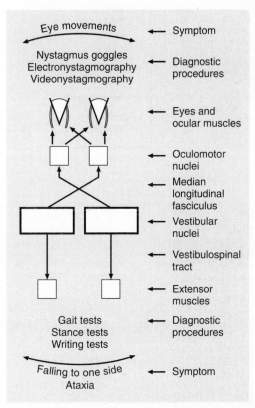

Fig. 1.**22** Efferent pathways arising from the vestibular nuclei. Symptoms and methods of examination

5. What *drugs or medication* (including caffeine, alcohol, and tobacco) has the patient used previously or at the time of the examination?
6. Is there a *history of head injury?*
7. Does the patient have any *systemic diseases* (circulatory, metabolic)?

Special Diagnostic Procedures

Vestibular and oculomotor disorders elicit eye movements such as nystagmus, and/or they can produce other effects via the vestibulospinal tract such as nondirectional ataxia or a tendency to fall to one side (Fig. 1.**22**). Eye

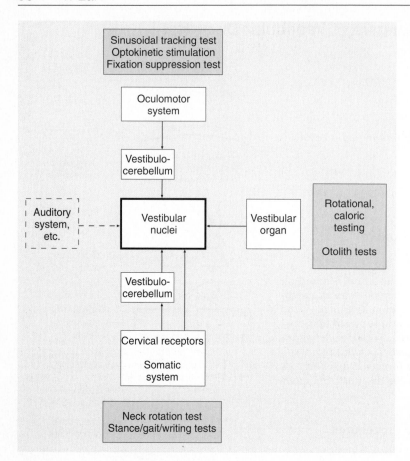

Fig. 1.**23** Afferent pathways to the vestibular nuclei and methods for their examination

movements are examined using Frenzel goggles, electronystagmography (ENG, or a videooculography (VOG). Gait, stance, and drawing tests are used to test the vestibulospinal system. In the following, those procedures available for examining the various afferent systems responsible for the maintenance of equilibrium will be described briefly.

Peripheral Vestibular Organs

Semicircular Canals:

○ *Caloric testing* involves the separate thermal stimulation of the vestibular labyrinths with water at 44° and 30 °C. This test yields an *absolute measure* of the responsiveness of each labyrinth and a *differential* measure between the right and left labyrinths.

○ *Rotating and pendular chair tests* provide a natural stimulation to both labyrinths. It is used to identify central vestibular disorders and assess the capacity for *central compensation* of a peripheral defect.

Otolith Organs

In the absence of external visual cues, the patient utilizes the afferent information from his or her otolith organs to adjust a straight luminous line to be parallel to the earth vertical.

○ Test of the *subjective vertical*.

○ *Test of circular vection:* These test methods are not yet standardized, and their clinical value has not been adequately established.

○ Caloric testing (as described above) also elicits a tonic torsional eye movement compo-

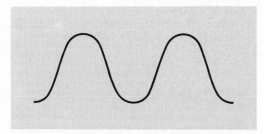

Fig. 1.**24a** Smooth pursuit of eyes tracking a swinging pendulum

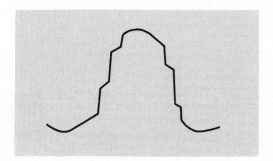

Fig. 1.**24b** Disruption of smooth pursuit by saccades due to vestibulocerebellar dysfunction

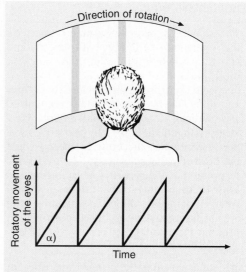

Fig. 1.**25** Experimental induction of optokinetic nystagmus. A striped drum rotating in a clockwise direction evokes a tracking movement of the eyes (slow phase of nystagmus) whose velocity depends on the rotational speed of the drum. The tracking movement is interrupted by a rapid corrective return movement (fast phase of nystagmus)

nent originating from the utricles. This component can be evaluated by videooculography.

Oculomotor System

○ *Slow voluntary pursuit system:* This can be examined easily by means of the performed *sinusoidal tracking test*. Normal ocular pursuit traces a smooth sinusoidal curve up to target speeds of 40°/s (Fig. 1.**24a**). At higher speeds, or if central vestibular dysfunction is present, saccades are observed (Fig. 1.**24b**).

○ *Optokinetic response system:* This system is best tested by using a visual surround stripes or a similar pattern that stimulates the full retinal field. Normal response to such optokinetic stimulation resembles a regular sawtooth pattern (i. e., optokinetic nystagmus see Fig. 1.**25**). In a pathologic response, the pattern shows irregular disruptions or nystagmus fatigue.

○ *Dominance of the visual system over the vestibular system:* A healthy subject is able to suppress vestibular nystagmus by visual fixation. The *fixation suppression test* assesses the degree to which an individual can suppress an experimentally induced nystagmus (Fig. 1.**26**).

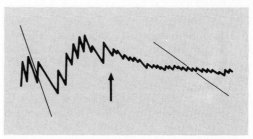

Fig. 1.**26** Fixation suppression: tests the ability to suppress an experimentally induced nystagmus. In this case the calorically evoked nystagmus is not adequately suppressed by visual fixation (starting at ↑)

Somatic System

o The somatic system has a major effect on the regulation of balance, both directly and via the vestibulocerebellum. At present there is no accurate, standardized method of evaluation, although *cervical nystagmus* and *arthrokinetic nystagmus* are recognized as somatically evoked eye movements. Cervical nystagmus is tested by the *neck rotation test* in which the body is rotated while the head remains stationary. The nystagmic response must be recorded both during and after rotation, and special attention should be given to the 30-s period in which the head is held stationary in the flexed position. At present, the examination is poorly standardized.

o The afferent somatic system and efferent vestibulospinal system are tested by *stance, gait, and drawing tests.* It should be noted that a peripheral disorder of the somatic system alters or reduces the transmission of afferent signals to the vestibular nuclei, whereas central vestibular disorders may not only alter signals arriving from the somatic system but also cause deterioration of the efferent signals to the extensor muscles. Since the pathways of the somatic system and the efferent vestibulospinal system have a fairly strictly lateralized arrangement, a *unilateral* disturbance (such as a unilateral loss of peripheral vestibular function) will produce a tendency to fall *toward the side of the lesion. Bilateral* peripheral disorders and most *central* disorders, on the other hand, are manifested by a *nondirected* falling tendency (ataxia).

  – *The Romberg test:*

    Technique: The patient stands with the feet close together, the ankles slightly apart. The arms hang to the side or are stretched forward. The eyes are closed.

    Test for feigning: The examiner traces a large number on the patient's back with his finger and asks the patient to name the number. This distraction tends to decrease sway in malingerers but increase it when true disease is present. In doubtful cases seek neurologic consultation!

    Normal limits cannot be specified reliably in the Romberg test.

  – *The Unterberger test:*

    Technique: With outstretched arms and blindfolded eyes, the patient is required to perform 50 paces on the spot. During each step, the thigh should be raised to the horizontal.

    Test for feigning: When the test is repeated several times with force platform, photo-optic or video recording feigning is easily recognized, as simulated pathology will not reproduce a similar pattern.

    Normal limits: 40° of rotation to the left, 60° of rotation to the right, and up to 1 m of forward deviation. The Unterberger stepping test can be observed directly, or it may be recorded photographically or by video camera for a more objective evaluation.

  – *Blindfold walking, tandem walking, and star-pattern walking* (backward and forward with eyes closed, Weil's test) offer no clinical improvements over the studies cited above.

  – *Symbol drawing test of Fukuda or Stoll:* Studies the effect of the vestibular system on the shoulder and arm musculature.

    Technique: The patient draws or prints symbols or letters in vertical columns. A normal subject can draw five columns of ten crosses from top to bottom without difficulty. The test is performed successively with eyes open and closed.

    Interpretation: Significant distortion of the symbols or lateral deviation of the vertical columns with eyes closed signifies the presence of disease.

    Normal limits: See W. Stoll et al. (1986).

Symptom   Vertigo

Vertigo refers to an altered or disturbed perception of the spatial environment by the patient (sensation of rotation, swaying, or floating). Vertigo may occur physiologically as a response to movements of the individual and of the environment or both. Pathologic vertigo results from disease of the peripheral or central vestibular systems, or the systems to which they are connected, predominantly the oculomotor and somatic systems. The various forms of vertigo are reviewed in Table 1.**49**).

Physiologic Vertigo

Vertigo is caused physiologically by the adequate stimulation of one or more sensor organs that connect directly or indirectly to the brain stem vestibular nuclei in the brain stem. This leads not only to a natural perception of the experienced or observed movement, due to the extensive connections within the central vestibular system, misinterpretation can also lead to morbid sensations (motion-induced vertigo, kinetosis, height vertigo) (Table 1.**50**).

Motion-induced Vertigo

Sensation of Motion
Perceived **During** a Movement

Definition: This involves a discrepancy between the sensation of movement and the actual movement. This type of sensation is of critical importance in aviation medicine, as it can induce a pilot to perform erroneous adjustment to his flight path according to his apparent motion perception.

Examples:
1. Linear acceleration in the horizontal plane stimulates the otolith receptors creating an illusion of reactive body tilt. Thus, a passenger sitting in an aircraft accelerating along the runway has the illusion that the plane is climbing (Fig. 1.**27**), while a passenger in a decelerating aircraft has the illusion of descending. Similarly, a person seated on a linear sled, which is being accelerated back and forth along the fronto-occipital

Table 1.**49** *Symptom* Vertigo

Synopsis
Physiologic vertigo
o Motion-induced vertigo
o Kinetosis
o Height vertigo
Pathologic vertigo
o Persistent vertigo
– Rotational vertigo
– Translational vertigo
– Dysequilibrium
– Phobic vertigo
o Episodic (paroxysmal) vertigo
– With auditory symptoms
– Without auditory symptoms
o Vertigo relating to movements and body positions
– Positional vertigo
– Postural vertigo
– Head-position-dependent vertigo

Table 1.**50** Physiologic vertigo

Synopsis
Motion-induced vertigo
– Sensation of motion during movement
– Sensation of motion after movement
Kinetosis
Height vertigo

axis, he will experience the illusion of moving backward and forward over a hillcrest (hilltop illusion).
2. Aircraft passengers notice a slow, sustained bank (e.g., to the right) only at the beginning (i.e. angular acceleration to the right) and end of the banking maneuver (i.e., acceleration to the left). This is because the semicircular canals can perceive only changes in angular velocity, i.e., acceleration. Without any visual cues, then, the passenger will perceive a long bank maneuver as two short rolls in opposite directions (Fig. 1.**28**).

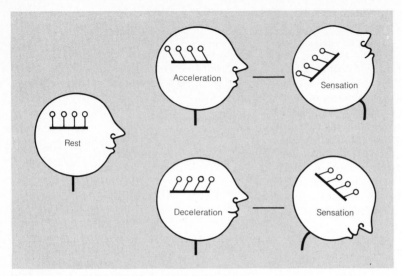

Fig. 1.**27**   Illusions induced by linear motion. Acceleration along a horizontal path creates the sensation of a backward head tilt (sensation of ascending flight in an airplane). Deceleration creates the sensation of a forward head tilt (sensation of descending flight in an airplane)

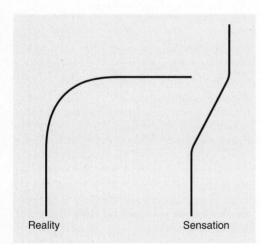

Reality   Sensation

Fig. 1.**28**   Spurious sensations induced by motion along a curved path. The vestibular organ responds only to angular acceleration. Movement on a gradually curving path, as during a banking maneuver in an airplane, is perceived only at the beginning and end points of the maneuver. Due to the opposite directions of acceleration at the onset and offset of the maneuver, the perceived path of motion differs from the actual path

3. Watching a moving visual stimulus for 10–20 s will cause the observer to experience an illusion of self motion, as illustrated by watching a flowing river from a bridge or watching a video presentation on a surround movie screen.

Sensation of Motion Perceived **After** a Movement

The components of the vestibular system have mechanical and neurophysiologic poststimulatory effects that may be evoked by natural as well as excessive or unphysiologic stimuli.

Examples:

1. *Turning sensation persisting after body rotation* (e.g., dancing a waltz). This is a mechanical phenomenon caused by the sudden cessation of body rotation, the endolymph in the semicircular canal continuing to move by its own inertia and pressing upon the cupula. The persistence of the aftersensation depends on the rate of rotation (e.g., up to 40 s after stopping from rotation at 90°/s). The sensation persists longer than the accompanying postrotatory nystagmus. Both

last longer than the eliciting cupula deflection because of an additional capacitor-like storage effect in the vestibular nuclei that undergoes a gradual, exponential decay (velocity storage mechanism).

2. *Turning sensation after watching a moving image:* This visually evoked aftersensation depends on the speed of the moving image and the stimulated area of the peripheral retina. Unlike the turning sensation following actual rotation of the observer, this lasts only a few seconds. The sensation is accompanied by optokinetic after nystagmus.

Kinetosis

Definition: Kinetosis refers to the various symptoms induced by excessive stimulation of a sensory receptor or by the simultaneous stimulation of more than one sensory receptor, and that produces conflicting signals (sensory conflict). The common terms "motion sickness" and "travel sickness" are misnomers because they refer not to a disease but a physiologic phenomenon.

Main symptoms: Kinetosis is marked by characteristic symptoms arising in a characteristic sequence (Table 1.51). Susceptibility to kinetosis varies widely among individuals and may increase or diminish with aging. The fact that it generally tends to increase with age has not been explained, although psychogenic factors play a significant role.

Many astronauts, after entering the weightlessness of space or returning to earth, experience an adaptation syndrome whose symptoms are very similar to those of kinetosis (Space Adaptation Syndrome, SAS). This is attributed to the adaptive modification that necessarily occurs after the loss of consistent otolithic stimulation by gravity. The asymmetry possible in the otolithic mass between the right and left labyrinths has also been proposed as a possible etiology. To date, it has not been proved that it is possible to predict the occurrence of an adaptation syndrome or kinetosis. Besides the *natural* variability of individual sensitivity to complex motions, there are individuals who have a *pathologic* sensitivity to mechanically induced body movements or moving images leading to an excessively rapid onset and progression of kinetosis. Psychic factors and, less

Table 1.**51** Symptoms of kinetosis (in order of occurrence)

Pallor
Fatigue (yawning)
Gastric fullness
Sweating
Nausea
Vomiting

commonly, traumatic or toxic (hallucinogenic) causes are to be considered.

Examples of sensory conflicts leading to kinetosis:

○ A passenger reading a newspaper in a moving car. The visual system signals a more or less stationary image while the vestibular system senses motion on curves and during acceleration or deceleration.

○ Rapid head movements during aircraft maneuvers. The visual system signals a stationary environment (airplane cabin) while the vestibular system senses the aircraft acceleration and the head movements.

Height Vertigo

Definition: Increased swaying and unsteadiness while standing on a precipice.

Physiologic mechanism: The visual system, particularly those components involved in spatial perception, plays a critical role in postural regulation. Loss of visual information (e.g., by closing the eyes) leads to increased body sway. Objects in the foreground of the visual field are assigned greater static importance than objects in the background. To the observer standing on an exposed precipice such as a mountain peak or tower, the foreground is absent, and an increased swaying tendency is experienced. While this effect occurs in *all* human beings, the psychological response is extremely variable and ranges from anxiety to extreme boldness.

Pathologic Vertigo

Any change in our vestibular and visual perception of the environment that does not arise from a body movement or movement of the environment is classified as pathologic vertigo. It is based on a disturbance involving the vestibular labyrinths and/or their central connections.

Persistent Vertigo

Definition: Vertigo with a slow or rapid onset that persists for several days or longer.

A useful criterion for differential diagnosis is whether the vertigo is directed or nondirected. Directed or *systematized* vertigo occurs when a malfunctioning peripheral organ delivers erroneous information to the CNS (like a faulty compass causing the ship's navigator to sail in circles). Systematized vertigo includes complaints involving sensations of rotation (semicircular canal dysfunction) and sensations of linear displacement (otolith dysfunction). It should be noted that systematized vertigo is often present only at the onset of disease. Later the pattern often becomes confused due to central compensatory processes. *Nonsystematized* vertigo is a common feature of disorders involving the central vestibular system, where all the afferent signals are processed. It includes disequilibrium and general disorientation.

Note: The classification of vertigo as directed or nondirected is useful only as a general guideline, as any number of transitional forms may occur.

Rotational Vertigo

Definition: A sensation that either the patient or his environment is rotating.

Main symptoms: Rotational vertigo in the horizontal plane is always associated with a horizontal spontaneous nystagmus. As the eyes rotate, the image of the environment drifts across the retina, producing a spinning sensation in which the patient feels that he is in motion or that objects are moving around him.

Causes: The cause of rotational vertigo is a continual imbalance of vestibular tone in the vestibular nuclei, similar to that which occurs when the body is actually rotated. Its usual cause is an *acute unilateral disease of the vestibular organ or of cranial nerve VIII.* There is an associated decrease (or occasionally increase) in the discharge rate in the afferent fibers of the vestibular nerve. If the change occurs rapidly or is pronounced, the rotational vertigo can subjectively be dramatic. Such an imbalance of vestibular tone may also occur with unilateral disease of the vestibular nuclei.

Acute Unilateral Vestibular Dysfunction

This has a variety of potential causes, which can be grouped according to broad differential diagnostic criteria (Table 1.**52**). Often, as in "idiopathic" sudden hearing loss or idiopathic facial paralysis, a specific disease cannot be found as the cause of the unilateral vestibular dysfunction. This has led to the use of the descriptive term *acute unilateral vestibular dysfunction.* Terms such as "vestibular neuronitis" or "vestibular neuropathy" are more limiting and therefore unsatisfactory.

The patient is very distressed because he or she cannot localize the focus of the disease unless associated auditory symptoms are present.

The course of acute unilateral vestibular dysfunction is so characteristic that the history often suffices for a diagnosis. The *initial stage* is marked by a spontaneous nystagmus toward the unaffected side, accompanied by a tendency to fall toward the side of the lesion. If *recovery* occurs, the nystagmus reverses its direction and beats toward the affected side. If the *dysfunction persists,* the spontaneous nystagmus is decreased by central compensation (Fig. 1.**29**). Residual symptoms such as head-shaking nystagmus may persist, depending on the degree of the dysfunction. Compensation can be hastened by vestibular training. It is hampered by a concomitant central vestibular or cervical disturbance, by bed rest, and by pharmacologic sedation.

Diseases that Can Cause Acute Unilateral Vestibular Dysfunction:

Inflammatory Processes

● **Viral Infections**

All neurotropic viruses are capable of causing vestibular dysfunction. Identification of the causative organism is rarely possible. Besides the viral diseases that incite a general polyneuritis, meningitis, or meningoencephalitis, there are viral infections that are readily classified on the basis of symptomatology:

○ *Zoster oticus*

   Main symptoms: Herpetiform eruptions on the auricle and in the external auditory canal, combined with multiple cranial neuropathies (V, VII, VIII) and otalgia (see pp. 4, 65).

   Cause: Infection with viruses from the herpes−varicella group.

○ *Influenzal otitis*

   Main symptoms: Severe to excruciating otalgia; blood blisters in the external auditory canal; hemorrhagic serotympanon: hearing impairment (see p. 10). Vestibular involvement is less common than cochlear involvement.

   Cause: Infection with type A, B, or C influenza virus.

● **Viral infections** that rarely affect the vestibular organ:

○ *Measles*

   Main symptoms: Typical exanthema, rhinitis, conjunctivitis. With neurogenic exacerbation, measles encephalitis becomes predominant. The vestibular system is affected in the setting of medullary involvement (see pp. 11, 66).

○ *Mumps*

   Main symptoms: Swelling of the parotid gland. Involvement of cranial nerve VIII usually leads to irreversible deafness from cochlear nerve damage (see pp. 65, 300). The pathogenesis of unilateral cochleovestibular dysfunction on the unaffected side remains unexplained.

○ *Tick-borne encephalitis*

− Spring−summer meningoencephalitis.

Main symptoms: Severe meningoencephalitis with multiple deficits.

Cause: Viral infection transmitted by the bite of the tick *Ixodes ricinus*.

Requires differentiation from spirochetal disease transmitted by the same tick:

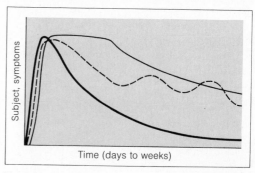

Fig. 1.**29**   Time course of the compensation of unilateral vestibular dysfuntion

▬▬▬▬	Normal course
− − − −	Delayed course due to central vestibular dysfunction
▬▬▬▬	Delayed course due to excessive bed rest at the start of the disease

Table 1.**52**   Causes of unilateral vestibular dysfunction

Synopsis
Inflammatory processes, see p. 104
Deficient blood flow, see p. 106
Traumatic disorders, see p. 107
Toxic disorders, see p. 107
Functional reduction of vestibular response, see p. 107
Neoplastic and destructive processes, see p. 108
Autoimmune disease, see p. 108
Brain stem lesions, see p. 108

− Lyme disease (erythema migrans).

Main symptoms: Erythema spreading outward from the area of the tick bite, with severe radicular pain and cranial nerve deficits (often affecting cranial nerve VII).

Cause: Infection with *Borrelia burgdorferi*, transmitted by the ubiquitous, contaminated *Ixodes* tick.

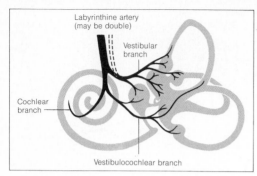

Fig. 1.**30**   Arterial blood supply of the inner ear

● **Bacterial Infections**

Bacterial Access to the Vestibular Organ:

○ Spread of infection *medially* from acute or chronic otitis media, e.g., via the bacterial colonization of a cholesteatoma (*Pseudomonas*), to produce a secondary labyrinthitis.

○ Spread of infection *laterally* from meningitis or meningoencephalitis. Cranial nerve VIII is affected primarily, but labyrinthitis can develop secondarily by the spread of infection through the internal acoustic meatus.

Main symptoms: Vertigo of more or less acute onset, initially with the signs of labyrinthitis (nystagmus toward the side of the inflammatory process) but with very rapid progression to labyrinthine failure (nystagmus toward the opposite side). The cochlea and, in cases of meningitis, the cochlear nerve are always affected.

Differentiation is required from a labyrinthine fistula caused by a destructive otologic process. The vertigo is of variable intensity and may occur episodically. There is fluctuating hearing loss. Labyrinthine fistula is readily distinguished from bacterial labyrinthitis by the fistula sign (Politzer balloon in the case of a tympanic membrane defect, Valsalva−Toynbee maneuver in the case of an intact membrane).

Deficient Blood Flow

Main symptoms: The labyrinthine artery is an endartery, and its occlusion produces an area of infarction whose size and associated symptoms depend on the site of the occlusion (Fig. 1.**30**).

○ Occlusion proximal to the origins of the anterior vestibular, vestibulocochlear, and cochlear arteries: Complete labyrinthine failure with deafness and paretic nystagmus toward the unaffected side. The prognosis is poor.

○ Occlusion of the anterior vestibular artery: Loss of the vestibular organ (with the exception of the macula sacculi, which is supplied by the vestibulocochlear artery) with paretic nystagmus toward the unaffected side and falling toward the affected side.

○ Occlusion of the cochlear artery: Sudden hearing loss due to loss of the cochlea excluding portions of the basal cochlear turn (low- to mid-frequencies).

○ Occlusion of the vestibulocochlear artery: Acute high-frequency hearing loss, occasionally combined with disequilibrium or a sensation of linear displacement and with vertical nystagmus due to loss of the macula sacculi.

○ The occlusion of more central arteries (e.g., the anterior or posterior inferior cerebellar artery) leads to multiple cranial nerve deficits, as in:

● *Wallenberg Syndrome*

Facial sensory disturbances; Horner syndrome; horizontal or sometimes torsional nystagmus away from the lesion with eyes open and toward the lesion with eyes closed. Involvement of caudal cranial nerves. Cause: Occlusion of the posterior inferior cerebellar artery.

Causes: Arteriosclerotic disease. Cardiac arrhythmias. Sludging of red blood cells, especially with primary and secondary polycythemia (elevated hematocrit, leukocytosis, thrombocytosis). Stress-induced vasospasm has also been postulated.

Differentiation is required from vertebrobasilar insufficiency in older people. The vertiginous symptoms are paroxysmal and are combined with drop attacks and other cranial nerve signs, especially visual disturbances.

Traumatic Disorders

Traumatic lesions of the peripheral vestibular system are easily diagnosed owing to the obvious correlation of the trauma history with a very characteristic set of symptoms (exception: cervical balance disturbances).

● **Transverse temporal bone fracture**
Main symptoms: Complete loss of vestibular function with nystagmus toward the opposite ear, falling to the affected side, deafness, and hematotympanon. Certain fracture patterns cause facial paralysis (see p. 39 ff.).

Differentiation is required from a longitudinal fracture, which is occasionally accompanied by vertigo due to cerebral concussion but is *not* accompanied by vestibular failure.

● **Labyrinthine concussion**
Main symptoms: Loss of vestibular and acoustic function on the side affected by a blunt head injury with no apparent fracture. There is no clear dividing line from a transverse fracture, since many temporal bone fractures, though present, are not manifest on radiographs (see p. 39 ff.).

Differentiation is required from cupulolithiasis. Benign paroxysmal positional vertigo (BPPV) is a common sequel to trauma in the ear region. It is attributed to the detachment of otoconia from the macula utriculi and their subsequent attachment to structures of the posterior semicircular canal (see p. 116).

● **Iatrogenic injury** of the vestibular organ or nerve during surgery on the ear or cerebellopontine angle.

● **Blast trauma:** Mechanical injury of the middle and inner ear combined with signs of labyrinthine failure (loss of vestibular and cochlear nerve) or with vertigo induced by loud noise (Tullio phenomenon, see p. 113). Special form: window rupture.

● **Acute noise trauma:** Chronic noise trauma is not associated with vestibular damage. Vertigo may occur with acute noise trauma but is nonspecific and reversible. It may result from an otolithic lesion. Tullio phenomenon is occasionally observed (see p. 113). Videooculography and the unilateral otolith tests (see p. 98) should improve the diagnosis of such peripheral vestibular disorders.

Toxic Balance Disturbances

● Due to **toxic breakdown products from bacteria or viruses** in the setting of otitis media.

● Due to **ototoxic drugs:** Ototoxic drugs damage both the vestibular organ and the organ of Corti to different degrees (see p. 67). The vestibular organ is affected mainly by streptomycin, gentamicin, sisomycin, netilmycin, and furosemide (Federspiel 1984). The main effects of ototoxic agents on the acoustic organ are summarized in Tables 1.**27**–1.**30**).

Main symptoms: *Unilateral* vestibular and cochlear dysfunction with nystagmus toward the unaffected side and rotational vertigo in patients receiving *local* treatment for Ménière disease or anti-inflammatory treatment with otic drops containing neomycin or gentamicin.

Parenteral ototoxic therapy leads to *bilateral* vestibulocochlear dysfunction. Rotational vertigo is absent because the symmetric influence does not produce a right–left disparity of vestibular tone in the vestibular nuclei. There is marked nondirectional ataxia, especially on standing with eyes closed and walking in the dark. Oscillopsia is common (up-and-down movement of the environment during gait).

Reduction of Vestibular Response due to Cervical Disfunction

It is likely that a disorder of the cervical afferents can produce a functional imbalance of vestibular tone in the vestibular nuclei accompanied by nystagmus and a diminished caloric response. There are several neurophysiologic mechanisms by which such an effect could be produced:
– Inhibition of activity in the lateral vestibular nucleus by the Purkinje cells of the cerebellum. These cells are activated by the sensory cervical afferents via mossy and climbing fibers.

– A modulation of signal weighting in the vestibular nuclei.
– A change in peripheral vestibular sensitivity through activation or inhibition of the efferent vestibular pathway.

Main symptoms: Fluctuating vertigo or episodic vertigo (see p. 113) of several seconds' duration, combined with restricted craniovertebral joint motion and foci of myegelosis in the short and long extensor muscles of the neck. Certain head movements (e. g., while hanging drapes) can precipitate such a vertigionous attack. Globus sensation, circumferential headache, nonspecific ocular symptoms, and pseudoparanasal sinus complaints are not uncommon.

Causes: Craniovertebral joint dysfunction, whiplash injury, postural defects.

Differentiation is required from vertebrobasilar insufficiency in older patients (see p. 113) and organic disease at the occipitocervical junction. Generally these disorders are likewise associated with vertigo induced by head movements.

Neoplasms

● **Acoustic neuroma**
Main symptoms: Acoustic neuroma generally causes a unilateral function deficit with little or no subjective vestibular symptoms. There is a unilateral, slowly progressive hearing loss combined with retrocochlear symptoms. With a rapidly enlarging tumor, there may be acute dysfunction of the vestibular apparatus or hearing organ (e.g., sudden hearing loss) due to intratumoral hemorrhage, compression of the labyrinthine artery, etc.

Other symptoms and special features: See pp. 29, 110 and 117.

● **Cholesteatoma**
Main symptoms: Slowly progressive suppuration, typical of cholesteatoma, leads to a gradual loss of cochlear and vestibular function. The extent of vestibular damage is generally equivalent to that manifested by sensorineural hearing loss. Accurate testing is not possible because bone destruction in the middle ear space precludes caloric stimulation with bilateral comparison of responses. Dysfunction

can occur *acutely* if a labyrinthine fistula develops (see pp. 24, 113, 117).

● **Glomus tumor**
Main symptoms: Pulsatile tinnitus. With erosion of the labyrinthine capsule, signs of cochlear *and* vestibular dysfunction appear. See also p. 29.

Differentiation is required from cervical disorders. Pulsatile tinnitus can result from the unilateral compression of nuchal arteries by areas of myogelosis. Functional cervical defects also can lead to vertigo. The otalgia and posterior neck pain that accompany the pulsatile tinnitus in cervical disorders serve to distinguish the cervical syndrome from a glomus tumor.

● **Carcinoma of the external auditory canal and middle ear**
Main symptoms: Fetid discharge from the ear canal, sequestrum formation, vertigo, and cochlear hearing loss due to erosion of the labyrinthine capsule.

Differentiation is required from cholesteatoma.

Autoimmune Diseases

The existence of vertigo brought on by autoimmune disease of the vestibular organ is likely but has not yet been definitely proved. Audiologic symptoms, with a progressive deterioration of hearing (stepwise reduction), are predominant (see p. 78).

Inflammatory Brain Stem Lesions

Main symptoms: As far as symptoms are concerned, it does not matter whether the damage occurs to the vestibular organ, the vestibular nerve, or to the brain stem at the nerve entry site. In all cases the lesion interrupts the flow of afferent signals to the vestibular nuclei, producing symptoms like those of a unilateral acute lesion of the vestibular organ with rotational vertigo and nystagmus toward the opposite side.

Causes: Localized foci of multiple sclerosis, tertiary syphilis, or residua of meningoencephalitis. Local ischemia can also produce such symptoms, which then are usually combined with other cranial nerve signs. This type of balance disturbance has been described as a primary manifestation of AIDS.

Differentiation is mainly required from other central disturbances associated with central vestibular symptoms rather than the signs of a unilateral vestibular lesion (disequilibrium, ataxia, etc.).

Translational Vertigo

Definition: Feeling of linear displacement (e.g., lift) floating or "walking on foam rubber." So far there is no single disease entity that has been associated with this symptom.

Cause: The symptom is probably based on a functional abnormality of the otolith organs.

Diagnosis: Newer techniques designed for the clinical evaluation of the otolith organs are not yet routinely employed, though developments are under way. Clinical examination may reveal a vertical nystagmus, but often this is obscured by blinking and may be missed by ENG. It is important to test upward and downward gaze during examination with the Frenzel goggles, as this will accentuate spontaneous nystagmus.

Differentiation is required from the "walking on foam rubber" sensation due to a bilateral peripheral sensory disturbance, as in polyneuritis.

Disequilibrium

Disequilibrium is the hallmark of central vestibular pathology. This is reasonable when we consider the extensive connections that link the vestibular nuclei with other basal portions of the brain. Moreover, the four vestibular nuclei on each side not only function as relay stations for the afferent signals from the vestibular end organs, oculomotor system, and somatic system to the main effectors (ocular and extensor muscles) but also possess integrating mechanisms in which the sensory information is weighted, stored, and coordinated.

Another characteristic of central vestibular dysfunction is the observation that complaints are often milder than would be expected on the basis of the observed nystagmus.

Table 1.**53**   Disequilibrium

Synopsis
Dysequilibrium in central disorders combined with
– Positional nystagmus
– Downbeating nystagmus, reduced vestibular response, and oculomotor dysfunction
– Dissociated gaze-induced nystagmus
– Unilateral labyrinthine failure and oculomotor dysfunction
– Other cranial nerve deficits
– Ocular tilt reaction
– Upbeating nystagmus, downbeating nystagmus
Dysequilibrium in peripheral disorders
– With unilateral peripheral defect
– With bilateral peripheral defect
– With an otolith lesion

The following symptoms associated with central vestibular disorders help to establish the site of the lesion (Table 1.**53**). It should be noted, however, that disequilibrium can occur in some cases of peripheral vestibular dysfunction, particularly in bilateral disorders and in the later stages of a unilateral disfunction.

Disequilibrium in Central Vestibular Disorders

Central disorders can produce symptoms that are characteristic of the location of the pathologic process. Such symptoms, and particularly combinations thereof, usually permit a *site-of-lesion determination* even if they do not furnish a diagnosis. Below is a listing of symptoms that are useful for identifying the site of the lesion and perhaps for making a diagnosis.

● **Disequilibrium combined with nonfatiguing convergent or divergent positional nystagmus**

○ **Disturbance of the vestibular nuclei near the midline. Diseases: multiple sclerosis, syringobulbia, tumors of the fourth ventricle.**

○ **Disturbances of the vestibulocerebellum near the midline, especially involving the inferior vermis and nodulus.**

○ **Toxic effects:**

Main symptoms: Narcotics, alcohol, and nicotine cause a disequilibrium, which is associated with a characteristic positional nystagmus, especially when narcotics or alcohol are used (see p. 117).

Causes: Positional alcohol nystagmus occurs when the lower specific gravity of alcohol ("light water") temporarily modifies the labyrinthine receptors, normally specialized for angular velocity, to function as gravity sensors.

● **Disequilibrium combined with occipital signs of increasing intracranial pressure**

Disease: Cerebellar abscess.

Main symptoms: A cerebellar abscess leads to rapidly progressive symptoms of rising pressure in the posterior cranial fossa including headache, meningism, altered head posture, disturbance of consciousness, and other brain stem and pontine signs such as vertical nystagmus (see also pp. 46, 129).

● **Disequilibrium combined with downbeating nystagmus, vestibular hypoexcitability, and impairments to ocular pursuit, optokinetic nystagmus, and fixation suppression**

Site of lesion: The vestibulocerebellum, especially the flocculus. A critical relay site in the vestibular system, the flocculus gathers information from the oculomotor system, the labyrinths, and cervical afferent fibers. Damage to the flocculus leads to the very characteristic set of findings noted above.

Causes: Vascular, inflammatory, and space-demanding lesions, atrophic lesions of the cerebellum.

Differentiation is required from Arnold–Chiari syndrome and from congenital disorders with vertical nystagmus, fixation nystagmus, and oculomotor dysfunction.

● **Disequilibrium combined with dissociated gaze-induced nystagmus** (see p. 128)

Disease: Multiple sclerosis.

Main symptoms: Intermittent, episodic course marked by remissions and exacerbations of neurologic complaints. Symptoms vary greatly according to the location of the pathologic foci and may coincide with one another or appear at separate times. It is typical for visual symptoms and disequilibrium to coincide with paresthesias. The incidence in females is about twice that in males, and peak age of onset is 20–40 years.

Causes: Foci of demyelination occurring mainly in the CNS. Numerous etiologies have been suggested ranging from overnutrition and undernutrition to metabolic disorders to the "slow virus" theory.

Differentiation is required from joint and muscle disorders in the area of the craniocervical junction. These may produce similar sets of symptoms, such as disequilibrium combined with temporal sensory abnormalities and visual defects. Differentiating signs include:

○ *Pain,* which is not a feature of multiple sclerosis.

○ *Fleeting symptoms in remote areas* (e.g., micturition difficulties), which do not occur with cervical dysfunction.

Basic rule of thumb: Suspect multiple sclerosis in patients with disequilibrium of changing intensity and sensory abnormalities.

● **Disequilibrium combined with progressive unilateral hearing deficit, unilateral vestibular failure, and oculomotor dysfunction**

Disease: Large acoustic neuroma compressing the brain stem.

Main symptoms: Slowly progressively, unilateral, retrocochlear sensorineural hearing loss with a slowly increasing, unilateral loss of vestibular function, which is *not* noticed because of ongoing compensation. Large and moderately large tumors may lead to a positional nystagmus whose amplitude is greater on the affected side than on the healthy side when the patient is lying down (Bruhn nystagmus). Smaller tumors also may cause a positional nystagmus that lacks the features of Bruhn nystagmus. Very large tumors that compress the brain stem additionally lead to oculomotor dysfunction. Also the lateral disparity of vestibular response decompensates, and disequilibrium appears or increases.

Diagnosis: Contrast-enhanced MRI.

Differentiation from other types of central vestibular dysfunction is based on the combination of retrocochlear impairment, positional nystagmus, lateral discrepancy of caloric response, and demonstrable expansion of the internal auditory canal.

● **Disequilibrium combined with other cranial nerve lesions (e.g., IX, X)**

Diseases: Disturbances of the lateral medulla oblongata, such as the Wallenberg syndrome (see Table 10.**16**), due to vascular disease. Localized foci of disseminated encephalitis.

● **Disequilibrium combined with an ocular tilt reaction**

Site of lesion: Tegmentum of midbrain.

● **Disequilibrium combined with upbeating nystagmus**

Site of lesion: Pontomedullary or pontomesencephalic tegmentum.

● **Disequilibrium combined with downbeating nystagmus**

Site of lesion: Floor of fourth ventricle or bilateral sites in the flocculus.

Disequilibrium in Peripheral Vestibular Disorders

Disequilibrium is not a prominent symptom of peripheral vestibular defects, although it may be caused by peripheral dysfunction in special cases or as a transitional symptom.

● **Disequilibrium in the late stage of an acute unilateral labyrinthine defect** (see p. 104, 109)

As compensation progresses, the initially directional (rotational) vertigo is superseded by an unsteady vertigo. The symptoms of a benign paroxysmal positional vertigo also may occur in this transitional stage.

● **Disequilibrium in the late stage of Ménière disease:** Multiple attacks of hydropic fluctuations in the inner ear lead to an irreversible change in function. The typical attacks of rotational vertigo subside and are replaced by permanent disequilibrium.

● **Disequilibrium as a sequel to a bilateral labyrinthine defect**

Diseases: Bilateral transverse temporal bone fractures. Labyrinthine failure due to drug ototoxicity.

Special case: Recklinghausen neurofibromatosis.

Main symptoms: Multiple neurofibromas of the peripheral nerve (progressive peripheral palsies), of the nerve root (radicular deficits), or involving the spinal canal (cord compression to complete lesion) or intracranial space, especially the vestibular nerve and optic nerve. Typical cutaneous signs appear in the form of extensive pigmentary anomalies (café-au-lait spots) and multiple dermal neurofibromas.

Involvement of the vestibular nerve in the internal auditory canal is marked by unilateral and bilateral, slowly progressive retrocochlear hearing losses and a reduced or abolished caloric response in one or both vestibular organs. Radiologically demonstrable expansion of the internal auditory canal is often absent in cases diagnosed early. Diagnosis is most reliably established by contrast-enhanced MRI.

Causes: The disease is included in the group of phakomatoses (CNS and skin diseases). The cause is unknown.

● **Disequilibrium caused by a disfunction of the otolith organs**

Little is known about this complex due to a lack of diagnostic options. It has not been associated with circumscribed disease entities.

Phobic Vertigo

Definition: Phobic vertigo generally occurs episodically, but sustained cases may occur. The primary manifestation occurs after periods of stress or disease with associated anxiety. Constant phobic vertigo can be difficult to distinguish from organic disease (Brandt and Dieterich 1986).

Episodic Vertigo

Episodic (paroxysmal) vertigo can be more difficult to evaluate than continuous vertigo, because frequently the patient is asymptomatic between attacks. In such cases, the diagnosis must rely on the history and, if possible, on the witnessing of an attack. Documentation of the symptoms is critical due to the profound effects of paroxysmal vestibular disorders on the patient's ability to work and drive a vehicle.

Table 1.**54** *Symptom* Episodic vertigo

Synopsis

Episodic vertigo with auditory symptoms in peripheral vestibular diseases

- With hearing loss and tinnitus: Ménière disease
- After hearing loss: Lermoyez disease
- Induced by loud noise: Tullio phenomenon
- With increased middle ear pressure: fistula sign

Episodic vertigo without auditory symptoms in central and cervical diseases

- In elderly patients with drop attacks: vertebro-basilar insufficiency
- Brief episodic vertigo: cardiac rhythm disturbance, cervical vertigo
- With "blackout": failure of blood flow auto-regulation, especially orthostatic disregulation
- With accompanying seizures or lapses of consciousness: epilepsy
- With occipital headache: basilar migraine, cervical vertigo
- In small children: migraine equivalent
- Induced by fatigue or prolonged reading: strabismus and other orthoptic disturbances
- Relation to sensory stimuli and social conflict situations: phobic vertigo

The accurate classification of vertiginous attacks requires attention to the "associated symptoms," which are reviewed in Table 1.**54**.

Clinical presentations: There are a great variety of diseases that cause episodic vestibular disorders. A very well-known and well-defined entity is Ménière syndrome. It tends to be overdiagnosed, because the full range of differential diagnostic possibilities is often not properly considered. This is particularly apparent in "the Ménière symptom complex," a catch-all diagnosis for cases that are insufficiently evaluated. A meticulous search for the correct diagnosis is particularly important from the standpoint of therapeutic implications. The various diseases that may underlie episodic vertigo are presented below, with brief commentaries and differential diagnostic possibilities.

Episodic Vertigo with Auditory Symptoms in Peripheral Vestibular Diseases

Vertiginous Attack with Unilateral Hearing Loss and Tinnitus

Disease: *Ménière disease.*

Main symptoms: Frequently there is an aura or prodrome consisting of unilateral headache and increased tinnitus, followed by a sudden, severe attack of vertigo accompanied by nausea and vomiting. There is concomitant unilateral hearing loss and unilateral tinnitus. Nystagmus may initially be toward the affected ear (irritative stage), but generally there is a paretic nystagmus toward the opposite side. The affected side is identified by a characteristic low-frequency hearing loss (see p. 81) and by the location of the experienced tinnitus. Vestibular response is highly variable, and in early stages the caloric response recovers fully between attacks. The duration of the vertiginous episodes is initially short, lasting minutes to hours, but later may increase to a period of days.

Causes: Though its exact cause remains unknown, Ménière disease is generally assumed to be based on a disturbance in the osmolar balance of the endolymph and perilymph. It is very likely that impaired metabolic processes, presumably involving the calcium in the melanin-carrying dark cells of the membranes of the endolymphatic system and in the endolymphatic sac, play a critical role. It is noteworthy that the disease occurs predominantly in white people.

As the disease progresses the endolymph becomes hyperosmolar, and endolymphatic hydrops develops. With distention of the membranous labyrinth, intracellular barriers become permeable to potassium at anatomic sites of predilection such as the cochlear apex, the ampullar wall, and the vestibule, where it causes depolarization of the nerve fibers culminating in acute failure of the vestibular organ and hearing loss with tinnitus.

Differential diagnosis: Not all patients exhibit the classic triad of episodic vertigo, unilateral hearing loss, and unilateral tinnitus. And while the course may be monosymptomatic, especially in the initial stage, it should always be questioned whether some other intercurrent disease might be responsible for the nonclassic pattern of findings.

Attacks of Vertigo bold **after** Brief Hearing Loss and tinnitus

(Symptoms same as in the Ménière syndrome, but with a different temporal pattern.)

Disease: *Lermoyez disease.*

These symptoms, too, are attributed to endolymphatic hydrops, but a difference in the severity of the hydrops and/or anatomic variations presumably account for the different temporal sequence of the symptoms. Lermoyez disease is thus regarded as merely a special form of Ménière disease.

Vertigo and Unsteadiness in Response to Loud Noise

Disease: *Tullio phenomenon.*

Main symptoms: Vestibular disorder with nystagmus and falling induced by exposure to noise louder than 90 dB. In extreme cases tapping the calvarium, touching the tragal cartilage, or tympanometry is sufficient to trigger a vertiginous attack.

Causes: Abnormally elastic connection between the middle ear space and labyrinth, allowing the transmission of low frequency sound waves into the vestibular organ where they stimulate the otoliths and/or semicircular canals. Tullio phenomenon may also be based on a loose stapes, an excessively long stapes prosthesis, or a spontaneous or induced semicircular canal fistula (see below). The duration and temporal course of the vertiginous attack is correlated to that of the precipitating noise.

Vertigo Induced by Pressure on the Tragus or a Rise of Pressure in the External Auditory Canal and/or Middle Ear

Disease: *Labyrinthine fistula.*

Causes:
- Destructive lesions, which generally arise in the middle ear and erode the labyrinthine capsule, as caused by cholesteatoma, carcinoma of the ear canal or middle ear, and glomus tumor. Symptoms: Vertigo induced by pressure on the tragus, which is transmitted by the cholesteatoma or tumor mass to the semicircular canals. Vertigo is also induced by raising the pressure in the middle ear with a Politzer bag (see p. 25).
- Spontaneous window rupture. Symptoms: Partial or total hearing loss with acute onset, which later becomes fluctuating (see p. 63), accompanied by vestibular disorder.

Differential diagnosis is straightforward with destructive lesions, since the middle ear findings and history (previous stapes operation, cholesteatoma surgery) are usually conclusive. A spontaneous window rupture can be difficult to distinguish from vascular or viral labyrinthine damage, however. Using newly developed rigid and flexible endoscopes, it is possible to explore the round window niche via the tympanic membrane or eustachian tube.

Episodic Vertigo without Auditory Symptoms in Central and Cervical Diseases

Disequilibrium in Elderly Patients, Occurring with Rapid Onset at Irregular Intervals, Combined with Drop Attacks

Disease: Vertebrobasilar insufficiency.

Other symptoms and special features: Attacks of vertigo may be accompanied by typical cortical visual disturbances with local scotomata or visual hallucinations. Other features are occipital headache, diplopia, sensory abnormalities, dysarthria, etc.

Cause: Vertebrobasilar insufficiency causing a recurrent, diffuse ischemia in the brain stem region, which affects *elderly* patients and does not cause permanent damage. It is especially common in patients with unilateral hypoplasia of a vertebral artery and accompanying insufficiency (arteriosclerosis) of the posterior portion of the circle of Willis.

Differentiation is required from:
- Episodic vertigo based on a circumscribed blood flow deficiency in the brain stem, vestibular nuclei, and cerebellum. This results in transient and persistent circumscribed insults with focal deficits that permit accurate localization of the ischemic area. Constant vertigo is generally present in these cases.
- *Subclavian steal syndrome* (see p. 396): Blood flow reversal in the vertebral artery caused by an occlusive lesion of the subclavian artery or brachiocephalic trunk. Use of the ipsilateral arm precipitates vertigo and obtundation.

Brief Episodic Vertigo

Vertigo Involving Brief Unsteadiness ("Soft Feet"), Generally Lasting Only Seconds, and Possibly Associated with Tightness in the Chest

Disease: *Cardiac rhythm disturbance.*

Main symptoms: Too little attention has been given to cardiac causes of vertigo. Rhythm disturbances that commonly lead to vertigo are listed in Table 1.**55**. Interruptions of the circulation for less than 5 s do not produce symptoms. More prolonged deficits are perceived as brief vertigo, syncope, or an Adams–Stokes attack, depending on the severity of the circulatory deficit.

Paroxysmal Vertigo Occurring after Rising in the Morning, Lasting for Several Hours, and Possibly Combined with Nuchal Headache

Disease: *Myogenic or arthrogenic dysfunction involving the craniovertebral joints* (usually C0–C1, less commonly C1–C2) (see pp. 107, 393).

Brief commentary: The receptors of the nuchal region are often characterized as an accessory sensory organ of balance. They supply information to the vestibular nuclei concerning the position of the head in relation to the neck and trunk. Cervical nystagmus is mediated by direct cervical afferent pathways to the vestibular nuclei concerning the position of the head in relation to the neck and trunk. Cervical nystagmus is mediated by direct cervical afferent pathways to the vestibular nuclei as well as indirect connections via the cerebellum. Cervical nystagmus is present in infants and in approximately 50% of all persons during rotation of the neck but is not present during static torsion of the neck. A unidirectional nystagmus in the neck rotation test when the head is held in a horizontally flexed position for 30 s (static torsion) may signify cervicogenic vertigo, or it may simply represent a form of induced nystagmus. A direction-changing nystagmus in the neck rotation test is, however, pathognomonic for cervicogenic vertigo.

Other symptoms and special features: High cervical syndrome caused by myogenic and articular dysfunction can lead to vertigo as well as hearing disorders. Often there are associated radicular symptoms with pain radiating to the temporal region with ocular complaints, to the maxillary region (pseudosinugenic headache), and to the neck region (globus sensation). Sensory abnormalities can also occur in these regions.

Causes: Postural defects and position faults in the vertebral column, whiplash injury, subluxation of vertebral bodies, cervical spine pathology, and anomalies of the occipital–cervical junction.

Differentiation is required from multiple sclerosis, migraine, and vertebrobasilar insufficiency. Differentiation is difficult because presentation of the cervical syndrome, in particular with sensory disfunction, is as diverse as that of multiple sclerosis. Occipital headache is also reported in cases of basilar migraine.

Vertiginous Attacks with "Blackout" Preceded by Disequilibrium or Rotational Vertigo

Disease: *Failure of blood pressure autoregulation.*

Definition: Failure of circulatory regulation in which the blood pressure falls below 100/70 mmHg. These disorders include primary sustained hypotension, orthostatic hypotension, secondary hypotension, and vagovasal reactions.

Causes: Insufficient adaptation of the cardiac output to physical demands (e.g., standing up quickly). Not enough attention is given to drugs that can cause secondary hypotension. These are listed in Table 1.**56**.

Attacks of Disequilibrium (Vaguely Described) at Irregular Intervals with Accompanying Convulsions or Lapses of Consciousness

Disease: *Epilepsy.*

Main symptoms: The complete picture of epilepsy includes disturbances of consciousness, convulsions, and tongue biting, although mild forms can present simply as episodes of disequilibrium.

Causes: Epilepsy represents a seizure disorder of the central nervous system. Attacks may be symptomatic of numerous conditions, including trauma.

Diagnosis: The diagnosis of epilepsy is established by EEG with provocation (photostimulation, hyperventilation, sleep deprivation).

Attacks of Disequilibrium Combined with Occipital Headache

Disease: *Basilar migraine.*

Main symptoms: While classic migraine consists of headache alone, a large percentage of migraine sufferers exhibit additional symptoms that fall under the heading of "complicated migraine." Forms include *ophthalmic migraine, migraine accompagnée* with paresthesias and motor monoparesis and hemiparesis, and *basilar migraine*. The latter is characterized by vertigo, gait ataxia, dysarthria, tinnitus, and bilateral paresthesias of the hands, head, and tongue.

Causes: Vasospasm. In the case of basilar migraine, the vertebral or basilar artery is affected.

Differentiation is required from craniovertebral joint dysfunction with incipient painful symptoms in the nuchal area and masticatory region accompanied by vertiginous complaints (see p. 113).

Table 1.**55** Causes of cardiac rhythm disturbances (from W. Stoll, D.R. Matz, E. Most: Schwindel und Gleichgewichtsstörungen. Thieme, Stuttgart 1986)

Coronary heart disease
Cardiomyopathies
Myocarditis
Congenital and acquired cardiac defects
Cardiac tumors
Thoracic trauma
Cardiac pacemaker dysfunction
Autonomic dysfunction and spontaneous arrhythmias with no apparent underlying disease
Endocrinopathies
Neuromuscular and CNS diseases
Drugs and environmental agents
Electrolyte abnormalities
Accessory conduction pathways in the heart

Table 1.**56** Hypotension-inducing drugs (after Most)

Classic antihypertensive agents (reserpine, methyldopa, clonidine, etc.)
Peripheral vasodilators (nitrates, sodium nitroprusside, dihydralazine, diazoxide, prazosin, etc.)
Calcium antagonists (verapamil, diltiazem, nifedipine, etc.)
Alpha-receptor blocking drugs
Beta-receptor blocking drugs
Converting enzyme inhibitors
Diuretics
Antiarrhythmic drugs
Tranquilizers
Barbiturates
Antidepressants
Anticonvulsants
Digitalis
Fibrinolytics (streptokinase, SK plasminogen)
Miscellaneous substances
– Alcohol
– Clomethiazol
– Insulin
– Isoniazide
– Nicotinic acid
– Piperazine
– Prostaglandins (PGE$_2$)

Table 1.**57** *Symptom* Vertigo during movements or certain body positions

Synopsis
Crescendo–decrescendo vertigo induced by position changes, turning over, or rapid body movements:
Benign paroxysmal positional vertigo (cupulolithiasis)
Symmetric positional vertigo:
Toxic alcohol-induced
Central disturbance
Asymmetric positional vertigo:
Acoustic neuroma
Positional vertigo in patients with otologic disease:
Positional fistula syndrome
Head-position-dependent vertigo:
Functional cervical dysfunction
Arnold–Chiari syndrome
Lax transverse ligament of the atlas
Dens fracture
Basilar impression
Arcuate atlantal foramen

Brief Episodic Vertigo (Lasting Seconds) Experienced as Brief Unsteadiness or Jerky Movements of the Environment

Disease: *Cervical vertigo* due to myogenic or articular dysfunction of the craniovertebral joints (C0–C2).

Episodic Vertigo in Children with Accompanying Headache

Disease: *Benign paroxysmal vertigo in children* represents a migraine equivalent. "Benign paroxysmal vertigo" is an unfortunate term in pediatric usage, as it does not correspond to the benign paroxysmal positional vertigo of adults (cupulolithiasis).

Increasing Unsteadiness over the Course of the Day due to Fatigue, or Prolonged Reading, often Combined with Frontal Headache

Disease: *Latent strabismus.*

Latent and overt strabismus are given too little attention in the diagnostic evaluation of vertigo. Typically, complaints increase during the course of the day. Frontal headache is also very common. The disease is diagnosed with the cover–uncover test and prism test. Latent strabismus is often demonstrated by Frenzel goggles as well. The headache is alleviated when one eye is closed.

Brief Episodic Vertigo in Erect Gait, Combined with a Sense of Impending Doom, Brought on by Particular Sensory Stimuli or Social Situations

Disease: *Phobic vertigo* (see p. 111).

Vertigo Related to Movements or Specific Body Positions

Definition: Vertigo induced by certain body or head movements (Table 1.**57**). The complaints and their symptoms are reproducible, with the reservations noted below.

Clinical Presentations

Very Severe Spinning Sensation with a Crescendo–Decrescendo Pattern Following Rapid Body Movements, Especially after a Position Change or Turning in Bed

Disease: *Benign paroxysmal positional vertigo (cupulolithiasis).*

Main symptoms: Symptoms and complaints appear after a latent period of up to 10 s, whereupon a very severe rotatory nystagmus becomes apparent. Reversing the movement leads to a reversal of the subjective rotating sensation and nystagmus.

Although symptoms are reproducible in about 90% of cases, they quickly become less intense with repeated provocation until they disappear — an effect that is utilized therapeutically.

The affected ear is the one toward which the greater nystagmus is directed in the lateral position. This ear also may exhibit sensorineural hearing loss.

Causes: Most likely a mechanical disturbance in the vestibular organ. It is theorized that calcite crystals from the macula utriculi detach from the macula and fall into the semicircular canal or ampulla of the posterior semicircular canal, coming to rest on the cupula and altering its oscillatory characteristics or being moved during head movement.

Ear surgery (e.g., stapedectomy or stapedotomy) and trauma could also dislodge "foreign bodies" into the vestibular organ.

A disturbance in the interaction of the organs of the otolith and semicircular canals has also been postulated as a causal mechanism.

Differentiation from cervical and vascular disorders is easily accomplished owing to the very characteristic pattern of symptoms, most notably the violent, rotational eye movements, the latent period, and the short duration of the symptoms. Nystagmus goggles are needed to establish the diagnosis, since pure rotatory eye movements cannot be evaluated by electronystagmography.

Positional Vertigo

Symmetric Positional Vertigo

Disease: *Toxic central vestibular dysfunction* (see p. 107).

Main symptoms: Divergent positional vertigo with rotation of the environment to the lowermost ear: PAN I (positional alcohol nystagmus) following alcohol ingestion (blood alcohol level >0.38 ppt). Convergent positional nystagmus (usually not noticed subjectively): PAN II, occurring after the blood alcohol level has fallen below 0.2 ppt.

Cause: Alcohol with a specific gravity less than water, diffuses into the labyrinth and transforms the cupula into a gravity sensor.

Asymmetric Positional Vertigo

Positional vertigo with a low-frequency, large-amplitude nystagmus while lying on the side of a sensorineural impairment, and a mid-frequency nystagmus of moderate amplitude while lying on the healthy side (Bruhn nystagmus).

Disease: Moderately large to large acoustic neuroma (see p. 110).

Positional Vertigo Combined with Destructive Ear Disease (e.g., Cholesteatoma)

Disease: *Positional fistula syndrome.*

Diagnosis: Fistula sign is tested with the Politzer bag (nystagmus toward the side of compression). With an intact tympanic membrane, the sign is tested by air insufflation through the tube or by the Valsalva maneuver (see p. 25).

Head-position-dependent Vestibular Disorder During Overhead Work (Hanging Drapes, Painting the Ceiling, etc.)

Disequilibrium is a more common subjective complaint than rotatory vertigo.

Diseases: *Cervical syndromes with myogenic or articular dysfunction.*

Main symptoms: Horizontal or rotational nystagmus of varying intensity, not consistently visible with Frenzel goggles and seldom reproducible (see pp. 107, 113 126).

Diagnosis: Neck rotation test. Interpretation is difficult.

Arnold-Chiari-Malformation

Main symptoms: In Arnold−Chiari malformation, hyperplastic cerebellar tonsils extend into the foramen magnum. They may become entrapped during head movements, leading to attacks of vertigo and an impaired oculomotor response.

Diagnosis: CT or MRI.

Other Organic Disturbances of the Cervical Spine or Malformations of the Occiput

See p. 393, Table 10.**2**.

Symptom   Nystagmus

Definition: Nystagmus refers to those reflex eye movements, which, among others, are elicited by the vestibulo-ocular reflex (VOR). Nystagmus consists of:
○ A slow phase which:
  a) is elicited by head movement, is of equal velocity to head movement, but is directed opposite to the head movement (vestibular nystagmus)
  b) is evoked by a moving visual image, is of near-equal velocity to the moving image, and moves in the same direction as the image (optokinetic nystagmus)
○ A fast phase representing a corrective return movement induced by the CNS (exhibits peak velocities of up to 700°/s.

Nystagmus occurs:
○ Physiologically during head movements, at the extreme limits of gazes, and often during rest ("physiologic spontaneous nystagmus").
○ Experimentally during optokinetic, or cervical stimulation, or stimulation of a vestibular sensor.
○ Pathologically due to disturbances of the sensory organs (peripheral nystagmus) or disease in the extensive central connections (central nystagmus).

The various forms are reviewed in Table 1.**58**.

Table 1.**58** *Symptom* Nystagmus

Synopsis
Physiologic nystagmus:
– Nystagmus during head movements
– End-point nystagmus
– Physiologic spontaneous nystagmus
Nystagmus induced by stimulation of a vestibular sensory organ
– Lack of response Caloric stimulation Rotatory stimulation
– Hyperactive response Caloric stimulation Rotatory stimulation
– Lateral disparity of response Caloric stimulation Rotatory stimulation
Nystagmus and eye movements induced by visual stimulation:
– Slow pursuit system
– Optokinetic nystagmus
– Visual suppression of nystagmus
Nystagmus induced by neck rotation
Pathologic nystagmus
Nystagmoid eye movements

Methods of Examination

Vestibular Nystagmus

Vestibular nystagmus can be suppressed by visual fixation. The nystagmus can be seen and recorded only if visual fixation is excluded, either by observing the eyes with illuminated Frenzel goggles (containing magnifying glasses, 20 dioptrin) or by recording the eye movements in total darkness. The following methods are clinically available:
○ Illuminated Frenzel goggles or similar device
○ Video goggles with infrared illumination
○ Electronystagmographic recording in darkness or with the eyes covered
○ Photoelectric nystagmography

Optokinetic Eye Movements

Optokinetic eye movements occur only when a moving environment is observed. They are visible to the naked eye, but electronic or video-based recording is necessary for an accurate quantitative assessment.
○ Electronystagmography
○ Video goggles with free field of view

Physiologic Nystagmus

Nystagmus During Head Movements

Definition: The neurophysiologic information required to produce this nystagmus comes from the vestibular organ (vestibular nystag-

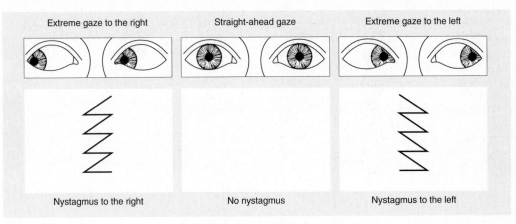

Fig. 1.**31** Gaze-evoked nystagmus induced by extreme lateral gaze

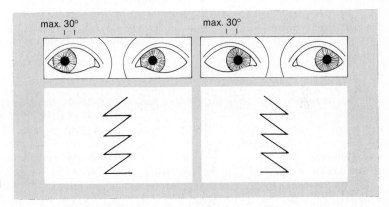

Fig. 1.**32** Gaze nystagmus induced by moderate lateral gaze (ca. 30°)

mus), from the visual system (optokinetic nystagmus), and from the neck receptors (cervical nystagmus). Owing to the fluid-mechanical properties of the semicircular canals and the otolith organs, vestibular nystagmus is elicited only by acceleration of the head. It persists longer than the cupula deflection that underlies the stimulus. The nystagmus may be horizontal, vertical, torsional or a combination thereof, depending on the direction of the acceleration. A constant, uniform head movement does not precipitate nystagmus. This is not true of nystagmus induced by oculomotor activity, which persists as long as the moving image is visually perceived.

When we move physiologically in nature with the eyes open and without benefit of assistive devices for locomotion, the associated reflex nystagmus is regulated by signals from the vestibular, oculomotor, and other systems that are processed and weighted centrally. If the head movement is faster than the ability of the balance system to maintain smooth pursuit, the visual image will become blurred.

Gaze-Evoked Nystagmus

Definition: Gaze-evoked nystagmus is a rhythmic, nonreflex eye movement induced by extreme lateral gaze (Fig. 1.**31**).

Cause: Muscular fatigue caused by the extreme eye position. The eye drifts slowly back toward the center of the orbit but then jerks back to the side when the fixation point moves too far from the fovea.

Differential diagnosis:
○ *Gaze-evoked nystagmus:*
Characteristics in brief: Moderate lateral gaze (approximately 30° is sufficient to induce this type of nystagmus (Fig. 1.**32**). It results from a disturbance of gaze mainte-

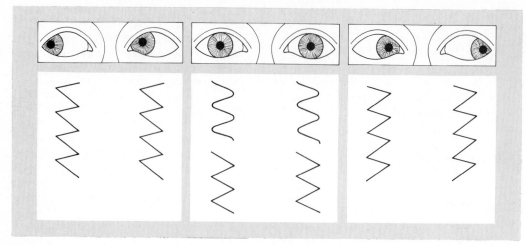

Fig. 1.**33** Congenital fixation nystagmus: Straight-ahead gaze is associated with pendular or jerky eye movements with approximately equal velocity in both phases. On lateral gaze these eye movements become nystagmus-like in the gaze direction whose intensity increases with the degree of lateral gaze

nance caused by a lesion in the pontine gaze center or cerebellum.

Causes: Pharmacologic cerebellar intoxication, systemic diseases causing cerebellar dysfunction.

o *Congenital or acquired fixation nystagmus:*
Characteristics in brief: This nystagmus consists of pendular eye movements that convert to a true nystagmus with increasing lateral gaze, the direction of the fast phase matching the direction of lateral gaze (Fig. 1.**33**). There is a point of minimal eye movements, which normally is not in the position of straight-ahead gaze. The patient will turn the head so that this "null point" is directed forward, resulting in a constant, typical angled head posture.

Cause: Damage to the oculomotor system in early childhood, disrupting its connections with the vestibular system. The disorder is commonly associated with visual impairment. Fixation nystagmas may also be acquired after severe disease of the central vestibular areas, see p. 127.

Physiologic Spontaneous Nystagmus

Definition: More than 50% of all healthy subjects will exhibit nystagmus without stimulation to any sensory organ. This spontaneous nystagmus can be recorded by ENG in complete darkness, but not by examination with illuminated goggles. This clearly distinguishes physiologic spontaneous nystagmus from pathologic spontaneous nystagmus, which is visible under Frenzel goggles. The question of whether the spontaneous nystagmus recorded by ENG is truly physiologic is controversial. Theories range from negligible asymmetries in the control circuitry to early trauma and sequelae to previous inflammatory changes. It should be emphasized that a spontaneous nystagmus detectable only by ENG must be considered pathologic if the history or associated symptoms are consistent with vestibular disease.

Nystagmus Induced by Stimulation of a Vestibular Receptor

Definition: Nystagmus occurring in response to adequate stimulation of a vestibular sensor (semicircular canals, otolith organs). The intensity of the nystagmus depends on the intensity of the stimulus. The question of whether the vestibular response is normal, hypoactive, or hyperactive is clinically important but is difficult to answer because of the very large variability. Norm statistics have been plotted for the response range of normal subjects to particular stimuli, but anyone using these curves must take care that their stimulation technique matches the stimulation and evaluation technique used by the source studies. In the sections that follow we shall either describe the technique or direct the reader to the appropriate reference.

Lack of Response

Caloric Stimulation

The caloric response may be absent bilaterally, unilaterally, or in one of the four steps of the test.

Bilateral Lack of Response

Artifacts:

- Lack of response may be artifactual if, for caloric testing, the head is placed in the position that is least favorable for the individual. There are some people who, in the "optimum" position described by Brünings (head elevated 30° in the recumbent subject), manifest their "pessimum" response.
- Incorrect stimulus temperature, with the water temperature too close to the body temperature (difference should be 7 °C). More artifacts occur when air is used rather than water.
- Bilateral obstruction of the external auditory canals (cerumen!).
- Sedation (e.g., with the antivertiginous drug dimenhydrinate).

Diseases:

- Prior use of ototoxic medications.
- Congenital absence or malformation of the vestibular organs (as in some deaf−mutism)
- Bilateral acoustic neuroma (Recklinghausen disease! Café-au-lait spots see pp. 111, 138).

Diagnostic adjuncts:

- Remove any wax from the external ear canal.
- Obtain the drug history.
- Repeat caloric testing in a different head position (find maximal response in trial irrigation by slowly moving the head forward and back while observing eye movements with illuminated goggles).
- Rotatory testing (a screening test can be performed using an office chair and Frenzel glasses). Lack of response implies complete loss of function of the vestibular organs. Normal response would indicate an erroneous caloric response.
- Stenvers radiographs and further radiographic studies to evaluate the morphology of the vestibular organs and internal auditory canals and exclude congenital anomalies.

Unilateral Lack of Response

Artifact: Unilateral ear canal obstruction (cerumen!).

Diseases:

- Combined with spontaneous nystagmus toward the opposite side: Acute loss of function of the vestibular organ.
- Without spontaneous nystagmus, but combined with head-shaking nystagmus toward the opposite side: Gradual or long-standing unilateral loss (acoustic neuroma!).
- As an isolated finding without complaints: Well-compensated congenital loss or loss acquired in early childhood (very rare but theoretically possible).

Lack of Response in One of the Four Steps of the Test

Artifact: Faulty irrigation technique. Repeat irrigation.

Disease: If warm stimulation of one side elicits little or no response while the responses to cold stimulation are equal on both sides, this signifies a pathologic hyporeactivity on that side with a directional preponderance to the opposite side.

Rotatory Stimulation

Lack of Response to Rotatory Stimulation in both Directions

Artifacts:

- Visual fixation of a visible or imaginary point (beware of malingering!)
- Head position corresponds to the individual

least favorable position for rotational testing, (e.g., 60° backward tilt, or pitch)
○ Sedative medication

Disease:
○ Bilateral loss of vestibular function

Diagnostic adjuncts:
○ Repeat the examination using ensuring correct head position (30° forward tilt)
○ If feigning is suspected, obtain separate d.c.
recording of both eyes or monitor the patient with infrared video

*Lack of Response to Rotatory Stimulation in
One Direction*

Since each of the labyrinths functions bidirec-
tionally lack of response in one direction cannot occur in patients with a unilateral, purely
peripheral lesion. This symptom can only occur in patients with central dysfunction, indicating that nystagmus cannot be generated in a
particular direction (very rare).

Hyperactive Response

Caloric Stimulation

A hyperactive caloric response may be detected on one or both sides. There are no set limits
defining a "hyperactive" response due to the
large interindividual variability. It may be assumed, however, that the response will be very
strong or excessive when the maximum slow
phase velocity is greater than 50°/s, and the
frequency of the nystagmus at maximum response is greater than 3.5 beats/s.

Bilateral Hyperactive Response

Artifacts:
○ Use of water that is too hot or too cold
○ Faulty calibration of ENG recording equip-
ment

Normal findings: There are healthy subjects
who develop a very intense nystagmus with a
slow phase velocity up to 80°/s and frequencies
greater than 4 beats/s.

Diseases:
○ Combined with disturbances in the oculomotor system: Lesion of the vestibulocere-

bellum, especially in the area of the flocculus. The hyperactive response then represents a disinhibition of the central vestibular
system.
○ Disinhibitory phase after alcohol ingestion.
As the blood alcohol level rises and falls,
the vestibular caloric response passes
through phases of different activity. Also,
lateral disparities may occur that were not
present before alcohol consumption.

Unilateral Hyperactive Response

More than a 1°C temperature difference in the
caloric stimulation of the lateral crus of the lateral semicircular canal will produce a unilateral hyperactive caloric response. This can occur:
− during irrigation of an ear that has under-
gone radical surgery
− during irrigation of an ear with an epithe-
lialized tympanic cavity

Rotatory Stimulation

Especially when combined with a reduced caloric response, a hyperactive response to rotatory stimulation may be artifactual or drug-induced. Physiologic and nonphysiologic stimuli
are affected to varying degrees by sedative
medications. Thus a patient may display a very
low caloric response while exhibiting a very
pronounced rotatory nystagmus.

Lateral Disparity of Responses

Caloric Stimulation

The normal range of variation for lateral differences in vestibular caloric response is shown
in Figure 1.**34**. The variation is calculated as
the sum of the responses of the left and right
labyrinths. The traditional formula for calcu-
lating the relative difference between the sides
($100\times$[right side − left side]/[right side + left
side]) is invalid when applied to biologic studies and is not recommended. The interindividual variability in normal subjects is very high,
i.e., there are healthy individuals who also exhibit little response on one side but a very
strong response on the other side. This has led
to the axiom that a lateral disparity of caloric

response is pathologic only if it is accompanied by clinical signs of disease.

Artifacts:
o Faulty irrigation technique
o External ear canal pathology (impacted cerumen, exostoses, etc.)

Diseases:
o Combined with spontaneous nystagmus toward the healthy side: Acute dysfunction of a labyrinth, vestibular nerve, or the brain stem at the entry site of the vestibular nerve (see pp. 104, 108).
o Combined with head-shaking nystagmus: Residual unilateral dysfunction. Spontaneous nystagmus has been eliminated by compensatory processes, but the lateral disparity remains.
o Combined with sensorineural hearing loss (may also present as sudden hearing loss): Slowly progressive, function-impairing lesion such as acoustic neuroma. The difficulty of interpreting caloric results in a patient with a gradually dwindling response can be illustrated by a case example: Assume that a patient, while healthy, had a right−left discrepancy of caloric response with a predominance of the left side (Fig. 1.**35**). He develops a left-sided acoustic neuroma, and his caloric vestibular response declines. During the course of this decline, there is a period in which the caloric responses of both sides are equal. Only later does a reduced vestibular response become apparent. Thus, *if a unilateral hearing loss raises the suspicion of acoustic neuroma, equal caloric responses in both ears do not disprove the existence of such a tumor. Follow-up studies are needed to reveal the declining vestibular response.*

Rotatory Stimulation

The variability of normal responses in the pendular chair test is illustrated in Figure 1.**36**. This was evaluated by Moser and Ranacher (1984) for a rotary deflection of 180° and a period of 20 s. Figure 1.**37a,b** shows the scatter in perrotatory and postrotatory tests using a rotating chair accelerated at 2°/s and brought to a sudden stop from a velocity of 90°/s.

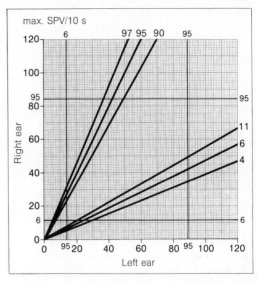

Fig. 1.**34** Normal variation of right−left disparity of vestibular response to caloric stimulation, with associated interquantile ranges. SPV = slow phase velocity of nystagmus (after Scherer)

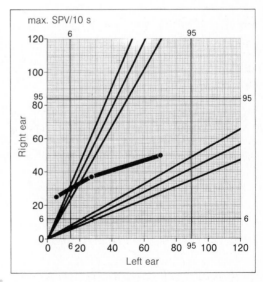

Fig. 1.**35** Regression of vestibular response during growth of a left-sided acoustic neuroma on the left side. The disease on the left side is concealed for some time by compensatory processes

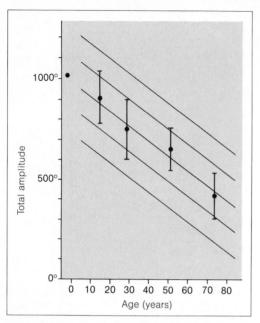

Fig. 1.**36**   Age dependence of the cumulated amplitude of sinusoidal rotatory nystagmus (after Ranacher)

A right−left disparity of response exists:
- In the initial stage of a peripheral vestibular dysfunction.
- In the late stage of an *uncompensated* peripheral dysfunction. Compensation is hampered by:
  - craniocerebral trauma
  - meningoencephalitis
  - cervical syndrome
  - bed rest
- As a central directional predominance of nystagmus. It is then combined with a directional preponderance in the caloric test. The normal range of variation of directional preponderance has not been established for rotatory testing, although Moser (1980) has published values for the torsion chair test. The normal range is 70−129% (calculated from the formula U(%)=right values/left values × 100).

Nystagmus and Eye Movements Induced by Visual Stimulation

The oculomotor system is comprised of:
- A slow pursuit system, stimulated by the *sinusoidal tracking test*. A slow ocular tracking movement is recorded (see Fig. 1.**24a**).
- A fast saccadic system, stimulated by *opto-*

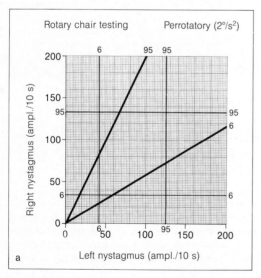

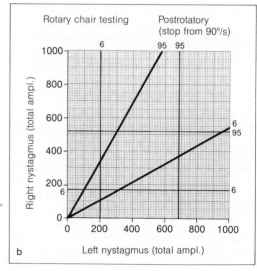

Fig. 1.**37 a,b**   Scatter of normal right−left differences in perrotatory (**a**) and postrotatory (**b**) responses with corresponding interquantile ranges (after Scherer)

kinetic testing. Optokinetic nystagmus is recorded (see Fig. 1.**25**).

The visual system cooperates with the vestibular system but is dominant over it. Thus, the central nervous command to fix the gaze on a point immobilizes the eye even if vestibular nystagmus is present, i.e., nystagmus initiated by the vestibular system can be suppressed by visual fixation. This phenomenon can be tested by the *fixation suppression test* (see Fig. 1.**26**).

The three main oculomotor examination techniques are described below.

Smooth Pursuit

Normally, smooth pursuit of an oscillating target is possible up to a target speed of 40°/s. The following abnormalities may be noted in the pendulum tracking test:

Ocular pursuit absent or fragmentary:
o Visual impairment
o Oculomotor paralysis (Fig. 1.**38**)
o Malingering

Smooth pursuit disrupted by saccades (see Fig. 1.**24b**):
o Central vestibular dysfunction
o Combined with hyperactive caloric, rotatory, and optokinetic nystagmus: lesion of the vestibulocerebellum (especially the flocculus)

Optokinetic Nystagmus

Observing a moving environment induces an optokinetic nystagmus whose gain factor (eye velocity/stimulus velocity) is a function of stimulus velocity. Figure 1.**39** shows the normal values reported by Pfaltz (1982) for stimulus velocities of 15, 30, and 60°/s. These values are not valid for every test apparatus. Besides normal findings, the following possibilities exist:

The Stimulus Response is Greater than the Stimulus

Unilateral:
o With equal caloric responses but unequal rotatory responses: central directional preponderance
o With unequal caloric and rotatory respon-

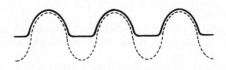

Fig. 1.**38**
———————— Smooth pursuit in left-sided abducens paralysis
– – – – Waveform in a healthy subject

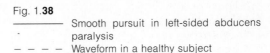

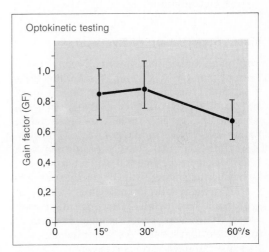

Fig. 1.**39** Normal values of optokinetic response (gain = eye velocity/stimulus velocity) for stimulus velocities of 15, 30, and 60°/s (after Pfaltz)

ses: *peripherally evoked directional preponderance,* i.e., *peripheral spontaneous nystagmus*

Bilateral:
Very rare; gain factor > 1. The patient reports motion sensations when looking at passing trains, etc.

Causes: Failure of suppression in the central vestibular system, such as that occurring with cerebellar dysfunction. *Caution:* If a hyperactive oculomotor response is noted as an isolated finding, and the finding occurs repeatedly, the stimulation and recording equipment should be checked for malfunction, or the examiner should establish his own baseline normal values.

The Stimulus Response is Weaker than that of Normal Subjects

Unilateral:
○ Lesion of the cerebellum on the side of the slow phase (usually associated with downbeat nystagmus)
○ Lesion of the parieto-occipital cerebrum (on the side of the fast phase)

Bilateral:
○ Visual impairment
○ Drug effect
○ Extensive brain stem lesion or symmetrical cerebellar lesion

Visual Suppression of Nystagmus

Vestibular nystagmus is normally suppressed by optic fixation. A screening test for this ability involves turning the patient rapidly back and forth on an ordinary examination stool while he fixes his gaze on his own outstretched thumb. Nystagmus should not occur. The visual suppression test is easily performed with ENG during experimental stimulation, e.g., by having the patient fixate on a light spot during an ongoing caloric nystagmus. The light spot should be presented after the culmination phase, in order to permit, manual evaluation, of the caloric response. An abnormal suppression test can have various causes:

Unilateral: Ipsilateral cerebellar (floccular) lesion or parieto-occipital cerebral lesion.

Bilateral: Strong suspicion of toxic influence, especially alcohol ingestion. Alcohol abolishes the normal dominance of the visual system over the vestibular system, so that an experimentally induced vestibular nystagmus will persist despite optic fixation. This phenomenon is a contributing factor in motor vehicle accidents involving drunken drivers. Alcohol use is also manifested clinically by positional alcohol nystagmus (PAN I and PAN II).

Nystagmus Induced by Neck Rotation

Defintion: Receptors in the muscles, joints, and tendons — especially in the upper portion of the neck — supply information to the vestibular system on the position of the head in

relation to the body. These receptors must be regarded as accessory sense organs that function as adjuncts to the vestibular labyrinth and oculomotor system. Accordingly, cervical nystagmus must exist as an entity along with vestibular and opto kinetic nystagmus. The intensity of cervical nystagmus is low. It is pronounced only if other systems are not yet fully functional (in infants) or have failed (functional loss of both labyrinths), in which case the nystagmus is physiologic. Cervical nystagmus also occurs when there is excessive activation of the cervical afferent fibers, e.g., due to dysfunction of the craniovertebral joints or lower cervical vertebral joints with associated muscular dystrophy (splinting). In this case the cervical nystagmus is pathologic.

A distinction is drawn between the first-degree cervical nystagmus that occurs during neck rotation (body rotated while head is stationary) and the second-degree cervical nystagmus evoked by holding the head in a lateral position. First-degree cervical nystagmus is present in approximately 50% of the healthy population, whereas second-degree cervical nystagmus is rarely present in healthy subjects.

Findings:
○ Unilateral nystagmus in the neck rotation test combined with directional preponderance on caloric and rotational testing: *spontaneous nystagmus evoked by the neck movement.*
○ Combined with an opposite spontaneous nystagmus before the examination: *cervical syndrome.*
○ Bilateral direction-changing nystagmus in the neck rotation test (95% divergent, 5% convergent): *cervical syndrome.* The d.c. recording must be performed to exclude gaze-induced nystagmus.
○ No demonstrable second-degree cervical nystagmus, but pronounced square-wave potentials in the neck rotation test: *probable cervical syndrome.* Repetition of the examination is advised.

Pathologic Nystagmus

Definition: *Pathologic* nystagmus differs from *physiologic* nystagmus in that it is not based on the adequate stimulation of a sensor that supplies afferent signals to the vestibular nuclei. It occurs:

- when any one of the sensory organs is in a pathologic state of irritation (typical of nystagmus due to cervical pathology, labyrinthitis, or at the onset of a Ménière attack)
- when an acute function deficit develops in one of the vestibular end organs (typical of nystagmus due to functional loss of a labyrinth)
- when there is a pathologic right−left disparity of neuronal activity in the central vestibular system (typical of localized lesions of the brain stem and vestibulocerebellum), as in multiple sclerosis (MS)

All pathologic nystagmus arising from the vestibular end organ corresponds in form and intensity to the nystagmus that is evoked by physiologic stimulation of those sensors. This pathologic nystagmus was discussed previously in connection with the differential diagnosis of vertigo (see p. 101). An exception is vertical nystagmus (see p. 129). Pathologic nystagmus arising from the central vestibular system generally has a different form, is markedly small or large, or the pattern of eye movements within the orbit is markedly limited (Table 1.**59**).

Fixation Nystagmus

Definition: Nystagmus or nystagmus-like pendular eye movements that are accentuated by optic fixation (unlike physiologic vestibular nystagmus, which is suppressed by optic fixation; see p. 118).

Causes: These eye movements, also known as "ocular nystagmus," probably arise from a congenital or acquired lesion of the central visual system. The *congenital form* of the disease has an X-linked recessive or occasionally dominant mode of inheritance. It appears during infancy and is often accompanied by primary visual defects. Congenital fixation nystagmus is caused by an oscillating instability of the ocular pursuit system activated by attempted visual fixation (Brandt and Büchele 1983).

The *acquired form* of the disease is rare. It results from damage to the brain stem and/or vestibulocerebellum caused by hypoxia or craniocerebral trauma.

Table 1.**59** Pathologic eye movements of central etiology

Congenital and acquired fixation nystagmus
Sensory deprivation nystagmus
Nystagmus due to latent strabismus
Gaze-peretic nystagmus
Dissociated gaze-induced nystagmus
Seesaw nystagmus
Upbeating and downbeating nystagmus

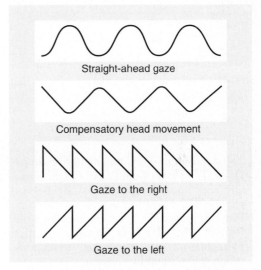

Straight-ahead gaze

Compensatory head movement

Gaze to the right

Gaze to the left

Fig. 1.**40** Patterns of ocular fixation nystagmus with associated compensatory head movements

Other symptoms and special features:

- The nystagmus presents a pendular, sinusoidal, or zigzag pattern on straight-ahead gaze (Fig. 1.**40** and 1.**33**). Thus, it typically cannot be resolved into a fast and slow phase.
- On gaze to the right or left, the nystagmus acquires a high-amplitude fast component in the direction of gaze. This component is slower, however, than the fast phase of vestibular nystagmus.
- As the gaze is directed farther laterally, the fast component of the nystagmus becomes increasingly rapid, and the amplitude becomes greater.
- Eye positions can be identified in which the fixation nystagmus is maximal or minimal.

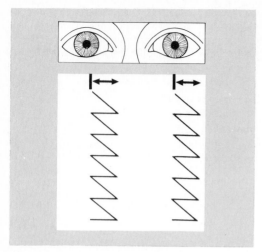

Fig. 1.**41**   Gaze-paretic nystagmus

casionally irregular—are present on straight-ahead gaze and convert to a right-beating or left-beating nystagmus when gaze is shifted to the right or left, respectively. Generally both the amplitude and the irregularity of the eye movements increase with the severity of the visual disturbance. Compensatory pendular head movements in the opposite direction are commonly present, especially if the patient attempts to read with his weakened visual system (Cogan 1966; Metz 1972; Gay 1974; Kornhuber 1974). Causes: Retinal damage, congenital cataracts, optic nerve atrophy, achromatopsia (color blindness), albinism.

Nystagmus Due to Latent Strabismus

This form of nystagmus exists in approximately 20% of patients with congenital strabismus (3% of the general population). It occurs only when one eye is covered, the fast phase beating toward the covered eye (see also p. 116).

Gaze-paretic Nystagmus

Gaze-paretic nystagmus results from lesions in the areas of the visual system that are responsible for conjugate eye movements. One particular direction of gaze is restricted (Fig. 1.**41**). The nystagmus is coarse and of low frequency. The fast phase beats in the direction of the restricted eye movement. With a unilateral lesion of the oculomotor nuclei, the nystagmus occurs only in the affected eye. In the case of a supranuclear lesion with bilateral gaze paresis, the nystagmus affects both eyes.

These positions vary among different patients. The point of minimal nystagmus usually does not correspond to straight-ahead gaze, but to a position slightly lateral to it.
○ Fixation nystagmus is accentuated by optic fixation. This clearly distinguishes fixation nystagmus from vestibular nystagmus, which is abolished by fixation.
○ Optokinetic nystagmus is frequently reversed. In 46% of patients, Kornhuber (1974) found that a pattern moving to the left evoked a left nystagmus (instead of a right nystagmus) while pattern movement to the right evoked a right nystagmus (instead of a left nystagmus).
○ When the eyes are closed, fixation nystagmus is greatly reduced and may alter its direction and beat pattern. This can only be demonstrated by ENG.
○ Vertigo is absent.

Sensory Deprivation Nystagmus

This type of nystagmus occurs in the presence of an afferent visual disturbance, which may be less severe than complete blindness. The ocular pursuit system lacks the ability to maintain foveal fixation of a target, or to track the target by means of corrective saccades. Pendular eye movements—usually regular but oc-

Dissociated Gaze-induced Nystagmus

(Internuclear ophthalmoplegia or medial longitudinal fasciculus syndrome)

This phenomenon is apparent only when gaze is directed laterally, the abducted eye manifesting an obvious nystagmus in the direction of gaze (Fig. 1.**42**). On experimental stimulation of the vestibular organ, markedly greater amplitudes are noted in the eye that is on the side of the fast phase. The lesion is located in the brain stem contralateral to the abducted eye. With bilateral disease, frequently there is multiple sclerosis involving the medial longitudinal fasciculus. With unilateral disease, there

Fig. 1.**42**   Dissociated
gaze-induced nystagmus

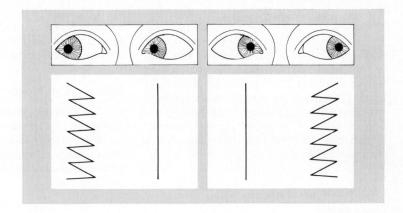

is usually a vascular disorder involving the brain stem. Dissociated gaze-induced nystagmus is a reliable early sign of multiple sclerosis.

Seesaw Nystagmus

This phenomenon is likewise marked by a dissociation of ocular movements. The nystagmus consists of one eye rising while the other falls. Sometimes this is associated with rotational movements of the eyes in opposite directions. The phenomenon is based on a lesion in the anterior part of the third ventricle or in the rostral midbrain (Brandt and Büchele 1983; Sano 1972). It also occurs with large sellar and parasellar tumors causing a bitemporal hemianopia.

Vertical Nystagmus

Vertical nystagmus occurs in response to stimulation not only of the semicircular canals, but also of the otolith organs (acceleration in the AP direction or head nodding) or an isolated loss of the otolith organs. Devices such as horizontal or vertical acceleration seats are not used for routine clinical testing. Also, isolated deficits of the otolith organs are extremely rare. Thus, *vertical nystagmus of peripheral origin has as yet very little clinical significance.* Vertical nystagmus due to *central vestibular dysfunction* of the coordinating centers for vertical gaze is a much more common finding.

Upbeating Nystagmus

The center for upward eye movement is the rostral interstitial nucleus of the medial longitudinal fasciculus. Lesions in this region as well as cerebellar lesions near the midline produce a tonus change with a slow downward eye movement followed by an upward saccade.

Causes: Brain stem tumors, disseminated encephalomyelitis, encephalitis, vascular disorders, pharmacologic side effect (Brandt and Büchele 1983).

Downbeating Nystagmus

The center for downward eye movement is in the pretectal area. A defect in the downward vertical pursuit system leads to a slow upward drift of the eyes followed by a downward saccade.

Causes: Lesion of the flocculus or pontomedullary brain stem. Besides the causes stated for upbeating nystagmus, particular attention should be given to abnormalities of the occipitocervical junction.

Nystagmoid Eye Movements

Periodic Alternating Gaze Deviations

These represent a rare disturbance of ocular motility, only recently discovered, characterized by spontaneous lateral eye movements having a square-wave pattern and a period of 1–2 s. Slow eyelid contractions may occur during the course of the deviation. The cause is attributed to potentially severe vascular lesions involving the tegmentum of the midbrain (especially the Darcchevich nucleus), which provides descending control of the vestibular nuclei. A lesion of the vestibulocerebellum can also produce this phenomenon (Cramon 1977).

Slow Pendular ("Roving") Eye Movements

These movements occur in superficial comatose states and during induction and recovery from general anesthesia. They also occur normally in stages I–III of sleep. The movements are usually horizontal with a very low frequency and large amplitude. Roving eye movements cannot be performed voluntarily.

Bobbing Eye Movements

"Ocular bobbing" consists of rapid, conjugate downward movements of the eyes, which drift slowly back to the primary position at once or after a delay. These eye movements occur in deep coma and often are present only as a preterminal event.

For a more detailed discussion of these and other nystagmus-like eye movements, see: Brandt and Büchele (1983); Gay et al. (1974); Leigh and Zee (1991); Brandt (1991) (1966, 1974); Schmidt and Löhe (1980).

2. Face

The facial region is the domain of various specialties, each having its own tasks and responsibilities. For success in differential diagnosis, the otolaryngologist must take into consideration at least the basic aspects of these neighboring specialties. Systemic diseases are also a potential cause of manifestations in the facial region (see Table 2.**1**) and should be included in the differential diagnosis.

Principal Diagnostic Methods

○ *Inspection* of the face not only supplies information on visible pathologic changes in this region but is an important key to evaluating the patient's overall personality.

○ The *history* and *palpation* convey information on diseases located on the surface of the face or in deeper facial tissues.

○ The *otorhinolaryngologic examination* (facial soft tissues, nose, paranasal sinuses, oral cavity, maxilla, mandible, and parotid region) provides the basic inventory that may demonstrate a need for further investigation by *biopsy*.

○ *Radiographic* options include *standard radiographs* of the facial region in various planes, various *tomographic* and especially CT techniques, and special imaging procedures (*angiography, radionuclide scanning*, etc.) for selected inquiries.

○ In the evaluation of morphologic defects and anomalies, radiography supplemented by *photography* in various projections will contribute to an accurate analysis of morphologic deviations and aid in the planning of corrective or reconstructive surgery.

○ MRI is essentially a soft-tissue modality, so it is not often used in evaluations of the face and facial skeleton (see footnote on p. 1).

○ *Sonography* (ultrasound) is useful in selected cases for the evaluation of subcutaneous changes in the facial soft tissues.

In some circumstances the changes that are identified may warrant consultation with an ophthalmologist, dermatologist, internist, neurologist, dentist, or oral surgeon.

General Facial Changes that May Be Important in Differential Diagnosis

See Table 2.**1**.

Table 2.**1**   Facial signs suggestive of disease (modified from F. J. Kessler. In: R. Ferlinz: Internistische Differentialdiagnostik. Thieme, Stuttgart 1989)

Sign	Suggestive of:
General facial appearance	
– Mask-like facies	Depression
	Generalized scleroderma
	Parkinsonism
– Oily, shiny facial skin	Parkinsonism
– Hippocratic facies (sunken cheeks and eyes, pinched nose, cold ears)	Gastric ulcer disease or other abdominal disease
– Risus sardonicus	Tetanus
– Coarse features	Acromegaly
– Bloated face	Nephrosis
Alteration of facial skin color	
– Red face (rubeosis)	Diabetes mellitus
	Essential hypertension
	Erythrocytosis
	Polycythemia vera
	Lupus erythematosus
	Alcoholism
	Metastatic carcinoid (flushes)
	Febrile diseases
– Dark red to purple skin color	Dermatomyositis
– Brownish-red skin color	Hemosiderosis (bronze diabetes)
– Café-au-lait color	Endocarditis lenta
– Reddened cheeks	Mitral stenosis (+ cyanotic lips)
– Cyanosis	Cardiac diseases such as "blue disease," right heart failure, mitral valve defects
	Pulmonary diseases such as cor pulmonale, pneumonia, chronic bronchitis, lung tumors
	Obstructive respiratory insufficiency (may also result from prepulmonary disease, see Table 6.**8**)
	Intoxication, e. g., prussic acid, CO, methemoglobinemia, etc.
	Endocrine pathology (Cushing disease)
	Polycythemia vera, symptomatic erythrocytoses
– Pallor	Anemia
	Shock, collapse
	Acute internal hemorrhage
	Renal disease
	Malignancy
	Tuberculosis
– Gray to yellowish skin color	Cirrhosis of the liver
	Vitamin A deficiency (ashen gray)
– Jaundice	Hepatobiliary disease
	Hemolytic disease
	Drug-induced icterus (does *not* involve the sclerae)
– Straw-colored skin	Pernicious anemia
– Yellowish-brown skin color	Carotenoderma (excessive intake of vitamin A and carotene-rich foods)

Table 2.**1**   (cont.)

Sign	Suggestive of:
– Mahagony skin color	Pellagra Melasma
– Bluish-gray skin color	Argyria (silver intoxication)
Alteration of facial skin turgor	Seen with hypo-, hyper- or isotonic dehydration of the organism
Diffuse facial edema/and or swelling	Cardiac (heart failure) Renal (nephritis, nephrotic syndrome) Hepatic (cirrhosis) Drug side effect Local lymphostasis (following neck dissection, tumor growth) Allergic or pseudoallergic Endocrine (myxedema, aldosteronism, Cushing disease) Hypoproteinemia (hunger) Hypokalemia "Idiopathic" (in women, related to menstrual cycle)
Pigmentary changes in the facial skin	Diabetes mellitus Autoimmune disease Addison disease Hepatic cirrhosis and chronic hepatic insufficiency Pregnancy Ovarian tumors Hyperthyroidism Arsenic poisoning (patchy or diffuse pigmentation)
Facial skin bleeding	Hemorrhagic diathesis (bleeding and coagulation disorders; hematologic or systemic diseases; thrombocytogenic, hemocytopoietic disorders; liver disease; sepsis)
Abnormal vascular markings	Telangiectasia in liver disease, spider nevi or stellate angiomas, Rendu–Osler disease, intestinal carcinoid
Facial erythema nodosum	Acute sarcoidosis, drug allergy or pseudoallergy, fungal infection, Crohn disease, ulcerative colitis
Eyelids	
– Xanthelasma	Suspected lipoproteinemia
– Edema of the eyelids	Nephrotic syndrome Myxedema
– Periorbital edema (possibly with exophthalmos)	Endocrine orbitopathy (hyperthyroidism)

(Cont. on next page)

Table 2.**1**   (cont.)

Sign	Suggestive of:
Conjunctiva and sclerae	
– Blue sclerae	Osteogenesis imperfecta Osteopsathyrosis
– Reddened sclerae	Alcoholism Allergy or pseudoallergy
– Yellow sclerae	Hepatobiliary or hemolytic jaundice
Pupils	
– Miosis	Opiate intoxication, morphine abuse, sleeping pill overdose
– Miosis with enophthalmos and ptosis	Horner syndrome (cervical sympathetic fibers)
– Mydriasis	Stroke, botulism, glaucoma attack, drug intoxication (e. g., atropine), alcohol use
– Unequal pupils	Intracranial disease
Exophthalmos	See Table 2.**3**

Symptom   **Change in Facial Morphology**

The face is freely exposed to analytic scrutiny, and morphologic abnormalities are readily apparent. There is never perfect symmetry between the two facial halves. Generally this is not a problem as long as all the facial contours and proportions are in harmonious relation to one another and to the face in general. There are well-established anthropometric and aesthetic guidelines for evaluating facial dimensions and proportions, but they are beyond the scope, of this book. Our present discussion is limited to obvious morphologic changes that have pathologic significance or are suggestive of specific disorders (Table 2.**2**).

Malformations

The morphologic prominence of malformations involving the facial region is extremely variable. The spectrum ranges from lateral and midline *clefts* to isolated nasal dysplasias and profound anomalies (e.g., *craniomandibulofa-*

cial dysostoses; craniosynostoses; otomandibular and otopalatinodigital anomalies; mandibulofacial dysplasia; maxillonasal, oculodental dysmorphias; hemimicrosomias, etc.). It would exceed our scope to describe these conditions in detail, particularly since most have already been diagnosed by a pediatrician and/ or geneticist by the time the patient sees an otorhinolaryngologist. The ENT physician, then, must be well-informed regarding the diverse clinical presentations and possible combinations. His principal task is to recognize and treat, surgically if necessary, the *functional disturbances* that commonly *result from these malformations.*

Table 2.**13** lists the more common facial malformations and the typical ear, nose, and throat dysfunctions that may accompany them. Dysplasias, dysgeneses, and deformities that are chiefly of rhinologic interest are listed in Tables 3.**23** and 3.**24**).

Table 2.**2**   *Symptom*   Change in facial morphology

Synopsis

Malformations

Injuries
  Facial fractures

Miscellaneous causes of circumscribed swellings

○ *Location: forehead and upper eyelid*
  Frontal sinusitis and complications, see pp. 179, 189, 210ff.
  Osteomyelitis of the flat cranial bones, see p. 212
  Abscess of the upper eyelid
  Mucocele and pyocele, see p. 180
  Pneumosinus dilatans, see p. 180
  Trauma and sequelae, see pp. 135, 180
  Neurofibromatosis (von Recklinghausen disease)
  Acromegaly (Pierre–Marie syndrome)
  Osteitis deformans (Paget disease)
  Encephalocele
  Glioma
  Benign and malignant tumors, see p. 214

○ *Location: orbit*
  Exophthalmos, see Table 2.**3**
  Rhinogenic orbital complications, see p. 210

○ *Location: maxilla, cheek, lower eyelid*
  Ethmoid and/or maxillary sinusitis and their complications, see pp. 179, 213
  Zygomatitis (otogenic), see p. 12
  Maxillary osteomyelitis
  Mucocele and pyocele (e. g., of the maxillary sinus), see p. 180
  Fibrous dysplasia
  Ossifying fibroma
  Dentogenic cysts

Inflammatory dental diseases, see Fig. 4.**1**
Dacryocystitis
Midfacial trauma, see pp. 136, 180
Angioneurotic syndrome (Quincke edema)
Benign and malignant tumors

○ *Location: lateral midface*
  Parotid diseases
  Zygomatic fracture
  Lymphadenopathy
  Temporomandibular joint disorders

○ *Location: external nose*
  See p. 208

○ *Location: lips*
  See p. 238

○ *Location: mandible and chin*
  Inflammatory dental diseases, see p. 237
  Dentogenic cysts, see pp. 142, 144
  Mandibular osteomyelitis
  Mandibular fracture, see p. 137
  Chin abscess
  Tumors, see p. 267ff.
  Masseter hypertrophy
  Paramandibular and/or submental lymph node swelling, see p. 400

Poorly circumscribed, diffuse facial swellings see Table 2.1

Injuries

Permanent changes in facial morphology that have been caused by trauma generally do not pose problems of differential diagnosis, because patients usually give a *history* of trauma spontaneously, while *inspection* and *palpation* disclose soft-tissue scars and/or circumscribed discontinuities, fracture lines, depressions, deviations, or deformities of the bony and cartilaginous facial skeleton, and *radiographs* (standard and special views of the cranium and face, including tomograms or CT scans) can document bony injuries not apparent externally.

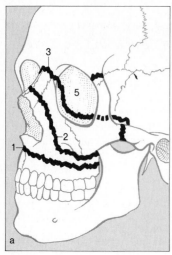 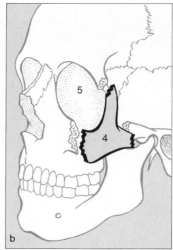 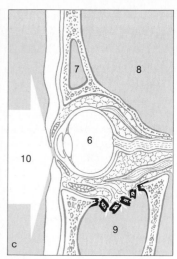

Fig. 2.**1a−c** Typical sites of facial fractures
a Medial facial fractures

 1 Le Fort I (low transverse maxillary fracture)
 2 Le Fort II (pyramidal fracture of the maxilla)
 3 Le Fort III (craniofacial dysjunction)

b Lateral facial fracture (zygomatic and/or zygomatic arch fracture)
 4 Isolated zygomatic fracture
 5 Orbit

c Orbital blowout fracture
 6 Eyeball
 7 Frontal sinus
 8 Anterior cranial fossa
 9 Maxillary sinus
 10 Direction of traumatic force

On the other hand, the differential diagnosis of facial injuries can be very difficult in cases of *recent blunt trauma* and is generally difficult in *injuries of the pediatric facial skeleton.*

The type of fracture that occurs depends on the nature and location of the trauma-producing impact (Figs. 2.**1a−c** and 3.**2**). The following *fracture types* are important to consider in the differential diagnosis of facial injuries:

○ *Frontal bone fracture:* Depressed fracture with lateral and/or posterior displacement of bone fragments in the area of the frontal bone and frontal sinus. Often there is a palpable fracture line or discontinuity. *Diagnosis:* See below. *Differential diagnosis:* Exclude a frontobasal fracture (see p. 178 and Fig. 3.**2a−c**) with injury of the dura and brain, concomitant injury of the ethmoid and sphenoid sinuses and of the orbit and its contents, and damage to cranial nerves I through VI.

○ *Midfacial fractures:* These fractures may be medial or lateral, isolated or combined with involvement of the maxilla, paranasal sinuses, orbit, nasal bone, or zygoma.
 − *Nasal fractures:* a) Simple *displaced fracture* with lateral displacement of the bony nasal pyramid and often the cartilaginous pyramid and nasal septum. b) *Depressed fracture and/or avulsion fracture* with flattening of the nose to the level of the surrounding face. The nasal skeleton is morselized and often avulsed in the glabellar region. This is always associated with significant intranasal destruction! c) Combination of (a) and (b).
 − *Maxillary fractures:* Transverse (Guerin) fractures are the most common (Fig. 2.**1a**).
 Le fort classification of *medial midfacial fractures:* a) *Le Fort I:* Low maxillary Guerin fracture with detachment of the superior alveolar crest, malocclusion, and

possible involvement of the maxillary sinus. b) *Le Fort II:* Pyramidal fracture with maxillary avulsion, the fracture line extending through the nasal bone, the frontal processes of the maxilla, the orbital floor, and the zygomatic−maxillary junction. The midface is displaced and driven inward with involvement of the maxillary and ethmoid sinuses, the orbits, and possibly the zygomas. c) *Le Fort III:* Detachment of the facial skeleton from the skull base, the fracture line extending along the nasofrontal, maxillofrontal, and zygomaticofrontal sutures and often involving all the paranasal sinuses, the anterior skull base, the orbits, and the zygomas.
Less common are *sagittal* (vertical) *fractures* that extend through the midline of the hard palate.

− *Lateral midfacial fractures:* a) *Zygomatic fracture* ("tripod" fracture) (Fig. 2.**1b**): The zygoma is displaced and rotated about its horizontal and/or vertical axis following fracture through the temporozygomatic and frontozygomatic sutures, zygomaticomaxillary process, orbit, infraorbital nerve canal, and often through the greater sphenoid wing. The depressed cheek contour produces lateral midfacial asymmetry. Restriction of mandibular movement is common, and there may be loss of infraorbital nerve sensation. A stepoff is palpable at the inferior and/or lateral orbital rim. b) *Isolated zygomatic arch fracture:* Usually a multiple-part fracture with depression of the arch fragments. Mandibular movement is often (though not always) restricted, and there is at least a palpable change in the zygomatic arch contour. c) *Orbital blow-out fracture* (Fig. 2.**1c**): Isolated fracture of the orbital floor, possibly with entrapment of orbital soft tissues in the fracture line, caused by the circumscribed application of a traumatic force to the orbital contents and/or to the zygoma. Symptoms include enophthalmos, diplopia, decreased ocular mobility, and infraorbital nerve loss. d) *Combinations* of (a)−(c).

○ *Mandibular fractures:* a) Fracture of the mandibular condyle and subcapital fracture (with detachment of the mandibular head). b) Fracture of the coronoid process (with involvement of the temporalis tendon). c) Fracture of the mandibular angle. d) Various fractures of the horizontal ramus (e.g., through the mental foramen). e) Midline and parasymphyeal fractures. f) Multiple fractures that are a combination of (a)−(e). Mandibular fractures are marked by malocclusion, abnormal mandibular mobility with a palpable step, and possible sensory disturbances about the chin and lower lip.

Main symptoms common to facial fractures: Swelling, hematoma, and other signs of acute trauma. Severe pain that gradually subsides. Bone and/or cartilage fractures are often obscured by soft-tissue swelling and, especially in children ("greenstick" fracture), often cannot be reliably detected or excluded by palpation!

Diagnosis:
• *Accurate* history with regard to the cause of the injury, the direction of the traumatic force, and previous injuries and operations.
• Inspection, palpation, and documentation (latter also important for forensic reasons!).
• Rhinoscopy. Inspection of the mouth and pharynx. Occlusal evaluation; dental consultation may be required.
• Radiographs: Standard biplane views of the facial skeleton supplemented by special views of the nasal framework and/or paranasal sinuses, depending on the injury. Tomograms and/or CT scans.
• Olfactory testing.

Miscellaneous Causes of Circumscribed Facial Swelling

See Table 2.**2**.

Location: Forehead and Upper Eyelid

Frontal Sinusitis (Including Extension to External Tissues)

Main symptoms: The initial symptom is edema of the overlying soft tissues with erythema and tenderness to pressure and percussion over the frontal sinus. Spread of infection to external soft tissues (possibly to the upper eyelid!) is marked by a boggy swelling over the forehead (see Fig. 3.**9b, c**). For further details see pp. 179, 189.

Differentiation is required from osteomyelitis of the frontal bone (rapid, diffuse spread beyond the limits of the sinus to the calvarium, very severe systemic symptoms), ethmoid sinusitis (swelling near the medial canthus of the eye), and malignant tumor extension (slow, nonpainful progression).

Osteomyelitis of the Flat Cranial Bones

See p. 212.

Abscess of the Upper Eyelid

Main symptoms: Painful swelling involving the entire lid; narrowing of the palpebral fissure. Preauricular lymph nodes and nodes at mandibular angle may be painful.

Cause: Infection, often rhinogenic or sinugenic.

Diagnosis: Detection or exclusion of a rhinogenic cause (sinusitis). Ophthalmologic consultation.

Differentiation is required from extension of a frontal or ethmoid sinusitis, chalazion, stye, a Moll gland retention cyst, dermoid, hemangioma, and malignancy.

Mucocele and Pyocele

See p. 180.

Pneumosinus Dilatans

See p. 180.

Trauma and Sequelae

See pp. 137, 178.

Neurofibromatosis (von Recklinghausen Disease) of the Face

Main symptoms: Multiple or solitary, painless, mobile, compressible nodules ("push-button

sign") and/or flat subcutaneous "pads" that slowly enlarge. Often associated with pigmented maculae (nevi, café-au-lait spots, etc.). Occasional plexiform neuromas and/or hemifacial elephantiasis ("drooping facial contour") as well as pigmented iris hamartomas.

Other symptoms: Involvement of the eyelids and/or the orbital contents (exophthalmos). Facial occurrence usually implies coexisting neurofibromas at other body sites (with possible involvement of the skeletal system, peripheral nerves, and CNS). Intellectual retardation is present in about 10% of cases. Malignant transformation is possible (approximately 10%).

Cause: Hereditary, polysymptomatic, neuroectodermal systemic disease (autosomal dominant inheritance).

Diagnosis:
● With clinical suspicion of neurofibromatosis, look for additional manifestations; exclude malignancy.
● Radiographic delineation may be helpful (cranial CT).
● Bipsy.

Differentiation is required from multiple fibromas or lipomas, metastatic malignancies, and other hereditary syndromes.

Acromegaly (Pierre–Marie Syndrome)

Main symptoms: Coarsening of the facial features with conspicuous enlargement of the frontal bones, supraorbital ridges, zygomatic arch region, nose, mandible, and chin. Onset after puberty.

Other symptoms: Radiographic enlargement of the frontal sinuses and sella (sphenoid sinus). Frequent headaches. Macroglossia. Increased levels of growth hormone (STH) in the blood. Possible bitemporal hemianopia and struma. Enlarged hands and feet.

Cause: Pituitary adenoma with excessive production of growth-hormone releasing factor (GRF).

Diagnosis: Radiography, internal medical evaluation, endocrinologic workup.

Osteitis Deformans (Paget Disease, Osteodystrophia Localisata)

Main symptoms: Increase in cranial circumference ("hat becomes too tight") and tumorous expansion of the facial skeleton (leonine facies). Oculomotor dysfunction, headache. Peak occurrence at 60–70 years of age.

Other symptoms: Bowing of individual long bones, spontaneous fractures. Elevated serum alkaline phosphatase. Hearing loss, see Table 1.**19**.

Diagnosis: Internal medical and radiographic evaluation (CT).

Encephalocele (Meningoencephalocele)

Main symptoms: Congenital protrusion, occasionally pulsatile, in the glabellar region with no signs of inflammation. Mass is soft, tense, and nontender on palpation.

Other symptoms and special features: The (meningo)encephalocele may present between the nasal process of the frontal bone and the nasal bone (= nasofrontal encephalocele), it may enter the orbit (= nasoorbital encephalocele), or it may be located on the nasal roof. An encephalocele may be *external* or *internal*.

Cause: Downward protrusion of dura and brain through a bone defect due to incomplete closure of the anterior neuropore.

Diagnosis:
● Inspection, palpation, and rhinoscopy.
● CT or conventional tomography.

Differential diagnosis: An *external* encephalocele requires differentiation from lipoma, fibroma, dermoid, and glioma. An *internal* encephalocele mainly requires differentiation from nasal polyposis. *Intraorbital* encephalocele requires differentiation from orbital tumor.

Glioma

Main symptoms: Soft, spherical tumor located in the area of the nasal root and dorsum, usually situated on the midline and, depending on location, covered by skin or mucous membrane. Some tumors extend high up into the nasal cavity. Pedunculated forms may occur!

Other symptoms and special features: Symptoms vary depending on whether the glioma is predominantly extranasal or intranasal and whether its connection with the brain is a tube containing brain tissue or an obliterated strand of connective tissue.

Cause: Presumably the same as for encephalocele (see above).

Diagnosis:
● Typical local findings.
● Radiographs (CT or conventional tomograms).
● Some cases require biopsy (frozen section, possibly with immediate definitive surgery).

Differentiation is required from meningoencephalocele, congenital nasal cyst, hemangioma, neurofibroma, fibroma, lipoma, etc.

Location: Orbit

Exophthalmos

Although exophthalmos is primarily a key symptom in ophthalmology, it often results from diseases originating in structures bordering the orbit, so it needs to be considered in rhinologic differential diagnosis. Table 2.**3** reviews the symptom of exophthalmos (and, for completeness, enophthalmos) from an otolaryngologic perspective.

Rhinogenic Orbital Complications
See p. 210.

Location: Maxilla, Cheek, and Lower Eyelid

Ethmoid and/or Maxillary Sinusitis

Main symptoms: Soft-tissue swelling occurs as collateral edema or signifies extension of infection from the ethmoid or maxillary sinus to external tissues. Extension from the ethmoid sinus causes initial circumscribed swelling at the medial canthus involving the lower eyelid (and sometimes the upper eyelid). Extension from the maxillary sinus causes more diffuse swelling in the medial cheek area and lower lid.

Table 2.**3**   Exophthalmos and enophthalmos

Type of exophthalmos	Special clinical aspects
Predominantly unilateral exophthalmos	
Rhinogenic orbital complications	See p. 210
Mucocele or pyocele	See p. 180
Orbital apex syndrome	Pathologic process in the orbital apex. Nerves and vessels traversing the optic foramen and superior orbital fissure may be affected. Cardinal symptoms: exophthalmos, visual deterioration, ptosis, diplopia, severe temporoparietal pain. Involvement of cranial nerves II, III, IV, V, VI. See also Table 1.**18**
Autochthonous intraorbital inflammation	E. g., due to myositis of eye muscles, tenonitis, orbital cellulitis, dacryoadenitis, etc.
Traumatic exophthalmos	Typical history. Usually bleeding within the orbit and its contents. Exopthalmos typically has a rapid onset. Pulsations may be palpable. Caused by orbital and globe injuries, by midfacial and basal skull fractures, or by surgery. Arteriosclerosis and hemophilia also can cause intraorbital bleeding
Traumatic orbital emphysema	Follows fractures of the paranasal sinuses, especially the ethmoid sinus
Intermittent exophthalmos	Caused by intraorbital varices. Eye reddens and protrudes (usually on one side) during bending, lifting, etc.)
Intraorbital pseudotumor	Nonspecific tissue proliferation that grows rapidly and episodically, displacing the globe and restricting its mobility
Pulsating exophthalmos	Aneursym between the cavernous sinus and internal carotid artery. Pulsatile bruit (strongest over the nasal root). Possible oculomotor palsy. Caused by trauma, arteriosclerosis, syphilis. Bone defect between the anterior cranial fossa and orbit ("open orbital roof")
Intra- and paraorbital neoplasms	Very slow progression of exophthalmos with no pain. Often coexisting collateral lid edema and restricted ocular mobility. Decreased vision
Predominantly bilateral exophthalmos	
Exophthalmos due to dysgenesis	Occurs in numerous forms of craniofacial dysplasia (e. g. Cruzon syndrome, Hurler syndrome). Less common: congenital cystic globe
Cavernous sinus syndrome	See p. 214
Endocrine exophthalmos (endocrine orbitopathy)	Observed in hyperthyroidism (Basedow disease), see p. 411. Bilateral exophthalmos with struma and tachycardia. Upper eyelid lags behind globe on downward gaze, infrequent blinking. Symptoms of thyrotoxicosis
Malignant exophthalmos	Same as above, but with increased ocular and endocrinologic symptoms. Lid edema, chemosis, conjunctival redness, lid closure incomplete or absent. Corneal ulcerations

Table 2.**3**   (cont.)

Type of exophthalmos	Special clinical aspects
Neoplasms of the skull base	Centrally located space-occupying lesion in the anterior or middle cranial fossa. Gradual development of bilateral exophthalmos is possible
Enophthalmos:	Horner syndrome (miosis, ptosis, enophthalmos) Orbital blow-out fracture Following ophthalmic or paranasal sinus surgery Following a perforating eye injury In severe dehydration

Swollen areas are tender to pressure (see Fig. 3.**9a**). For further details see p. 179.

Zygomatitis

Main symptom: Painful swelling over the zygomatic arch or possibly the entire zygomatic bone.

Other symptoms and special features: Otitis media with osseous complications involving the pneumatic system of the zygomatic bone. For further details see p. 12.

Maxillary Osteomyelitis

Main symptoms: Buccal swelling and redness. Severe facial pain. Fever. Laboratory findings consistent with inflammation.

Other symptoms and special features: Possible escape of pus to the outside or into the oral cavity with fistula formation.

Causes: Dentogenic, less commonly hematogenous or traumatic. May also result from sequestrum formation after radiation therapy (radionecrosis) or, very rarely, a general infectious disease (measles, typhus).

Diagnosis:
- Rhinoscopy and possibly paranasal sinus endoscopy.
- Radiographs of the facial skeleton, paranasal sinuses, and maxillary teeth.
- Blood count and ESR.
- Dental consultation.

Differentiation is required from extension of maxillary sinusitis or antral tumor, actinomycosis, osseous tuberculosis (hematogenous), and tertiary syphilis.

Maxillary Osteomyelitis in Infants

Main symptoms: Buccal swelling of rapid onset. Abscess formation, usually with breakthrough into the oral cavity. Presumptive cause: infected tooth germ.

Mucocele and/or Pyocele of the Maxillary Sins

See p. 180.

Fibrous Dysplasia

Main symptoms: Very slowly increasing, painless midfacial swelling, usually limited to one side and involving the nasal and/or zygomatic region. Later stages are marked by maxillary deformity and function impairment (with displacement of the globe, possible encasement of the optic nerve and/or − individual trigeminal nerve branches, and involvement of the nasolacrimal duct). Peak occurrence at 10−30 years of age.

Other symptoms and special features: Extension into the skull base can lead to temporal bone involvement with encasement of the internal auditory canal. Involvement of other skeletal regions (ribs, femur, etc.) is possible (approximately 30%).

Causes: Unknown. May relate to hyperparathyroidism, hyperthyroidism, or pituitary disorders.

Diagnosis:
- Radiographs: standard paranasal sinus projections. CT.
- Biopsy.

Differentiation is required from ossifying fibroma; generalized, polyostitic fibrous dysplasia; epulis (peripheral granuloma); Paget disease (very rare in the maxilla and mandible!). Idiopathic hyperostoses. Albers-Schönberg osteopetrosis (see Table 1.**19**). Maxillary cyst. Eosinophilic granuloma. True maxillary tumors such as adamantinoma, giant cell tumor, osteoma, and fibrosarcoma.

Ossifying Fibroma

Main symptoms: Solitary, slowly progressive hypertrophic bone growth, chiefly affecting the mandible and less commonly the frontal bone, ethmoid bone, or lateral skull base. Expansive growth within the facial skeleton. Unlike fibrous dysplasia, monostotic occurrence is the rule. Peak incidence is 15–30 years of age, with a preponderance of females.

Causes: Unknown. Some authors equate the lesion with fibrous dysplasia, but this has not been generally accepted.

Diagnosis: Same as in fibrous dysplasia.

Differential diagnosis: Fibrous dysplasia is frequently polyostotic (see Fibrous Dysplasia) and chiefly affects the maxilla. On radiographs, ossifying fibroma appears more uniform and sharply circumscribed, while fibrous dysplasia appears less homogeneous and has less well-defined boundaries. There are marked histologic differences as well.

Dentogenic Cysts

Main symptoms: Smooth protrusion in the oral vestibule, on the nasal floor, or on the palate with no signs of inflammation and with associated prominence of the upper lid and/or cheek. Slow-growing. Consistency is initially hard and later elastic, sometimes with a "parchment crackle."

Other symptoms and special features: Development toward the nose causes elevation of the alar wing and/or lateral displacement of

the nasal base. Also displaces the antral lumen. Possible secondary infection of the cyst contents with fistula formation.

Causes: Two forms may occur: The *radicular* cyst (three times more common than the follicular), composed of an inflammatory root granuloma, and the *follicular* cyst, a malformed tooth bud that includes dental elements (Malassez epithelial cell nests).

Diagnosis:
- Exclude a rhinogenic cause (rhinoscopy, paranasal sinus radiographs).
- Panorex jaw films and dental spot films. Possibly tomograms and CT scans.
- Dental consultation.

Differentiation is required from maxillary sinusitis with incipient complication and nondentogenic cysts such as dermoid cyst, nasolabial cyst, median palatal cyst, or posttraumatic cyst.

Inflammatory Dental Diseases

Main symptoms: Swelling and redness around the tooth on the alveolar ridge, sometimes with collateral edema or spread of inflammation (apical granuloma, periapical abscess, pulpitis) to facial soft tissues. Tenderness to pessure, dentalgia (see Fig. 4.**1**).

Dacryocystitis

Main symptoms: Inflammatory swelling and redness at the medial canthus of the eye, possibly with fluctuation. Pressure may extrude a purulent discharge from the lacrimal point. There is accompanying edema of the eyelids and lateral nose.

Other symptoms and special features: Possible fever. Regional lymphadenitis in the preauricular area or on the mandibular border. Symptoms tend to recur.

Cause: Inflammation of the duct system, usually secondary to chronic ductal injury.

Diagnosis: Typical site of occurrence along the lacrimal drainage system. Purulent discharge expressed from a lacrimal point. Ophthalmologic consultation.

Differentiation is required from a malignant tumor at the medial canthus (carcinoma, basal cell carcinoma) or an abscess of the lower eyelid.

**Angioneurotic Syndrome
(Quincke Edema)**

Main symptoms: Paroxysmal firm, nontender, edematous facial swelling, particularly affecting the lips and eyelids, appearing suddenly and regressing in 1−3 days. Marked tendency to recur.

Other symptoms and special features: Feeling of facial tension. Itching. Sometimes headache and vomiting. Possible involvement of the tongue, mouth, and pharynx. Peak incidence in 3rd and 4th decades with a 2:1 ratio of males to females.

Causes: Allergic "angioneurotic" subcutaneous edema based on an anaphylactic type of allergic response or possibly a pseudoallergic process. Precipitated by oral or parenteral administration of the allergen, which may be a drug (e.g., salicylate, penicillin), iodinated contrast medium (see Table 3.**15**), or animal venom (insect sting). May be acquired or hereditary. See also p. 249 ff.

Diagnosis: Most patients have a history of previous episodes. If hereditary edema is suspected, test for serum $C1_q$ esterase deficiency. Patient should undergo allergy testing when symptoms are absent.

Differentiation is required from other diseases associated with acute edema such as urticaria, nephritis, nephrosis, the Melkersson−Rosenthal syndrome (see p. 153) and the Ascher syndrome (see pp. 241 and Table 4.**26**).

Benign and Malignant Tumors

The more common benign and malignant tumors that may produce facial swelling are listed in Table 2.**5**.

Main symptoms: Besides causing visible facial swelling, most tumors present as a slow-growing, painless, nondisplaceable mass. There may be associated mass effects or gradual functional deficits (e.g., affecting various anterior cranial nerves).

Diagnosis:
- Endoscopic examination of the nose, paranasal sinuses, mouth, and pharynx.
- Radiographic workup may include cranial survey films, and CT scans depending on the location and extent of disease.
- Biopsy.

Location: Lateral Midfacial Region

The parotid gland and excretory duct, the zygoma, and the temporomandibular joint are common sites in which lateral midfacial swelling originates. Another frequent but banal cause is acute soft-tissue injuries with accompanying hematoma.

Parotid Cyst
See p. 302.

Parotitis
See p. 299.

Sialolithiasis of the Parotid Gland
See p. 300.

Sialadenosis of the Parotid Gland
See p. 304.

Injury of the Parotid Gland
See p. 299.

Tumors of the Parotid Gland
See p. 305 ff.

Zygoma
See p. 138.

Facial Swelling Caused by Lymph Node Disease

The only truly "facial" lymph nodes in the strict sense are the preauricular nodes, but the clusters situated on and below the mandibular border are of major clinical importance, and both mandibular sites should be considered "facial" because they drain the facial region (see Fig. 10.**2**).

The characteristic diseases (inflammatory lesions and tumors) that are consistently associated with lymph node enlargement, their symptomatology and differential diagnosis are discussed in context on p. 397ff.

Lateral Midfacial Swelling Caused by TMJ Disease

Underlying disorders include:
○ Acute arthritis
○ Osteomyelitis of the ascending ramus of the mandible
○ Fracture of the mandibular head
○ TMJ involvement by an adjacent suppurative process (otogenic, parotid gland, soft-tissue cellulitis)
○ TMJ involvement by adjacent tumor

Main symptoms: Swelling and redness over the TMJ. Associated symptoms (point tenderness, pain on movement of the mandible [chewing], radiographic findings, history, regional symptoms) generally lead rapidly to a diagnosis (see also p. 17).

Location: External Nose

Diseases that lead to swelling of the external nose are discussed on p. 208ff. and in Table 3.**2**.

Location: Lips

Diseases that cause lip swelling are discussed on p. 238ff.

Location: Mandible and Chin

Inflammatory Dental Diseases
See p. 235.

Dentogenic Cysts

Most cysts occurring in the mandible are of the follicular type (also wisdom tooth cysts). The symptoms noted on p. 142 for dentogenic maxillary cysts also apply in essence to mandibular cysts.

Mandibular Osteomyelitis

Main symptoms: Swelling, redness, and exquisite tenderness of facial soft tissues over the inflamed bone. Constant, severe pain. Fever and occasional chills. Pain on mastication, frequently with trismus.

Other symptoms and special features: Coexisting dental disease. History of trauma, surgery, or radiotherapy in the mandibular region. Percussive tenderness and looseness of *multiple* teeth in the affected area. Abscess formation with breakthrough of pus to the oral cavity or to external soft tissues with fistula formation and the formation of mandibular sequestra. In *chronic* stage: Abatement of pain, persistent draining fistula(e) with purulent discharge, expulsion of necrotic bone fragments. Risk of spontaneous mandibular fracture with nonunion.

Causes: Infection of the mandibular bone and its medullary cavities. Frequent causes: Extension of periapical osteitis or periodontitis; infection of an extraction wound, cyst, or jaw fracture; sequestration following radiotherapy.

Diagnosis:
● Dental and/or oral surgical consultation.
● Special radiographic views (Panorex); typical bone destruction and demarcation are not apparent until 1−2 weeks after the onset of disease.

Differentiation is required from actinomycosis, tumor with secondary infection, recurrent tumor, and tuberculosis of the mandibular bone (hematogenous).

Fracture of the Mandible
See p. 137.

Abscess of the Chin

Main symptoms: Swelling, redness, and tenderness of the chin. Often accompanied by disease of the lower incisors and their roots. Occasional rupture of a (dentogenic) abscess with fistula formation.

Diagnosis: Dental consultation. Some cases require needle aspiration or excision.

Differentiation is required from lymphadenitis or abscess formation involving the submental lymph nodes, actinomycosis, inflamed midline cervical cyst, and Ludwig angina.

Mandibular Tumors

See p. 267 ff.

Diagnosis: History, local findings, radiographs (including tomograms and/or CT scans), and possibly MRI. Biopsy is essential for diagnosis.

Masseter Hyperplasia

Main symptoms: Marked unilateral or bilateral prominence of the mandibular angle (in the area of the masseter muscle), most obvious during jaw closure and chewing ("square face"). Generally no pain. Impairment of jaw opening and chewing, also transient painful swelling of the parotid gland.

Cause: Attributed to unphysiologic loading of the "stomatognathic system."

Diagnosis: Palpation of the masseter muscle belly from the oral vestibule and cheek with the thumb and index finger while asking the patient to repeatedly open and bite down. The swelling disappears when the mouth is open, but on biting the masseter muscle belly becomes very prominent and its borders clearly palpable.

Differentiation is required from lipoma, fibroma, myositis of the masseter muscle, (organized) hematoma, cavernous angioma in the masseter muscle area, parotid diseases, mandibular diseases.

Diffuse Facial Swelling

See Table 2.**1**.

Symptom   **Change in the Facial Skin**

A variety of cutaneous lesions may be apparent in the facial region, which may be the only site where the change is manifested or one of multiple sites. It is not our intention to offer an exhaustive dermatologic differential diagnosis, particularly since evaluation by a dermatologist will furnish a definate diagnosis in a great many cases. However, several skin diseases are relevant to the ENT specialist owing to their relatively common and typical occurrence in the facial region or their special diagnostic and therapeutic relationship to otorhinolaryngology. To facilitate a more complete differential diagnosis, Table 2.**4** includes a number of diseases that belong exclusively to the realm of dermatology or internal medicine and are not commented upon further in this context.

Skin diseases that commonly affect the *external nose* are listed separately in Table 3.**2**.

Skin diseases affecting the *lips* are discussed in connection with lesions of the oral mucosa (see p. 238).

Tumors Arising from the Facial Skin

See Table 2.**5**.

Benign Tumors

Most benign skin tumors of the face can be quickly diagnosed with reasonable confidence from the characteristic appearance of the lesion, its typical location and palpable qualities (mobility, consistency), absence of pain, typical absence of functional disability, and long history. Doubt can be resolved by dermatologic consultation and, if necessary, biopsy. A special case is posed by the various types of *ne-*

Table 2.**4**   Common (nonneoplastic) skin diseases of the face (after Braun-Falco, Plewig, and Wolf)

Synopsis	
Caused by viruses – Herpes simplex, see p. 239 – Herpes zoster, see p. 245 – "Acute infectious diseases" (measles, rubella, scarlet fever; infectious erythema)* **Caused by bacteria** – Contagious impetigo, see p. 238 – Furuncle, carbuncle, see p. 208 – Chronic staphylogenic folliculitis, see p. 238 – Erysipelas, see p. 173 – Chronic pyodermias* – Acne vulgaris* – Specific inflammatory diseases (tuberculosis, syphilis, leprosy, rhinoscleroma), see p. 191 **Caused by protozoans** – Leishmaniasis **Caused by fungi** – Dermatomycoses (trichophytosis), see pp. 175, 190, 249 and Table 4.**28** **Eczema** – Contact eczema* – Microbial eczema* – Seborrhoic eczema* – Atopical eczema* **Drug-induced exanthemas,** see pp. 186, 249	**Urticaria*** **Caused by physical or chemical agents** – Burn, see p. 4 – Frostbite, see pp 4, 18 – Electrical injury, see p. 4 – Caustic injury* – Other chemical injuries (e. g., tar, pharmacologic agents, etc.)* – Radiodermatitis* – Phytodermatoses* – Photodermatoses* – Artifacts* **Benign pigmentary disorders*** – Freckles – Melasma – Toxic melanodermatitis – Perioral and peribuccal melanosis – Perfume pigmentation – Lentiginosis – Nevi (pigmented nevus, nevus cell nevus, nevus flammeus) **Caused by connective tissue diseases** – Lupus erythematosus, see pp. 210, 255, 291 – Congenital cutaneous atrophy* – Diffuse elastoma* – Progressive systemic scleroderma, see p. 255

* No further commentary

vi, which tend to require dermatologic evaluation to avoid confusion with malignant melanoma. Nevi are by definition intermediate between malformation and tumor, and this can be a source of diagnostic and occasionally therapeutic difficulties.

Angiomas

For therapeutic reasons, these tumors require special differential diagnostic consideration: They are true *vascular neoplasms*, conspicuous, sometimes causing function impairment, and potentially dangerous in some locations (risk of hermorrhage or asphyxia). The most common sites of occurrence of head and neck angiomas are the skin and mucous membranes. Lesions are classified histologically as *cavernous* or *capillary*, which occur in various types and combinations.

Main symptoms: Flat or sligthly prominent, painless tumor area, generally with associated discoloration and irregularity of the overlying skin, often present at birth or appearing shortly thereafter. Angiomas in the mucosa usually produce a deep red or purple discoloration. In the distended state the tumor is soft, tense, and easily compressible. On exertion (straining, crying), the tumor may produce a very prominent swelling, which subsides again with rest. Hemangiomas may regress spontaneously in the first 3–4 years of life. Peak occurrence is

Table 2.**5**   Neoplasms that are common in the facial region (selection)

Synopsis	
Pseudotumors*	**Precancerous lesions**
– Atheroma	– Cutaneous horn
– Dermoid cyst and epidermoid	– Actinic cheilitis, see p. 241
– Milia	– Senile keratoma
– Colloid milium	– Actinic keratosis ("farmer's skin")
	– Keratoses in xeroderma pigmentosum
Benign epithelial tumors*	– Lentigo maligna
– Sebaceous adenoma	– Bowen disease and erythroplasia, see p. 257
– Hidradenoma (eyelid)	– Radiokeratosis
– Keratocanthoma	
– Melanocanthoma	**Malignant epithelial tumors**
– Vascular spider	– Basal cell carcinoma
– Sebaceous nevus	– Basal cell nevus syndrome
– Verrucous nevus	– Spindle-cell carcinoma
– Nevus cell nevus	– Secondary skin carcinoma (metastatic)
– Papilloma	– Malignant melanoma
– Pigmented nevus	
– Trichoepithelioma	**Malignant mesenchymal tumors**
– Verruca vulgaris	– Malignant lymphoma of the skin
– Xanthelasma	– Leukemic manifestations in the skin
	– Malignant histiocytosis of the skin
Benign mesenchymal tumors	– Kaposi syndrome (with or without HIV infection)
– Angioma (hemangioma, less commonly lymph-angioma)	
– Fibroma	**Neoplasms that involve the face secondarily**
– Granular cell tumor	– Nose and paranasal sinuses, see p. 214
– Keloid	– Oral cavity, see p. 267
– Lipoma	– Maxilla and mandible including the dentition, see p. 267 ff.
– Neurofibroma	– Parotid gland, see p. 305 ff.
	– Aural region, see p. 28

* No further commentary

in infants and small children, but lesions may persist and enlarge in adolescence and adulthood, possibly during active growth spurts. Multifocal occurrence is possible. Sites of predilection are the facial skin and scalp, lips, oral mucosa, tongue, cheek, and palate. The pharyngeal and laryngeal mucosae are less frequent sites, but the parotid gland and its immediate surroundings are very commonly affected. See also pp. 308, 405.

Other symptoms and special features: A relatively common lesion besides cavernous angioma ("blood-filled sponge") is "racemose angioma," a more or less prominent, large, coarse-contoured, violet or ruby-red mass of tangled vessels, which may pulsate and cause

significant deformity. Sites of predilection are the lip, tongue, and cheek. The triad of large —mostly—cavernous hemangioma, thrombocytic purpura, and consumptive coagulopathy in infants is called the *Kasabach−Merrit syndrome*.

Causes: Familial occurrence is not uncommon with angiomas. A continuum exists from congenital dysplastic vessel wall changes (nevi) to true (vascular) neoplasms.

Diagnosis:
● Typical history and palpable findings.
● Especially with very large hemangiomas, attempt to define the extent of the lesion and its feeding and draining vessels by superselective

angiography. CT or even MRI may be appropriate for some lesions.

● Some cases may require biopsy, preferably a complete excisional biopsy.

Differentiation is required from lymphangioma (much less common, with no propensity for spontaneous regression), congenital skin changes (nevi), and dysplasia-associated diseases such as the Klippel−Trénaunay−Weber syndrome, the Sturge−Weber syndrome, and the Hippel−Lindau syndrome.

Precancerous Lesions of the Facial Skin

See Table 2.**5**. The possibility of a precancerous lesion or incipient malignant change should always be considered in patients with long-standing, innocent-appearing, and possibly recurring superficial skin changes. Dermatologic evaluation and biopsy (possibly encompassing the whole lesion with histologic examination and confirmation of clear margins) establish the diagnosis. See also pp. 215, 256.

Malignant Tumors

See Table 2.**5**.

Basal Cell Carcinoma (Basal Cell Epithelioma)

Main symptoms: Slowly growing, superficial induration in previously normal-appearing but usually sun-damaged skin, gradually assuming a nodular shape and often covered by a small, recurring crust of blood. The lesion matures in months or years to a firm, painless nodule of a waxy color with teleangiectasias, often with central umbilication and a pearly border. There is increasing ulceration ("rodent ulcer") with a hermorrhagic eschar. Peak occurrence is in the 6th−7th decades; both sexes are affected equally.

Other symptoms: Gradually progressive ulceration and destruction of adjacent skin areas and underlying connective tissues including cartilage and bone with corresponding function deficits. Site of predilection: in the face *above* a line between the angle of the mouth and the base of the auricle; very rare in the lower third of the face. Basal cell carcinoma is the most common tumor of the external nose!

It is also relatively common on the auricle (posterior surface, helix, concha, preauricular area). These tumors do *not* tend to metastasize, and transformation to squamous cell carcinoma is rare, but "degenerative" basal cell carcinomas are known to occur, especially after radiotherapy.

Causes: Radiation exposure (ultraviolet, roentgen), genetically determined increase in radiosensitivity of skin, local carcinogenic exposure (e.g., arsenic, tar). Basal cell nevus syndrome.

Diagnosis:
● Local findings and very slow, largely asymptomatic course usually lead rapidly to a presumptive diagnosis.
● Biopsy. Differentiation from spindle cell carcinoma can be difficult (e.g., with "metatypical" basal cell carcinoma).

Differentiation is required from precancerous lesions and squamous cell carcinoma.

Squamous Cell Carcinoma (Spinocellular Carcinoma)

Main symptoms: Usually starts as a fast-growing nodule in previously damaged or altered skin. The lesion ulcerates relatively quickly, usually forming a crater-like border. Initially there is no pain. The tumor is poorly mobile on underlying tissues. There is rapidly progressive destruction of surrounding and deep tissues with increasing functional deficits (nose, eye, paranasal sinuses, oral cavity, etc.) and onset of pain. Lymphogenous metastasis to regional nodes (submandibular, preauricular, intraparotid) is relatively common. Basal cell carcinoma is approximately five times more prevalent than squamous cell carcinoma in the facial region. Site of predilection: *lower* third of the face.

Other symptoms and special features: Distant metastasis depends on the differentiation and growth rate of the tumor. Light erosive bleeding is not unusual. Ulceration is usually followed by superinfection with fetor!

Causes: Radiation damage to the skin, other chronic skin irritations, precancerous lesions, chemical carcinogenesis. Fair-skinned individuals are predisposed.

Table 2.**6**   Factors to be considered in the differential diagnosis of suspected malignant melanoma

Alternative lesions

Angioma (teleangiectatic and/or thrombosed)	Nevoid lentigo
Benign juvenile melanoma	Nevus cell nevus (activated melanocytic nevus)
Blue nevus	Pigmented actinic keratosis
Pyogenic granuloma	Pigmented apocrine cystadenoma
Halo nevus	Pigmented basal cell carcinoma
Histiocytoma	Pigmented seborrheic keratosis
Keratoacanthoma	Pigmented spindle-cell nevus
Lentigo simplex, lentigo senilis	Verruca vulgaris

Warning signs

- Rapid growth: diameter >5 mm
- Irregular pigmentation: blue, black, red discoloration
- Surface scaly, eroded, and/or blood-tinged

- Outline irregular, prominent, exophytic
- Sensitivity: itching, possible slight pain
- Surroundings: reddish border, satellites
- Frequent: longstanding skin blemish ("liver spot")

ABCD rule for melanoma: A = **A**symmetry
                              B = **B**orders (irregular)
                              C = **C**oloration (mottled or uneven)
                              D = **D**iameter (>5 mm)

Risk of metastasis (after Braun-Falco and Schmöckel)

- Approximately 5% if *diameter* <15 mm and *height* <1 mm
- Approximately 75% if *diameter* >15 mm and *height* >4 mm

- <10% if *tumor thickness* <0.75 mm and *mitotic index* <5 mitoses/mm^2
- Approximately 70% if *tumor thickness* >3.0 mm and *mitotic index* >13 mitoses/mm^2

Diagnosis:
- History (usually brief) and palpable findings, including regional lymph nodes.
- Biopsy.
- Tumor extent is established by radiographs of the skull and paranasal sinuses in various planes. Tomography or CT is indicated for some situations.

Differentiation is required from actinic keratosis, keratoacanthoma, basal cell carcinoma, and amelanotic melanoma.

Special Form:

Carcinoma of the Lip

Main symptoms: Most commonly affects the lower lip (lateral third) and is very rare in the upper lip. Peak occurrence is in the 7th–8th decades with a 10:1 preponderance of males.

Predisposition: Outdoor occupations involving prolonged ultraviolet exposure of the lower lip; also tar workers, glassblowers, smokers, alcoholics, and persons with poor oral hygiene. *Carcinoma of the lower lip* (usually well-differentiated squamous cell carcinoma) generally starts as a painless, slow-growing lesion that does not metastasize early. *Neoplasms of the upper lip* are more often basal cell carcinomas than squamous cell carcinomas, although the latter grow relatively swiftly on the upper lip, are occasionally painful, cause early function impairment, show relatively early regional metastasis, and have a poor prognosis.

Other symptoms and special features: Initially flat, adherent scale below which a gradually increasing induration of the lip tissue can be felt. There is relatively early superficial ulceration, but with a hard base. Lesions often develop on a background of leukoplakia. The affected lip is enlarged, and the mouth becomes distorted and difficult to close. Speech is impaired.

Causes: Besides other putative causes of cancer formation, those on the lip include actinic damage to skin and mucosae, tarry substances (smoking), rust, glassblowing work, and presumably poor oral and dental hygiene.

Diagnosis: Same as for basal cell carcinoma (see above).

Differentiation is required from leukoplakia, basal cell carcinoma (especially on the upper lip), keratoacanthoma, verruca vulgaris, Bowen disease, and syphilis chancre.

Malignant Melanoma

Main symptoms: Increase in the diameter, prominence, and/or dark coloration of a long-preexisting pigmented nevus. Also may develop as a small, dark (deep brown to bluish-black) macule on previously unblemished skin. "Satellite" lesions form in the area immediately surrounding the original pigmented spot. Swelling of regional lymph nodes. No pain. Twice as common in females as in males.

Other symptoms and special features: Malignant melanoma of the head region may occur on the scalp, ear, or neck. It is rare on the external nose but slightly more common in the nasal interior, especially the anterior septum.

Malignant melanomas also occur on the oral and pharyngeal mucosae. The rare amelanotic melanoma lacks the characteristic dark coloration, so conspicuous hyperpigmentation is not a strict criterion for malignant melanoma! Peak occurrence is in middle age (20–60 years).

Causes: Unknown. Many melanomas (about 30%) develop from a nevus cell nevus, about 20% from lentigo maligna, and some 10–20% arise in normal skin. Sunburn also may promote the development of malignant melanoma. A genetic predisposition is assumed.

Diagnosis:
* Dermatologic consultation should be sought at once if malignant melanoma is suspected!
* Biopsy is not advised, as it may promote metastasis.
* Prognosis and treatment depend critically on the diameter and depth of invasion of malignant melanoma. *The Clark level of invasion* was initially used to define prognosis, but the *Breslow thickness* appears to be more reliable.

Differential diagnosis is left to the dermatologist, because there are numerous pigmented skin tumors that are not malignant and because biopsy is contraindicated for malignant melanoma. The cutaneous lesions of greatest differential diagnostic importance are listed in Table 2.**6.**

Symptom   **Facial Paralysis**

The facial nerve (motor) and trigeminal nerve (mainly sensory) are responsible for innervation of the facial region in the strict sense. In a broader sense the facial innervation includes the cranial nerves responsible for the eye and its functions: II (optic nerve), III (oculomotor nerve), IV (trochlear nerve), and VI (abducens nerve). These nerves can have major differential diagnostic importance in otolaryngology by virtue of their close proximity.

Motor Paralysis and Other Functional Disturbances in the Facial Region

Facial Nerve

The *facial nerve* supplies *motor fibers* to the mimetic musculature, the auricular muscles, the posterior belly of the biventer muscle, the stylohyoid muscle, and the platysma. The sep-

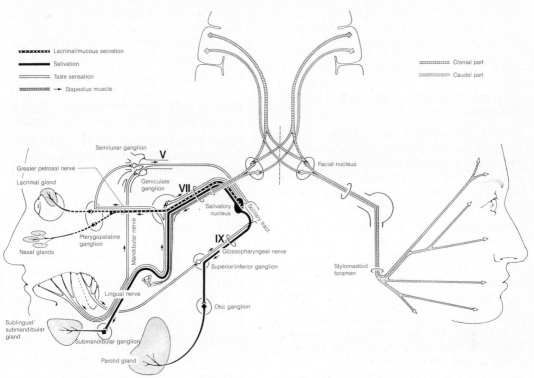

Fig. 2.**2**   Anatomy of the facial nerve (schematic) (from M. Mumenthaler: Neurologic Differential Diagnosis, 2nd ed. Thieme, Stuttgart 1992)

arate fiber bundle of the *nervus intermedius* supplies preganglionic, parasympathetic, secretomotor fibers to the lacrimal gland, nasal mucosal glands, and the submaxillary/sublingual salivary glands as well as gustatory fibers to the ipsilateral anterior two-thirds of the tongue. The course of these fibers is shown schematically in Figure 2.**2**, which shows the morphologic basis for the topognostic differential diagnosis of facial nerve lesions.

Facial paralysis may be classified by *degree* as *incomplete* or *complete*, by *duration* as *transient* or *permanent*, and by *site of lesion* as *peripheral* or *central*.

In central (supranuclear) paralysis, the frontal division of the facial nerve remains functionally intact because the *rostral* facial nucleus, responsible for upper facial movements, is supplied by *both* cortical fields whereas the *caudal*

nucleus, responsible for the middle and lower face, is supplied by the contralateral motor center only (Fig. 2.**2**).

In *peripheral* paralysis, it is clinically useful to distinguish between lesions located in the *intratemporal* portion of the facial nerve and those involving the *extratemporal* portion (see Fig. 2.**2**). Cases can be further classified by onset of paralytic symptoms as *sudden and complete* or *gradually progressive*, and pathologically according to the stage and severity of the nerve damage:

1. *Neurapraxia* (axons not disrupted. Reversible functional deficit: "conduction block").

2. *Axonotmesis* (partial or complete disruption of the axons with preservation of the connective tissue sheaths, i.e., the epineurium, perineurium, and endoneurium. Functional deficit is largely but not wholly reversible).

3. *Neurotmesis* (complete disruption of axons and their sheaths. Function loss is irreversible without surgical repair).

Principal Diagnostic Options in Facial Paralysis

Several physiologic and electrophysiologic methods are available for *functional testing* of the facial nerve. Generally these tests are performed in the sequence indicated to determine the site of the facial nerve lesion and assess its severity and prognosis:

○ *Peripheral/central differentiation:* With a central lesion, the frontal branch of the facial nerve is functionally intact (see above); with a peripheral nerve lesion proximal to the pes anserinus, all branches are generally affected.

○ *Test of the mimetic musculature:* Right and left sides are compared as the patient frowns, closes the eyes, whistles, bares the teeth, and wrinkles the nose.

○ a) *Taste testing* (see p. 293 for method): The chorda tympani provides the sensory innervation for the anterior two-thirds of the tongue. Corresponding loss of taste sensation implies a lesion above the origin of the chorda tympani in the fallopian canal, while preservation of function implies a lesion in the descending nerve segment peripheral to the second genu.
  b) *Salivary flow testing* has the same anatomic and physiologic rationale, for the submandibular and sublingual glands are likewise supplied by fibers from the chorda tympani. A small plastic tube is threaded into the submandibular duct (of Wharton) on each side, and the salivary output is separately collected and measured (with and without stimulation).

○ *Schirmer test:* Quantitative test of lacrimal secretion (using [litmus] filter paper strips). Reduced lacrimal secretion implies involvement of the greater petrosal nerve (origin of the lacrimal anastomosis in the geniculate ganglion) in the lesion (see Figs. 2.**2** and 4.**4**). A difference of 30% or more between the sides is considered pathologic.

○ *Stapedius reflex testing:* Loss of stapedius muscle function implies a lesion above the origin of the stapedius nerve (see Fig. 2.**2**). Method: see p. 57.

○ *Orbicularis oculi reflex:* If facial nerve function is intact, tapping the forehead with a finger or reflex hammer will evoke bilateral contraction of the orbicularis oculi muscle.

○ *Nerve excitability test (NET):* Determines the minimum current level (in mA) of 0.3-ms electrical impulses needed to elicit a muscle twitch. Two healthy facial nerves have approximately equal thresholds (about 0.4 mA), so a difference of 3.5 mA or more between the sides is considered pathologic. An increase in the threshold signifies progressive degeneration of the nerve fibers and implies a progressive axonotmesis. A valid result can be obtained 72−96 h after the injury. (*But*: Even with a complete nerve disruption, normal excitability may be registered in the peripheral nerve segment during the first 2−3 days!).

○ *Electromyography (EMG):* Muscle action potentials are recorded with needle electrodes during voluntary facial movement. The results of EMG are not rewarding before 12−14 days after the onset of paralysis, since denervation potentials do not appear before that time.

○ *Electroneurography (ENoG)* measures the summation action potentials of the facial muscles evoked by a contraction during maximal faradic stimulation. Comparison of the summation action potentials of the healthy and affected sides provides an approximate (quantitative) assessment (in %) of the number of damaged nerve fibers. The test is valid 24−48 h after onset of paralysis.

○ Adjunctive parameters (not routinely assessed):
  − *Determination of rheobase:* The rheobase is the lowest current level (in mA) that still evokes a visible muscle twitch. The rheobase is increased (or infinite) when axonotmesis is present (see p. 151).
  − *Determination of chronaxy:* The chronaxy is the shortest electrical impulse (in ms) that can evoke a visible muscle twitch at a constant current level (= twice the

rheobase value). The chronaxy is prolonged (or infinite) when axonotmesis is present. The test is valid from the very onset of paralysis.

Idiopathic Facial Paralysis (Bell Palsy, "Rheumatic" or "Cryptogenic" Facial Paralysis)

Main symptoms: Complete or incomplete, generally unilateral peripheral facial nerve paralysis developing within hours. About 50% of patients have initial and/or accompanying pain in the mastoid region (tenderness at the stylomastoid foramen). Paralysis that is incomplete initially, may become complete within a few days. Some 30% of cases show disturbance of taste sensation or some degree of of fine hearing impairment (dysacusis or hyperacusis). There is no fever or malaise.

Other symptoms and special features: Peak occurrence is in middle age. Complete paralysis is marked by inability to wrinkle the forehead, close the eye, and purse the lips. On attempted eye closure, the eye rolls upward (The Bell phenomenon). Orbicularis oculi reflex is absent. The corner of the mouth sags on the affected side, and the patient has difficulty drinking, eating, and speaking.

Cause: Poorly understood; presumably relates to disturbances of the microcirculation secondary to neurotropic viral infection. A diabetic metabolic state or hypertension is often present as an "accompanying" disorder.

Diagnosis:
- Typical negative history. Exclude an otogenic (see p. 36) or neurologic cause (see Table 2.7).
- Site-of-lesion determination (see Table 2.8).
- Electrodiagnostic baseline examination and follow-ups.

Differentiation is required from otogenic and all symptomatic peripheral facial nerve palsies (see Table 2.7). Also from tumors involving or adjacent to the nerve, and late paralysis following temporal bone fractures.

Melkersson–Rosenthal Syndrome

Main symptoms: Triad of recurrent facial nerve paralysis (usually complete), ipsilateral facial swelling (especially the upper lip, cheilitis), and fissured tongue.

Other symptoms and special features: Often there is severe facial pain, especially during development of the edematous phase. Later there is complete recovery of nerve function, followed in recurrent cases by increasing signs of permanent residual effects (concomitant movements and contractures). Familial occurrence.

Cause: Unknown.

Diagnosis: Verification of the characteristic triad (occasionally accompanied by hyperhidrosis and megacolon!) and electrodiagnostic facial nerve testing.

Traumatic Facial Paralysis

Main symptoms: Incomplete or complete peripheral paralysis following (immediately or after an asymptomatic interval of 1–10 days) a basal skull fracture, especially a transverse or longitudinal temporal bone fracture (see p. 39, Fig. 1.4, and Table 1.12). Also may result from mandibular fractures, blast injuries, gunshot injuries, stab wounds, lacerations, or surgical trauma (ear or parotid surgery). Blunt or sharp soft-tissue injuries of the face, unless concentrated in the parotid region, usually affect only *individual* facial nerve branches.

Diagnosis:
- Detailed, comprehensive documentation of cranial injuries including complete cranial nerve status.
- Imaging studies: Radiography (skull base and ear region). Delineation of the intratemporal facial nerve course using high-resolution CT; occasionally MRI may be helpful (see Fig. 1.3).
- Electrodiagnostic facial nerve testing (see p. 152 ff.) with detailed documentation of initial findings. Many cases of traumatic facial paralysis are missed on initial examination!

Infectious Facial Paralysis (Nonotogenic)

Approximately 60% incidence following *(herpes) zoster infection* (see p. 4) (herpetic vesicles may not be confined to the ear region, but

Table 2.**7** *Symptom* Paralysis or other functional disturbance of the facial nerve

Synopsis	

Peripheral paralysis

"Idiopathic" facial paralysis (Bell palsy)

Melkersson–Rosenthal syndrome

(Post)traumatic paralysis (including surgical injury to the intra- or extratemporal portion of the facial nerve)

Otogenic paralysis, see p. 36 and Table 1.**11**

Infectious (*non*otogenic) paralysis

- Viral infections, e.g., coxsackie, measles, mumps, rubella, EBV, herpes simplex, herpes zoster, varicella
- Bacterial infection, e.g., meningitis, encephalitis
- Lyme disease, see pp. 66, 155

Parotitis and parotid tumors, see p. 298 ff.

Paralysis due to acute and chronic polyneuropathies*

Paralysis due to metabolic disorders (diabetes, uremia, hyperthyroidism)*

Paralysis due to various diseases such as polyarteriitis nodosa, Wegener granulomatosis, sarcoidosis (Heerfordt syndrome), Paget disease, osteopetrosis (Albers-Schönberg syndrome), amyloidosis, porphyria, malignant hypertension

Paralysis due to space-occupying and/or destructive lesions in perineural soft-tissues of the face, lateral cranium, and upper neck

Paralysis due to space-occupying and/or destructive extra- or intracranial lesions

Congenital paralysis (also occurring as central paralysis, e.g., in Moebius syndrome)

Bilateral occurrence in:
- Cranial polyradiculitis (Guillain–Barré)*
- Cephalic tetanus*
- Meningeal diseases (inflammation, carcinosis)*
- Head trauma (severe bilateral basal fracture)
- Multiple sclerosis
- Neuritis multiplex (e.g., leprosy)*

Central paralysis (*) due to:
- Cerebral insult
- Head trauma
- Encephalitis
- Intracranial tumor

Possible *bilateral* occurrence in
- Poliomyelitis
- Progressive paralysis
- Moebius syndrome (congenital)

Special forms

Involuntary facial movements

Facial spasm

Blepharospasm

Facial tic

Psychogenic paralysis

Facial myokymia

Faciobuccolingual dystonia*

Chorea*

Poverty of facial expression

Parkinsonism*

Depression*

Pseudobulbar paralysis*

Loss of facial muscle tone (bilateral)

Myopathy*

* No further commentary

---

also may occur on the oral mucosa and/or tongue).

If cranial nerves other than the facial nerve are involved by the (herpes) zoster infection (e.g., cranial nerves V, VI, VIII, IX, X, or XII) the *Ramsey–Hunt syndrome* (herpes geniculatum syndrome) is said to be present. *Peak occurrence:* 5th–7th decades. CSF examination in the acute stage shows mild to moderate pleocytosis (several 100/3 cells; see Table 1.**15**). Peripheral facial paralysis occurs in other *viral diseases* such as coxsackievirus, rubella, infectious mononucleosis (EBV), and herpes simplex. The same applies to *bacterial* and *other microbial inflammations* that spread to the nerve from nearby tissues.

Table 2.**8**   Site-of-lesion determination in facial nerve paralysis (from D. Schmidt, J.-P. Malin: Erkrankungen der Hirnnerven. Thieme, Stuttgart 1986)

Site of lesion	Clinical manifestations (see Fig. 2.**2**)
Periphery (distal to pes anserinus)	Loss of individual facial nerve branches marginal branch, zygomatic branches, buccal branches, frontal branch)
Distal to stylomastoid foramen	Paralysis of facial muscles without taste disturbance, auditory dysfunction, or salivation disturbance (chorda tympani not involved)
Proximal to origin of chorda tympani and distal to origin of stapedius nerve	Paralysis of facial muscles with disturbance of taste and salivation (involvement of chorda tympani)
Proximal to origin of stapedius nerve and distal to origin of greater petrosal nerve	Paralysis of facial muscles with disturbance of taste, salivation, and (mild) auditory dysfunction (stapedius nerve involvement)
Proximal to geniculate ganglion and origin of greater petrosal nerve	Paralysis of facial muscles with disturbance of taste, (mild) auditory dysfunction, and marked disturbance or loss of lacrimal and salivary gland secretions (involvement includes afferent parasympathetic fibers of the foregoing nerves)
In the pons or intradural facial nerve segment	Complete facial paralysis with involvement of additional cranial nerves. With pyramidal tract involvement in pons region: complete facial nerve paralysis with contralateral hemiplegia (hemiplegia alternans, Gubler's paralysis)
Central paralysis	Paralysis of the facial muscles *sparing* the upper face (see p. 151 and Fig. 2.**2**), usually combined with ipsilateral hemiplegia (lesion in the internal capsule)

Miscellaneous Causes
(see also Table 2.**7**)

Facial nerve paralysis may develop secondary to *basal meningitis* and *brain abscess*. The meningeal or intracranial symptoms in these cases are unmistakable. Unilateral or bilateral facial nerve paralysis is not unusual in *viral meningits* and *viral encephalitis* (secondary to rubella, measles, mumps, or varicella). This is also true of lymphocytic *meningoradiculitis*, caused by ticks and spirochetes (Lyme disease, see p. 66).

A number of *neurologic* diseases are associated with facial paralysis, including carcinomatous or leukemic *metastases* in the basal CSF spaces, acute and chronic ascending polyneuropathies (the *Guillain–Barré syndrome*), poliomyelitis, and syphilis.

Peripheral facial paralysis occasionally occurs as a manifestation of a *diabetic, porphyric,* or *"idiopathic" polyneuropathy*, or of polyneuropathy due to *drug toxicity* (alcohol, DDT, thalidomide, thallium, trichloroethylene, vincristine, etc.).

Congenital Facial Paralysis

This may result from obstetric trauma or from a true anomaly in the course of the facial nerve (see Table 1.**19**).

Facial Paralysis Caused by Tumors

The paralysis may be caused by a neuroma located in the nerve itself, by the pressure or infiltration of an adjacent tumor, or by tumor metastatizing to the facial nerve from a distant primary. Examples:

○ Facial nerve neuroma (see p. 39)
○ Acoustic neuroma (see p. 29)
○ Glomus jugulare tumor (see p. 29)
○ Meningioma, chordoma, etc.
○ Primary true cholesteatoma (epidermoid)
○ Various grades of carcinoma and sarcoma
○ Paget disease, fibrous dysplasia, von Recklinghausen disease (osteitis fibrosa)
○ Cereberal tumors

Special Form

Involuntary Facial Movements

Facial Spasm

Main symptoms: Paroxysmal, spasmodic, tonic–clonic muscle twitches limited strictly to the mimetic muscles supplied by the facial nerve. Bilateral occurrence is not uncommon. Symptoms tend to increase over time, possibly with irreversible contractures and paresis.

Other symptoms and special features: There may be prolonged asymptomatic intervals (weeks and months) or remissions, or the intervals between attacks may last only a few hours. Spasms may even occur during sleep. Peak occurrence is in the 5th–7th decades, with females predominating.

Cause: Unknown. Probably based on a central innervation disturbance of cranial nerve VII or mechanical irritation of the intracranial nerve segment by adjacent blood vessels (cerebellopontine angle).

Diagnosis:
● Typical history and clinical presentation.
● Function testing of the facial nerve.
● Neurologic consultation.

Differentiation is required from blepharospasm and facial tic.

Blepharospasm

Main symptoms: Spasmodic contraction of the orbicularis oculi muscle, generally bilateral, varying in degree from a mild "winking tic" to a persistent, spastic, bilateral lid closure.

Other symptoms and special features: Blepharospasm may be combined with buccofacial dyskinesias *(The Meige syndrome)* and thus may resemble facial spasm.

Causes: An extrapyramidal lesion is assumed.

Diagnosis: Established mainly by electromyography (spontaneous, synchronous, rhythmic, or arhythmic series of single or clustered discharges). Workup includes EMG measurement of the orbicularis oculi reflex.

Facial Tic

Main symptoms: Involuntary muscle contractions occurring at varying sites on the face.

Causes: presumably psychogenic, as it is most commonly observed in nervous or neurotic individuals.

Facial Myokymia

Main symptoms: Involuntary periorbital muscle contractions of varying location and intensity; may affect the entire half of the face. Undulating contractions continue during sleep. They are not limited to muscles supplied by the facial nerve!

Cause: Unknown. May occur in setting of multiple sclerosis, also in patients with polyneuropathies and brainstem tumors.

Diagnosis: Electromyography shows typical double discharges of motors units ("doublets") at a regular frequency. The interference pattern is normal during voluntary movement.

Sensory Disturbances in the Facial Region

Trigeminal Nerve

In contrast to the most common functional disturbance, *trigeminal neuralgia* (see p. 159), other paresthesias, dysesthesias, anesthesias, and trophic and motor disturbances of the trigeminal nerve (trigeminal neuropathy) are relatively rare and usually have less prominent clinical features. For the most part, these disorders fall within the domain of the neurologist. They may be important in otolaryngologic diagnosis, however, so the most important aspects are mentioned here and the most frequent causes are listed in Table 2.**9**. The sensory component of the trigeminal nerve (taste) is considered in the section on Anomalies of Taste (see p. 291). See also Figures 3.**1** and 4.**4**.

Procedures for Testing Trigeminal Nerve Function

○ *Sensory testing* (touch, temperature [warm and cold], superficial pain; test and compare both sides!) on the face; may include the tongue, nasal mucosa, and nasopharynx.

○ *Corneal reflex test* (touching the inferior border of the cornea with a cotton wisp from the side should evoke eyelid closure). Loss of the reflex implies damage to the first division of the trigeminal nerve.

○ *Orbicularis oculi reflex* (when the facial and trigeminal nerves are functionally intact, tapping the forehead with a finger or reflex hammer evokes bilateral contraction of the orbicularis oculi muscles).

Table 2.**9**   Trigeminal neuropathy

Possible causes or antecedents of trigeminal neuropathy:
- Acoustic neuroma (<1%)
- Multiple sclerosis (approximately 2%)
- Lesion of gasserian ganglion (surgery, trauma, infection, etc.)
- Damage by adjacent vessels (intracranial portion of nerve)
- Facial injuries
- Surgical procedures (on the face, nose, or paranasal sinuses, intraoral)
- Dental procedures
- Alcohol injection into the nerve or gasserian ganglion
- Tumors of the skull base and facial skeleton

Trigeminal neuropathy can also occur *idiopathically* and in the setting of a *polyneuropathy* (e. g., due to intoxication, encephalitis, herpes zoster, etc.)

○ *Masseter reflex* (tapping the chin while the mouth is open evokes reflex contraction of the masseter muscles).
○ *Electromyography* may be used for the objective assessment of masseter innervation.

In all cases the results should be confirmed by a neurologist and interpreted within the framework of the neurologic consultation.

Symptom   **Facial Pain and Headache**

Drawing a strict distinction between *facial pain* and *headache* is problematic because both symptoms frequently overlap and may have a common cause. Another difficulty is that the face is part of the head, and "facial" pain can coexist with pain elsewhere about the head (e.g., the oral cavity, pharynx, ear, etc.).

Given the multitude of potential causes of facial pain and headache, our present scope calls for a selection of causative disorders that is tailored to the needs of the otolaryngologist but also takes into account aspects and relationships that are "outside" the ENT specialty.

The *nomenclature* and *classification* of headache are poorly standardized,* although several terms are used with universal comprehension: *neuralgia* for paroxysmal pain corresponding to a specific nerve distribution; *localized pain* for pain that cannot be assigned to a

---

* A classification published by the International Headache Society in 1988 still requires more practical testing and general acceptance. Thus we chose not to use it in this presentation, especially since it disregards the Bing–Horton syndrome and other terms employed in clinical use.

specific nerve but whose boundaries are well-defined; *referred pain* for pain that is perceived at a site other than that in which it originates; and *prosopalgia* for facial neuralgia that strikes paroxysmally with a highly variable incidence and is accompanied by marked vasomotor–autonomic symptoms.

Principal Diagnostic Methods

Unless headache symptoms are clearly referable to a cause in his field, the otorhinolaryngologist evaluating headache or facial pain must consider a broad and diverse diagnostic spectrum that includes many disorders in neighboring specialties, as shown in Table 2.**10**. Our present scope limits the depth of our exploration of differential diagnoses in other specialties, but we can appreciate the far-reaching interrelationships by taking note of cardinal symptoms and basic diagnostic options.

o A very thorough *history* is essential in the evaluation of head and facial pain. It can lead to a correct diagnosis more quickly than the concentrated but indiscriminate application of many "high-tech" studies! Questions should focus on the *total duration* of the patient's symptoms; the *frequency*, *timing*, and *duration* of attacks (when pain is episodic); the *location, character, dynamics*, and *intensity* of the pain; objective and subjective *associated symptoms*; *external factors* that precipitate, accentuate, or mitigate the symptoms; the patient's *occupational*, private, and family *situation*; previous or accompanying diseases; *drug use* (including prescription drugs, alcohol, tobacco, and caffeine); and whether there is a *family history of headache*.

o The otorhinolaryngologist then proceeds with a thorough *ENT clinical examination* focusing on the nose, paranasal sinuses, and ear. The examination includes *radiographs* of the paranasal sinuses, petrous pyramid, and possibly cranial films and cervical spine views. *Tomography, CT* and/or *MRI* may be needed for the complete evaluation of some cases.

o The workup includes testing for *tenderness at nerve exit sites* on the skull (including the occipital nerves!), *blood pressure*, standard laboratory tests *(urinary sugars, ESR, blood*

count), palpation of the temporal arteries, and possibly *olfactory testing*.

o with negative ENT findings, the examiner can look for additional symptoms by following the sequence in Table 2.**10**, unless the symptoms accompanying the pain clearly point in a particular direction.

The use of *electroencephalography, echoencephalography, radionuclide brain scanning, CSF examination* (cell count, protein, sugar, immune-specific constituents; CSF scintigraphy, etc.), *sonography*, and *arteriography* is generally determined by the result of neurologic consultation. Consultation with other specialists (internist, ophthalmologist, dentist or oral surgeon, etc.), if indicated, will similarly determine the need for more specific diagnostic procedures.

Ear, Nose, and Throat Diseases

Relevant otorhinolaryngologic disorders are discussed elsewhere, as indicated by the page references in Table. 2.**10**.

Dental and Jaw Diseases

See Table 2.**10**.

Inflammatory Diseases of the Teeth, Periodontium, Jaws, and Surrounding Soft Tissues

Main symptoms: Tenderness and/or temperature sensitivity of individual teeth, localized pain (momentary, transitory, or sustained). History, local findings, radiographs.

Temporomandibular Joint Disorders

Main symptoms: Pain in the TMJ radiating to the face and temple. Possible crepitation on jaw movement, usually bilateral. Palpable and radiographic findings.

Costen Syndrome (TMJ Arthropathy)

Main symptoms: Unilateral attacks of pain in the preauricular area, over the TMJ, or in the ear. Malocclusion and occlusal dysfunction. Radiograph shows "set-back condyle."

Myoarthropathies

See p. 17.

Ophthalmic Disorders

(See Table 2.**10**)

Asthenopia and Disturbances of Accommodation

Main symptoms: Dull ache around the eyes with lacrimation, burning, and fatigue, tends to follow strenuous use of the eyes (reading, etc.). Blurred vision or diplopia. Frontal headache.

Inflammatory Eye Diseases

Acute Glaucoma

Main symptoms: Severe, paroxysmal headache and ocular pain, often commencing toward evening; red, painful eye; increased intraocular pressure; severe malaise; vomiting. Visual impairment. Fixed pupil. Tense globe.

Chronic Glaucoma

Main symptoms: Concentric narrowing of visual field, occasional headache.

Optic Neuritis

Main symptoms: Decreased vision, pain on eye movement, pain in the orbit, forehead, and temple. Decreased pupillary response.

Ophthalmoplegic Migraine

Main symptoms: Attacks of facial pain preceded or accompanied by flittering scotomata for approximately 10–20 min. Photophobia.

Tolosa–Hunt Syndrome (Ophthalmoplegia)

Main symptoms: Constant, severe retrobulbar pain radiating to the forehead and temple. Palsy of eye muscles.

Ocular Myositis

Main symptoms: Combination of ptosis, exophthalmos, lid endema and/or chemosis; severe ocular pain, conjunctival irritation.

Neuralgias

(See Table 2.**10**)

Trigeminal Neuralgia

Main symptoms: Sudden, very intense, lancinating pain with a tearing, stabbing, and boring quality (unilateral) in the distribution of the maxillary (second) or mandibular (third) division of the trigeminal nerve. Pain involves the ophthalmic (first) division in only 5% of cases. Attack is brief, lasting seconds to minutes, and is precipitated by stimulation of typical trigger zones (skin of cheek, oral mucosa, nasolabial groove, corner of mouth).

Other symptoms and special features: Between attacks there is generally no pain or, rarely, a constant, dull pain. Peak occurrence is in the 6th–8th decades, and women are more commonly affected. Most patients experience many attacks per day, but remissions lasting months or years may occur. "Tic douloureux" refers to the twitches and distortions of the mimetic muscles that occur during attacks. The affected area is always the same but may enlarge over time to involve multiple trigeminal nerve divisons. There is an anxious "favoring" of facial and oral musculature!

Causes: Not fully understood for the *idiopathic* (true) form. The *symptomatic* form is secondary to diseases of the paranasal sinuses, teeth, and jaws; central lesions that irritate the nerve divisions, roots, or semilunar ganglion; and posttraumatic nerve lesions.

Diagnosis:
● Otorhinolaryngologic examination to exclude rhinogenic disease (including evaluation of jaws and dentition).
● Radiographs of the paranasal sinuses, jaws, and teeth. Consider the Gradenigo syndrome!
● Neurologic examination is usually normal between attacks, but typical symptoms occur during an attack, or after an attack has been

Table 2.**10** *Symptom* Facial pain and headache (causes)

Synopsis

Ear, nose, and throat diseases

○ *Nose and paranasal sinuses*

Inflammatory conditions of the external nose (furuncle, herpes zoster, etc.) see p. 173 ff.

(Massive) intranasal obstruction (e.g., septal deformities, turbinate hypertrophy, polyposis, adhesions, foreign bodies), see p. 199 ff.

Acute and chronic rhinopathies (inflammatory, vasomotor, allergic), see p. 182

Disturbances of ventilation and/or drainage in the paranasal sinus system (positive or negative pressure), see pp. 179, 180

Sinusitis (maxillary, ethmoid, frontal, sphenoid) and other paranasal sinus diseases, see pp. 179, 189

Posttraumatic state, see p. 180

Rhinogenic suppurative complications, see p. 210

Atrophic rhinitis and ozena, see p. 206

Tumors (benign and malignant) of the paranasal sinuses, see p. 214 ff.

○ *Ear*

Inflammatory conditions of the external ear and external auditory canal, see p. 3 ff.

Various forms of otitis, see p. 8 ff.

Gradenigo syndrome, see p. 14

Otogenic suppurative complications, see p. 40

Tumors (benign and malignant), see p. 28 ff.

Otalgias (nervus intermedius, facial nerve, glossopharyngeal nerve, vagus nerve, greater auricular nerve) see p. 15

Sluder syndrome, see p. 162

○ *Mouth and pharynx*

Tonsilitis and peritonsillar abscess, see pp. 229, 233 ff.

Tonsillogenic complications, see p. 262

Neuralgias (e.g., of nerves IX and X), see p. 162

Styloid syndrome (stylalgia, Eagle syndrome), see p. 234

Dentogenic pain, see p. 235

Tumors (including nasopharyngeal tumors), see pp. 214, 218

○ *Salivary gland diseases*, see Table 5.**1**

Dental and jaw diseases

Inflammatory diseases of the teeth, periodontium, and surrounding tissues; difficult dentition; denture pressure sores, etc., see p. 237

Maxillomandibular osteitis or osteomyelitis, see pp. 141, 144

Mandibular arthritis, see pp. 17, 13

Osteoarthritis

Costen syndrome (dysfunctional), see p. 158

Myoarthropathy (dysfunctional), see p. 17

Tumors (benign and malignant), see p. 214

Ophthalmic disorders

Asthenopia (refractive error), e.g., hyperopia, astigmatism, anisometropia

Muscular asthenopia (extraocular muscle strain, e.g., due to latent strabismus, faulty convergence, fusion disturbances)

Disturbances of accommodation, e.g., presbyopia, accommodative paralysis or spasms

Ocular disorders in the strict sense such as corneal foreign body, keratitis, iridocyclitis, glaucoma, scleritis, optic neuritis, ophthalmoplegic migraine. Also ophthalmic zoster, Tolosa–Hunt syndrome (ophthalmoplegia), myositis of eye muscles

Table 2.**10**   (cont.)

Synopsis

Neuralgias

Trigeminal neuralgia

Nasociliary neuralgia (Charlin syndrome)

Pterygopalatine ganglion neuralgia (Sluder syndrome)

Geniculate ganglion neuralgia (nervus intermedius) (Hunt neuralgia), see p. 15

Auriculotemporal neuralgia, see p. 16

Glossopharyngeal neuralgia

Vagus neuralgia (including superior laryngeal nerve)

Neuralgia of occipital nerves

Atypical facial pain ("sympathalgia")

Neck, Nuchal Area, and Occiput

Occipital pain, see p. 163 and Table 10.**2**

Dysgenesis (platybasia, basilar impression), see p. 18

Vertebragenic or spondylogenic pain and cervical syndromes, see p. 393

Whiplash injury including trauma to cervical spine, see p. 392

Tension headache

Intracranial causes

o *Vasomotor phenomena*

Vasomotor headache

Posttraumatic (postconcussional) status

"Ice cream," "hot dog," and "Chinese restaurant" headache

(True) migraine

Erythroprosopalgia (cluster headaches, Bing–Horton neuralgia)

o *Vascular anomalies* (dysgeneses, abnormal vascular courses, aberrant vascular loop syndrome, aneurysms)*

o *Pressure changes*

Head trauma

Intracranial edema

Intracranial hemorrhage (epidural, subdural, subarachnoid, tumoral hemorrhage, aneurysms, massive hemorrhage)*

Meningitis. diffuse encephalitis, brain abscess, sinus thrombosis, see p. 40ff.

Ischemia (stroke)*

Intracranial tumors*

Impaired CSF circulation (production disturbance or fistula formation with low CSF pressure; outflow obstruction,e. g., hydrocephalus, posttraumatic, postoperative)

o *Organic brain diseases of varying etiology**

Miscellaneous causes

Temporal arteritis (cranial arteritis, giant cell arteritis)

Carotidynia

Intoxication and drug intolerance (see Table 2.**12**)

Symptoms accompanying medical disorders such as infectious diseases, febrile states, hematologic disorders, disturbances of circulatory regulation (especially hypertensive crises but also hypotension), hepatogenic headache, metabolic disorders (e. g., hypoglycemia)*

Altitude sickness*

Alcohol abuse*

Nicotine abuse*

Caffeine withdrawal*

Overexertion*

Sleep deficit*

Psychic factors, psychoses, neuroses, neoplasms and their background symptoms*

Working conditions

* No further commentary

incited by stimulating a trigger zone (chewing, talking, moving the tongue, touching the facial skin, washing, laughing, etc.).

Differentiation is required from the Charlin syndrome, sluder neuralgia, auriculotemporal neuralgia, and possibly glossopharyngeal neuralgia. Multiple sclerosis, brain stem or cerebellar lesions.

Nasociliary (Charlin) Neuralgia

Main symptoms: Paroxysmal, unilateral pain in the lateral nose (external and internal) and sometimes in the eye near the medial canthus, combined with swelling of the ipsilateral nasal mucosa, conjunctival irritation, and lacrimation. Possible erythema in the medial canthal area. Spontaneous ocular pain and tenderness. *Ophthalmic symptoms are predominant.*

Other symptoms: Triggers zones (medial canthus of eye, nasal interior) are sometimes identifiable.

Cause: Not definitely known. Presumably based on a lesion of the ciliary ganglion.

Diagnosis:
● First exclude disease of the nose, paranasal sinuses, eye and orbit.
● Typical symptoms during the attack. An attack can sometimes be stopped by dabbing the nasal mucosa in the area of the agger nasi with a 5% procaine solution.

Differentiation is required from trigeminal neuralgia, Sluder neuralgia, and sinusitis.

Pterygopalatine Ganglion Neuralgia (Sluder Syndrome, "Lower Half Headache")

Main symptoms: Similar to those of nasociliary neuralgia (see above), but affecting a larger area on one side of the face. Pain, occurring mostly at night, radiates from the nasal dorsum and root and the nasal interior across the orbit and maxilla, sometimes extending to the temple and mastoid. Also sneezing (characteristic!) and ipsilateral coryza. *Rhinologic symptoms are predominant.*

Other symptoms and special features: Profuse lacrimation; females are more commonly affected.

Cause: Presumably based on irritation of the pterygopalatine ganglion, e.g., by inflammatory processes in neighboring tissues (paranasal sinuses, orbit). See Figure 3.**4**.

Diagnosis:
● First exclude rhinologic and ophthalmologic disease.
● Similar problems as in Charlin neuralgia. A pain attack in the sluder syndrome can sometimes be stopped by anesthetizing the nasal mucosa adjacent to the ganglion in the posterior portion of the middle meatus of the nose (confirms diagnosis!).

Differentiation is required from trigeminal neuralgia, nasociliary neuralgia, and sinusitis.

Geniculate Ganglion Neuralgia (Hunt Syndrome)

See p. 15.

Auriculotemporal Neuralgia

See p. 16.

Glossopharyngeal Neuralgia

Main symptoms: Very severe, paroxysmal, lancinating pain in the area of the pharynx, the base and border of the tongue, the tonsils, and the soft palate. An attack, lasting up to 30 s, is triggered by stimulation of the hypopharynx (eating, talking, etc.). Most common in older patients. See Figure 3.**1b**.

Other symptoms and special features: Radiation of pain to the lower jaw and ear ("pain strikes like a flame from the ear"). The head is typically canted toward the *healthy* side! See also stylalgia, p. 234. There may be concomitant involvement of vagus-innervated areas (cardiac arrhythmia, syncope, epileptiform attacks).

Causes: Unclear.

Diagnosis: Characteristic symptom pattern, obvious trigger zone. Normal neurologic findings between attacks.

Differentiation is required from mandibular and auriculotemporal neuralgia, Hunt neuralgia, organic lesions of the lower cranial nerves, and stylalgia (the Eagle syndrome).

Vagus Neuralgia

Main symptoms: Similar to glossopharyngeal neuralgia (both nerves are closely intertwined). The sensory portions of the vagus nerves (superior laryngeal nerve and auricular branch) are chiefly affected with corresponding pain over the lateral neck from the ear to the sternum. Pain may occur in attacks lasting seconds or as a more prolonged ache. Marked tenderness is noted at the entry point of the superior laryngeal nerve in the hypothyroid membrane.

Other symptoms and special features: Radiation of pain to the ear. Pain is paroxysmal, tends to occur at night, and may be triggered by swallowing, coughing, or yawning. See Figure 3.**1b**.

Causes: Unknown. *But:* Neuralgiform symptoms of irritation of the auricular branch of the vagus nerve (otalgia) are common with pharyngeal and laryngeal tumors!

Diagnosis:
● Typical tenderness of the laryngeal nerve in the hyothyroid membrane and of the deep lateral cervical soft tissues anterior to the sternocleidomastoid muscle at the level of the greater cornu of the hyoid bone. (Tenderness at the latter site is often more pronounced than at the former.) Normal neurologic findings between attacks.
● Very through endoscopic examination to exclude a neoplasm of the pharynx, larynx, or esophagus!

Differentiation is required from symptomatic neuralgias (inflammatory lesions, malignant tumors of the pharynx, larynx, or esophagus), glossopharyngeal neuralgia, and Hunt neuralgia.

Occipital Neuralgia

Main symptoms: Pain, usually of long duration, radiating from the occiput over the top of the head to the forehead and eyes. Occasionally pain is confined to the occiput and nuchal area. Marked tenderness is noted at nerve exit site(s).

Causes: Unclear. Occipital neuralgia is often confused with vertebragenic pain or "tension headache" (see p. 164).

Diagnosis:
● The cardinal symptom is marked tenderness at occipital nerve exit points.
● Exclude vertebragenic headache (see p. 393) and subtentorial organic disease.
● Diagnostic aid: Pain is abolished by injecting procaine into the nerve exit points.

Differential diagnosis: See Tables 2.**11** and 10.**2**.

Atypical Facial Pain ("Sympathalgia")

Main symptoms: Deep, prolonged pain in the facial musculature, mainly at night. The pain cannot be localized to specific anatomic structures and is aggravated by states of exhaustion.

Other symptoms and special features: Vague symptomatology.

Causes: Variable. "Psychoautonomic lability" or endogenous depression is often a contributing factor.

Diagnosis: Exclusion of typical neuralgia or a localized organic cause. Neuropsychiatric consultation.

Differentiation is required from trigeminal neuralgia, the Sluder or Charlin syndromes, migraine, erythroprosopalgia, paranasal sinus diseases, and diseases of the teeth and jaws.

Neck, Nuchal Area, and Occiput

See Tables 2.**10**, 2.**11**, 10,**1**, 10.**2**, and 10.**3**.

Occipital Pain

Occipital pain can be caused by a variety of disorders, most notably *lesions of the cervical spine* and its musculotendinous structures, *tension headache, dysplasias of the craniocervical junction* (see p. 18), *subtentorial* organic diseases, and (less often than diagnosed) *occipital neuralgia* (see above). See also Table 2.**11**.

Vertebragenic (Spondylogenic) Headache

See p. 393.

Table 2.**11**   Differential diagnosis of occipital headache (from M. Mumemthaler, F. Regli: Der Kopfschmerz. Thieme, Stuttgart 1990)

Headache	Cause	Characteristics	Precipitating factors	Findings
Spondylogenic	Spondylosis, cervical discopathy, joint subluxations, anomaly at craniocervical junction	From occipital to frontal, often unilateral, possibly with brachalgia	Faulty posture, trauma	Decreased range of head motion, fixed position, tenderness of paravertebral muscles
"Occipital neuralgia"	Mechanical root irritation of C1 or C2; existence is questionable	Lightning-like onset, brief duration	Spontaneous	Localized tenderness at greater occipital nerve
Tension headache	Abnormal sustained contraction of nuchal muscles	Dull, deep pain that is increased by active postural maintenance and decreased by recumbency	Prolonged maintenance of faulty head posture; psychic tension	Tenderness of paravertebral nuchal muscles and their attachments; possible psychic conflict situation
Space-occupying lesion in the posterior cranial fossa	Tumor	More or less constant headache, intracranial pressure signs	Aggravated by straining	Cerebellar signs, signs of increased intracranial pressure

See also Table 10.**2**

Whiplash Injury and Other Cervical Spine Trauma

See p. 392.

Tension Headache ("Muscle Contraction" Headache, "Psychogenic" Headache)

Main symptoms: Dull, aching, nonpulsating pain usually starting in the occipitonuchal area and radiating to the frontotemporal areas and lasting for 1–6 days (though chronic cases may last months or years). The pain may feel like a clamp or constricting band around the head ("hatband" headache) and may be bilateral or confined to one side. Headache is typically present on waking in the morning.

Other symptoms: Irregular occurrence; brought on by physical and mental exertion, prolonged maintenance of an awkward body posture (job-related), as well as stress, excessive demands, emotional tension, and depres-

sion. Tenderness is most pronounced at the insertions of the nuchal muscles. Peak occurrence is from 15–40 years of age, with females predominating. The condition is very prevalent and may be accompanied by nausea, hypersensitivity to noise, photophobia, vomiting, etc. Recumbency tends to alleviate the pain.

Causes: Sustained contraction of the scalp and nuchal muscles due to various (somatic and psychological) causes. Neurotic or endogenous depression is frequently present as an underlying disorder.

Diagnosis:
● Exclude an ENT disorder and organic neurologic disease. Tenderness is noted along lines of muscular insertion and at pressure points (exit points of the occipital nerves; see also occipital neuralgia, p. 163, which can be very difficult to distinguish from tension headache!).
● Neurologic findings, laboratory results, radiographs, and EEG are usually normal.

• Sites of spasticity, myalgia, and myogelosis are identifiable in the neck and shoulder muscles. EMG shows sustained acitivity in the mimetic musculature.

• Analysis of patient's personality type and occupational and/or family situation may be rewarding. Psychiatric consultation is appropriate in some cases.

Differential diagnosis: See Table 2.**11**.

Intracranial Causes

(See Table 2.**10**)

Several types of *headache due to intracranial causes* can be identified on the basis of their course and underlying pathology:

○ *Vascular type:* Paroxysmal, sometimes throbbing, dull headache, mostly unilateral, with variable pain-free intervals. History spans a period of years. Associated vasomotor phenomena are often noted in the face. Examples: migraine, Bing–Horton syndrome, vasomotor headache.

○ *Hemorrhagic type:* Very severe, "bursting" headache of abrupt onset, often radiating down the neck and associated with nausea, vomiting, and nuchal stiffness. Impairment of consciousness is common but not always present. Example: subarachnoid hemorrhage.

○ *Mass type:* Dull, diffuse headache of consistent character and location, which gradually increases in severity and may increase acutely with a rise in intracranial pressure (e.g., changing the head or body position). Examples: brain tumor, brain abscess, "chronic" subdural hematoma).

Vasomotor Headache

Main symptoms: Chronic "hangover" headache, i.e., deep, diffuse pain localized mainly in the forehead, behind the eyes, in the temples, but possibly involving the whole cranium ("ring around the head"). Pain is aggravated by bending, straining, and physical exertion and becomes throbbing. Symptoms are terminated by sleep.

Other symptoms and special features: Intense pain is usually felt in the morning. Peak oc-currence is from 10–40 years of age (most common type of headache in school-age children!); 3:1 ratio of females to males. Headache is exacerbated by noise, shaking, prolonged sun exposure, and strenuous physical exertion. Frequently combined with other autonomic disturbances (circulatory, digestive, etc.).

Causes: Dysregulation of the intracranial vessels (dilatation) caused by exposure to various injurious agents.

Diagnosis: Neurologic and internal medical consultation are sought after exclusion of ENT disease. Vasomotor headache is closely related to, and on a continuum with, true migraine (see below) and tension headache.

Differentiation is required from true migraine, tension headache, sinusitis, hypertensive and hypotensive headache; drug abuse.

Posttraumatic (postconcussional) *headache* not based on a demonstrable organic lesion belongs to the same group, which also includes "foehn sickness" (headache and weariness brought on by "foehn" wind conditions in Central Europe).

Additional, rare forms of headache belonging to the vasomotor category are: a) *"ice cream" headache* occurring within 30 s after cold exposure of the palate and pharynx; b) *"hot dog" headache* caused by the ingestion of sodium nitrite; and c) *Chinese restaurant headache* caused by the ingestion of monosodium glutamate.

(True) Migraine

Main symptoms: Often preceded by an aura. Episodic, pounding headache, usually synchronous with the pulse, mostly affecting one side but at times changing to the opposite side. An attack may last hours to days. Photophobia, nausea, hypersensitivity to noise. Meteorotropia. Severe incapacitation.

Other symptoms and special features: Symptoms are very diverse and may involve the eyes, gastrointestinal tract, brain, etc. Positive family history is obtained in 60% of cases. Females predominate by a 4:1 ratio. Attacks often begin during puberty.

Table 2.**12**   Drugs and other chemical substances that frequently cause headache (selection)

Vasoactive drugs		**Miscellaneous drugs**	
– Carbenoxolone	– Nicotinic acid	– Amitriptyline	– MAO inhibitors
– Clonidine	– Nitrates (including oc-	– Barbiturates	– Meprobamate
– Caffeine	cupational exposure)	– Benzodiazepines	– Resochin
– Dipyramidol	– Nitrites (including oc-	– Iron compounds	– Saponins
– Ergotamine	cupational exposure)	– Glycosides	– Sulfonamides
(overdose)	– Norepinephrine	– Indomethacin	– Vitamins A and D
– Histamine	– Papaverine	– Isoniazide	
– Hydralazine	– Reserpine		
– Nifedipine	– Theophylline		

Hormones

- Contraceptives
- Progestins
- Androgens
- Glucocorticoids

Industrial toxins

- E.g., arsenic, lead, bromine, mercury, carbon monoxide, manganese, nitro compounds, hydrogen sulfide, carbon disulfide, thallium
- Also organic solvents such as benzine, benzol, xylene, carbon tetrachloride, chloroform

Central stimulants

- Metaphetamine
- Phenmetrazine
- Methylphenidate
- Pemoline
- Propylhexedrine
- Metrotonine

Other organic substances

- Ethyl and methyl alcohol
- Acetanilid
- Plant toxins
- Insecticides

Analgesics (with misuse)

- Phenacetin
- Pyrazol derivatives
- Pentazocine
- Mixed analgesics
- Acetylsalicylic acid and derivatives

Causes: Presumably based on faulty autonomic–humoral regulation of the intracranial vessels (serotonin, histamine, plasma kinins) with vasoconstriction in the prodromal phase and vasodilatation in the headache phase.

Diagnosis: Internal medical and neurologic consultation are sought after the exclusion of ENT disease ("symptomatic migraine").

Differentiation is required from vasomotor headache, tension headache, vertebragenic headache, erythroprosopalgia, and migrainoid headache based on organic disease.

Erythroprosopalgia (Cluster Headaches, Bing–Horton Neuralgia)

Main symptoms: Recurrent attacks (lasting 20–120 min) of very severe, boring or stabbing, unilateral pain of sudden onset localized to the orbit and temporal region and radiating to the frontal region and ear. Hypersensitivity of the scalp; redness of the ipsilateral eye and upper face and forehead.

Other symptoms: Lacrimation, rhinorrhea, nasal obstruction. Partial Horner symptom complex. Peak occurrence is from 20–40 years of age; males predominate by a 6:1 ratio. Attacks tend to commence at night (!) and occur in temporal clusters followed by remissions that may last for years. Attacks are precipitated by histamine or nitroglycerin.

Causes: Unclear. Upper cervical root compression is thought to be causative in some cases.

Diagnosis:
- Exclude ENT disease (which may function as a "trigger").

● Cranial radiographs, exclusion of orbital apex syndrome (see Table 1.**18**).

Differentiation is required from trigeminal neuralgia, migraine, and vasomotor headache (which is closely related nosologically to cluster headaches).

Intracranial Pressure Changes

See also Table 2.**10**. Headache may be a cardinal symptom of *increased intracranial pressure* due to an inflammatory, neoplastic, hemorrhagic or other cause. It can also be an important symptom of *reduced intracranial pressure* (abnormality of CSF production or circulation). Because characteristic neurologic symptoms dominate the clinical picture and the course of the disease in all these situations, it is unnecessary to discuss the individual relevant disorders in this context. The same applies to many organic nerve and brain disorders that are associated with headache and fall within the domain of the neurologist.

Miscellaneous Causes

Temporal Arteritis (Cranial Arteritis, Giant Cell Arteritis)

Main symptoms: Severe, sustained, dull, boring pain in the temporal region, usually undulating or throbbing, generally starting on one side and spreading to involve both sides. With disease of the temporal artery, the latter is very prominent, tortuous, hard, extremely tender, and nonpulsatile.

Other symptoms and special features: Other arteries of the head also may be involved, so there may be associated facial nerve paralysis and inner ear symptoms. Usually there is severe malaise, which may include fever and anemia. Peak occurrence is from 55–80 years of age, and females are more commonly affected than males. Episodic course. Rheumatoid polymyalgia is an occasinal precursor. High risk of blindness (opticomalacia!).

Causes: Generalized inflammatory vascular disease (giant cell panarteritis), presumably with an autoimmune basis (see Table 4.**29**).

Diagnosis:
● Condition is easily diagnosed by palpation when the temporal artery is affected.
● Biopsy of the vessel wall confirms the diagnosis.
● Associated findings: Generally there is marked elevation of the ESR with leukocytosis and often anemia. Involvement of other vessels (ophthalmic artery, occipital artery, subclavian artery, etc.) is demonstrable by Doppler sonography, digital subtraction angiography, etc.
● Serum electrophoresis: increase in α-2 globulin and β globulin, fall of albumin.
● Ophthalmologic and/or neurologic consultation may be indicated.

Differentiation is required from otologic disease, protracted migraine, arteriosclerosis, and intracranial disease.

Carotidynia

Main symptoms: Throbbing pain along one side of the neck from lower jaw to clavicle, lasting from minutes to several hours. Tenderness over the carotid artery, which may show increased pulsations. Females predominate. A rare disorder!

Intoxication and Drug Intolerance

Headache is a relatively constant feature of a number of acute and especially chronic intoxication with organic and inorganic substances. It is also a common symptom of drug intolerance or abuse. Because all patients have associated neurologic (mainly central nervous) symptoms and most have visceral symptoms that dominate the clinical picture, the otorhinolaryngologist rarely plays a pivotal role in the diagnosis of intoxication in headache patients. Nevertheless, there are a number of insidious, oligosymptomatic cases of intoxication in which headache represents an early warning sign, so it is important that this cause be considered and excluded in the otorhinolaryngologic differential diagnosis. "Thinking of it" can be half the diagnosis!

Medications and chemical substances that frequently cause headache are listed in Table 2.**12**.

Headache and Working Conditions
(After Müller—Limmroth)

○ Unfavorable working posture of the head and neck (e.g., during prolonged keyboard or monitor work and during work in unaccustomed positions) (see Tension Headache, p. 164)
○ Insufficient or improper lighting at the workplace
○ Excessive noise levels
○ Unfavorable room climate (humidity, O_2 deficiency, temperature, drafts)
○ Air impurities (vapors, gases, suspended particles, etc.)
○ Sustained stressful situation
○ Intellectual overload

Syndromes Involving the Facial Region

The more common *malformation syndromes* of the facial region are reviewed in Table 2.**13**.

Other *non-dysgenetic syndromes* in the facial region:

○ Angioneurotic syndromes (Quincke edema), see p. 143
○ Orbital apex syndrome, see Table 1.**18**
○ Bing—Horton syndrome (erythroprosopalgia), see p. 166

○ Heerfordt syndrome, see Table 5.**8**
○ Hunt syndrome (geniculate ganglion neuralgia), see p. 15
○ (Pierre—)Marie syndrome (acromegaly), see p. 138
○ Melkersson—Rosenthal syndrome, see p. 153
○ Raeder syndrome, see Table 1.**18**
○ Cavernous sinus syndrome, see Table 1.**18**

Table 2.**13**   Common facial malformation syndromes (after Leiber and Olbrich)

Name of syndrome	Classification	Typical ENT deficits	Other symptoms and comments
Apert syndrome	Acrosphenosyndactyly	Hypertelorism, oxycephaly, possible choanal atresia and/or nasal cleft; exophthalmos; possible conductive hearing loss (stapes ankylosis); micrognathia, possible cleft palate	Syndactyly, "spoon" hand and foot. Possible debilitation
Binder syndrome	Arhinencephaloid midfacial hypoplasia, maxillonasal hypoplasia	Short, flat-bridged nose with narrow nostrils; pseudoprogenia	
Chotzen syndrome	Cranio-oculodental syndrome	Asymmetry of cranium and face, ptosis, strabismus. Hypertelorism, maxillary hypoplasia. Low-set ears	Syndactyly
Christ–Siemens–Touraine syndrome	Hypotrichotic anhidrosis with hypodontia	Dry skin and mucosae. Hypofunction of mucous glands. Features of atrophic rhinitis	Dysplasia and aplasia of teeth. Aplasia of nails. More common in males

Table 2.**13**   (cont.)

Name of syndrome	Classification	Typical ENT deficits	Other symptoms and comments
Crouzon syndrome	Craniofacial dysostosis	Frontotemporal broadness, acrocephaly, parrot nose, maxillary hypoplasia, dental position abnormalities, cleft palate. Conductive or occasional mixed hearing loss	Oxycephaly. Divergent strabismus. See alsoTable 1.**43**
Down syndrome	Mongolism, trisomy 21	Typical facial morphology, typical facial expression, epicanthus, button nose, scrotal cheilitis, possible sialorrhea. Frequent auricular dysplasia with conductive hearing loss. Sensorineural hearing loss may occur. Macroglossia	Often combined with mental retardation, brachycephaly
Franceschetti–Zwahlen (Treacher Collins) syndrome	Mandibulofacial dysostosis	Lateral coloboma of eyelid, antimongoloid position of palpebral fissure, bird facies. Microtia and ear canal atresia. Hypoplastic zygoma. Possible choanal atresia. Macrostomia, microgenia	Second most common facial anomaly, see Table 1.**43**
Gardner syndrome (but also see Table 4.**26**!)	Hereditary mesenchymal dysplasia (inherited as dominant trait)	Multiple osteomas and osteofibromas chiefly affecting the jaws, nose, paranasal sinuses, and flat cranial bones	Multiple atheromas and dermoid cysts, fibromas. Colonic polyps, multiple nevi. Symptoms do not appear before 10 years of age
Goldenhar syndrome	Oculoauricular dysplasia (autosomal recessive auriculo-oculo-vertebral dysplasia)	Unilateral facial hypoplasia, macrostomia. Malformation of eye and ear. Atresia of external auditory canal. Preauricular appendages	Astigmatism, epibulbar dermoid, frequent deformity or aplasia of the cervical spine
Greig syndrome	Familial hypertelorism	Extreme increase in interorbital distance. Flat, broad nasal root	Growth retardation. Microcephaly. Malformations of the hands and/or feet
Grob syndrome	Linguofacial dysplasia	Nasal dysplasia, median cleft of upper lip, fragmentation of anterior tongue. Abnormalities of palate and dentition	Limb anomalies, low IQ
Hallermann–Streiff syndrome	Oculomandibulofacial dysmorphia	Dyscephaly with bird face. Hypoplasia of nasal cartilages. Microgenia. Dental anomalies	Growth retardation. Congenital cataract

Table 2.**13**   (cont.)

Name of syndrome	Classification	Typical ENT deficits	Other symptoms and comments
HMC syndrome (*H*ypertelorism, *M*icrotia, facial *C*lefting)	Multiple midfacial and cranial malformations	Hypertelorism; lateral facial cleft (cleft lip, alveolus, and palate). Microgenia. Auricular dysplasia	Microcephaly. Cardiac and renal anomalies
Lateral facial cleft syndrome	Probably based on multicausal developmental disturbances of midfacial formation	Very diverse malformations involving the lip, jaws, and/or palate. Secondary involvement of auditory function is common!	See p. 271. The most common facial malformation syndrome
Lejeune syndrome (cri du chat syndrome)	Group B chromosome abnormality	Characteristic round face with hypertelorism, antimongoloid lid position, low-set ears, microgenia. See also Table 1.**43**	Typical high-pitched stridor ("cat's cry") in newborns and infants. Females predominate by 5:1
(de) Myer syndrome	Midfacial cleft syndrome with hereditary basis	Hypertelorism with midfacial clefts of variable extent (3 clinical types)	Closely related to Greig syndrome
Nager–de Reynier syndrome	Mandibular dysostosis	Dysplasia of the mandibular ascending ramus and TMJ. Severe microgenia. Maxillary hypoplasia. Auricular and ear canal anomalies	Dysplasias of the hand and arm. Rib and vertebral anomalies. Similar to Franceschetti syndrome but without lid anomalies
Peters–Hövels syndrome (maxillofacial syndrome)	Combined midfacial malformations (inherited as recessive trait)	Narrow lower face, antimongoloid position of palpebral fissure, very slender nose, flattened frontonasal angle. Zygomatic hypoplasia. Open bite. Hearing impairment	Oligophrenia, growth retardation
Von Pfaundler–Hurler syndrome (gargoylism)	Dysostosis multiplex (hereditary thesaurismosis)	Gargoyle-like facies. Enchondral dysostoses in the face and throughout the skeleton. Hearing impairment (in some cases)	Asmmetric growth retardation. Paw-like hands. Micropolysachariduria. Corneal clouding
Pyle syndrome	See table 1.**43**		
(Pierre) Robin syndrome	Combined dysplasia of mouth, jaws, and tongue	Severe microgenia, cleft palate, glossoptosis. Danger of mechanical respiratory impairment! Eustachian tube dysfunction	Dysplasias may also affect other body regions and organs. High mortality due to risk of mechanical aerodigestive obstruction!

Table 2.**13**   (cont.)

Name of syndrome	Classification	Typical ENT deficits	Other symptoms and comments
Von Romberg syndrome	Progresive facial hemiatrophy	Unilateral atrophy of facial soft tissues and bone (sometimes including cervical organs, larynx, and tongue). Possible associated coup de sabre (linear atrophic zone)	
Rubinstein syndrome	Craniomandibulofacial dysmorphia and limb anomalies	Microcephaly. Beaked nose. Hypertelorism. Frequent nevus flammeus on the forehead	Growth retardation. Oligophrenia. Hand and foot dysplasia. Strabismus
Sturge–Weber syndrome	Encephalofacial neuroangiomatosis	Unilateral nevus flammeus on the face (often confined to area over first trigeminal nerve division) or on the head	Unilateral glaucoma, buphthalmos. Epileptiform seizures. May be combined with other organ malformations
Ulrich–Scheye syndrome	See Table 1.**43**		
Waardenburg syndrome	Dyscephalosyndactyly	Oxycephaly, microgenia. Dental anomalies. Parrot beak nose. Hypertelorism. Malformations of the external ear. Asymmetric sensorineural hearing loss. Reduced vestibular response. Possible facial clefts	Syndactyly. Ocular malformations. Growth retardations. Combination of Apert and Crouzone syndrome. See also Table 1.**43**
Wildervanck (II) syndrome	Zygomaticomaxillomandibulofacial dysostosis	Multiple dysplasias of the cranium, face, and eyes. Hypoplastic zygoma. Auricular dystopia. Nasal hypertrophy ("old man's face"). Malposition of teeth. Sensorineural hearing loss. Reduced vestibular response. Microgenia and micrognathia	Blepharophimosis. Oligophrenia. Vertebral dysmorphias. There are 2 Wildervanck syndromes. Wildervanck I is associated with severe conductive hearing loss and often with sensorineural hearing loss of variable degree. See also Table 1.**43**

3. Nose, Paranasal Sinuses, and Nasopharynx

The Symptoms

○ Pain and dysesthesia, p. 173

○ Nasal discharge (rhinorrhea), p. 182

○ Epistaxis, p. 193

○ Nasal airway obstruction, see p. 199

○ Dry nose, p. 207

○ Nasal fetor, p. 208

○ Morphologic change (swelling, tumor), p. 208

○ Malformation, p. 221

○ Olfactory dysfunction, p. 224

○ Common syndromes, p. 222

Principal Diagnostic Methods

○ *History taking* should be thorough and systematic, because paranasal sinus symptoms can be vague, ambiguous, and misinterpreted by the patient. Multidisciplinary aspects often must be considered in the differential diagnosis.

○ *External inspection and palpation.*

○ *Anterior and posterior rhinoscopy.*

○ *Nasal endoscopy* (including the meati) using a rigid and/or flexible fiberoptic scope; inspection of the nasopharynx with a magnifying endoscope.

○ *Rhinomanometry* or *rhinorheography* for the objective assessment of nasal airflow, i.e., the resistance to nasal respiration. Usually the spontaneous air flow is recorded.

○ *Diagnostic irrigation* of a suspect paranasal sinus: The maxillary sinus is irrigated through the inferior meatus ("sharp" technique) or middle meatus ("blunt" technique); the frontal sinus is irrigated using the (Kümmel–)Beck trephine technique; and the sphenoid sinus is irrigated through its ostium. The irrigating solution can be recovered for bacteriologic or mycologic (and possibly cytodiagnostic) analysis. In selected cases with corresponding symptoms, the instruments can be modified to *combine* diagnostic irritation with sinus endoscopy.

○ *Paranasal sinus endoscopy* is most commonly performed on the maxillary sinus (*"antroscopy"*), less commonly on the frontal sinus, and rarely on the sphenoid sinus. Sinus endoscopy is particularly useful in the diagnosis of chronic paranasal sinus disease.

○ *Sonography*: Ultrasound is widely used for examinations of the maxillary sinus, frontal sinus, and even the anterior ethmoid bone. Its main application is in the diagnosis of sinusitis, where it offers a simple, low-cost procedure for screening and follow-up. It cannot replace diagnostic radiography, however.

○ *Radiographic evaluation*: Conventional radiographic examination; standard workup: nasal skeleton (lateral), paranasal sinuses (occipitomental, occipitofrontal, axial, bitemporal, Rhese projection), and biplane skull films (for trauma, neoplasms, etc.). Tomograms, preferably CT scans are indicated for the differentiation of local findings and relationships difficult to appreciate on conventional radiographs (e.g., fracture lines, relationships of adjacent structures, etc.). See also footnote on p. 1.

○ *Arteriography, digital subtraction angiography*, and *superselective angiography* are indicated for special studies of mass effects (vascular displacements), vascular relationships to neoplasms, posttraumatic states, etc.

o *Radionuclide scanning* can furnish various kinds of information, including the identification of areas with different metabolic activities.

o *Investigation of discharges and smears:* Bacteriologic, mycologic, cytodiagnostic.

o *Allergic evaluation*: Besides the *determination of IgE in the nasal discharge*, which is currently the most reliable method for the detection of allergic rhinitis, other special allergic tests are useful and necessary for an accurate differential diagnosis, e.g., *skin tests* (prick, scratch, intradermal, patch), *provocative tests* (intranasal, conjunctival test), and *laboratory tests* such as the PRIST (paper radioimmunosorbent test) and especially the RAST (radioallergosorbent test). Also: determination of immunoglobulins A and G in the serum and discharge.

o *Serology*: e.g., syphilis serology; titer determinations for suspected Epstein–Barr virus, HIV (AIDS), or other clinically relevant viral diseases; suspicion of rare (e.g., tropical) infectious organisms, etc.

o *Laboratory screening*, e.g., for suspected bleeding or coagulation disorders, etc.

o *Biopsy* is the differential diagnostic mainstay for any suspected malignancy as well as other neoplasms, indeterminate inflammatory causes, etc.

Symptom   **Pain and Dysesthesia (Itching, Tension, or Fullness)**

Rhinogenic pain and dysesthesias can be extremely challenging in terms of differential diagnosis—first because of the frequent ambiguity of symptoms, which often are poorly localized and confused, and second because the head and face encompass many structural and functional systems that are mutually interdependent.

Often these difficulties call for close interdisciplinary cooperation in pursuing the differential diagnosis. Moreover, the vagueness with which many patients describe their illness underscores the importance of a precise, systematic history that includes specific questions on details such as the *character of the pain* (superficial or deep), the *onset* and previous course, the *location* of the pain, its *temporal pattern*, the presence of *underlying* or *associated diseases*, and how the pain is influenced by *external factors*. When this is done and appropriate diagnostic methods are employed, there should be little difficulty in demonstrating or excluding an organic "rhinogenic" cause. Even if findings are obviously negative, it still behooves the specialist to make at least a presumptive diagnosis so that further diagnostic investigations can be selectively planned and economically carried out (Table 3.**1**).

Pain and dysesthesia in the nasal region are often the result of diseases that involve both the external and the internal nose. Despite the frequent overlaps, we shall attempt in this section to highlight distinctions by differentiating between disorders that chiefly affect the *external nose* and diseases that have primarily an *intranasal* localization.

External Nose

Diseases that cause pain and other abnormal sensations involving the external nose (excluding physical damage such as burns and frostbite) are listed in Table 3.**2**. The diseases that can pose the greatest problems of differential diagnosis are erysipelas, perichondritis, tinea faciale (trichophytosis), and lupus erythematosus.

Facial Erysipelas

Main symptoms: Sudden onset, usually with high fever and possible chills. Sharply demarcated, rapidly spreading red lesion with raised borders and associated skin tension and tenderness (nose and midface).

Other symptoms and special features: Regional lymph nodes are swollen and painful; significant malaise. Rarely: vesiculation and gangrenous course. Propensity for recurrence. Wom-

Table 3.**1** *Symptom* Pain and dysesthesia (itching, tension, or fullness)

Synopsis	
Nasal origin	
Inflammatory lesions (and functional disturbances)	Chronic rhinopathy
– *External nose:*	Nasal polyposis
Disease of the integument and supportive structures (see Table 3.**2** for specific diseases)	Atrophic rhinopathy and ozena
– *Internal nose:*	Trauma and its sequelae
Acute rhinitis or rhinopathy, coryza	– Isolated nasal and/or facial injury, see pp. 135, 199 ff.
Allergic rhinitis (see p. 184)	– Frontobasal fracture
Vasomotor rhinopathy (see p. 186)	Intranasal foreign bodies, see p. 192
Anterior rhinitis sicca	Intranasal tumors, see pp. 181, 214
Origin in paranasal sinuses	
Inflammatory lesions	Trauma and its sequelae
– Acute sinusitis	– Paranasal sinus fractures, see pp. 178, 180
– Chronic sinusitis	– Barotrauma
– Rupture of abscess into soft tissues, see p. 137	Special disease entities
– Osteomyelitis of the flat cranial bones, see p. 212	– Frontal sinus aplasia
– Orbital complications, see p. 210	– Pneumosinus dilatans
– Intracranial complications, see p. 213 ff.	– "Vacuum sinus"
	– Mucocele and pyocele
	Tumors of the paranasal sinuses
Origin in nasopharynx	**Neuralgias**
Nasopharyngeal	See Table 2.**10**
– Inflammatory lesions	
– Tumors	

en are affected more commonly than men. Erysipelas of the auricle, see p. 5.

Causes: Streptococcal infection (usually with group A; see p. 5). Portal of infection: superficial skin wounds.

Diagnosis: Patient is acutely ill with a high fever, leukocytosis, and a markedly elevated ESR. Increased antistreptolysin titer is demonstrable after about a week.

Differentiation is required from nasal furunculosis, Quincke edema, acute (contact) dermatitis, and herpes zoster.

Perichondritis of the Nasal Framework

Main symptoms: Severe pain, redness of soft-tissue envelope of anterior nose, diffuse swelling; subperichondrial abscess with an external draining fistula. Fever.

Other symptoms and special features: Concomitant involvement of the septal cartilage is common (septal abscess; see p. 201).

Causes: Exogenous infection (trauma, surgery).

Diagnosis:
● History. Typical clinical picture.
● Laboratory findings consistent with acute inflammation.
● If necessary, wound decompression and antibiotic sensitivity testing.

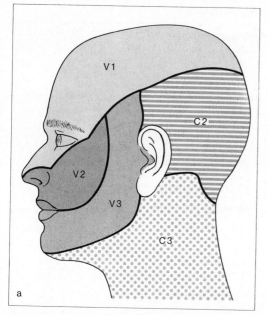
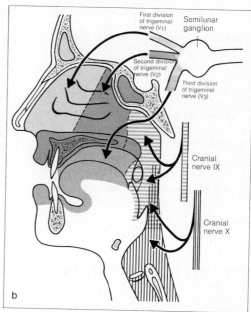

Fig. 3.**1a,b** Sensory innervation of the scalp and facial skin (**a**) and of the nasal, oral, and pharyngeal mucosae (**b**) (auricle see Fig. 1.**1**)

Differentiation is required from folliculitis (sycosis), nasal furuncle, erysipelas, and rhinophyma.

Tinea Faciale (Dermatomycosis)

Main symptoms: Redness and scaling of the facial skin with vesicles or pustules at the border of the affected area. Lesions resolve centrally and spread at their periphery.

Other symptoms: Sharply defined borders, central resolution.

Cause: Various *Trichophyton* species.

Diagnosis: Identification of the causative fungus.

Differentiation is required from eczema, psoriasis, and lupus erythematosus.

Sarcoidosis (Besnier–Boeck–Schaumann Disease)

Main symptoms: Swelling of the nasal tip area with bluish-red to brownish nodules. Feeling of tension but no pain. Very slow course. See p. 255 for further details.

Differentiation is required from rhinophyma, lupus, gumma, and neoplasms.

Leishmaniasis (Cutaneous Leishmaniasis, Espundia)
See p. 191 and Table 4.**28**.

Lupus Erythematosus
See p. 210.

Table 3.**2**   Diseases of the nasal skin and supporting framework (selection)

Cutaneous diseases of diverse etiology

- Acne rosacea*
- Acne vulgaris*
- Erysipelas, see p. 173
- Nasal introital folliculitis and furuncles, see p. 238
- Impetiginous eczema*
- Rhinophyma, see p. 210
- Tinea faciale

Secretory disturbances of the skin glands

- Granulosis rubra nasi*
- Hyperhidrosis*
- Seborrhea*

Viral etiology

- Nasal herpes, see p. 239
- Nasal zoster, see p. 245

Patchy lesions (redness, erythema)

- Solar erythema (sunburn)*
- Lupus erythematosus, see p. 210

Infiltrates

- Tuberculosis (lupus), see pp. 191, 247
- Sarcoidosis
- Perichondritis
- Leishmaniasis, see p. 191
- Malleus, see p. 191
- Rhinoscleroma, see p. 192

Ulcerative lesions (nonmalignant)

- Tuberculosis, see pp. 191, 247
- Gumma, see p. 248
- Leishmaniasis, see p. 191
- Leprosy, see p. 191
- Trauma sequelae, see p. 177
- Malleus, see p. 191
- Blastomycosis, see Table 4.**28**
- Trophoneurotic ulcer of the nasal ala (after trigeminal sclerotherapy), see p. 156

Unknown etiology

- Wegener granulomatosis, see p. 192
- Midline granuloma, see p. 192
- Remitting perichondritis, see p. 174

Benign tumors, see p. 214

- Fibroma
- Lipoma
- Hemangioma
- Lymphangioma
- Keratoacanthoma
- Neuroma
- Neurofibromatosis

Precancerous lesions, see pp. 148, 215

- Senile keratoma
- Cutaneous horn
- Lentigo maligna (circumscribed preblastomatous melanosis)
- Xeroderma pigmentosum

Malignant tumors

- Basal cell carcinoma, see p. 148
- Squamous cell carcinoma, see p. 148
- Malignant melanoma, see p. 150
- Malignant lymphoma, see p. 408 and Table 10.**13**
- Kaposi sarcoma (association with HIV infection), see p. 245

Facial skin diseases (nonneoplastic), see Table 2.**4**
Facial neoplasms (selection), see Table 2.**5**

* No further commentary

Internal Nose

Acute rhinitis can cause dysesthesia, local pain, or even general headache, especially in the initial phase. These symptoms are not predominant in this group of diseases, however (see p. 182).

Rhinitis Sicca Anterior

Main symptoms: Itching and dry sensation in the anterior nose, sometimes with crusting. Epistaxis provoked by scratching is frequent but *always very mild.* An anterior septal perforation with crusted edges may form in later stages (see p. 202).

Causes: No specific known cause; may relate to mechanical and/or climatic influences (dust, heat, chemical irritants, etc.).

Diagnosis: Typical local changes in the skin and mucosa of the anterior nasal septum (dry, fragile area at the mucocutaneous junction; also metaplastic squamous epithelial plaques on the mucosa). See Table 3.**7**.

Differentiation is required from chemical damage to the mucosa (e.g., in chromate workers), iatrogenic damage (following septal surgery or excessive cauterization), cocaine sniffing, and lupus.

Chronic Rhinopathies

These conditions, like *nasal polyposis*, can cause a feeling of pressure in the head and facial area or even true headache, but nasal obstruction generally coexists as the predominant symptom (see p. 199 ff.).

Atrophic rhinitis (atrophic rhinopathy) is associated with a vague feeling of midfacial pressure in its early stage. As the condition more closely approaches a state of fully blown ozena, (dull) headache becomes a more prominent feature. See p. 206 for details.

Virtually *all infections and inflammatory Conditions involving the nasal cavities* can produce abnormal sensations in the nasofacial region that vary in quality and degree among different individuals and may occasionally present as true headache; clinically overt sinusitis need not be present (see Fig. 3.**3**).

Trauma and Sequelae

Main symptoms: Pain occurring at highly variable sites in the nasofacial region and perceived as a constant ache, dull pressure, or paroxysmal neuralgiform pain. Patients generally give a history of trauma, head surgery, or a self-inflicted injury correlating with the onset of pain. See also p. 180.

The **diagnosis** is made from the history, inspection, nasal endoscopy, and, if necessary, radiographic findings.

Differentiation is required from true neuralgias (see p. 159), which, incidentally, may themselves be caused by trauma. Neurologic consultation may be required.

Frontobasal Injury (Rhinobasal Skull Fracture)

Main symptoms: Usually there is a history of a motor vehicular accident or occupational injury. Possible CSF rhinorrhea. A soft-tissue wound, often inconspicuous, may be found on the upper face or forehead. Monocle or eyeglass hematomas; extensive facial swelling and/or hematomas; possible profuse bleeding from the nose, wound, or pharynx, with or without exophthalmos; possible vision loss.

Other symptoms and special features: Concussion or contusion; anosmia (in 75%); involvement of other cranial nerves (II−VI). External soft-tissue wounds are absent in about 20% of cases! Potential for early or late intracranial complications (see p. 210).

Causes: Skull fractures in the area of the upper face or forehead with possible involvement of the upper paranasal sinuses (frontal, ethmoid, sphenoid), the cribriform plate, the anterior and middle cranial fossae (Fig. 3.**2a−c**), the adjacent dura, and often the adjacent brain.

Diagnosis:
● Careful history with reconstruction of the mechanism of the fracture.
● Inspection of the injury and, if possible, nasal endoscopy.
● Radiography: General biplane skull films; standard paranasal sinus views; CT scans to demonstrate the fracture lines. At least standard tomograms of the paranasal sinuses and skull base should be obtained.
● Olfactory testing.
● Confirmation or definitive exclusion of CSF rhinorrhea (see Table 1.**6**).
● Symptoms and findings may warrant consultation with a neurosurgeon, neurologist, or ophthalmologist or both.

Intranasal Foreign Bodies
See p. 192.

Intranasal Tumors

A feeling of pressure or typical headache is generally a late feature of benign and malignant intranasal tumors (see p. 214).

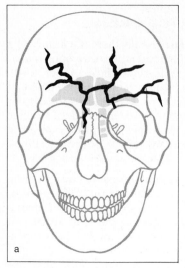 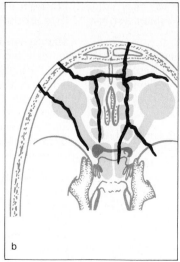 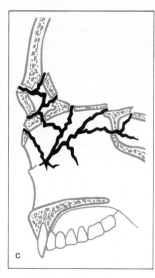

Fig. 3.**2a–c** Typical patterns of frontobasal fractures

a Fracture involving the frontal calvarium, frontal sinuses, and ethmoid bone (generally combined with **b**)
b Frontobasal fractures (involving the paranasal sinuses, visual organ, dura, and often the brain) (transverse section)
c Frontobasal fracture lines (sagittal section)

Paranasal Sinuses

The paranasal sinuses, unlike the nasal cavity, are a very common and important source of severe headache (cardinal symptom!), which is usually associated with a typical pattern of symptoms.

Inflammatory processes in a sinus are not the only cause of significant rhinogenic headache and/or facial pain. Even relatively slight deviations from normal atmospheric pressure in a sinus (by as little as $20-50\ mmH_2O$) are sufficient to cause severe pain. By this mechanism, even apparently trivial *abnormalities of sinus drainage and ventilation* that produce minimal objective signs may be responsible for alarming symptoms.

Acute Sinusitis

Common main symptoms: Pain in the facial skeleton or cranial interior, usually well-circumscribed but not always localized to the affected sinus (see Fig. 3.**3**); may become severe with acute inflammation. Characteristically

the pain is aggravated by bending, lifting, or straining, i.e., by acts that raise the intrasinus pressure. Relatively pain-free intervals alternate with periods of severe pain (hours). Sinugenic pain has a stabbing, boring, throbbing character. Tenderness to pressure or percussion is often noted over the affected sinus. Further symptoms see p. 189 and Figure 3.**3**.

Characteristics of Pain Associated with Specific Sinuses

○ *Maxillary sinus:* Maxillary sinus pain is generally referred to the midfacial area but may also radiate to the forehead. With dentogenic maxillary sinusitis, dental pain may obscure the sinusitic pain. The area over the maxillary sinus (cheek) may be tender to pressure or percussion. A typical symptomatic trigeminal neuralgia of the maxillary nerve is common.

○ *Ethmoid sinus:* Pain may radiate to the medial canthus, nasal root, or temporal region, sometimes producing only a sensation of pressure or fullness. There is typical ten-

Fig. 3.**3** Typical pain reference points associated with various points of irritation in the nose and paranasal sinuses (after McAuliffe; Goodell; Wolff and Stevenson)

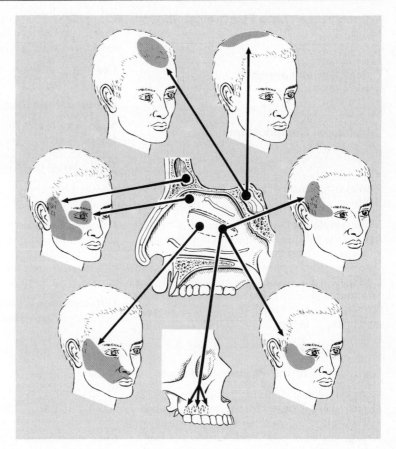

derness at the medial canthus. Ethmoid pain is generally less intense than maxillary or frontal sinus pain. This can easily cause an ethmoiditis to be missed, especially if the disease takes a chronic course with nonspecific symptoms.

○ *Frontal sinus:* Frontal sinus pain is usually very severe and typically localized above the eyes but is sometimes felt over the temporal region, accompanied by deep pain in the forehead; pain may be felt even on the uninvolved side! Tenderness to pressure and percussion is noted over the forehead.

○ *Sphenoid sinus:* Usually dull, nonspecific pain localized within the cranium or radiating to the vertex and occiput (see Sig. 3.**3**) or even to the ear. Sphenoid sinus pain may be so diffuse and poorly localized that the cause is difficult to ascertain (especially in patients with small sphenoid sinuses that do not show marked opacity on routine radiographs!).

Further details on acute sinusitis are given on p. 189.

Chronic Sinusitis

In all *chronic* forms of *sinusitis*, the symptom of pain is less distinct and of diminishing intensity, the patient complaining more of a feeling of pressure and fullness than of significant pain.

Osteomyelitis of the Flat Cranial Bones
See p. 212.

Orbital Complications
See p. 210.

Intracranial Complications
See p. 213 ff.

Paranasal Sinus Trauma, Posttraumatic State

Main symptoms: Onset of headache correlates temporally with trauma. Endoscopy may show granulation tissue that bleeds easily or scar tissue. Radiographs show abnormal contours and contrasts in the cranial region (especially the face and skull base). Foreign bodies also may be demonstrated (shell or safety glass fragments, etc.). See pp. 135, 177 for further details.

Barotrauma of the Paranasal Sinuses

Main symptoms: Sudden, lancinating pain in the paranasal sinuses (frontal, maxillary) during and after exposure to large pressure gradients. Mainly affects fliers, divers, and parachutists.

Other symptoms and special features: Epistaxis, subsequent sinusitis. Nasal airway obstruction (with dysfunction of the sinus ostia) is often present as an associated finding (septal deviation, polyps, chronic rhinitis, etc.).

Diagnosis:
● Nasal endoscopy: Nasal mucosa swollen and erythematous on the affected side. Possible nasal cavity obstruction due to structural change. Nasal discharge is initially blood-tinged and becomes increasing mucopurulent during subsequent days.
● Radiographs show clouding of the affected sinus(es). Sonography is helpful in some cases.

Frontal Sinus Aplasia

Main symptoms: Long-standing, more or less persistent frontal headache that may be quite severe and is unresponsive to treatment. Radiographs show aplasia of the frontal sinus(es). *But:* Every case of frontal sinus aplasia is not associated with headache.

Cause: Unknown.

Pneumosinus Dilatans

Main symptoms: Abnormal enlargement of a frontal sinus with bulging of the anterior sinus wall and, in many cases a feeling of pressure. Maxillary sinus involvement is extremely rare.

Cause: Unknown. Antecedent cranial trauma has been proposed.

Diagnosis: Based on clinical and radiographic findings. In contrast to mucocele, the sinus is aerated, so the excretory duct is patent. Sinus boundaries are sharply defined on radiographs.

Differentiation is required from mucocele and bone tumor (osteoma).

"Vacuum" Sinus

Main symptoms: Aching head or facial pain, mostly unilateral, which may be constant or intermittent. Rhinoscopic findings are generally normal.

Causes: Transient or permanent obstruction of a sinus ostium, with a consequent fall of pressure within the affected sinus.

Diagnosis:
● Rhinoscopy.
● Standard radiographic projections of the paranasal sinuses.
● If above findings are normal, proceed with trial decongestion of the mucosa of the suspect ostium or probational puncture of the sinus. With a "vacuum" sinus, either trial procedure will abruptly relieve pain.

Differentiation is required from sinusitis, neuralgia, and neoplasms. See also Table 2.**10**.

Mucocele and Pyocele

Main symptoms: Smooth-bordered swelling that usually starts at the medial canthus of the eye (ethmoid bone, frontal sinus) and enlarges very slowly, displacing the globe laterally and inferiorly. Palpation may disclose a "parchment crackle" or "tennis ball" consistency. The mass is *nontender*. Lesions that reach considerable size produce in increasing feeling of pressure and mass effects.

Other symptoms and special features: Restriction of eye movements; diplopia is unusual even with marked ocular displacement. Rarer still are optic nerve atrophy and amaurosis. *Sphenoid sinus mucoceles* can cause an orbital apex syndrome (see Table 2.**3**). *Maxillary sinus mucocele* causes bulging of the cheek and upward displacement of the globe.

Causes: Obstruction of the excretory duct of the affected sinus(es). The frontal sinus, sphenoid sinus, and maxillary sinus are affected in order of decreasing frequency.

Diagnosis:
● Rhinoscopy.
● Standard paranasal sinus films show clouding and indistinct margins of the affected sinus. Options include tomography and CT, sonography, and diagnostic aspiration.

Differentiation is required from an early inflammatory complication, meningocele, and a malignant tumor.

Tumors of the Paranasal Sinuses

Main symptoms: Benign and malignant tumors are more likely to cause a feeling of pressure and fullness in the affected sinus than pain, at least initially. A persistent feeling of pressure (e.g., in the frontal region with osteoma) warrants further investigation until a diagnosis is reached!

Paranasal sinus tumors cause facial pain and headache when sensitive structures (nerves, vessels, dura) have become involved by tumor growth (and accompanying inflammation) (e.g., a carcinoma reaching the dura) or have become irritated by expansile growth (e.g., maxillary neuralgia secondary to fibrous dysplasia). See also p. 214.

The **diagnosis** is made from the clinical and radiographic findings (possibly including CT scans, or MR images for better soft-tissue contrast).

Nasopharynx

Pain caused by *inflammatory processes* in the nasopharynx rarely presents as headache or facial pain. Most patients describe an unpleasant sensation "behind the nose"; some describe diffuse pain radiating to the ear or localized in the neck. Nasopharyngeal inflammatory conditions may also produce a vague, poorly localized foreign-body sensation.

Benign and malignant tumors of the nasopharynx are usually associated with nonspecific symptoms in their early development. Because the nasopharynx is a relatively difficult region to examine, a (vague) sensation of pressure or pain in the skull, "behind the nose," or in the neck always warrants a *careful and thorough endoscopic evaluation of the nasopharynx!*

Malignant Tumors of the Nasopharynx

Advanced nasopharyngeal malignancies cause typical headache, which is usually perceived as a very severe pain in the central portion of the skull base region or occasionally in the ear (see Table 3.**22**). Pain is often the *only cardinal symptom* in these cases. Other alarming symptoms are nasal airway obstruction, refractory conductive hearing loss ("tubal catarrh"), lymph node swelling at the mandibular angle (often bilateral and occurring early!), and recurrent epistaxis (e.g., in Burkitt lymphoma, malignant lymphoma, plasmocytoma, rhabdomyosarcoma). Neurologic deficits generally supervene as the disease progresses (see p. 218 and Table 1.**18**).

Other symptoms and special features: Nasal fetor, rhinophonia (usually rhinolalia clausa), neuro-ophthalmologic deficits, symptomatic trigeminal neuralgia, dysphagia ("continuous angina"), and pain on swallowing. Loss of cranial nerves II−VI; possible Horner syndrome (cervical sympathetic trunk). Typically there is early lymphogenous seeding, accompanied later by hematogenous spread. See also p. 218.

Diagnosis:
● Rhinoscopy and nasopharyngeal endoscopy (with or without velotraction), giving special attention to the pharyngeal recess (Rosenmüller fossa) and adjacent areas!

- Standard radiographs of the paranasal sinuses and an axial projection of the skull base. CT scans. Digital subtraction angiography is useful in some cases.
- Local findings may necessitate one or more biopsies. The primary tumor can be very difficult to locate!
- Audiologic evaluation.
- Findings may justify neurologic and ophthalmologic consultation.

Differentiation is required from an inflammatory ulcerative process (tuberculosis, HIV [AIDS], actinomycosis, candidiasis, lymphogranulomatosis). Various common nasopharyngeal tumors (see Table 3.**22**). In children, adenoid hyperplasia.

Neuralgias Manifested in the Nose, Paranasal Sinuses, and/or Nasopharynx

Trigeminal neuralgia (first and second divisions): see p. 159
Sluder neuralgia: see p. 162
Charlin neuralgia: see p. 162
Glossopharyngeal neuralgia: see p. 162
Horton neuralgia: see p. 166
Stylalgia: see p. 234

Symptom   **Rhinorrhea (Nasal Discharge)**

Although mucous drainage is important for maintaining the diverse protective functions of the intranasal mucosa and is an essential prerequisite for a "healthy" nose, spontaneous fluid drainage from the nose is a pathologic sign if the *quantity, consistency, color,* or *odor* of the fluid differs from that of the normal nasal discharge.

Nasal discharge may be characterized as watery, mucoid, purulent, or sanguinolent (blood-tinged). It may be fetid or normal-smelling, unilateral or bilateral, acute or chronic, constant or intermittent (Table 3.**3**).

Acute Rhinitis (Coryza, Common Cold)

Main symptoms: "Dry" prodromal stage with systemic symptoms (chills alternating with sensation of heat, headache, anorexia, occasional slight temperature elevation initially) and with burning, tickling, and a dry sensation in the nose and (naso)pharynx. Sneezing. The "catarrhal" stage supervenes within hours, marked by increasing watery discharge and/or nasal airway obstruction. Increasing malaise. Progression to "mucous" or "mucopurulent" stage occurs several days later, marked by a thicker, yellowish discharge and abatement of symptoms.

Other symptoms and special features: Transient hyposmia or anosmia, lacrimation, rhinophonia clausa. Bacterial superinfection is signaled by purulent rhinitis, possibly with sinusitis and a protracted course. The severity of illness can range from slight malaise to incapacitation, depending on the virulence of the infecting organism and the individual constitution. If the disease does not resolve within a week, the diagnosis of "common cold" should be reconsidered.

Causes: Rhinoviruses (of picornavirus group), also coronaviruses, adenoviruses, and other viral species. Bacterial infection (staphylococci, streptococci, *Haemophilus influenzae*, etc.) is rarely primary and more commonly is acquired secondarily.

Diagnosis: Typical clinical presentation, often relating to climatic influences ("cold outbreaks" during cold, wet seasons). Virologic tests are indicated only if the symptoms surpass the features of a common cold.

Differentiation of common cold is required from "generalized" viral infection, the onset of an acute exanthematous disease, influenza (virologic or serologic testing), vasomotor or allergic rhinitis, and (in small children) foreign bodies.

Table 3.**3** *Symptom* Rhinorrhea (nasal discharge)

Synopsis

Predominantly watery discharge

Acute rhinitis (coryza, common cold)	"Eosinophilic" rhinopathy
Influenza (true viral influenza)	Rhinitis medicamentosa
Coryza initiating a biphasic viral disease	– Pharmacotoxic
Coryza in infants and small children	– Side effect
– Infantile coryza	– Allergic
– Coryza in congenital syphilis	– Pseudoallergic
– Gonorrheal coryza	Vasomotor rhinitis
– Staphylococcal coryza	Posttraumatic
– Diphtheritic coryza	Posttraumatic CSF leak
– Foreign-body coryza	
Allergic rhinitis	
– Seasonal (pollinosis, hay fever)	
– Perennial	

Predominantly mucoid discharge

Chronic rhinopathy, see p. 202	Rhinitis of pregnancy, see p. 203
Toxic rhinitis, see p. 204	Nasal polyposis, see p. 203
Occupational rhinitis, see p. 204	Cystic fibrosis (mucoviscidosis)

Discolored discharge

Bacterial rhinitis	Fungal infection
Infantile coryza	Rare rhinologic infections (diphtheria, tuberculosis, syphilis, leprosy, malleus, leishmaniasis, etc.)
Sinusitis	
Pediatric sinusitis	

Bloody discharge

Wegener granulomatosis	Foreign bodies
Midline granuloma	Neoplasms

Acute rhinitis may be an early feature of viral diseases that later produce symptoms in other organs (e.g., acute exanthemas, tracheobronchial system, gastrointestinal tract, endocranium, musculature, etc.). This cannot be determined at the onset of the rhinitis, but the complete, definitive symptom complex of these *"biphasic viral diseases"* generally unfolds within a few days, making diagnosis easier.

An important differential diagnostic entity in this setting is *true influenza* (see below), which often is not distinguished from coryza with sufficient clarity.

Influenza ("True Viral Influenza," Uncomplicated Influenza)

Main symptoms: Sudden onset with sneezing and itching, rapid temperature elevation, and severe malaise with headache, vertigo, nausea, sweating, and possibly diarrhea. Within 12–24 h the full picture develops with fever, coryza, or nasal obstruction, and a puffy, flushed face. The nasal and oropharyngeal mucosae are hyperemic. Also: headache and limb pain. Epidemic spread.

Other symptoms and special features: Epistaxis (in some cases). Anorexia. Palatal enanthema. Possible features are dry cough, stiff neck, and herpes labialis. Swollen lymph nodes at the mandibular angle. The course of the disease is 3–5 days. Numerous disorders may coexist or supervene: peritonsillar abscess, otitis media, sinusitis, pharyngolaryngotracheobronchitis, myocarditis, myositis, pneumonia, pyelonephritis, meningoencephalitis, etc.

Cause: Infection with an influenza virus.

Diagnosis:
● Characteristic local (speculum) and systemic findings.
● Viral detection in nasal or pharyngeal smears (immunofluorescence; ELISA). Serologic tests are positive only after symptoms have subsided.

Coryza in Infants and Small Children

"Infantile Coryza"

Infants tend to present a more severe symptom complex than adults, with a higher rate of complications (otitis media, nutritional disturbance, high fever, severe systemic illness with bronchopneumonia). The pathogens are often RS (respiratory syncytial) viruses. The course tends to become increasingly mild after 1 year of age.

The following forms, though rare today, can still occur:

Coryza in Congenital Syphilis

Onset in the 3rd week of life: Fetid nasal discharge with crusting. Lymph nodes at the mandibular angle are firm and enlarged. Usually associated with typical syphilitic mucosal changes (e.g., intraoral plaques) and cutaneous lesions. See also p. 248.

Gonorrheal Coryza

Gonococcal organisms can be recovered from a greenish nasal discharge present immediately after birth. There is associated intranasal crusting and conjunctival involvement.

Staphylococcal Coryza in Infants

A purulent nasal discharge commences within days after birth (infecting organism is generally *Staphylococcus aureus*). A serious disease!

Diphtheritic Coryza

This form is marked by blood-tinged rhinorrhea, crusts, and rhagades in the nasal vestibule generally appearing after 6 months of age. Gray coatings adhere to the lining of the nasal cavity and nasopharynx (site of origin!). *Corynebacterium diphtheriae* is identifiable in smears.

Foreign-body Coryza

Unilateral rhinorrhea, initially watery or bloody, later becoming yellowish and foul-smelling. This form of coryza can occur at *any* age.

Allergic Rhinitis

Main symptoms: Seasonal or perennial manifestation (depending on the causative allergens). Paroxysmal or prolonged (spring, summer, fall), significant itching and tickling in the nose with a profuse, bilateral watery discharge. Nasal obstruction. Often there is accompanying conjunctivitis and/or pharyngitis. Feeling of pressure, irritation, or pain in the head. Malaise varies from case to case but often is severe.

Other symptoms and special features: Anorexia, hyposmia or anosmia, various associated neuroautonomic disturbances, photophobia. The rhinitis may coexist or alternate with spastic bronchitis and asthma. With *pollinosis*, symptoms are ameliorated by damp weather, an ocean voyage or trip to the mountains (less pollen in the air), and usually by aging (>55 years). Onset in childhood or adolescence (>6 years).

Causes: Antigen–antibody reaction (type I) incited by various antigens. *Seasonal allergic rhinitis:* pollen and molds (see Table 3.**4**). *Perennial allergic rhinitis:* numerous inhalation allergens (mold spores, animal epithelial cells, animal saliva, danders, house dust, downs, plants, woods, flour, etc.) as well as food allergens and microbial and parasitic allergens; also drugs and "occupational" allergens (see Tables 3.**15** and 3.**16**).

Diagnosis:
● Typical history and symptoms.
● Rhinoscopy in acute cases shows maximal redness and swelling of the nasal mucosa; ob-

Table 3.**4**   Differentiating features of acute rhinitis, vasomotor rhinitis, and allergic rhinitis

Criterion	Acute rhinitis, common cold	Allergic rhinitis	Vasomotor rhinitis
Cause	Viral infection, possibly combined with bacterial superinfection	Antigen–antibody reaction in the nasal mucosa to specific antigens such as pollen (grasses, trees), house dust, animal dander, downs, molds, etc., also foods, drugs, occupational allergens	Pathologic neurovascular response to various physical or chemical stimuli acting on the nasal mucosa. Also dependent on stress and psychic factors. Parasympathetic predominance
Age group	No age predilection	Onset usually at preschool age. Symptoms tend to diminish after about 60 years of age	Onset usually in middle age (>20 years). Symptoms do not abate with aging
Subjective complaints	Sneezing, nasal airway obstruction, head fullness, possible mild fever, rhinorrhea, initially marked malaise	Pruritus of the nose, eyes, and pharynx with attacks of sneezing. Nasal obstruction. Head fullness. With *seasonal* AR, symptoms show seasonal variations; with *perennial* AR, severity varies individually with degree of sensitization, exposure, and antigen	Very profuse, clear, watery rhinorrhea. Sneezing attacks may not occur. The paroxysmal rhinorrhea usually causes little subjective distress. Generally there is no pain or fullness in the head; there is transient nasal obstruction
Duration	4–8 days	*Seasonal:* approximately 2 months (pollination season of various plant groups). But patients allergic to early- and late-flowering plants may be symptomatic from spring to fall! *Perennial:* depends on allergens, exposure, and degree of sensitization	Duration of an attack: minutes (rarely hours). Some patients may have several attacks daily in critical periods
Sense of smell	Usually markedly reduced or abolished at the height of the disease	Reduced or abolished in full-blown cases	Usually not affected
Nasal discharge	Initially watery, then mucopurulent	Watery, low in protein, very profuse. Also mucopurulent with superinfection	Very profuse, clear, watery, low in protein
Diagnostic options and findings	Possible identification of the causative organism. Usually there is an obvious clinical presentation and typical history. Bacteriologic and/or mycologic smear may be helpful if the course is unusually prolonged	Typical history. Exposure/elimination trials. Prick, scratch, intradermal testing. Screening tests. Intranasal provocation test. Lab tests: PRIST and RAST. Markedly increased IgE level in nasal discharge (>10 I.U.)	History. Attempt to identify the precipitating factor. All allergy tests are negative. IgE is not increased in nasal discharge (<10 I.U.)

Table 3.**4**   (cont.)

Criterion	Acute rhinitis, common cold	Allergic rhinitis	Vasomotor rhinitis
Eosinophilia in nasal discharge	Negative	Positive in fewer than 50% of allergic rhinitis patients	a) In classic, *noneosinophilic vasomotor* rhinitis there is profuse rhinorrhea but only slight to moderate nasal obstruction and normal olfaction (accounts for about two-thirds of VR cases) b) In *"eosinophilic" vasomotor* rhinitis there is moderate but significant nasal airway obstruction and hypo- or anosmia (approx. one-third of VR cases). Aspirin intolerance is usually associated with eosinophilic form of VR

struction of the nasal cavity; profuse watery discharge. Mucosa appears pale to livid between attacks. *Special situation*: Patients suffering from nasal house dust allergy generally show a dry nasal mucosa.

● Important screening test: The *IgE level in the nasal discharge* is elevated (> 10 I.U.) in allergic rhinitis.

● The specific allergen can be identified by the prick test, intradermal test, epicutaneous test, or possibly the intranasal test (provocative test) with rhinomanometric documentation.

● Serum IgE level: RAST (radioallergosorbent test), PRIST, and/or ELISA. A diagnosis of allergy can be established in more than 90% of cases; the allergen itself is far more difficult to identify.

● Eosinophilia *need not* be present in the nasal discharge or blood!

Eosinophilia in the nasal discharge is demonstrable in fewer than half of *confirmed cases of allergic rhinitis*. On the other hand, eosinophilia may be detected in the nasal discharge of patients with allergic rhinitis symptoms even when all allergy tests are negative. The cause of this phenomenon is not yet understood (prostaglandin deficiency?). The term *"eosinophilic rhinitis"* or *"eosinophilic*

form of vasomotor rhinitis" has been applied to this condition.

The practical clinical relevance of differentiating cases into NARES (*n*onallergic *r*hinitis with *e*osinophilia *s*yndrome) or nasal *mastocytosis* has yet to be determined.

Drugs can incite a *true allergic rhinitis* in rare cases or, more commonly, a *pseudoallergic rhinopathy*. The symptoms are very similar, differing only in certain pharmacologic aspects (see Table 3.5) and in the results of specific allergy tests. Drugs that commonly lead to rhinopathies with allergy-like symptoms are listed in Table 3.**15**.

Allergic rhinitis and pseudoallergic rhinitis medicamentosa *should not be confused* with *pharmacotoxic rhinopathy* caused by drug abuse, drug overdose, or drug side effects (see p. 204 and Table 3.**15**).

Differentiation is required from vasomotor rhinitis, pseudoallergic rhinitis, acute common cold, and infective allergy.

Vasomotor Rhinitis (Vasomotor Rhinopathy)

Main symptoms: Profuse, bilateral, watery rhinorrhea with severe nasal airway obstruction;

Table 3.5 Differential diagnosis of undesired drug effects on the mucosae of the upper aerodigestive tract (based in part on the tables of Fleischer and Zenner)

Type	Time dependence	Dose dependence	Clinical picture	Individual disposition	Allergy testing	Remarks
Allergic	*Initial* use: latency (sensitization); *repeated* use: no latency	None	Symptoms consistent with immune responses, unrelated to the pharmacologic and toxicologic profile of the administered drug	Generally a prerequisite	Strong positive reaction	Extreme manifestation: anaphylactic shock
Pseudoallergic	Generally no latency, even on initial exposure	Generally present (in varying degrees)	Exogenous allergy imitation that is unexpected and independent of the pharmacologic profile of a given drug	A genetic disposition is presumed	None	Extreme manifestation: anaphylactoid reaction
Pharmacotoxic	No latency except with accumulation	Very strong	Individual, nonimmunologic reaction with a symptom complex determined by pharmacologic and toxicologic properties	Generally insignificant, but a genetic disposition (e.g., enzyme defects) is possible	None	Normal drug "toxicity" can be harmful depending on the dose
Intolerance	No latency	Generally none	Individual, nonimmunologic hypersensitivity to a *normal* drug dose	Prerequisite or intolerance	None	Concept of intolerance overlaps with "pseudoallergy"
Idiosyncratic	No latency	None	Individual, nonimmunologic hypersensitivity to a normal drug dose, with symptoms going beyond the predictable spectrum of drug action	Prerequisite for idiosyncrasy	None	Concept of idiosyncrasy overlaps with "pseudoallergy"

possible attacks of sneezing. Occasional head fullness. Abrupt cessation of nasal symptoms, which closely resemble those of allergic rhinitis.

Other symptoms and special features: Usually the patient feels well during attacks but is bothered by their unpredictability (concert, theater, social occasions, etc.). Allergens are *not* identifiable! Rhinoscopy: Between attacks the nasal mucosa appears pale or livid; during attacks the mucosa is deep red and markedly swollen, especially in the region of the turbinates. Clear, watery, profuse nasal discharge. Conjunctival involvement is possible.

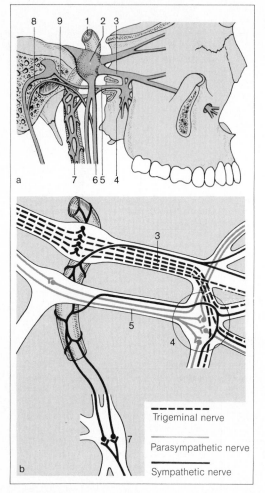

Fig. 3.**4 a,b** Innervation of the nasal mucosa (from Becker, Naumann, Pfaltz)

a General lateral view (schematic)
b Fiber course and pterygopalatine ganglion (circle)
1 Internal carotid artery (with sympathetic plexus)
2 Semilunar (gasserian) ganglion
3 Maxillary nerve (V2)
4 Pterygopalatine ganglion
5 Nerve of pterygoid canal
6 Mandibular nerve
7 Sympathetic plexus with superior cervical ganglion
8 Facial nerve
9 Greater petrosal nerve

Causes: Faulty regulation (hyperreactivity) of the autonomic innervation of the nasal mucosa (predominance of parasympathetic flow). See Figure 3.**4a,b**. Attacks can probably be triggered by a great variety of physical, chemical, climatic, and emotional factors.

Diagnosis:
● Typical history. Give special attention to the circumstances of the attacks!
● Rhinoscopic findings.
● Before allergy testing, determine IgE in the *nasal discharge*. Values < 10 I.U. are consistent with vasomotor rhinitis, values > 10 I.U. with allergic rhinitis! If doubt exists, proceed with allergy tests (intradermal, epidermal, prick tests; intranasal test; antibodies in serum and nasal discharge, RAST), which are consistently negative in vasomotor rhinitis. See also p. 184 ff.

Differentiation is required from allergic rhinitis, toxic rhinitis, intranasal foreign bodies (especially in children), and incipient cold.

CSF Leak

Main symptoms: Discharge of a watery fluid from one side of the nose or into the nasopharynx, usually following cranial trauma or surgery about the rhinobase but also occurring spontaneously (with no history of surgery or trauma). The discharge is rarely bilateral (depending on the location and extent of the dural defect). CSF leak is frequently but not always provoked or aggravated by bending, straining, certain head positions, and by the Queckenstedt maneuver.

Other symptoms and special features: Since a dural defect always poses a risk of meningitis, signs of meningeal irritation may be present at a subthreshold level or may become increasingly apparent. Often a CSF leak is suspected when light spots with sharp borders are noticed on the bed pillow.

Causes: A dural defect in the region of the anterior (or possibly the middle) cranial fossa, generally caused by trauma.

Diagnosis:
● History of cranial trauma. Rhinoscopy reveals a watery "track" only if the CSF leak is profuse.

● Screening tests for identifying the fluid as CSF: glucose positive, protein content increased (relative to nasal mucous); other methods are noted in Table 1.**6**.

● Diagnostic imaging: Demonstration of the fracture site by tomography and/or CT.

Differentiation is required from vasomotor rhinitis, allergic rhinitis, and coryza.

Chronic Rhinitis
See p. 202.

Pharmacotoxic Rhinopathy
See p. 204.

Occupational Rhinitis
See p. 204.

Rhinitis of Pregnancy
See p. 203.

Nasal Polyposis
See p. 203.

Cystic Fibrosis (Mucoviscidosis, Cystic Fibrosis of the Pancreas)

Main symptoms: Copious, viscous, glue-like, glassy, white to yellow secretion that obstructs the nasal lumen. Concomitant sinusitis, usually with associated nasal and sinus polyposis. Progressive bronchial obstruction, bronchiectasis, pneumothorax, and abdominal symptoms (pancreatic enzyme deficiency and pancreatic fibrosis, diabetes mellitus, chronic diarrhea, hepatic cirrhosis, occasional rectal prolapse).

Other symptoms and special features: Rhinologic findings may be the first symptom noted in infants and small children. Increased chloride and sodium levels are measured in sweat and saliva, with excessive viscosity of the secretions. Forms range from severe to abortive. Chronic cough.

Causes: Most common congenital disease of childhood. Based on widespread exocrine gland dysfunction transmitted as an autosomal recessive trait.

Diagnosis:
● Bronchopulmonary and abdominal symptoms are usually predominant. The viscous discharge from the nose and tracheobronchial region, together with rhinologic findings (polyposis, sinusitis), raise suspicion of cystic fibrosis.

● Laboratory values: Elevated sweat electrolytes (sodium and chloride levels >45 mEq/L in infants, >50 mEq/L in children, >70 mEq/L in adults are evident for diagnosis.

● Paranasal sinus and chest radiographs.

● Bronchoscopy may be required.

Differentiation is required from immune deficiency syndrome.

Bacterial Rhinitis

It is common for bacterial superinfection to develop secondary to an upper respiratory viral infection, manifested by a yellow to greenish discoloration of the nasal discharge. The leading bacterial pathogens are pneumococci, *Haemophilus influenzae*, hemolytic streptococci, staphylococci, and colibacilli, and mixed infections are common.

Acute bacterial rhinitis is a particularly important disease in infants and small children.

Infantile Coryza
See p. 184.

Sinusitis

Main symptom: An initially colorless mucoid discharge, often unilateral, which later turns yellow or green and is accompanied in the acute stage by potentially severe headache and/or facial pain (see p. 179). The purulent discharge has a variable consistency (creamy, doughy, gritty, crumbly, etc.). The odor is usually bland but may be foul or fetid (dentogenic cause!). Rhinoscopy shows "pus tracks" at typical sites (Fig. 3.**5**) and on the posterior pharyngeal wall.

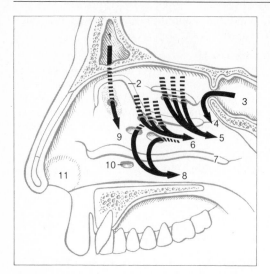

Fig. 3.**5** Characteristic drainage routes from the sinus ostia (the three nasal turbinates have been resected at their base) (from Becker, Naumann, Pfaltz)

1 Frontal sinus
2 Bony base of middle turbinate
3 Sphenoid sinus
4 Drainage from the sphenoid sinus
5 Drainage from the posterior ethmoid cells
6 Drainage from the anterior ethmoid cells
7 Base of the inferior turbinate bone
8 Drainage from the maxillary sinus
9 Drainage from the frontal sinus (shaded area = infundibulum)
10 Excretory orifice of the nasolacrimal duct
11 Nasal vestibule

Other symptoms and special features: Nasal airway obstruction on the affected side—although bilateral sinusitis is not uncommon. Hyposmia or anosmia; also cacosmia, especially with chronic sinusitis or a dentogenic cause. Children are especially likely to have accompanying conjunctivitis (due to eye wiping) and eczema of the nasal vestibule. Systemic symptoms include lethargy and fever; the latter is most common in children and in patients with severe systemic infection or an incipient rhinogenic complication.

Causes: Viral and/or bacterial infection, possibly combined with mycosis. Anaerobes may be present with a dentogenic cause! Incompetence of sinus ostia and its pathologic seque-

lae; also, spread of infection to the sinus from the nose or less commonly by the hematogenous route (Fig. 3.**6**).

Diagnosis:
● Anterior and posterior rhinoscopy or endoscopy: purulent tracks characteristic of the affected sinus(es) (Fig. 3.**6**).
● Radiographic examination: Standard paranasal sinus projections. Tomograms and/or CT scans for special inquiries.
● Sonography is useful for screening and follow-up of the maxillary sinuses, frontal sinuses, and anterior ethmoid bone.
● Other options are diagnostic irrigation, with or without paranasal sinus endoscopy, and microbiologic examination of the sinus discharge with sensitivity testing.
● Findings may warrant biopsy or surgical exploration of the sinus.

Differentiation is required from chronic rhinitis, nasal polyposis, mucocele or pyocele, cysts, benign or malignant tumors, "vacuum" sinus (see p. 180), neuralgias, barotrauma, and facial pain or headache of other etiology.

"Pediatric" Sinusitis ("Occult" Sinusitis)

Main symptoms: Dry cough, sniffing, "lingering cold" (although "dry" sinusitis can occur). Anorexia, failure to thrive. In some cases the symptoms may be like those of "adult" sinusitis.

Other symptoms and special features: Chronic catarrhal course with *few symptoms.* Peak occurence is from 7 to 12 years of age. An allergic basis is common (type IV). Radiographs confirm the diagnosis.

Fungal Infections of the Nose and Paranasal Sinuses

Main symptoms: Chronic coryza with a greenish, yellow, grayish, or occasionally blood-tinged discharge and few subjective complaints. Paranasal sinus involvement produces the features of chronic sinusitis. See p. 249 for further details.

Other symptoms and special features: Fungal infections are most likely to occur when host defenses are impaired (e.g., in tumor patients,

Fig. 3.**6** Pathogenic mechanisms of sinusitis (from Becker, Naumann, Pfaltz)

1 Nasal cavity
2 Maxillary sinus
3 Ethmoid cells
4 Frontal sinus (sectioned far posteriorly)
5 Orbit
6 Maxillary tooth
7 Oral cavity
8 Anterior cranial fossa

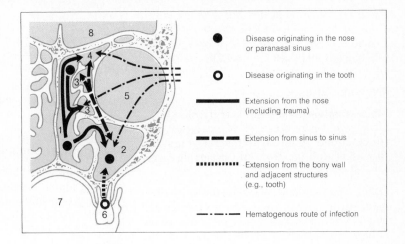

● Disease originating in the nose or paranasal sinus

○ Disease originating in the tooth

▬▬▬ Extension from the nose (including trauma)

▬ ▬ ▬ Extension from sinus to sinus

▪▪▪▪▪▪▪▪▪▪ Extension from the bony wall and adjacent structures (e.g., tooth)

▬ · ▬ · ▬ Hematogenous route of infection

following immunosuppressive or antibiotic therapy, in diabetics, or in AIDS patients; see p. 245 for details). Three forms of fungal infection can occur: a) noninvasive mycosis, b) invasive mycosis, or c) allergic mucosal inflammation caused by contact with fungal spores.

Causes: Infection with *Aspergillus, Candida albicans*, or rarely with tropical species (see Table. 4.**28**).

Diagnosis:
● Detection of fungi in sinus washings or discharge (*Aspergillus, Candida,* various *Blastomyces [Paracoccidioides]* species, and phycomycetes such as *Mucor* or *Rhinospiridium seeberi*).
● Standard radiographic projections of the paranasal sinuses.
● Some cases require biopsy (fungal hyphae in the mucosa!).

Rare Rhinologic Infections

Discolored nasal discharge is a *cardinal symptom* of several bacterial or parasitic nasal diseases that are rare in the United States and Central Europe, including:
○ *Diphtheria* (mainly in children over 6 years of age; see p. 233).
○ *Intranasal tuberculosis*, an ulcerating mucosal tuberculosis producing a discolored, greasy, sometimes blood-tinged discharge.

Rhinoscopy: mucosal ulcerations on the septum or turbinates with a greasy coating ("moth-eaten"). Organisms are identifiable in bacteriologic smears or biopsy specimens. *Nasal lupus*, see p. 247.
○ *Intranasal syphilis.* Secondary: yellow, sticky discharge, rhinoscopy showing unilateral nasal obstruction. Tertiary: fetid, greasy, discolored discharge, possibly *without* pain. Rhinoscopy: firm infiltrates and ulcerations within the nasal cavity. Identification of causative organism, serologic tests, biopsy. *Syphilitic* ulceration and necrosis generally involve the *skeletal* portions of the nose, while tuberculous (lupus) lesions involve the *cartilaginous* nose. See also p. 247.
○ *Intranasal leprosy:* Profuse, serous or mucoid discharge that may be blood-tinged. Fetid crusting. Intranasal obstruction, especially at the onset of disease. Specific lesions are found at other body sites. Identification of the causative organism, see Table 4.**28**.
○ *Malleus:* Purulent, foul-smelling, usually profuse discharge, followed later by intranasal granulations. See also Table 4.**28**.
○ *Leishmaniasis (espundia):* Months to years after healing of the primary cutaneous lesions ("boils") of leishmaniasis, the secondary stage commences with involvement of the nasal, oral, and/or pharyngeal mucosae (granulations and ulcerations with viscous, occasionally bloody and fetid discharge and

crusts). Isolation of the causative organism. Other options: intradermal test with leishmania antigen, biopsy. See also Table 4.**28**.
○ **Rhinoscleroma**, see Table 4.**28**.

Wegener Granulomatosis

Main symptoms: Chronic, slightly bloody catarrh with heavy crusting. Nasal airway obstruction and epistaxis. Intranasal granuloma formation with necrosis, also occurring in paranasal sinuses.

Other symptoms and special features: Involvement of the rest of the respiratory tract and lung parenchyma. Possible involvement of the kidney, liver, joints, nervous system, eye, and ear. Symptoms change frequently! Peak incidence in the 3rd–5th decades.

Cause: Necrotizing vasculitis belonging to the class of collagen diseases (see Table 4.**29**).

Diagnosis: Because the disease generally originates from the nasal region or upper respiratory tract, the otolaryngologic findings (nose, pharynx, larynx, trachea) are of key importance.
● Radiographs (depending on location). CT scans of the neck or MRI may contribute to the evaluation.
● Identification of the autoantibody against cytoplasmic antigens in granulocytes and monocytes (= ACPA).
● Single or multiple biopsies.
● Due to consistent involvement of other organs and organ systems, consultation with an internist, ophthalmologist, or dermatologist is always indicated.

Differentiation is required from periarteritis nodosa, other granulomatous lesions (bacterial, fungal, foreign, body), malleus, gumma, scleroma. Sarcoidosis. Malignant tumors. Also midline granuloma (see below).

Midline Granuloma
(Midline Lethal Granuloma)

Main symptoms: Much like those of Wegener granulomatosis, except that midline granuloma is a *unifocal* disease resulting in the gradual destruction of the *midfacial tissues*.

Causes: Not fully understood. May be closely related or identical to T-cell lymphoma.

Diagnosis: Rhinoscopy. Biopsy. ACPA (autoantibody detection): negative.

Differential diagnosis same as for Wegener granulomatosis (see above).

Foreign Bodies in the Nose or Paranasal Sinuses

Main symptoms: Unilateral nasal discharge, which gradually becomes purulent and finally putrid. Recurrent unilateral epistaxis is also possible. Acute cases show significant symptoms of pain and irritation that subside within days or weeks.

Foreign bodies in a paranasal sinus are rare. Residues from intrasinus drug administration or dental filling residues may occur in the maxillary sinus, or foreign objects (shell fragments, etc.) may be driven into sinuses as a result of trauma.

Diagnosis:
● Rhinoscopy (or endoscopy) after nasal decongestion. Probing of the nasal cavity.
● Radiography: Metallic foreign bodies and "rhinoliths" are well-displayed by radiographs. Sinus foreign bodies can be demonstrated with contrast medium or by tomography (or CT).

Tumors

Malignant tumors of the nose or paranasal sinuses are most conspicuous as far as the symptom of *nasal discharge* is concerned: They are marked by a fetid discharge, initially unilateral in most cases, that is increasingly blood-tinged or associated with transient epistaxis. Gradual unilateral nasal obstruction. See p. 214 for further details.

Diagnosis:
● Rhinoscopy.
● Radiography: Standard projections *and* CT scans.
● Biopsy.

Symptom   Epistaxis (Nosebleed)

Nosebleed is a very common symptom (Table 3.6). Most cases have an innocuous cause and pursue a mild, self-limiting course. In other cases, however, epistaxis may result from a life-threatening disease or may itself be life-endangering and pose considerable diagnostic difficulties. There are two age categories in which nasal bleeding is particularly common: a) children and adolescents, and b) persons over 60 years of age. Males are affected about twice as frequently as females.

The source of epistaxis in more than 80% of cases is the Kiesselbach plexus (Fig. 3.7). This bleeding site is easily localized. Bleeding from tumors and profuse bleeding from the posterior nasal cavity or paranasal sinuses can be considerably more difficult to evaluate. In many of these cases the bleeding site cannot be localized, and the epistaxis must be managed "blindly" by packing the nasal cavity and/or by ligation or embolization of the larger supply vessels.

Epistaxis may be due to *local causes* (i.e., a bleeding site in the nose) or it may be *symptomatic* of an underlying disorder that is extrinsic to the nasal region.

Epistaxis Due to Local Causes

Idiopathic, Spontaneous Epistaxis

Main symptoms: Usually mild, unilateral nosebleed that has no apparent cause, generally

Table 3.**6**   *Symptom*   Epistaxis (causes)

Synopsis	
Local causes	
Idiopathic, "constitutional"	Occupational damage to the nasal mucosa, see p. 204
Rhinitis sicca anterior, see p. 176	Environmental or climatic insult, see p. 203
Perforating septal ulcer, see p. 202	Trauma or foreign bodies, see pp. 192, 199
Vascular injury ("microtrauma" to the Kiesselbach plexus), see Table 3.**7**	Bleeding septal polyps, intranasal granulomas and granulomatoses
Vascular injury (larger vessels inside the nose or in a sinus), see Table 3.**7**	Neoplasms of the nose or paranasal sinuses
Specific inflammatory lesions of the nasal mucosa, see p. 191	Neoplasms of the nasopharynx – Juvenile nasopharyngeal fibroma – Other nasopharyngeal tumors, see p. 218
Symptomatic forms	
Systemic disorders such as – Infectious diseases – Vascular and circulatory diseases – Pheochromocytoma – Vicarious epistaxis – Epistaxis in pregnancy	– Other endocrine causes – Bleeding and coagulation disorders – Uremia – Hepatic insufficiency Hereditary hemorrhagic telangiectasia (Rendu–Osler disease)
Pseudoepistaxis	
Pulmonary hemoptysis, see p. 273ff. Injury of the internal carotid artery* Bleeding esophageal varices, see p. 379	Tumor bleeding from the pharynx, larynx, trachea, see p. 274 Hematemesis, see p. 385

* No further commentary

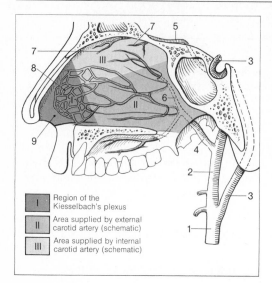

Fig. 3.**7** Blood supply to the internal nose (from Becker, Naumann, Pfaltz)

1 Common carotid artery
2 External carotid artery
3 Internal carotid artery
4 Maxillary artery
5 Ophthalmic artery
6 Sphenopalatine artery
7 Anterior and posterior ethmoidal arteries
8 The Kiesselbach plexus
9 Nasal vestibule

ceases within a short time or is easily controlled by minor local therapeutic measures. Very common in children and adolescents. Propensity for recurrence, at least in subsequent weeks or months.

Other symptoms and special features: This type of bleeding also results from "microtrauma" of the nasal membranes (caused by nose picking, washing, noseblowing, etc.), i.e., from a definable mechanical insult to the very delicate and vulnerable mucosa of the anterior nasal septum. There is no pain and no effects on the blood count or hemoglobin.

Diagnosis: Rhinoscopy (generally the bleeding site is easily localized to the Kiesselbach plexus; Table 3.**7**).

Rhinitis Sicca Anterior and Perforating Septal Ulcer

See pp. 176, 202 and Table 3.**13**.

Intranasal Foreign Bodies

See p. 192.

Bleeding Septal Polyp and Other Intranasal Granulomas

Main symptoms: Recurrent, unilateral epistaxis, usually of moderate intensity. No pain. *Septal polyp:* Red, globular mass (millet- to pea-size) attached to the anterior septum on a broad base; bleeds easily when touched (angioma-like granuloma, pyogenic granuloma). *Granuloma:* Granulating tissue projecting farther into the nasal cavity from the septum or turbinate; includes Wegener granulomatosis (see p. 192).

Diagnosis: Excisional biopsy.

Differentiation is required from true neoplasms, Wegener granulomatosis, midline granuloma, leishmaniasis, and other fungal and parasitic infections.

Tumors of the Nose and Paranasal Sinuses

Benign tumors (chiefly angiomas) and especially malignant tumors (see Table 3.**21**) of the nose and paranasal sinuses can cause severe epistaxis. The associated symptoms depend on the location, type, and extent of the neoplasm.

Diagnosis:
● Anterior and posterior rhinoscopy and endoscopy.
● Radiography: Standard projections, and CT scans. Angiography (superselective) is helpful in some cases.
● Biopsy.

Tumors of the Nasopharynx

These tumors occupy a special position in this context, because they can lead to life-threatening hemorrhage from the nose and pharynx (see Table 3.**22**).

Table 3.**7**   *Diagnostic investigation of epistaxis*

1. History

2. Localization of the bleeding site and identification of the cause:
   - *Anterior* epistaxis: Digital trauma, idiopathic epistaxis, rhinitis sicca anterior, perforating septal ulcer, epistaxis accompanying infectious diseases, etc. (see p. 193 ff.)
   - *Posterior or midnasal* epistaxis: Hypertension, arteriosclerosis, fractures, tumors
   - *Diffuse* epistaxis: Hemorrhagic diathesis, coagulation disorder (see Table 3.**9**), Osler disease

3. Blood pressure measurement and circulatory assessment

4. Bleeding and coagulation analysis (see p. 195)

In selected cases:

5. Radiographs of the skull, nose, and paranasal sinuses (standard projections, possibly supplemented by tomograms or CT scans)

6. Exclusion of underlying internal diseases as a cause of the epistaxis (see Table 3.**6** and p. 195)
   (See also Table 3.**8** [hemostaseologic screening tests])

Angiofibroma of the Skull Base (Juvenile Nasopharyngeal Fibroma, Basal Fibroid)

Main symptoms: Severe, spontaneous bleeding from the nose and/or pharynx. Nasal airway obstruction. Rhinophonia clausa. Endoscopy shows a smooth-walled, mostly lobulated mass causing variable nasopharyngeal obturation. Occurs almost exclusively in teenage males.

Other symptoms and special features: Purulent rhinosinusitis (due to damming back of secretions), eustachian tube dysfunction (conductive hearing loss), eventual expansion of the lateral face ("frog face"), and proptosis. Secondary anemia. Very hard consistency on palpation. Juvenile nasopharyngeal fibromas are said to generally (but not always!) regress spontaneously after 20 years of age.

Causes: Very vascular tumor arising from the roof of the nasopharynx; histologically benign but clinically malignant because of its aggressive, expansile growth.

Diagnosis:
● Anterior and posterior rhinoscopy and endoscopy (smooth, globular surface, hard consistency).
● Radiography: Biplane tomograms of the skull base, nasopharynx, nasal cavities, and paranasal sinuses. CT (to exclude intracranial involvement). Possibly MRI. Angiography of the external carotid artery and, with extensive disease, the internal carotid artery as well. Superselective angiography (feeding and draining vessels).
● With intracranial extension, neurologic or neurosurgical consultation is required.
● Biopsy is done *strictly* as an inpatient procedure so that immediate tumor removal can be carried out if heavy bleeding occurs.

Differentiation is required from choanal polyp, adenoid hyperplasia, lymphoma, chordoma, teratoma, and carcinoma.

Other Nasopharyngeal Tumors
See p. 218 and Table 3.**22**

Symptomatic Epistaxis

○ *Brief summary:* Epistaxis is the *primary symptom* of many infectious diseases such as acute exanthemas in children, influenza, coryza and other systemic viral infections, and severe bacterial systemic infections such as typhus and spotted fever. It is also a feature of life-threatening *generalized infections* such as sepsis. This form of epistaxis results from parching of the nasal mucosa, increased vulnerability of the mucosal vessels (due

Table 3.**8** Screening tests to exclude abnormalities of hemostasis

Minimum list	Normal limits
Bleeding time	2–6 min
Clotting time	4–10 min
Partial thromboplastin time (PTT)	25–35 s
Quick test (prothrombin index)	70–120%
Platelet count	150 000–300 000/mm^3
With suspected consumption coagulopathy: Fibrinogen (Clauss test)	150–300 mg/dL
Fibrin breakdown products	up to 10 µg/mL
Euglobulin lysis time	120–480 min
Fibrinopeptide A	0.5–3.0 ng/mL
Plasminogen	70–125%

If just *one* value is pathologic, and this is confirmed by retesting, a comprehensive hemostatis workup should be performed!

to mucosal drying or toxic factors), and from the occasionally abnormal bleeding and coagulation status of the patient. It generally poses no problems of differential diagnosis as a prodromal or syndromal process.

Epistaxis is an *accompanying symptom* or at times the *cardinal symptom* of other *underlying organic diseases*. It is a cardinal symptom of *hypertension* and *hypertensive crises* and also of *arteriosclerosis*. This bleeding has a spurting, pulsatile character and is unilateral, though discharge through the opposite choana can mimic bilaterality. The farther posterior the bleeding site is in the nose, the more profuse the epistaxis. Most cases occur in persons over 60 years of age, and there is a high rate of recurrence. A rare tumor associated with hypertensive crises and catecholamine secretion, *pheochromocytoma*, also belongs in this category. In this disease, caused by a hormonally active paraganglioma, sustained or paroxysmal hypertension is usually but not invariably present. Additional features are headache and autonomic lability. Other forms based on hormonal factors are *vicarious epistaxis*, occurring in place of menstruation, and *epistaxis during pregnancy*.

Epistaxis is common in the setting of *bleeding and coagulation disorders*, which is understandable given the vascular anatomy of the nasal mucosa. The principal screening tests for these disorders are listed in Table 3.**8**, and the most common diseases of this group are shown in Table 3.**9**.

It should be added that *certain antibiotics can interfere with blood coagulation* by inhibiting *platelet function* (e.g., azlocillin, cephalothin, mezlocillin, penicillin G, piperacillin, ticarcillin), by reducing the *platelet count* (e.g., cephalothin, chloramphenicol, penicillin G, rifampin, streptomycin, tetracycline), or by affecting *vitamin K production* (e.g., ampicillin, azlocillin, carbenicillin, cephalotin, cefamandole, mezlocillin, ticarcillin) (Preyer and Luckhaupt).

Additional systemic causes of epistaxis are *metabolic emergency situations* such as *renal failure* and *hepatic insufficiency*.

General diagnostic evaluation of acute epistaxis:

See Table 3.**7**. It must be determined whether the nature of the bleeding (quantity, location, etc.) permits a thorough evaluation of the *cause of the bleeding prior to* emergency treat-

Table 3.**9**   Bleeding and coagulation disorders that are important in otolaryngology

Group	Disease	Type of bleeding	Typical laboratory findings (see also Table 3.**10**)
Thrombocyto-penia	Werlhof disease (idiopathic thrombo-cytopenic purpura, essential thrombope-nia); allergic or toxic thrombocytopenia	Petechiae in the mucosa and skin. Epistaxis, bleed-ing gums, etc.	Thrombocytopenia (<130000). Leukocytes normal. Bleeding time: prolonged; clotting time: normal
Thrombocyto-pathy	von Willebrand–Jürgens	Proneness to epistaxis or petechial mucosal hemor-rhages in response to mi-crotrauma. Petechial or more widespread cutane-ous hemorrhages. Propens-ity for postoperative bleed-ing. Severe hemorrhagic diathesis in some cases	Platelet count: normal or per-haps slightly low. Platelet mor-phology: normal. Bleeding time: prolonged. Clotting time: normal. Platelet adhesiveness: impaired. Thromboelastogram: marked reduced. Rumpel–Leede: negative
	Glanzmann syndrome	Ecchymoses on the skin and mucosae. Excessive bleeding from cuts, extrac-tion sites, and other wounds. Epistaxis	Platelet count: normal. Abnor-mal platelet morphology (pyc-nosis, anisocytosis, deficient granulation, giant platelets). Absent or delayed agglomera-tion. Bleeding time: normal. Clotting time: normal. Throm-boelastogram: markedly re-duced. Rumpel–Leede: posi-tive
Congenital coagulopathy	Hemophilia A and B	Extensive bleeding in response to minor trauma (cuts, tooth extractions, sur-gical procedures). Disease is manifested only in males	Deficiency of factor VIII or fac-tor IX activity. Bleeding time: normal. Clotting time: pro-longed. PTT prolonged. Quick value: normal
Acquired coagulopathy	Vitamin K deficiency (hepatobiliary disease)	Proneness to extensive bleeding	Quick value: reduced (<10). Decrease in factors II, VII, IX, X. Platelet count: low
	Anticoagulant ther-apy (coumarin, etc.)	Diffuse bleeding sites. Postoperative bleeding	Same as above
	Consumption coagu-lopathy		Thrombocytopenia. Fibrinogen reduced. Quick value: re-duced. Thrombin time: pro-longed. Hyperfibrinolysis + fi-brin cleavage products de-monstrable. PTT: prolonged. Factor V reduced
Vascular abnormalities	Schoenlein–Henoch purpura, scurvy, in-fections, cryoglobu-linemia, Osler dis-ease, drug-induced vascular damage	Urticaria, petechiae, and purpura	Coagulation status: normal. Hy-pertension. Hematuria (in some cases). Rheumatoid factor may be positive. Diagnosis made from general clinical picture

Table 3.**10** Typical patterns of hemostaseologic findings (after Kaboth and Heilmann)

Principal findings	Diseases to be considered in differential diagnosis
Prolonged bleeding time with thrombocytopenia	Werlhof disease, symptomatic thrombocytopenias, metabolic disorders (hepatic, renal, storage diseases). Toxic injury (e.g., by drugs); dys- and paraproteinemias
Prolonged bleeding time with normal platelet count	Glanzmann syndrome, von Willebrand–Jürgens syndrome, associated finding in all forms of severe thrombocytopenias and hemorrhagic thrombocythemias. May be present in bleeding disorders due to vascular abnormalities
Hypofibrinogenemia	Congenital forms, hyperfibrinogenolysis. Consumption coagulopathies severe hepatic diseases
Reduction of factors II, V, VII, X	Congenital reduction of these factors, acquired depression of the factors of the prothrombin complex. Vitamin K deficiency. Severe liver damage. May occur in consumption coagulopathies and hyperfibrinolysis. Uremia, leukoses, pernicious anemia. Anticoagulant therapy
Prolonged partial prothrombin time (PTT)	Congenital reduction of factors V, VIII, IX, X, XI, XII; von Willebrand–Jürgens syndrome. Immune-inhibitor hemophilia. Associated finding in congenital hypoprothrombinemias, during treatment with vitamin K antagonists, in the presence of antithrombins, in all forms of consumption coagulopathy and hyperfibrinolysis
Prolonged thrombin time	Generalized hyperfibrinolysis, endogenous and exogenous hyperheparinemias. May occur in local hyperfibrinolysis, paraproteinemia, liver damage, collagen disorders, and uremia
Decreased capillary resistance	Congenital or acquired vascular defects. Generalized toxic capillary damage in severe infectious diseases, rheumatoid disorders (Schoenlein–Henoch purpura) or following exposure to exogenous toxic or allergic agents

ment, or whether differential diagnostic measures must be deferred until *after* the bleeding has been controlled. Except for innocuous localized bleeding from the Kiesselbach plexus, all severe and recurrent nosebleeds require a thorough differential diagnostic evaluation that includes the history, localization of the bleeding site, and identification of the cause:
● History (bleeding episode[s], organic diseases, cranial trauma, surgery). Rhinoscopic and endoscopic scrutiny of the nasal cavity and nasopharynx.
● Radiography: Standard paranasal sinus projections. According to symptoms: biplane skull films; CT scans; digital subtraction angiography of the external and internal carotid arter-

ies; superselective angiograms (also as a prelude to embolization).
● Internal medical consultation.
● Laboratory findings: complete blood and coagulation status (Table 3.**10**).

Hereditary Hemorrhagic Telangiectasia (Rendu–Osler Disease)

Main symptoms: Relatively mild but frequently recurrent, *chronic* nosebleed, usually commencing in youth and becoming more severe in middle age. Predominantyl unilateral, but tends to change sides. Asymptomatic periods lasting for weeks alternate with periods of constant light or heavy epistaxis. Marked or even severe anemia can follow prolonged bleeding episodes. Rhinoscopy shows red speckling of the septal and turbinate mucosae with tiny, tortuous capillary clusters that are slightly raised above the mucosal surface and may bear crusted deposits.

Other symptoms and special features: Similar teleangiectases are usually seen on the mucosal surfaces of the mouth, lips, palate, and on the face. They are less common on the trunk and extremities. Similar angiomatous changes occur in the gastrointestinal tract, liver, lung, or CNS and may coexist with a−v anastomoses (lung). Clinical manifestation sites of the vascular changes: nose 73%, lips 68%, facial skin 60%, tongue 45%, fingers 30%.

Cause: Autosomal dominant disease of the capillary walls (teleangiectasia).

Diagnosis:
● Personal and family history; typical endoscopic findings, possibly with analogous cutaneous changes on the face, limbs, and trunk.
● Blood and coagulation status.
● In doubtful cases, biopsy of a typical vascular nodule.
● With suspicion of gastrointestinal bleeding: consultation with an internist.

Simulated Nosebleed

This occurs when the bleeding source is extrinsic to the nose and the blood merely drains or is removed through the nose, as in hemoptysis, injury to the internal carotid artery (drainage via the nasopharynx or eustachian tube), bleeding esophageal varices, or bleeding from a pharyngeal, laryngeal, tracheal, or bronchial neoplasm.

Symptom   **Nasal Airway Obstruction**

An obstructed or "stuffy" nose is an invariably troublesome condition, which can have a variety of causes (Table 3.**11**). The obstruction may be unilateral or bilateral, transient or permanent, partial or complete, or based on functional or structural causes. The results of obstructed nasal breathing, besides significant subjective discomfort, may include permanent injury (e.g., to the respiratory organs) if the obstruction is of long standing. The potential consequences are summarized in Table 3.**12**.

Short History

Folliculitis and Eczema of the Nasal Vestibule
See p. 238.

Nasal Furunculosis
See p. 208.

Acute Rhinitis and Sinusitis
See pp. 179, 182, 184.

Allergic Rhinitis
See p. 184.

Vasomotor Rhinitis
See p. 186.

Sluder Neuralgia
See p. 162.

Trauma

Isolated nasal injuries, such as injuries of the midface and anterior cranial fossa (rhinobase), are generally associated with unilateral or bilateral impediment of nasal respiration. This obstruction of the nasal cavity (or cavities) may be caused purely by mucosal and soft-tissue edema, by hematoma formation (especially septal hematoma), or by displaced fracture fragments. The symptoms vary accordingly:

Traumatic Edema

Main symptoms: Boggy swelling of injured mucosae and soft tissues, possibly with reddish

Table 3.**11** *Symptom* Nasal airway obstruction

Synopsis

Nasal vestibule, nasal cavity, paranasal sinuses

Short history

- Vestibular folliculitis and eczema
- Nasal furuncle, see p. 208
- Acute rhinitis and sinusitis
  - Infectious, see p. 182
  - Vasomotor, see p. 186
  - Allergic, see p. 184
- Feature of Sluder neuralgia, see p. 162

Long history

- Alar collapse (flaccid nares)
- Vestibular stenosis; "valvular" stenosis; narrow nose
- Scar formation (synechiae) and/or insufficiently corrected posttraumatic states
- Rhinitis sicca anterior, see p. 176
- Septal perforation with crusting
- Septal deviation or subluxation, septal ridge or spur
- Chronic rhinopathy including turbinate hyperplasia and/or enlarged posterior ends
- Chronic sinusitis, see pp. 179, 189
- Nasal polyposis
- Bullous concha
- Rhinitis medicamentosa

- Drug side effects
- Occupational or climatic injury to the nasal mucosa
- Cystic fibrosis, see p. 189
- Bleeding septal polyp, see p. 194
- Foreign body or rhinolith, see p. 192
- Atrophic rhinitis and ozena
- Wegener granulomatosis and other granulomas
- Rhinoscleroma, see Table 4.**27**
- Intranasal tumors, see p. 214
- Choanal atresia
- Malformations and deformities of the nasal framework

In infants

- Dysgenesis, see Table 3.**23**
- Septal hematoma
- Other head trauma during or after birth

- Septal deviation
- Turbinate hyperplasia

Nasopharynx

Short history

- Pharyngeal (retronasal) angina, see p. 231 Retropharyngeal abscess, see p. 266

Long history

- Adenoid hyperplasia, possibly combined with hyperplasia of the palatine tonsils in children and adolescents, see p. 262
- Juvenile nasopharyngeal fibroma, see p. 195

- Choanal polyp, see p. 204
- Synechia between the soft palate and posterior pharyngeal wall*
- Nasopharyngeal tumors, see p. 218

* No further commentary

or pale discoloration. Tenderness to pressure but no fresh bleeding.

Diagnosis:

● Establish whether there is simple mechanical soft-tissue irritation, or whether there is a fracture of the bony and/or cartilaginous nasal framework (palpation: crepitation and abnormal motion).

● Rhinoscopy, endoscopy. Probing as required.

● Radiographs if a fracture is suspected.

Differentiation is required from nasomidfacial fracture and hematoma.

Hematoma and Septal Abscess

Main symptoms: Hematomas usually develop on the anterior nasal septum due to accumulation of blood between the mucoperichondrium and septal cartilage. A tense, compressible swelling of the nasal septum forms a pouch between the mucoperichondrium and its substrate. Frequently bilateral. Nonpainful. Infection leads to a septal abscess with (severe) pain, fever, and gradual liquefaction of the septal cartilage (result: "duckbill" nose).

Diagnosis: See above.

Differential diagnosis is accomplished by needle aspiration (with subsequent therapeutic drainage).

Fracture

Main symptoms: Nasal airway obstruction, intranasal deformity, bleeding soft-tissue defects, tenderness of the nasal pyramid, palpable edge or stepoff, displacement of the nasal pyramid, and swelling of external nasal soft tissues. See p. 135 ff.

Diagnosis:
- Palpation of the nasal pyramid (crepitus and abnormal motion).
- Rhinoscopy; probing as required.
- Radiographs: Lateral projection of the nasal pyramid. Exclude involvement of the paranasal sinuses and rhinobase.

Differentiation is required from hematoma, midfacial fracture, and basal skull fracture (see p. 178).

Intranasal Foreign Bodies
See p. 192.

Long History

Alar Collapse (Alar Flaccidity)

Main symptoms: Visible indrawing ("collapse") of the nasal alae during forcible inspiration. Nasal breathing is significantly improved by placing a small cotton wad into the dome of the nasal vestibule to prevent alar collapse.

Table 3.**12**   Potential consequences of long-term nasal airway obstruction

Disturbance or impairment of the dependent respiratory system including the lungs
Eating difficulties
Sleep disturbance
Snoring
Development of obstructive apnea syndrome
Head pain or fullness
Hyposmia or anosmia
Increased susceptibility to upper respiratory infections such as pharyngitis, laryngitis, and bronchitis
Predisposition to paranasal sinus disease
Strain on the heart and circulation
Speech difficulties
Other possible effects in children:
Maxillary growth disturbance ("pointed palate")
Positional abnormalities of teeth
Anorexia
Thoracic deformity
Failure to thrive
Physical and intellectual retardation
Increased susceptibility to otogenic and rhinogenic diseases

Causes: Insufficient rigidity of the alar cartilages.

Diagnosis: Inspection of the anterior nose during respiration, palpation of the nasal alae, rhinoscopy.

Differentiation is required from valvular stenosis, septal deviation, and airway obstruction due to organic intranasal causes.

Nasal Vestibular Stenosis, Valvular Stenosis, (Extreme) Narrow Nose, Posttraumatic State

Main symptoms: With *vestibular stenosis* in the strict sense, there is insufficient patency for nasal airflow due to deficient cross-sectional area of the naris and/or the nasal vestibule. *Valvular stenosis* is similar to (and may coexist with) alar collapse in that inspiration produces narrowing or collapse of the nasal valve — the slit-

Table 3.**13**   Causes of septal perforation

Traumatic
- Microtrauma (fingers, dust, chemicals, etc.)
- Frequent cauterizations, cryosurgery, or laser treatments for recurrent epistaxis
- Following septal abscess
- Sharp nasal or mucosal injury
- Long-term transnasal intubation
- Cocaine sniffing, heroin inhalation
- Occupational mucosal injuries (dust, cement, mercury, arsenic, lead, tar, heat, etc.; see Table 3.**16**)

Infections
- Specific inflammatory conditions (tuberculosis, lupus, sarcoidosis tertiary syphilis, leprosy)
- Rare tropical infections (blastomycosis, leishmaniasis, etc.), see p. 191 and Table 4.**28**
- Fungal infections

Granulating mucosal diseases
- Wegener granulomatosis
- Midline granuloma

Neoplastic

Septal Perforation (Perforated Septal Ulcer)

Main symptoms: Recurrent epistaxis, nasal airway obstruction by crusting.

Other symptoms and special features: Whistling sound during inspiration and expiration. Typical of small perforations in the anterior part of the septum.

Causes: See Table 3.**13**.

Diagnosis: Nasal endoscopy.

Differential diagnosis: See Table 3.**13**.

Septal Deviation, Septal Dislocation, Septal Spurs and Ridges

Main symptoms: Unilateral or bilateral, constant or variable impediment of nasal respiration, depending on the site and severity of the septal deformity. Hyposmia is rarely present. Headache can result from pressure of a septal spur against a turbinate or, more rarely, from a tension septum, i.e., a septum that is under tension because it is too large relative to surrounding structures.

Other symptoms and special features: Septal deviations are frequently combined with morphologic abnormalities of the external nose (e.g., deviated nose). Compensatory turbinate hypertrophy is often present on the concave side of the deviated septum. Occasional proneness to epistaxis and rhinitis sicca anterior ("baffle" during inspiration). Snoring.

Causes: Developmental defect or trauma.

Diagnosis: Rhinoscopy. Often the nasal mucosa must be decongested before septal deformities can be diagnosed! Rhinomanometry is helpful in some cases.

Differentiation is required from chronic rhinitis and intranasal mass lesions. With sleep-associated respiratory problems, consider obstructive sleep apnea.

like opening between the caudal end of the lateral cartilage and the nasal septum.

Causes: *Vestibular stenosis:* dysgenesis or trauma. *Valvular stenosis:* malposition of the anterior border of the lateral cartilage or of the anterior septal border, creating a deficient lumen at what is normally the narrowest portion of the nasal airway.

Similarly, nasal breathing can be impeded by an *extremely narrow* nose (usually the result of a faulty rhinoplasty), by the inadequate treatment of nasal trauma,, or by poor intranasal surgical technique (synechia formation).

Diagnosis: Rhinoscopy, palpation of the nasal framework. Rhinomanometry is helpful in some cases.

Differentiation is required from alar collapse, septal deviation, septal dislocation, and other intranasal organic causes of airway obstruction.

Rhinitis Sicca Anterior
See p. 176.

Chronic Rhinopathy

Main symptoms: Chronic "runny nose" with a viscous, mucoid, usually colorless discharge. Initially intermittent and alternating nasal obstruction, later becoming constant and usually bilateral. Accompanied by annoying postnasal drainage. Rhinophonia clausa. Habitual throat clearing and sniffing. Snoring. Rhinoscopy shows dark red or pale livid, swollen turbinates. Vasoconstricting nosedrops initially provide transient shrinkage of the mucosal "pad" (*chronic rhinitis simplex*) but later produce no appreciable decongestive effect (*chronic hyperplastic rhinitis*). Swelling most commonly affects the heads of the inferior and/or middle turbinates and possibly the posterior ends. Increasing coarsening of the mucosal surface ("mulberry turbinates"). Occasional polyp formation. Posterior rhinoscopy shows enlarged, pale, glazed, raspberry-like posterior ends of the turbinates (especially the inferior turbinates).

Other symptoms and special features: Headache or pressure from the nasal obstruction. Secondary dacryocystitis, epiphora, conjunctivitis, and/or pharyngitis. Lethargy. In severe cases: sleeplessness and impaired physical and mental performance.

Causes: Very heterogeneous causal factors (Table 3.**14**).

Diagnosis:
● Detailed history is required! Look for causative exogenous agents.
● Rhinoscopy: See above. Intranasal and nasopharyngeal endoscopy is recommended!
● Histologic examination shows an edematous mucosa with vascular alterations and typical changes in the epithelium, glands, and lamina propria ("mucous dyscrinism"); also perivascular infiltrates.

Differentiation is required from sinusitis, specific mucosal inflammatory conditions (see p. 191), allergic rhinitis, enlarged adenoids, Wegener granulomatosis, intranasal neoplasms (suspicion warrants biopsy!), CSF rhinorrhea, and foreign bodies.

Rhinitis of Pregnancy

Increasing bilateral nasal airway obstruction, especially in the second half of pregnancy, caused by marked swelling of the turbinate mucosae and increased, usually very troublesome nasal discharge. Symptoms subside during the postpartum period.

Table 3.**14**   Causes of chronic rhinopathy

Predominantly exogenous factors
Inflammatory conditions
– Recurrent common infections, frequent colds, diseases of adjacent tissues (e.g., paranasal sinuses), specific infections
Physical and/or chemical injury to the nasal mucosa
– Unfavorable climate
– Unfavorable working conditions (work space, air conditioning, etc.)
– Air impurities (e.g., combustion gases, tobacco smoke, organic solvents, wood preservatives, insecticides, impregnation sprays, detergents, cleansers)
– Occupational injury
Drugs and the nasal mucosa
– Pharmacotoxic rhinitis
– Side effects of drugs not used for rhinologic indications
– Drug allergy or pseudoallergy
Mixed exogenous and endogenous factors
Sequelae of a mucosal allergy
– Recurrent reactions of the immediate type (I, humoral)
– (Recurrent) reactions of the delayed type (IV, cell-mediated or T-cell-dependent)
– "Infective allergy" (?)
Predominantly endogenous factors
Immunopathies of the nasal mucosa (e.g., IgA deficiency, inhibitor deficiency, nasal mastocytosis (Connell), functional deficits involving previously unidentified protective mechanisms of the nasal mucosa
Endocrine dysfunctions
Disturbed neuroautonomic regulation of the nasal mucosa (also subject to psychoneurologic influences)
Organic lesions of the nasal mucosa
Genetically determined ("constitutional") functional disturbances of the nasal mucosa
Anatomic intranasal disease-promoting factors
Systemic diseases affecting the nasal mucosa

Chronic Sinusitis
See pp. 179, 189.

Nasal Polyposis

Main symptoms: Increasing unilateral or bilateral nasal airway obstruction (stuffy nose), occasionally varying in intensity. Hyposmia or anosmia is common in severe cases. Head fullness. Rhinoscopy: glazed, smooth-walled, whitish or reddish, soft, localized excrescence of the nasal mucosa, presenting a broad or pedunculated base (site of predilection: middle and/or inferior meatus). Usually multiple and bilateral. Soft and mobile on probing.

Other symptoms and special features: Epiphora, mucoid or mucopurulent nasal discharge. Rhinophonia clausa, snoring. Often coexists with chronic sinusitis, usually of the ethmoid sinus but also affecting other sinuses (often pansinusitis with intrasinus polyposis).

Causes: Inflammatory; allergic cause is demonstrable in about 25% of cases.

Diagnosis:
• Anterior *and* posterior rhinoscopy.
• Paranasal sinus radiographs.
• Olfactory testing. Rhinomanometry and allergy tests may be rewarding (see p. 185 ff.).

Differentiation is required from turbinate hyperplasia, meningoencephalocele, intranasal neoplasms (especially malignancies); also intranasal extension of an intracranial tumor.

Choanal Polyp

Solitary polyp that produces variable obstruction of the choana and/or nasopharynx, frequently arises on a pedicle in the maxillary sinus, and causes nasal airway obstruction and rhinophonia clausa.

Differentiation is required from nasopharyngeal fibroma and other nasopharyngeal tumors.

Bullous Concha

Main symptoms: Partial, usually unilateral impediment of nasal respiration. Rhinoscopy: markedly expanded head of the middle turbinate partially obstructing the nasal lumen and usually impinging on the septum. A bony resistance on probing distinguishes the bullous concha from the soft consistency of a nasal polyp.

Cause: Large, pneumatized ethmoid cell in the head of the middle turbinate.

Diagnosis: Rhinoscopy, probing. Diagnosis may be aided by radiographs in the AP projection.

Differentiation is required from nasal polyps and intranasal tumor (especially ethmoid malignancy).

Rhinitis Medicamentosa

Main symptoms: Partial or complete, bilateral nasal airway obstruction, sometimes with olfactory impairment. Excessive rhinorrhea or nasal dryness.

Causes:
○ Long-term local use of decongestant nosedrops or other locally administered agents (= toxic rhinitis, Table 3.**15**).
○ Undesired side effect of systemic drugs or other agents (Table 3.**15**).
○ Individual allergic or pseudoallergic drug reaction. Differentiating criteria, see Table 3.**5**.

Rhinoscopy: Usually red, hypertrophic, sometimes "granular" nasal mucosa; less commonly, pale livid mucosal discoloration.

Occupational Rhinopathy

The injurious effects of occupational agents on the nasal mucosa may incite a chronic or allergic form of rhinopathy or, less commonly, an atrophic rhinitis or rhinopathy. Symptoms may include nasal airway obstruction, chronic or recurrent coryza, dryness and crusting, or even recurrent epistaxis. The rhinitis may be caused by:
○ mechanical
○ chemical
○ physical, or
○ biological agents

The more common causative agents of occupational rhinopathy are listed in Table 3.**16**.

Bleeding Septal Polyp
See p. 194.

Foreign Bodies and Rhinoliths
See p. 192.

Table 3.**15**   Rhinologic disturbances caused by drugs (selection)

Pharmacotoxic rhinitis (long-term local application, overdosage)

- Imidazoline and catechol derivatives
- Factors causing ciliary damage (pH, osmotic pressure)
- Sensitizing drugs (see below)
- Tachyphylaxis and rebound effect

Drugs causing mucosal dryness

- Atropine
- Belladonna
- Imidazoline and catechol derivatives
- Glucocorticoids
- Centrally acting psychotropic drugs (e. g., dopamine antagonists, hydantoin, lithium salts, phenothiazines)
- See also Tables 4.**8** and 5.**7**

Drugs causing nasal stuffiness (mucosal swelling; combination of allergic and pseudoallergic reactions, see below)

- Acetylsalicylic acid and derivatives
- Antihistamines
- Antihypertensive drugs (e. g., alpha-methyl-dopa, guanethidine, hydralazine, phentolamine, prazosin, reserpine)
- Antithyroid drugs (e. g., mercaptoimidazole, thiouracil)
- Ephedrine (rebound effect)
- Hydantoin
- Hydralazine
- Iodides
- Estrogens
- Paracetamol
- Paraminosalicylic acid
- Phenothiazines
- Tetraethylammonium
- Antiarrhythmic drugs (e. g., disopyramide, propafenone)
- Nonsteroidal antirheumatic drugs (e. g., indomethacin, ibuprofen, phenylbutazone, dextroproxyphene, paracetamol, mefenamic acid, pentazocine)

Drugs causing epistaxis (by various mechanisms)

- Phenylbutazone
- Isoniazid
- Sulfonamides
- Anticoagulants
- Semisynthetic penicillins, cephalosporins, etc.

Less commonly:
- Clofibrate, bezafibrate
- Chloroquine
- Sodium valporate
- Penicillin and related compounds
- Estrogens
- Platelet-aggregation inhibitors
- Cyclo-oxygenase inhibitors
- Cytostatic drugs

Drugs inciting allergic or pseudoallergic reactions

- Acetylsalicylic acid and derivatives
- Antihistamines
- Cephalosporins
- Chloramphenicol
- Chlorpromazine
- Clometiazol
- Codeine
- Formaldehyde
- Griseofulvin
- Indomethacin
- Isoniazid
- Isocyanates
- Colloidal plasma expanders
- Local anesthetics
- Metamizol
- Morphine
- Muscle relaxants
- Narcotics
- Nitrofurantoin
- Estrogens
- Papaverine
- Penicillin and related compounds
- Platinum salts
- Pyrazolone and derivatives
- Radiographic contrast media
- Streptokinase
- Streptomycin
- Sulfite
- Sulfonamides
- Tetracyclines

Table 3.**16** Common occupational agents that can cause rhinopathy (after Manz and Schwab)

Physical agents
- Coarse dust (particle size >5 μm)
- Dusts that are highly water-soluble, strongly corrosive, and/or sensitizing
- Nontoxic dusts such as iron, lead, nickel and its compounds, plaster, calcium cyanamide, copper, coal, talc, quartz, cement, ground basic slag, glass wool, flax, hemp, jute, textiles

Chemical agents
- Sulfur dioxide (leading agent, representative of atmospheric pollutants), hydrocarbons, carbon monoxide, ozone
- Chlorine, bromine, ammonia, sulfur dichloride, phosphorus chlorides, formalin, acrolein, hydrofluoric acid, hydrochloric acid
- Isocyanates, cyanides, epoxy resins, and casting resins
- Chemical irritants: arsenic, chromium, chromates, cadmium, carbon disulfide, hydrogen sulfide
- Iodine, mercury, aluminum

Biological agents
- Inhalation allergens, e.g., dust in poultry plants; feed concentrates, wheat flour, raw cotton, dust in lumber mills and woodworking shops; hemp, straw, silage dust, tobacco dust Dust containing animal epithelial cells or insect parts, library dust, grain dust, pollen
- Food allergens, e.g., milk, chocolate, wheat, citrus fruits, eggs, bananas, tomatoes, corn, peas, beans, coffee, tea; alcohol. Dyes and preservatives
- Other substances that act as complete antigens or haptens such as parasubstituted aromates, materials used in synthetic resin production, detergents, paraphenyldiamine, gum arabic, drugs such as acetylsalicylic acid, phenacetin, quinidine, papain, numerous antibiotics, fungicides, and pesticides

Climatic agents
- Work in an exceptionally hot or cold environment. Direct exposure to infrared radiation. A warm, damp work environment. Rapid temperature changes

Atrophic Rhinopathy and Ozena

Main symptoms: Although the nasal cavities are widely patent, there is a sensation of nasal obstruction. Headache is common. Olfaction is absent or diminished. In *ozena*, a foul, fetid nasal odor is *the* cardinal symptom. Rhinoscopy: The nose is filled with greenish-yellow to dark brown, hard, firmly adherent crusts interspersed with a scant, viscous, purulent discharge. After cleansing, the very wide nasal cavity affords an excellent view of the posterior wall of the pharynx. Loss of sensibility of the nasal mucosa (degeneration of maxillary nerve fibers). The nasal membranes, and often those of the pharynx and/or larynx, are atrophic, dry, and leathery.

Other symptoms and special features: Incidence is generally low, with a 3:1 female preponderance. Onset is usually in puberty. The face is often broad and flattened, the nose small and wide ("Slavic" facies).

Causes: Not fully understood. Today a very rare disease. Presumably multifactorial (endogenous and exogenous) with a genetic basis. "Symptomatic atrophic rhinitis" occurs after destructive trauma and/or surgery of the nose.

Diagnosis: Rhinoscopic findings.

Differentiation is required from intranasal foreign bodies, chronic sinusitis, syphilis (tertiary), mucosal tuberculosis, malleus, and AIDS.

Intranasal Tumors
See p. 214 and Table 3.**20**.

Choanal Atresia

Main symptoms: Complete unilateral or bilateral nasal obstruction. Persistent purulent coryza on the obstructed side; inability to blow the nose.

Other symptoms and special features: Symptoms are present from birth, except in acquired (posttraumatic) cases due to scarring. Olfaction is absent on the affected side. Bilaterality is not uncommon, and both sides may be affected in different degrees (i.e., stenosis on one side, atresia on the other). Unilateral choanal atresia is five times more prevalent than bilateral; girls predominate by a 5:1 ratio. *Bilateral* choanal atresia in *newborns* poses an acute risk of asphyxiation! These cases are marked by cyanosis and gasping, arrhythmic, stridorous respirations. The symptoms are exacerbated by feeding!

Causes: Presumably transmitted as a dominant trait. Secondary atresia will follow a history of prior damage (trauma, surgery) to the internal nose.

Diagnosis:
- In emergency situations (risk of asphyxiation in infants or newborns): Try using a Politzer bag or similar device to force air into the pharynx through the nose, or try passing a thin rubber or plastic catheter through the nose into the pharynx.
- Even in nonemergent situations, these techniques can be effectively combined with anterior and posterior rhinoscopy and nasopharyngeal endoscopy.
- Radiographic visualization (after instilling contrast medium into the obstructed side in the supine patient). Tomograms are useful in some cases.

Differentiation is required from all other lesions causing nasal obstruction (e.g., polyposis, previous trauma, foreign bodies, meningoencephalocele, neoplasms).

Malformations and Deformities of the Nasal Framework or Face

These are not unusual as causes of nasal airway obstruction (see Table 3.**23**). It is rarely difficult to identify the anatomic and functional relationships underlying the obstruction.

More difficult are malformations that are not readily visible (e.g., choanal atresia, see above) or do not bear an obvious relationship to nasal pathology (e.g., cleft palate and alveolus, typically associated with significant septal deviation toward the cleft side). See details on p. 221.

Deformities of the nasal pyramid (saddle nose, deviated nose, etc., see Table 3.**23**) can also cause nasal airway obstruction. The diagnosis is based on rhinoscopy and, in some cases, rhinomanometry.

Juvenile Nasopharyngeal Fibroma
See p. 195.

Choanal Polyp
See p. 204.

Nasopharyngeal Tumors
See p. 218.

Symptom   **Dry Nose**

The symptom of nasal dryness may be caused by exogenous as well as endogenous influences. The most common and clinically important causes are listed in Table 3.**17**.

Table 3.**17** *Symptom* Dry nose

Synopsis	
Exogenous causes	Typical drug action (e. g., atropine, belladonna, glucocorticoids, imidazole and catechol derivatives, sympathomimetics, etc.)
Unfavorable climatic conditions	
Occupational exposure to heat or cold	
Work in a dusty environment (plaster, granite, lime, coal, cement, wood, arsenic, nickel carbonyl, etc.), see p. 204 and Table 3.**16**	Pharmacotoxic rhinitis, see. p. 204
	Side effect, especially of drugs used for the treatment of organic and/or psychiatric disorders (rauwolfia, psychotropic drugs), see Table 3.**15**
Prolonged stay in an excessively dry "climatized" area (relative humidity <50%)	
Previous nasal trauma and/or surgery	
Previous therapeutic radiation to the head	**Endogenous causes**
Initial stage of acute rhinitis	"Dry" constitution ("sympathicotonic type" with relatively low eccrine glandular activity)
Bacterial, fungal, or parasitic chronic mucosal inflammation (e. g., tuberculosis, tertiary syphilis, leishmaniasis, mycosis)	Endocrine, e. g., in Basedow disease, also in endemic cretinism and adrenocortical hyperfunction (interrenalism)
Chronic febrile and consumptive systemic diseases	Sjögren disease (sicca syndrome)

Symptom   **Nasal Fetor** (Table 3.**18**)

Table 3.**18** *Symptom* Nasal fetor (causes)

Synopsis	
Atrophic rhinopathy with fetor (ozena)	Malleus
Nasal and paranasal sinus tumors	Tertiary syphilis (gumma)
Purulent rhinitis	Intranasal foreign bodies and rhinoliths
Purulent sinusitis	Nasopharyngeal tumors
Dentogenic sinusitis	Pharyngeal bursitis (Tornwaldt disease)
Nasal diphtheria	
Tuberculosis of the nasal mucosa	
Leishmaniasis and other rare infections	

Symptom   **Morphologic Change (Swelling, Tumor)**

Some of the diseases associated with this symptom have been discussed elsewhere. Page references to these disorders are included in the synopsis given in Table 3.**19**.

Nose and Paranasal Sinuses

Nasal Furunculosis

Main symptoms: Tender swelling. Edema and redness of the nasal tip (especially in the tip pouch), columella, and upper lip. Feeling of tension throughout the anterior nose. Resolves by demarcation and sloughing of a central necrotic plug.

Other symptoms and special features: Severe systemic illness with fever. Infection may spread to the angular vein (lateral nasal pyramid) and cavernous sinus (cavernous sinus thrombosis, see p. 214).

Causes: Pyoderma arising from the hair follicles in the nasal vestibule or upper lip (usually staphylococci).

Diagnosis:
● Typical appearance of a furuncle with a central yellow plug, always located in the *skin*.
● Option: bacteriologic smear with sensitivity testing.

Differentiation is required from carbuncle (multiple necrotic foci), perichondritis, erysipelas, and trichophytosis (tinea).

Erysipelas
See p. 173.

Perichondritis
See p. 174.

Trauma and Its Sequelae
See pp. 135, 177.

Chilblains (Pernio)

Main symptoms: Bluish to livid nodules of a firm consistency in the soft tissues of the nasal tip. Develop during cold season and are initially painless. Exposure to warm environment provokes intense itching and/or burning.

Other symptoms and special features: A rare condition, most commonly affecting adolescent females.

Causes: *Not* true frostbite, but the result of a constitutionally deficient adaptative capacity of the microcirculation to low temperatures.

Differentiation is required from Boeck disease, lupus erythematosus, and granulosis rubra nasi.

Table 3.**19**   *Symptom*   Morphologic change (swelling, tumor)

Synopsis
Nose and paranasal sinuses
Hyperplasias, inflammatory conditions, injuries, etc.
– Nasal furuncle
– Erysipelas, see p. 173
– Perichondritis, see p. 174
– Trauma, see pp. 135, 177
– Chilblain
– Rhinophyma and rosacea
– Lupus erythematosus
– Chronic and specific inflammatory conditions (tuberculosis, syphilis, sarcoidosis), see pp. 191, 255
– Granulomas and granulomatoses, see pp. 192, 255
– Cysts and celes, see p. 180
– Dentogenic maxillary cysts, see p. 142
– Inflammatory rhinogenic complications
– Orbital complications
– Osteomyelitis of the flat cranial bones
– Epidural abscess
– Subdural abscess
– Rhinogenic sinus thrombosis
– Rhinogenic brain abscess
Benign tumors
Precancerous lesions
Malignant tumors
Systemic neoplasias
– Eosinophilic granuloma of the skull
– Plasmocytoma (extramedullary)
Nasopharynx
Hyperplasias, inflammatory conditions, trauma sequelae
Benign and malignant tumors
– Juvenile nasopharyngeal fibroma, see p. 195
– Teratoma
– Chordoma
– Craniopharyngeoma (Erdheim tumor)
– Glomus tumor, see p. 29
– Nasopharyngeal carcinoma

Rhinophyma

Main symptoms: Coarsening of the anterior nasal contour with firm, lobular, bluish-red to reddish-brown outgrowths ("potato nose"). No pain, slow growth. In later stages there is severe disfiguration with possible breathing and eating difficulties.

Other symptoms and special features: Peak occurrence is in middle age, with about a 20:1 preponderance of males. Often combined with rosacea and/or seborrhea.

Causes: Pseudotumor produced by hyperplasia of sebaceous glands and overgrowth of stroma. A causal relationship with rosacea is controversial.

Diagnosis: Unmistakable clinical presentation with regard to symptoms and localization.

Lupus Erythematosus (LE)

Main symptoms: Cutaneous erythema showing a "butterfly" distribution on the nose, forehead, and cheeks. Skin becomes coarse and thickened; formation of scales and plaques. Culminates in atrophy of the affected skin areas.

Other symptoms and special features: Mainly affects middle-aged women (4:1 preponderance over males). Possible sites of involvement are the ear region and the orolabial mucosae (see p. 255). Lymph node involvement (about 50%) and joint symptoms (70–90%) are common. Cutaneous LE (discoid LE, chronic LE) is distinguished from visceral (systemic) LE.

Causes: Autoimmune disorder plus exposure to injurious exogenous agents ("collagen disease" with immune vasculitis). See Table 4.**29**.

Diagnosis:
• Typical cutaneous lesions, detection of LE cells in the blood. Immunofluorescent detection of antinuclear factors and autoantibodies.
• Blood count in systemic LE shows leukopenia, thrombopenia, and anemia. Positive LE cell phenomenon.
• When LE is suspected, dermatologic consultation is required!

Differentiation is required from seborrhea, erysipelas, psoriasis, lupus vulgaris, photodermatosis, rosacea, and tinea facialis.

Specific Inflammatory Conditions (Tuberculosis, Syphilis, Sarcoidosis)
See pp. 191, 255.

Granulomas and Granulomatoses
See pp. 192, 255.

Cysts and Celes
See p. 180.

Dentogenic Maxillary Cysts
See p. 142.

Symptoms of Inflammatory Rhinogenic Extracranial and Intracranial Complications

Table 3.**20** and Figures 3.**8**–3.**10** illustrate the proximity of the paranasal sinuses to the orbit, face, skull base, and brain and to the principal structures located in those areas. Inflammatory paranasal sinus complications can be classified accordingly, and by pathologic criteria, as follows:
○ Soft-tissue abscesses in the forehead or cheek
○ Orbital complications
○ Osteomyelitis of the flat cranial bones ("frontal bone osteomyelitis")
○ Epidural abscess (external pachymeningitis)
○ Subdural abscess (internal pachymeningitis)
○ Thrombosis of a large dural sinus
○ Meningitis (leptomeningitis)
○ Diffuse encephalitis and circumscribed encephalitis (brain abscess)

Abscess Rupture into the Soft Tissues
See Tables 2.**2** and 3.**20**, Fig. 3.**9**

Orbital Complications

Main symptoms: Initial circumscribed lid and orbital edema (periostitis), then progression to

Table 3.**20**   Proximity of the paranasal sinuses to surrounding structures

	Maxillary sinus	Frontal sinus	Ethmoid cells	Sphenoid sinus
Anterior cranial fossa, dura, brain	–	+	+	(+)
Middle cranial fossa, dura, brain	–	–	(+)	+
Orbit and globe	+	+	+	(+)
Optic nerve	–	(+)	+	+
Internal carotid artery	–	–	–	+
Superior sagittal sinus	–	+	–	–
Cavernous sinus	–	–	–	+
Supraorbital nerve (V$_1$)	–	+	–	–
Infraorbital nerve (V$_2$)	+	–	(+)	–
Eye muscles and their nerves	+	+	+	+
Facial soft tissues	+	+	+	–
Maxillary teeth	+	–	–	–
Pterygopalatine fossa	+	–	(+)	+

+   = Direct proximity (in all cases)
(+) = Proximity depends on individual anatomic structures
–   = Not directly adjacent

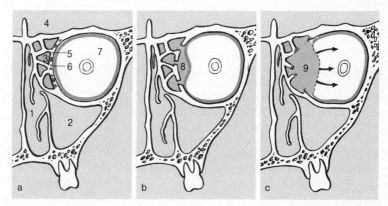

Fig. 3.**8a–c**   Various stages in the progression of an orbital complication arising from the ethmoid bone (after H. Marx)

a Orbital periostitis
b Subperiosteal abscess
c Orbital cellulitis
   1 Nasal cavity

2 Maxillary sinus
3 Ethmoid cells
4 Anterior cranial fossa
5 Carious orbital plate

6 Orbital periosteum
7 Globe
8 Erosion of abscess through ethmoid wall to orbit
9 Extension of suppuration to the globe

subperiosteal abscess and finally to orbital cellulitis. Accompanied by acute (or sometimes chronic) purulent, ipsilateral sinusitis. Severe pain and systemic illness with fever. See details on p. 138, 139.

Other symptoms and special features: Elevated ESR and left shift in the white blood count. Redness and tenderness of the swollen eyelid and, increasingly, of the globe. Possible development of a lid abscess (see p. 138). Typical

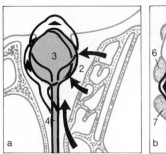

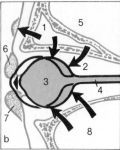

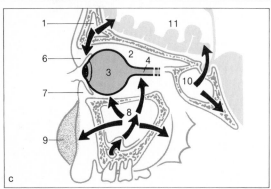

Fig. 3.**9a–c** Inflammatory complications of sinusitis (schematic) (from Becker, Naumann, Pfaltz)

a Transverse section through the orbit and surrounding structures

b Parasagittal section through the orbit and surrounding structures

c Parasagittal section through the facial skeleton
1 Extension of infection from the frontal sinus to the soft tissues of the forehead
2 Extension of infection from the frontal sinus to the orbit
3 Globe
4 Optic nerve
5 Anterior cranial fossa
6 Upper lid with inflammatory swelling
7 Lower lid with inflammatory swelling
8 Spread of infection from the maxillary sinus to the orbit, cheek, and retromaxillary space; the infection may be dentogenic (arrow)
9 Spread of infection from the maxillary sinus to the soft tissues of the cheek
10 Extension of suppuration from the sphenoid sinus to the intracranial space or bony skull base
11 Brain

progression in stages: orbital edema (prodrome)—orbital periostitis—subperiosteal abscess with periorbital edema and displacement of the globe (usually laterally and/or inferiorly, sometimes anteriorly)—orbital cellulitis with severe proptosis and decreased ocular mobility. Rapid visual deterioration. Lid and orbital edema (collateral edema) develop very rapidly in small children.

Cause: Extension of purulent sinusitis into the orbit (Fig. 3.**8a–c**).

Diagnosis:
- Rhinoscopy.
- Diagnostic imaging. Radiographs: Standard paranasal sinus projections, possibly augmented by CT, and MRI.
- Sonography is helpful in some cases.
- Ophthalmologic consultation.

Differentiation is required from mucocele or pyocele (indolent course with no pain or fever) and from intraorbital mass lesions (slow growth, usually without pain initially; radiographic and sonographic findings).

Osteomyelitis of the Flat Cranial Bones

Main symptoms: Diffuse, doughy swelling ("puffy tumor") with tense, glossy skin over the frontal bone. High fever, chills, severe headache. Tenderness to percussion over the affected portion of the cranium (generally over the frontal sinus and surrounding bone).

Other symptoms: Most cases take a fulminating course with rapid physical debilitation, clouding of consciousness, and the development of intracranial complications (see sections below).

Cause: Usually an infection spreading rapidly from an infected frontal sinus (rarely metastatically) to involve the diploic layer of the skull, with a potential for intracranial spread. See Figure 3.**10**.

Diagnosis:
- Rhinoscopy.
- Diagnostic imaging: Radiographs of the forehead and calvarium (osteolytic areas are not visible until 10–14 days after onset!). CT

scans. Radionuclide imaging. MRI for identification of intracranial abscess formation.

● Blood count shows a left shift with a markedly increased ESR.

Differentiation is required from uncomplicated frontal sinusitis, erysipelas, and other diseases that take a septic course. Overt *intracranial* complications (extradural abscess, bacterial meningitis, diffuse or circumscribed encephalitis).

Epidural Abscess

Main symptoms: Very nonspecific. Headache (in some cases), subfebrile temperatures. Symptoms of a fulminating or protracted frontal, ethmoid, or sphenoid sinusitis with relatively mild systemic illness. Often discovered only during surgical exploration of the adjacent sinuses.

Cause: Extension of paranasal sinus suppuration into the adjacent epidural space.

Diagnosis:
● Rhinoscopy with observation of sinus drainage.
● Radiography: Standard projections of the paranasal sinuses, CT scans, especially of the anterior cranial fossa and facial skeleton.
● Neurologic and ophthalmologic findings are generally normal (*no papilledema*, no neurologic deficits, normal CSF).

Differentiation is required from other intracranial complications (see Tables 1.**13** and 1.**16**) and from epidural hematoma.

Subdural Abscess

Main symptoms: Headache and potentially marked temperature elevation. Usually significant malaise. Increasing signs of meningeal irritation, though these may be absent. As the disease progresses, intracranial symptoms increase with somnolence, possible seizures, (lower limb) palsies, and other neurologic disturbances, especially signs of increased intracranial pressure.

Causes: Erosion of suppurative sinus infection through the bone and adjacent dura into the subdural space. Progression to diffuse meningitis or encephalitis can occur at any time.

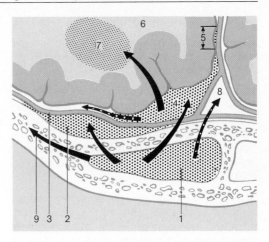

Fig. 3.**10** Potential intracranial complications of sinusitis (schematic) (from Becker, Naumann, Pfaltz)

1 Frontal sinus
2 Epidural abscess
3 Dura
4 Large subdural abscess (broken arrow = tracking of pus along dura = meningitis)
5 Small, encapsulated subdural abscess
6 Brain
7 Circumscribed encephalitis (brain abscess)
8 Superior sagittal sinus
9 Spread of infection into the medullary spaces of the cranial bone (osteomyelitis)

Diagnosis:
● History and rhinoscopic findings. Confirmation of sinusitis, observation of sinus drainage.
● Radiography: Standard paranasal sinus projections. Tomography and/or CT (anterior cranial fossa and face). Possibly MRI.
● Laboratory findings: Markedly increased ESR; blood count shows leukocytosis with a left shift. CSF: Generally only a moderate increase in cellularity (granulocytes). Elevated protein, increased pressure. CSF sugars normal. Fluid may have a floccular appearance.
● EEG (electroencephalography) and other neurodiagnostic procedures according to neurologic consultation.

Differentiation is required from other intracranial inflammatory processes and subdural hematoma. See also Tables 1.**13** and 1.**16**.

Rhinogenic Sinus Thrombosis

This is a rare complication chiefly affecting the *cavernous sinus* and less commonly the superior sagittal sinus.

Main symptoms: Lid edema, proptosis, chemosis, decreased ocular motility, visual deterioration. Chills and septic temperatures. Headache, papilledema, increasing somnolence, and features of meningitis and septic metastasis (see also Table 1.**18** and cf. Fig. 3.**10**).

Causes: Extension of sphenoid sinusitis or frontal bone osteomyelitis to the adjacent dural sinus. But there are many other potential sources and routes of infection, especially in the case of the cavernous sinus: Extension of thrombophlebitis from a furuncle of the nose and upper lid (angular vein), septal abscess, orbital cellulitis, petrositis, tonsillogenic complication.

Diagnosis:
- Complete ENT status.
- Ophthalmologic consultation.
- *Radiography:* Standard paranasal sinus views, tomograms, CT scans. Other options: DSA, MRI.
- *Laboratory findings:* Markedly increased ESR, leukocytosis with a left shift in the white blood count; attempted recovery of infecting organism from the blood; urinalysis. Increased CSF pressure with elevated protein and mild pleocytosis.
- Internal medical and neurologic consultation (septic metastasis, e.g., spleen, lung, brain).

Differentiation is required from orbital cellulitis, dentogenic or tonsillogenic cellulitis and septis, otogenic sinus thrombosis.
In cases of rhinogenic *superior sagittal sinus thrombosis* (very rare!) and confirmed *sinusitis* (frontal), the *main symptoms* are parietal pain, meningism, and limb palsies. There is eventual progression to meningitis and/or brain abscess.

Meningitis
See p. 42.

Rhinogenic Brain Abscess

Main symptoms: The great majority of rhinogenic brain abscesses occur in the frontal lobe. They exhibit the four classic stages of brain abscess and the classic symptom groups: a) systemic symptoms, b) intracranial pressure signs, and c) focal symptoms. The focal signs of frontal lobe abscess are nonspecific: psychic changes such as euphoria; compulsive joking (witzelsucht); logorrhea; increased excitability; and disturbances of drive. Possible contralateral ataxia, abnormal grasp reflex, and turning of the gaze and head toward the unaffected side (see also Table 1.**17**). *Suggestive signs* may include malaise, fever, dull or boring headache, tenderness to percussion over the calvarium, nausea, and vomiting. Slowing of the pulse ("pressure pulse"). Papilledema (in some cases), possible unilateral anosmia. Intellectual impairment and altered mentation. Individual cranial neuropathies (I, III, VI).

Causes: Extension of sinusitis (usually frontal sinusitis, less commonly ethmoid sinusitis) to the frontal bone. Hematogenous spread is also possible.

Diagnosis:
- Complete endoscopic and neurotologic ENT workup.
- Eye examination (papilledema, ipsilateral mydriasis, optic neuritis).
- Diagnostic imaging. Standard paranasal sinus views, CT, possibly MRI. Carotid angiography, possibly radionuclide scanning, etc.
- Neurologic consultation. May initiate further studies such as EEG, echoencephalography, and CSF examination (see Table 1.**14**).

Differentiation is required from stroke, brain trauma, brain tumor, viral encephalitis, infectious diseases, etc. (see also Tables 1.**13** to 1.**17**).

Tumors of the Nose and Paranasal Sinuses

Benign Tumors

A discussion of the specific types of benign tumor occurring in this region would be of limited value, because benign tumors of the nose and paranasal sinuses are relatively rare, and an essentially constant diagnostic algorithm is followed for all neoplasms, which generally are diagnosed by biopsy. Accordingly, the present sections deals only with *common* diagnostic aspects. The most frequently encountered benign nasal and paranasal sinus tumors* are listed in Table 3.**21**. See also Table 2.**5**.

Main symptoms: Generally very slow tumor growth with no pain. Mass effects in later stages may cause a feeling of pressure in the face or head. Examination of sensory or motor cranial nerves shows corresponding functional deficits. Bleeding is unusual except with very vascular tumors. Intranasal growths cause gradual impairment of nasal function (airway obstruction, olfactory impairment) and paranasal sinus function (impaired aeration and drainage, displacement or destruction of adjacent structures). Tumor extension into facial soft tissues causes visible protrusions and deformities.

Diagnosis:
● Long history with few symptoms. Rhinoscopy, possibly endoscopy (including paranasal sinuses).
● Sonography is useful for some tumor locations.
● Radiographs: Standard films (paranasal sinuses, axial skull base), also CT scans. Angiography is indicated for selected cases, e.g., suspected intracranial extension.
● Olfactory testing; some cases warrant complete cranial nerve status.
● Neurologic, ophthalmologic, or dental consultation may be required.
● Biopsy.

Differentiation is required from chronic inflammatory processes including complications, cysts, muco/pyoceles, bullous concha, and congenital anomalies of the facial bones (Table 3.**21**).

---

* The *tumor classification* of the WHO is widely accepted as the international standard for pathoanatomic nomenclature. It says little, however, about the important criterion of *clinical prevalence*. For our present purposes, then, we did not simply reproduce the WHO lists but chose to provide survey tables (3.**21**, 3.**22**, 4.**18**, 5.**3**, 6.**4**, 6.**5**, 7.**6**, 8.**11**, 10.**6**) that present a *selection* geared mainly toward clinical prevalence.

Precancerous Lesions

Precancerous lesions of the *external nose* include *senile keratoma* and *cutaneous horn* (cardinal symptom: circumscribed hyperkeratosis with increasing yellowish-brown pigmentation and a flat to irregular, verrucous surface = *senile keratoma*). Excessive thickening of the lesion can produce a solitary horny excrescence of the skin (= *cutaneous horn*). *Lentigo maligna* can be a precursor of malignant melanoma (cardinal symptom: irregular, brownish-black macula with irregular borders; long history, female preponderance). The foregoing skin lesions generally appear in persons over 60 years of age. By contrast, *xeroderma pigmentosum* ("senile" skin changes with abnormal, mottled pigmentation and keratoses) usually begins in childhood. Dermatologic consultation is necessary for the differential diagnosis of these lesions.

The essential premalignant lesions of the *internal nose* (and paranasal sinuses) are *leukoplakia* and *inverted papilloma*.

Leukoplakia
See p. 256.

Inverted Papilloma

Main symptoms: Nasal airway obstruction, mostly unilateral; occasional light epistaxis. Rhinoscopy shows a fleshy, cauliflower-like growth, usually arising from the septum but sometimes forming in the nasal vestibule.

Other symptoms and special features: Relatively rare nasal tumor, grossly indistinguishable from "normal" exophytic nasal papilloma. May involve not just the nasal passages but also the paranasal sinuses (especially the maxillary sinus and ethmoid cells). Only inverted papillomas exhibit signs of malignant transformation (in about 20% of cases)! High rate of recurrence!

Diagnosis:
● Rhinoscopy; nasal and paranasal sinus endoscopy.
● CT scans.
● Biopsy.

Table 3.**21**   Tumors of the nasal cavity and paranasal sinuses (selection)

Benign
- Osteoma (approximately 50%)
- Chondroma
- Fibroma
  Ossifying fibroma
  Paget disease
- Myxoma
- Giant-cell tumor
- Lipoma
- Histiocytoma
- Hemangioma
- Lymphangioma
- Papilloma
- Teratoma (dermoid)
- Adenoma
- Cystadenolymphoma
- Pleomorphic adenoma
- True cholesteatoma (heterotopic epithelium)

- Odontoma
- Adamantinoma (ameloblastoma)
  (approximately 4% malignant)
- Ameloblastic fibroma
- Dentinoma
- Cementoma
- Neuroma, neurinoma
- Neurofibromatosis
- Olfactory neuroblastoma (esthesio-
  neuroblastoma) (secondary)
- Glioma
- Meningioma (secondary)
- Chordoma (may be benign or highly malignant)
- Chloroma

Precancerous lesions
- Inverted papilloma (malignancy rate approximately 20%)

Malignant
- Basal cell carcinoma (spreading secondarily to
  the nasal interior)
- Squamous cell carcinoma (approximately 60%
  of malignant tumors at this location)
- Adenocarcinoma (approx. 10%)
- Adenoid cystic carcinoma (formerly "cylindro-
  ma") and mucoepidermoid carcinoma (approx.
  5%)
- Verrucous carcinoma
- Undifferentiated carcinoma
- Odontogenic carcinoma
- Malignant melanoma (approx. 2%), see p. 150
- Eosinophilic granuloma
- Other forms of histiocytosis X
- Malignant lymphoma, see p. 408 and
  Table 10.**12**

- Extramedullary plasmocytoma (benign and
  malignant forms occur)
- Various types of sarcoma, e. g.,
  ○ Lymphoreticular sarcoma (approx. 10%), see
    p. 408
  ○ Lymphosarcoma
  ○ Kaposi sarcoma (HIV correlation)
  ○ Fibrosarcoma
  ○ Rhabdomyosarcoma
  ○ Malignant hemangiopericytoma
  ○ Carcinosarcoma
  ○ Osteo- and chondrosarcoma (may occur in
    setting of Paget disease)
  ○ Odontogenic sarcoma
  ○ Ewing sarcoma (predominantly in children)

Occasional distant metastases from:
- Hypernephroma
- Osteogenic sarcoma
- Hemangioendothelioma

- Seminoma
- Breast carcinoma
- Metastasizing struma

Pseudotumors
- Plasma cell granuloma
- Fibrous dysplasia, see p. 141
- Bone cyst, see p. 142

- Meningoencephalocele, see p. 139
- Bleeding septal polyp, see p. 194
- Pyogenic granuloma

See also Tables 3.**2** and 3.**22**

Malignant Tumors

Malignant tumors of the internal nose and paranasal sinuses are much more common than benign tumors at these sites, but they are uncommon compared with malignant tumors in other body regions (<1% of all malignancies). Approximately 50% of nose and paranasal sinus malignancies arise in the maxillary sinus, 20% in the ethmoid sinus, and 25% in the nasal cavity. Specific tumors cannot be discussed fully in the present context. The diagnostic algorithm is the same for the entire group (see below). The malignant tumors of greatest clinical importance are listed in Table 3.**21**.

Main symptoms: *Tumors of the external nose,* see Tables 2.**5** and 3.**21**.

Intranasal tumors: Unilateral, fetid coryza. Increasing sensation of pressure in the face and/or head; severe (e.g., neuralgiform) pain in the early stage is rare. Malignant tumors of the internal nose and/or paranasal sinuses are often clinically silent in their initial stages! Neurologic deficits and lacrimation may provide a relatively early suggestive sign, depending on the tumor site and direction of spread. Other warning signs are epistaxis or blood-tinged rhinorrhea and nasal fetor.

Other symptoms and special features: *Intranasal* and/or *transsinus extension* causes nasal airway obstruction. Often there is expansion of adjacent facial structures (cheek, medial canthus, proptosis). Intranasal tumor growth is usually easy to detect by rhinoscopy. But small malignancies still confined within a sinus can be detected only (if at all) by endoscopy! There is rapid destruction of adjacent structures such as the orbit and its contents, intracranial structures, the pharynx, and the oral cavity (loosening of maxillary teeth). Regional lymph nodes are involved in 20–25% of cases! Adenocarcinomas of the internal nose are particularly common in woodworkers (beech and oak).

Diagnosis:
Malignancies of the external nose: Delineation with respect to intranasal structures and underlying bone; also biopsy.

Malignancies of the internal nose:
● Rhinoscopy (possibly augmented by endoscopy).

● Diagnostic imaging. Radiography: Standard projections of the paranasal sinuses and skull base, and CT scans. An additional option is MRI.
● Biopsy, which may be combined with exploration of the suspect sinus.
● With suspected intracranial involvement (very severe "dural" headache), a complete cranial nerve examination is indicated! Malignancies of the nose and anterior paranasal sinuses can involve individual branches of the trigeminal nerve as well as cranial nerves I, II, III, or IV. Malignancies of the posterior sinuses and nasopharynx may involve cranial nerves III, IV, V, VI, IX, X (and possibly XI and XII). See also Table 1.**18**.
● Neurologic consultation. Ophthalmologic consultation is also required when orbital involvement is suspected.

Differentiation is required from inflammatory conditions and complications of the paranasal sinuses, benign tumors, malignant granuloma, gumma, and tuberculoma.

Systemic Neoplasias

Eosinophilic Granuloma of the Skull

Main symptoms: Headache, usually diffuse or unilateral. Inspection and palpation reveal a flat or crater-like, retracted tumor with a tense consistency, frequently tender to pressure, in the head region. Tumor location determines whether symptoms are scant (e.g., tumor at the skull base) or whether early organic symptoms arise (e.g., otologic symptoms with disease of the petrous bone, ophthalmic symptoms with periorbital disease). Cerebral deficits also occur!

Other symptoms and special features: Multifocal lesions are relatively common, affecting numerous bones in addition to the skull (e.g., femur, pelvis, ribs, vertebral bodies). Peak occurrence is in the 1st–2nd decades.

Causes: A distinction is drawn between *eosinophilic granuloma of bone*, which occurs *mainly in children* and causes bone destruction in the cranium and mandible, and *facial eosinophilic granuloma*, which mainly affects adults and produces lesions of the facial skin and oral mucosa. Eosinophilic granuloma is one form of *histiocytosis X*, which also includes *Hand—Schüller—Christian disease*. The symptoms of the latter include multiple bone involvement, especially in the cranial region ("map-like skull"), exophthalmos, and soft-tissue involvement of the lymph nodes, hypothalamus, and neurohypophysis (diabetes insipidus). It chiefly affects *older children* and *adults*.

Diagnosis:
● Complete ENT status including audiologic and neuro-otologic evaluation.
● Radiography: Cranial survey films and spot films (sharply circumscribed osteolytic foci). CT scans. Radionuclide imaging also may be considered.
● Laboratory findings are usually nonspecific.
● Neurologic and ophthalmologic consultation may be required.

Differentiation is required from Abt—Letterer—Siwe disease, Hand—Schüller—Christian disease, other bone tumors, and osteomyelitis.

Malignant Lymphoma

See p. 408 and Table 10.**12** A special manifestation is plasmacytoma.

Plasmacytoma of the Head and Neck (Extramedullary Plasmacytoma)

Main symptoms: Chiefly affects the mucosae of the nose, paranasal sinuses, or nasopharynx, accounting for about 4% of nonepithelial tumors at these sites. Endoscopy shows a yellowish or reddish, smooth-walled, nonulcerating lesion with a broad or pedunculated base. Possible involvement of the underlying bone. Head and neck plasmacytomas are multiple in an estimated 15% of cases. May be manifested clinically by nasal airway obstruction, obstructed nasal and paranasal sinus drainage, dysphagia (pharynx), or dyspnea and hoarseness (larynx).

Other symptoms and special features: Slightly more than half of these neoplasms remain well-localized; the rest spread aggressively to adjacent bone and soft tissues and associated lymph nodes.

Causes: Manifestation of an extranodal non-Hodgkin lymphoma (see p. 408). Progression to multiple myelomas is possible.

Diagnosis:
● Endoscopy.
● Biopsy.
● Radiographic delineation of the tumor with respect to bone and soft tissues (CT and/or MRI).
● Oncologic consultation.

Differentiation is required from pseudoneoplastic plasma cell granuloma (especially in the oral cavity), from other types of plasma cell tumor (solitary bone plasmacytoma ([femur, pelvis, vertebrae]), multiple myeloma (jawbones), other lymphomas, and other rare tumors.

Tumors of the Nasopharynx

Tumors of the nose and paranasal sinuses, especially malignancies, may well spread to involve the nasopharynx. Tumors in that area pose no special problems of differential diagnosis if their origin from the nose or paranasal sinuses is apparent. On the other hand, there are neoplasms and other form-altering diseases that are characteristic *only* of the nasopharynx. Accordingly, these lesions are considered separately in terms of differential diagnosis (Table 3.**22**).

Juvenile Nasopharyngeal Fibroma
See p. 195.

Teratoma

Main symptoms: Nasal airway obstruction. Nasal endoscopy shows a hair-bearing mass of irregular shape based broadly or by pedicle on the wall of the nasopharynx and exhibiting a firm consistency.

The **diagnosis** of this rare congenital tumors is made histologically (conglomerate tumor composed of skin, hair, fatty and/or nervous tissue, cartilage, etc.).

Differentiation is required from choanal polyp, angiofibroma, and adenoid hyperplasia.

Chordoma

Main symptoms: Obstruction of the nasopharynx and nasal airway. Neuro-ophthalmologic symptoms are common due to destruction of the skull base. Rhinoscopy shows a smooth-walled mass more or less filling the nasopharynx. Peak incidence is from 20–40 years of age. A rare neoplasm.

Cause: Blastoma composed of elements of the embryonic notochord.

Diagnosis:
● Rhinoscopy.
● Radiographic evaluation of the nasopharynx, skull base, and cervical spine including, CT, and/or MRI. Biopsy.

Differentiation is required from choanal polyp, juvenile nasopharyngeal fibroma, teratoma, and other malignant tumors.

Craniopharyngioma (Erdheim Tumor)

Main symptoms: Nasal airway obstruction and pressure or pain in the head. Usually diagnosed in childhood or adolescence.

Other symptoms and special features: Symptom pattern consistent with damage to the pituitary, sella turcica, optic chiasm, and diencephalon (growth disturbances!) Occasional hydrocephalus. Cystic tumor is prone to calcification. Nasal endoscopy shows bulging of the mucosa of the posterosuperior nasopharyngeal wall.

Cause: (Cystic) neoplasm arising from the Rathke pouch or the craniopharyngeal duct.

Diagnosis:
● Rhinoscopy and nasopharyngeal endoscopy.
● Radiography: CT of the skull base and nasopharynx in two planes (typically show a capsule of calcific density!).
● Evaluation may be aided by MRI. Pneumoencephalography may be considered as an adjunct.
● Neurologic consultation; endocrinologic consultation may also be required.

Differentiation is required from juvenile nasopharyngeal fibroma and adenoid hyperplasia. Mucocele of the sphenoid sinus should be considered in adults.

Table 3.**22**   Common tumors of the nasopharynx (involving the nasopharynx primarily or by extension from adjacent structures)

Benign
− Juvenile nasopharyngeal fibroma, see p. 195
− Pleomorphic adenoma, see p. 305
− Hemangioma, see pp. 146, 308, 405
− Lymphangioma, see p. 406 ff.
− Hemangiopericytoma (prone to malignant transformation)*
− Chondroma*
− Neurinoma*
− Chordoma
− Craniopharyngioma (Rathke pouch tumor)
− Glomus tumor (chemodectoma), see p. 29
− Hair-bearing nasopharyngeal polyp
− Nasopharyngeal teratoma

Malignant
− Squamous cell carcinoma
− Anaplastic carcinoma (Schmincke–Regaud lymphoepithelial tumor)
− Adenoid cystic carcinoma
− Adenocarcinoma
− Malignant lymphomas, see p. 408
− Sarcomas
− Malignant melanoma
− Distant metastases (e. g., hypernephroma)

Tumors chiefly affecting the pediatric age group
− Juvenile nasopharyngeal fibroma, see p. 195
− Leukemic manifestation
− Malignant lymphoma
− Lymphosarcoma
− CNS tumor
− Neuroblastoma
− Rhabdomyosarcoma
− Burkitt tumor

Rare
− Histiocytosis X (eosinophilic granuloma, Hand–Schüller–Christian disease, Abt–Letterer–Siwe disease), see p. 217
− Wilms tumor
− Ewing sarcoma (bone sarcoma in children)

Pseudotumors
− Meningoencephalocele, see p. 139

* No further commentary

Glomus Tumor

See p. 29.

Nasopharyngeal Carcinoma

Main symptoms: Nasal airway obstruction. Eustachian tube dysfunction (conductive hearing loss, tubotympanic effusion). Purulent, blood-tinged rhinorrhea or massive epistaxis. Nasal fetor. Ipsilateral headache located deep in the skull base. Later involvement of the soft palate is signaled by bulging and/or rigidity. Nasal endoscopy shows an ulcerating mucosal lesion (often located near the pharyngeal orifice of the eustachian tube).

Other symptoms and special features: Involvement of cranial nerves III−VI and IX−XII is possible in advanced stages. Early lymphogenous spread (lymph nodes at both mandibular angles!); nodal involvement may be the key early symptom leading to tumor detection! Peak occurrence: 40−60 years of age. Males predominate by 3:1.

Nasopharyngeal tumors in *children* are mostly malignant lymphomas, plasmacytomas, or rhabdomyosarcomas. Burkitt lymphoma (Epstein−Barr virus) is relatively common in certain regions (especially in Africa).

Typical neurologic deficit syndromes associated with nasopharyngeal tumors are listed in Table 1.**18**. One or more of the following cranial nerve deficits present as *cardinal symptom(s)* in approximately one-third of nasopharyngeal malignancies: anosmia, diplopia, ptosis, trigeminal neuralgia, dysphagia, dysar-

thria, hoarseness. Extension from the nasopharynx is by way of the foramina lacerum, ovale, or spinosum or via the carotid canal.

Diagnosis:
● These tumors can be *very* difficult to detect by routine rhinoscopy or even endoscopy, often appearing merely as a small, flat, roughened mucosal defect (frequent submucous growth). Site of predilection: the Rosenmüller fossa (in doubtful cases obtain multiple mucosal biopsies!).
● Radiography: CT scans. Angiography also may be helpful.
● Biopsy.
● Immunologic tests can be used to detect antibodies against EBV capsid antigens (IgA−VCA).
● Regional lymph nodes can be assessed by palpation and biopsy. Look for hematogenous metastases.
● Symptoms may warrant neurologic and ophthalmologic consultation.

Differentiation is required from other types of malignancy such als malignant lymphoma, sarcomas, etc.; also pituitary tumors and specific inflammatory conditions such as tuberculosis, mycoses, diphtheria, etc.

Undifferentiated carcinoma of the (naso)pharynx (synonyms: *anaplastic carcinoma, lymphoepithelial tumor* [Schmincke−Regaud]) occupies a special clinical category. It is closely related pathogenically to Epstein−Barr virus and has a markedly higher radiosensitivity and thus a more favorable prognosis than the ordinary solid squamous cell carcinomas.

Symptom   Malformation of the Nose, Paranasal Sinuses, Nasopharynx

Given the complex ontogeny of the face, it is understandable that a great variety of malformations can occur in the nasal region. While most of these anomalies are conspicuous and easily detected, their further diagnostic evaluation always requires a complete otolaryngologic workup (including endoscopy and function tests!) as well as a pediatric examination (and basic care), which in most cases has already been provided. Differential diagnosis and treatment require the concerted efforts of multiple specialties, including a geneticist, depending on the specific regions and organs involved.

The most clinically important malformations of the nasal region are reviewed in Table 3.23.

In patients with *craniofacial dysplasias* and *premature fusion of cranial sutures,* the diagnostic role of otolaryngology goes beyond assigning the case to a particular type of malformation. Besides aesthetic deformity, these anomalies often cause very severe, life-threatening functional disturbances. These may result from intracranial abnormalities (increased pressure, involvement of the encephalon and of the somatic and autonomic nervous systems) as well as disproportionality between individual morphologic elements (e.g., maxilla to mandible to hyoid bone) within a given region or between different segments of the upper aerodigestive tract. The *diagnostic responsibilities* of the attending ENT physician include not only a careful endoscopic examination of these systems, but also a potentially long-term and detailed functional evaluation (e.g., observation during sleep!) and the identification of any remedial measures that may be required. The differential diagnosis of life-threatening *acute respiratory disturbances* in *newborns* (and small infants) is summarized in Tables 6.9 and 6.10.

The immediate postnatal period is especially critical and hazardous for the child with a significant craniofacial anomaly. Once this period has been safely bridged, the evaluating physician must proceed with a comprehensive diagnostic "inventory," particularly since many patients will have multiple or combined malformations affecting sites all over the body!

Table 3.23 *Symptom* Malformation. Rhinologically important malformations of the nose, paranasal sinuses, and nasopharynx

Synopsis
Nasal anomalies (in newborns)
Choanal atresia and choanal stenosis, see p. 206
Septal deviation, see p. 202
Dermoid cysts*
Encephalocele and meningoencephalocele, see p. 139
Glioma, see p. 139
Cleft lip, cleft alveolus, cleft palate and their combinations, see p. 271
Cleft nose*
Anterior, middle, and posterior nasal atresia*
Craniofacial dysplasias
Arhinia*
Hypoplasia or aplasia of the nasal bones*
Agenesis of the nasal turbinates*
Rhinodymia (true duplication of the nose, partial or complete)*
Proboscis lateralis ("trunk nose")
Cysts of the nasal vestibule, see p. 142
Nasal fistulae and dermoids*
Midline facial clefts*
Hypertelorism*
Midline nasal cleft*
Transverse or oblique facial cleft*
Nasal deformities associated with cleft lip and palate*
Deformities
Septal spur, ridge, deviation, see p. 202
Nose: hump nose, saddle nose, short nose, long nose, large nose, wide nose, flat nose, deviated nose, drooping nasal tip*
See also Table 2.13
* No further commentary

Malformations of the head region that are relatively common and are associated with significant respiratory impairment which may pose an acute risk of asphyxiation (e.g., during sleep) are reviewed in Table 3.24.

Table 3.**24** Common dysontogenic causes in the head region for disturbances of the upper aerodigestive tract

Dysgenesis:

Franceschetti–Zwahlen (Treacher Collins) syndrome, see Tables 1.**43** and 2.**13**

Crouzon syndrome, see Tables 1.**43** and 2.**13**

Apert syndrome, see Table 2.**13**

Pierre–Robin syndrome (micrognathia, glossoptosis, cleft), see Table 2.**13**

Hypothyroidism, myxedema, see p. 410

Aplasia of a nasal bone*

Bilateral choanal atresia, see p. 206

Unilateral choanal atresia

Stenosis or atresia of the anterior naris (or nares)

Midline facial clefts*

Cleft lip, alveolus, palate (unilateral or bilateral), see p. 271

Retroposition of the midface (retrognathia), as in Franceschetti disease, Crouzon disease, Apert disease

Meningoencephalocele, see p. 139

Glioma, see p. 139

Glossoptosis

Macroglossia, see p. 260

Collapse of the anterior nasal cartilages, see p. 201

Space-occupying lesion in the nasopharynx (encephalocele, glioma, cysts, atlas prominence)*

Intranasal dentition*

Intranasal cysts and celes, see p. 142

Septal deformities (especially in the presence of clefts), see p. 202

Thyroglossal duct cyst, see p. 403

Struma of tongue base, see p. 410 and Table 4.**13**

Ocular disturbances*

Lesions of cranial nerves IX, X, XII, see Table 1.**19**

Cardinal symptoms:
– Stridorous respiration
– Apneic episodes
– Open mouth (mouth breathing can also result from severe malocclusion)
– Eating difficulties (swallowing, mastication)

Associated symptoms:
– Sinusitis
– Otitis media
– Recurrent respiratory tract infections
– Cor pulmonale

* No further commentary

Syndromes Involving the Nose and Paranasal Sinuses

Table 3.**25**   Rhinologically important syndromes not due to dysontogenic causes (selection) (after Leiber and Olbrich)

Syndrome	Classification	Typical ENT deficits	Remarks
Charlin syndrome	Neuralgia of ciliary nerve	See p. 162	
Pterygopalatine fossa syndrome	Associated feature of maxillary sinus or nasopharyngeal tumors	Severe deep facial pain and parietal headache. Impaired mandibular movement or trismus. Displacement of lower toward upper dental arch	

Table 3.**25**   (cont.)

Syndrome	Classification	Typical ENT deficits	Remarks
Godtfredsen syndrome (sinonasopharyngeal tumor syndrome)	Associated feature of paranasal sinus or nasopharyngeal tumors	Unilateral trigeminal neuralgia (2nd and/or 3rd division). Abducens paralysis, joined later by paralysis of cranial nerves II, III, IV. Visual deterioration	Very similar to Jacod syndrome (see Table 1.**18**)
Horton syndrome (Bing–Horton syndrome, erythroprosopalgia)	Irritation of the pterygopalatine ganglion	See p. 166	
McBride–Stewart syndrome	Progressive ulcerogangrenous process in the midfacial region	Bloody catarrh with intranasal granuloma formation and nasal airway obstruction. In later stage, nasal fetor. Necrosis of nasal skeleton and palate. Most common in males aged 30–45	Corresponds to midline granuloma, see p. 192
Kartagener syndrome	Congenital familial malformation syndrome	Sinusitis plus nasal and sinus polyposis	Combined with visceral transposition and bronchiectases
Lateral niche syndrome	Associated feature of lateral nasopharyngeal tumors	Unilateral trigeminal neuralgia; concomitant eustachian tube obstruction (hearing loss) and ipsilateral lymph node metastases at the mandibular angle or in the cervical nodes	
Sinopulmonary syndrome	Coordinated occurrence of chronic sinusitis and bronchitis	Chronic or recurrent sinusitis	Combined with chronic or recurrent bronchitis or circumscribed bronchopneumonia. All authors do not recognize the syndrome nature, based on a common mucosal weakness in the sinonasal and bronchial systems
Sluder syndrome	Neuralgia of the pterygopalatine ganglion	See p. 162	
Trotter syndrome	Associated feature of nasopharyngeal tumors	Unilateral neuralgiform pain in the mandible, tongue, and ear. Conductive hearing loss. Ipsilateral protrusion of the soft palate. Trismus may supervene. Nasal airway obstruction	

Symptom   **Olfactory Dysfunction**

H. Scherer

Anatomic Principles

A knowledge of the olfactory fields in the nose and of the olfactory pathway is important in the differential diagnosis of peripheral and central olfactory disturbances. The basis anatomy of this sensory system is reviewed below:

The olfactory areas of the nasal mucosa are located in the anterior septum and in the adjacent mucosa of the lateral nasal wall. An impediment of airflow to these sites creates a *respiratory* olfactory disturbance. The two olfactory fields in each side of the nose, each with an area of approximately 2.5 cm^2, contain the distal ends of some 10−20 million bipolar receptor cells. These structures have an expanded, club-like shape and bear sensory hairs. The sensitivity of the olfactory sense depends on the length of these sensory cilia. Organisms possessing the sense of smell may be categorized as micro-osmatic or macro-osmatic, with humans belonging to the former group. The sensory cilia lie in the olfactory mucus, which contains no proteolytic enzymes that could alter the chemical composition of odorous molecules. Damage to the olfactory field leads to *epithelial* olfactory dysfunction.

The proximal process of the bipolar cells are collected in the fila olfactoria, which pass through the cribriform plate to the bulb of the olfactory tract. Damage in the area of this first olfactory neuron leads to *neural* olfactory dysfunction. The second neuron of the olfactory pathway passes via the olfactory tract to secondary olfactory centers in the rhinencephalon. The projection to the *olfactory cortex* (olfactory tubercle and temporobasal cortical structures) is clinically important for the perception of smells and their association with other sensory impressions. Also important is the projection to the *limbic system*, where the olfactory pathway connects with the autonomic olfactory centers in the thalamus and hypothalamus. These pathways are responsible for the emotional content of olfaction and the associated affective mechanisms.

Principal Diagnostic Methods

○ Odorous substances can be classified into three main groups:
  a) Substances that predominantly stimulate the olfactory nerve. These include numerous spices, alcohol-free perfume, coffee, and tea.
  b) Substances that stimulate the olfactory nerve and terminal branches of the trigeminal nerve in the nasal mucosa. These include ethereal substances such as camphor, all acids (e.g., acetic acid), and alcohol solutions.
  c) Substances that stimulate the olfactory nerve and the terminal branches of the glossopharyngeal nerve at the base of the tongue, such as chloroform (sweet) and pyridine (bitter).

○ *Screening examination:* Sniff test on bottles containing a sample from each of the above groups.

○ *Subjective but quantitative examination:* Sniff test using Elsberg bottles containing a designated amount of the dissolved substance. Serial dilutions are used to determine the subjective olfactory thresholds for the various substances. The true olfactory threshold (of detection) is distinguished from the threshold of perception, at which the subject can perceive the odor but cannot identify the substance.

○ *Objective, semiquantitative examination using evoked olfactory cortical potentials:* The computer-controlled presentation of olfactory stimuli and the artifact-free recording of EEG potentials is difficult and, for the present, is offered at only a few centers.

Definitions

In 1987 Fikentscher et al. introduced a concise and convenient nomenclature for olfactory dysfunction that will be used in the sections below.

Normosmia

The ability to detect an odorous substance within the limits of the normal olfactory threshold. The latter depends on the state of hunger and thus is subject to significant daily fluctuations.

Dysosmia

Quantitative Dysosmias

The olfactory impairment may be general or restricted to particular stimuli (specific dysomia). To date more than 80 specific dysosmias have been identified, some of which are inherited, such as the inability to smell isobutyric acid (sweat), N-butylmercaptan (skunk), and hydrogen cyanide (bitter almond).

● **Anosmia:** Complete absence of the sense of smell or components of it (specific anosmia).
● **Hyposmia:** Diminished sense of smell.
● **Hyperosmia:** Heightened sense of smell.

Qualitative Dysosmias

● **Parosmia:** Sensation of an odor that the subject knows is not present, at least in the form perceived.
● **Pseudosmia** (olfactory illusion). Illusory perception of an actual odor under the influence of strong emotions. A particular personality structure is required, and the subject can be convinced of his error. Pseudosmia has no pathologic significance as an isolated entity

and becomes important only when it occurs in the setting of psychiatric disorders.

● **Phantosmia** (olfactory hallucination): Olfactory impression having an objective character, but perceived in the absence of an olfactory stimulus. Like other types of hallucination, the experience is both cognitive and sensory. Due to the authentic quality of the sensation, the patient does not complain of an olfactory disturbance and cannot be convinced of his error, seeking, rather, to locate the source of the presumed odor.

Causes include schizophrenia, organic brain disorders, and epilepsy.

● **Agnosmia:** Loss of the ability to recognize a familiar odor, analogous to psychic blindness and deafness.

Causes: Cortical lesions.

Diseases and Causes

See Table 3.**26**.

Olfactory Dysfunction Due to Nasal Airway Obstruction and Obstructive Processes (Respiratory Dysosmias)

Transient Mucosal Swelling

Olfactory dysfunction occurs in both acute rhinitis and recurrent allergic rhinitis when the swollen nasal membranes occlude the superior meatus (olfactory cleft). Chronic mucosal swelling like that in pharmacotoxic rhinitis (see p. 187, 204) leads to hyposmia and less commonly to anosmia. The diagnosis is established by the improvement of olfaction in response to decongestive therapy.

High Septal Deviations

These can occlude the superior meatus on both sides, especially if the middle and upper turbinate mucosae are chronically swollen as a result of chronic paranasal sinus infection, which is not uncommon with high deviations.

Bullous Concha

Excessive pneumatization of the middle turbinate can completely choke off the upper nasal portion.

Table 3.**26** *Symtom* Olfactory dysfunction

Synopsis
Olfactory dysfunction due to nasal airway obstruction and obstructive processes inside the nose
Olfactory dysfunction due to changes in the mucosa
Olfactory dysfunction due to trauma
Olfactory dysfunction due to central nervous disorders

Nasal Polyposis

Nasal polyps based on chronic rhinitis are often located in the middle meatus. Objective hyposmia is demonstrable. Postoperatively patients consistently report a markedly improved sense of smell. If polyps obstruct the superior meatus, the patient complains of significant olfactory impairment.

Tumors

Tumors in the superior meatus (adenoid cystic carcinoma, adenocarcinoma) constrict the olfactory field before becoming externally apparent by expanding the nasal root. Hyposmia or anosmia may be the initial sign of tumor growth, therefore. Differential diagnosis must distinguish a tumor from a posttraumatic septal hematoma and from scar tissue following corrective septal surgery.

Laryngectomy and Tracheostomy

These procedures consistently lead to anosmia by diverting the respiratory air away from the nasal passages.

Olfactory Dysfunction Due to Changes in the Mucosa (Epithelial Dysosmias)

Atrophic Rhinitis

A mucous blanket is essential for proper function of the olfactory mucosa, because the olfactory cilia degenerate in a dry milieu. Thus, an atrophic rhinitis that involves the superior portions of the nasal passages leads to hyposmia or even anosmia. Anosmia is consistently present in ozena.

Ozena

In this disease the respiratory mucosa undergoes a structural transformation to squamous epithelium.

Mucosal Changes Caused by Exposure to Exogenous Agents

Numerous chemical and pharmacologic agents can damage the olfactory mucosa, including all lacquers and solvents (benzene, trichloroethylene, etc.) and all caustic substances (acetic acid, nitric acid, etc.). Some of these substances, especially the heavy metals, can probably cause direct damage to the receptors.
Toxic injury is a known effect of chromic acid, cadmium, osmium tetroxide, and zinc. With some agents (e.g., butylene glycol, benzoic acid, putrescent gases, chemical weapons), a single contact is sufficient. A single inhalation of, e. g., hydrogen selenide is sufficient to produce anosmia. The local use of cocaine, procaine, tetracaine, and neomycin is also known to damage the olfactory mucosa or receptors.

Endocrine Disorders

Hyposmia or anosmia is observed in the Cushing syndrome, hypothyroidism, and diabetes mellitus. Anosmia is present congenitally in the Kallmann syndrome (hypoplasia of the olfactory system, combined with hypogonadotropic eunuchoidism) and in the chromosomal anomaly of the Turner syndrome (primary hypogonadism).

Deficiency Disease

Pernicious anemia.

Drug-induced Olfactory Dysfunction

Olfactory dysfunction has been described in connection with the oral or parenteral administration of centrally acting drugs:
o Centrally acting drugs (amphetamines, dopamine antagonists, imipramine, meprobamate, morphine, phenothiazine)

○ Antibiotics (kanamycin, neomycin, strepto-
mycin)
○ Antirheumatic drugs (penicillamine)
○ Thyreostatic drugs (thiamazol)
○ Anticoagulants (coumarin derivatives)

Olfactory Dysfunction Due to Trauma

There are three mechanisms by which trauma
can produce olfactory dysfunction:
● **Comminuted nasal bone fracture** with mechanical obstruction of the superior meatus by
bone fragments or a septal hematoma.
● **Frontobasal fracture** running through the
cribriform plate of the ethmoid bone (especially in Le Fort III fractures).
● **Avulsion of the fila olfactoria** at the ethmoid plate by tangential trauma (frontal,
occipital, or less commonly temporal contact
trauma; never from contact trauma at the vertex).

Olfactory Dysfunction Due to Central Nervous Disorders (Central Dysosmias)

Hyposmia or anosmia always signifies a peripheral olfactory lesion. This may be a lesion
of the first or second neuron, i.e., the pathway
up to the end of the olfactory tract (including
the olfactory bulb). Farther centrally the olfactory signals are coordinated and relayed to the
olfactory cortex. Lesions in this region lead to
olfactory hallucinations and other forms of altered perception. Typically, additional central

nervous symptoms are present. Unilateral central nervous disorders (central to the olfactory
tract) *never* cause olfactory impairment.

Olfactory hallucinations (phantosmias) are a
feature of:
○ Temporal lobe tumors or abscesses (olfacto-
ry aura, uncinate seizures)
○ Productive psychoses
○ Psychomotor seizures
○ Schizophrenic psychoses

Traumatic Central Olfactory Dysfunction

Contusion of the temporal lobe or traumatic
hemorrhage.

Infectious Central Olfactory Dysfunction

○ Secondary to an influenzal infection ("flu
anosmia")
○ Frontal lobe abscess
○ Meningitis
○ Syphilis

Neoplastic Central Olfactory Dysfunction

This occurs with:
○ Frontal lobe tumors
○ Olfactory meningioma
○ Vascular tumors
○ Sellar tumors
○ Parasellar tumors

4. Mouth and Pharynx

The Symptoms

- Pain and dysesthesia, p. 229
- Mucosal lesions of the lip, p. 238
- Mucosal lesions of the oral cavity, p. 243
- Mucosal lesions of the tongue, p. 257
- Diseases of the lymphoepithelial organs, p. 260
- Diseases with predominantly pharyngeal symptoms, p. 264
- Morphologic change (swelling, tumor), p. 267
- Malformation, p. 271
- Oral fetor, p. 272
- Blood in the sputum, p. 273
- Disturbance of salivation, pp. 275, 309
- Paralysis involving the mouth and/or pharynx, p. 276
- Trismus, p. 277
- Dysphagia (oropharyngeal), p. 279
- Airway obstruction in the mouth and pharynx, p. 281
- Disturbance of speech, see p. 353
- Disturbance of taste, p. 291
- Common syndromes, p. 281

The symptomatology of the oropharyngeal region is very diverse due to the large number of organs and structures in the region, many of which blend together with no obvious morphologic or functional line of demarcation.

The *crossing of the upper respiratory and digestive tracts* in the oropharynx and hypopharynx gives rise to very heterogeneous circumstances, relationships, and diagnostic criteria that must be considered in making a differential diagnosis. For clinical purposes, then, it is convenient to consider the entire pharynx (naso-, oro-, and hypopharynx) and the oral cavity as a structural and functional unit from the standpoint of differential diagnosis.

Principal Diagnostic Methods

- *Inspection* (including "indirect" mirror examination) and a *detailed history* are still the foundation for diagnostic evaluation of the mouth and pharynx.
- The *palpation* of suspect or pathologic areas in the mouth and pharynx that are accessile to finger or probe is very rewarding. Palpable findings often furnish decisive clues for differential diagnosis, especially if simultaneous internal *and* external bimanual palpation can be performed.
- For special inquiries and when findings are equivocal, indirect findings are supplemented by *endoscopic techniques:*
  - The rigid *magnifying endoscope* with an angled viewing/illumination axis and variable magnification significantly enhances the visual inspection of areas that are otherwise difficult to see (e.g., the nasopharynx, hypopharynx, tongue base, etc.). Small-caliber *flexible endoscopes* can be used in similar fashion. A rigid 30° rod-lens telescope (2.7 mm diameter) can be passed transnasally to evaluate the nasopharynx and oropharynx while the mouth is closed (e.g., in questionable sleep apnea).

− The *operating microscope* can be used in conjunction with mirrors if desired.

○ *Soft palate retraction* ("velotraction"), combined with magnifying endoscopy and palpation, permits a very detailed examination of the nasopharynx after the administration of topical or general anesthesia. It also facilitates selective biopsy. Today it is increasingly being replaced by flexible endoscopes in combination with extraction instruments.

○ Various instrumental methods (*hypopharyngoscopy* using a tongue blade or hypopharyngoscope, *self-retaining endoscopy*) permit the meticulous inspection (and biopsy) of the hypopharynx, piriform sinuses, tongue base, and other structures that are otherwise difficult or impossible to inspect.

○ *Diagnostic imaging.*
   − *Radiography:* Evaluation of the *oral cavity* includes standard projections of the maxillary sinuses and nasal floor to demonstrate the bony roof of the oral cavity as well as special views of the mandible and its articulations. These films can be supplemented by *CT scans*, which are excellent for delineating inflammatory osteitis, osteomyelitis) and neoplastic lesions and defining the extent of trauma. The teeth and alveolar ridges can be evaluated by single radiographs, orthopantomography, and other specialized techniques.
   − *Magnetic resonance imaging* (MRI), plain or enhanced with gadolinium DTPA, has proven very informative for oropharyngeal studies. See also p. 1 (footnote).

− *Radionuclide bone scanning* is useful for applications such as the detection of metabolically altered bone tissue.

− *Superselective angiography* and *digital subtraction angiography* of the carotid and vertebral artery systems are mainstays in the diagnosis of highly vascular oropharyngeal tumors.

− The *pharynx* can be evaluated by conventional soft-tissue radiography in multiple planes and by various tomographic techniques. Contrast radiographs and CT are also frequently used (e.g., in choanal atresia, for evaluating the hypopharynx and esophagus, etc.).

− Various *ultrasound* techniques are rewarding in the oropharyngeal and neck region: the *A scan* for demonstrating cavities, cysts, abscesses, etc., their boundaries and their contents; the *B scan* for discriminating soft-tissue planes and defining their extent; and *Doppler ultrasound* for determining the velocity and direction of blood flow.

○ The examination of *smears* from the mucosal surfaces of the oral cavity and pharynx is still an important differential diagnostic tool in *microbiologic investigations*. Cytodiagnosis is very rarely indicated in the oropharyngeal region, which generally is readily accessible for *biopsy*.

○ *Taste tests* are discussed on p. 291 and *phoniatric function tests* on p. 336.

Symptom   **Pain and Dysesthesia in the Mouth and Pharynx**

In the interest of clarity and conciseness, this section focuses on painful disorders that have site-specific causes in the oropharyngeal region and manifest pain or discomfort as their characteristic *cardinal symptom*. In the following synopsis, a simple page reference is given for painful oropharyngeal diseases in which other symptoms tend to be predominant (Table 4.**1**).

Throat Pain

Acute Tonsillitis

Main symptoms: Burning throat pain of acute onset. Pain on swallowing (odynophagia) becomes very severe and usually radiates to the ear. Fever, chills, severe malaise. Mirror examination shows deep redness of both palatine

Table 4.**1** *Symptom* Pain and dysesthesia

Synopsis	
Throat pain	**Intraoral pain**
Acute tonsillitis (lingual tonsillitis, adenoiditis, infection of lateral pharyngeal bands)	Cheilitis, see p. 240
	Stomatitis, see p. 243 ff.
Infectious mononucleosis	Other mucosal inflammatory conditions, see p. 252 ff.
Plaut–Vincent angina (ulceromembraneous angina), p. 260	Burns of the tongue
Herpangina	Diseases of the dental system
Scarlet fever	Osteitis and osteomyelitis of the jaws, see pp. 141, 144
Syphilitic tonsillitis, see p. 261	Salivary gland diseases, see p. 298
Agranulocytosis	Trauma
Tonsillitis in diphtheria	Neoplasms, see p. 267
Tonsillitis in leukemia, see pp. 262, 408	
Peritonsillar abscess	**Paroxysmal pain**
Retropharyngeal abscess, see p. 266	Neuralgia of the trigeminal nerve and its branches, see p. 159
Abscess of tongue (base) and oral floor	Neuralgia of the nervus intermedius, see p. 15
Epiglottitis and epiglottic abscess, see p. 316	Neuralgia of the glossopharyngeal and vagus nerves, see pp. 162, 163
Stylalgia (Eagle syndrome)	Trotter syndrome, see Table 3.**25**
Stylokeratohyoid syndrome	
Carotidynia	**Painful swallowing and dysphagia**
Acute pharyngitis	See pp. 279, 380, Table 4.**25**, and Table 8.**8**
Trauma (including burns, caustic lesions, and foreign bodies)	
Neoplasms	

tonsils and their immediate surroundings (*catarrhal tonsillitis*). Yellow stipples (*follicular tonsillitis*) or yellow spots (*lacunar tonsillitis*) may be visible on the tonsils themselves.

Other symptoms and special features: Mild to moderate trismus with significant speech and eating impairment is not uncommon. Airway obstruction is occasionally present due to inflammatory swelling of the faucial isthmus. Cervical lymph nodes at the mandibular angle are swollen and painful. Possible accompanying diseases and sequelae include acute rheumatoid arthritis (in about 3% of patients with inadequately treated streptococcal tonsillitis), acute glomerulonephritis, focal nephritis, endocarditis, myocarditis, pericarditis.

Causes: Infection (systemic!) with ß-hemolytic streptococci, less commonly with staphylococ-

ci, *Haemophilus influenzae*, or pneumococci. Viral tonsillitis can also occur.

Diagnosis:
● Mirror examination shows typical findings.
● Temperature check(s). Elevated ESR, left shift in white blood count, Urologic status.
● Referral for cardiovascular examination and renal function testing may be indicated.

Differentiation is required from diphtheria (uncommon, smear); infectious mononucleosis (common, typical hematologic findings); agranulocytosis; leukemia; secondary syphilis; herpangina; aphthous angina. With *unilateral* disease: Plaut−Vincent angina, peritonsillar infiltration or abscess, tuberculous tonsillitis, tonsillar tumors.

Special Forms:

Lingual Tonsillitis

Inflammation localized to the *lingual tonsil* at the base of the tongue. Symptoms include swelling, redness, yellow deposits, and severe pain.

Adenoiditis (Acute Retronasal Tonsillitis)

Symptoms are mainly localized to the *adenoid.* Most common in childhood: Burning throat pain followed by mucoid and/or purulent coryza, usually with significant or complete nasal airway obstruction.

Infection of the Lateral Pharyngeal Bands (Angina lateralis)

The lymphoepithelial tissue located in the area of the *tubopharyngeal plicae* (lateral pharyngeal bands) shows swelling, redness, and yellow stippling and causes tonsillitis-like complaints, especially after a previous tonsillectomy ("substitute" inflammation in tonsillectomized patients).

Infectious Mononucleosis (Pfeiffer Disease, Glandular Fever)

Main symptoms: Usually severe sore throat, severe odynophagia, bouts of high fever. Chalky fibrinous deposits on the tonsils. Severe bilateral swelling of cervical nodes. Severe malaise. Children and adolescents are principally affected.

Other symptoms: Monocytosis, splenomegaly, possible hepatomegaly. Involvement of pharyngeal mucosa, possible involvement or oral and nasal mucosae. Occasional skin eruptions (> 10%). Generalized lymphadenopathy may ensue (see Table 10.5).

Cause: Attributed to infection with the Epstein–Barr virus (herpes virus), probably transmitted by droplet infection.

Diagnosis:
● Characteristic tonsillar findings and cervical lymphadenopathy.

● Characteristic blood count: Initial leukopenia followed by leukocytosis (20 000–30 000 cells or more) with up to 80–90% monocytes and atypical lymphocytes.
● Positive Monospot test, Paul–Bunnell test (for heterophilic serum antibodies, positive when titer exceeds 1:128). Wöllner differential agglutination test. Elevated antibody titers against EB viruses.
● A sore throat unresponsive to antibiotics generally signifies infectious mononucleosis!

Differentiation is required from diphtheria (smear), Plaut–Vincent angina (smear), scarlet fever, syphilis, rubella, agranulocytosis, leukemia, toxoplasmosis, listeriosis, and tularemia.

Plaut–Vincent (Ulceromembranous) Tonsillitis
See p. 260.

Herpangina

Main symptoms: Sore throat, odynophagia, high fever, headache, severe malaise, debility, anorexia. Chiefly affects children and adolescents. Initial stage is marked by very fleeting, milky-white vesicles with red halos located on the anterior faucial pillar and adjacent to the tonsils or on the tonsils themselves.

Other symptoms and special features: Usually the tonsils are only *slightly* red and swollen. The vesicles about the tonsils range to lentil-size and show a typical "string of beads" arrangement. Vesicles may also occur on the palate or buccal mucosa. The disease runs a brief course (usually <1 week) and is most prevalent in the summer and fall.

Cause: Infection with coxsackievirus A.

Diagnosis:
● Detection of vesicles (only in initial stage!) by mirror examination.
● Blood count: left shift with moderate leukocytosis.
● Identification of causal organism in pharyngeal washings, elevated serum antibody titer. Detection of causative organism in the stool.

Differentiation is required from aphthous or ulcerative stomatitis (Table 4.2), Plaut–Vin-

Table 4.**2** Differentiating features of herpangina and herpetic gingivostomatitis (aphthous stomatitis) (after T. Nasemann)

	Herpangina	Gingivostomatitis
Etiology	Coxsackievirus A	Herpes simplex virus
Occurrence	Epidemic, sometimes sporadic	Sporadic and epidemic
Season	Late summer, fall	Perennial, frequent in winter
Pain, fetor	Slight pain on swallowing	Very painful, salivation, oral fetor
General appearance	Mild pharyngitis	Oral and pharyngeal mucosae red and swollen
Lymph nodes	Occasional slight enlargement	Regional lymph nodes are swollen and tender
Eruptions	Grayish-white vesicles with areolae, later flat ulcers	Vesicles, pale yellowish aphthae (slightly raised), thin red halos
Number of lesions	2–20	Often very numerous, up to 50 or more
Duration	3–7 days	10–14 days

cent angina, streptococcal tonsillitis, measles (Koplik spots), varicella, eruption, diphtheria, and candidiasis.

Scarlet Fever

Main symptoms: Sudden onset with fever (chills), sore throat, and pain on swallowing. Tonsils are deep red and swollen and may be stippled or coated. Strawberry tongue; purple eruptions on the uvula, palate, and pharyngeal mucosa. General malaise. Typical scarlet fever rash generally appears after 24 h (starting on the upper body).

Other symptoms and special features: Facial redness that spares the perioral skin ("white beard" pattern). Skin desquamation commences in about the 2nd–4th week. A flare-up of manifestations, mainly in the pharynx, occurs in about the 3rd–4th week (pseudodiphtheria). Scarlet fever has become *very rare*!

Causes: Infection with group A hemolytic streptococci (concomitant viral infection has been suggested).

Diagnosis:
● Mirror examination shows typical intense redness of the tonsils and pharyngeal mucosa and a strawberry tongue.
● Leukocytosis with a left shift; eosinophilia is present by the 5th day.

● Typical scarlet fever rash; desquamation starts after 8 days. Rumpel–Leede phenomenon (petechiae). Schultz–Charlton reaction, Dick test.

Differentiation is required from diphtheria (smear), secondary syphilis (dark-field dab smear), viral infection, and drug rash.

Syphilitic Tonsillitis (Lues II)
See pp. 248, 261.

Agranulocytosis

Main symptoms: Severe sore throat and odynophagia, chills, high fever, severe systemic signs. Ulceration and necrosis of the tonsils and pharyngeal mucosa, sometimes with blackish coatings.

Other symptoms and special features: Oral fetor, copious salivation. Most common in middle-aged and elderly individuals. Regional lymphadenopathy is *absent*, but splenomegaly and/or hepatomegaly is observed.

Causes: Damage to the hematopoietic system (by cytostatic drugs, benzene, irradiation, or drugs such as aminopyrine, phenylbutazone, antibiotics [chloramphenicol], sulfonamides, sedatives, hypnotics, psychotropic drugs, anticonvulsants, antihistamines, antidiabetics, diuretics).

Diagnosis: Indirect findings in the pharynx, blood count (white blood cells $< 500/mm^3$ with absence of granulocytes).

Differentiation is required from diphtheria, infectious mononucleosis, Plaut–Vincent angina, and acute leukemia.

Acute Tonsillitis (and Pharyngitis) in Diphtheria

Main symptoms: Usually begins with relatively mild sore throat, slight pain on swallowing, and moderate fever ($< 39 °C$). The tonsils and pharyngeal mucosa are moderately red and swollen and are coated with a thick, grayish-white, adherent membrane that later turns dusky. The extratonsillar extent of the confluent membrane distinguishes it from that of simple acute tonsillitis! Cervical lymph nodes are markedly swollen, hard, and tender.

Other symptoms and special features: Sweet, stale breath odor ("acetone"). Pulse rate is often very high! Course is variable depending on the etiologic agent, some cases showing involvement of the heart and circulation, the CNS, and even the kidneys. Airway obstruction can occur (edema, membranes, etc.; see also p. 316). Risk of descending laryngeal involvement. Late changes appear in the 2nd–3rd week (paralysis of the soft palate, eye muscles, and diaphragm; paralytic dysphagia).

Diptheria has become *very rare* but is still endemic in some regions.

Causes: Infection with *Corynebacterium diphtheriae* (usually the mitis type, which produces a very potent toxin). Infection is transmitted by droplets or contact.

Diagnosis:
● Local indirect findings.
● Bacteriologic smear (for immediate *screening*), culture (*confirmatory* within about 10 h), and isolation of the causative organism (*establishes* the diagnosis in 2–8 days).

Differentiation is required from infectious mononucleosis, streptococcal tonsillitis, Plaut–Vincent angina, and peritonsillar abscess.

Tonsillitis in Leukemia
See pp. 262, 408.

Peritonsillar Abscess

Main symptoms: Rapidly increasing, typically unilateral throat pain, which can become quite severe and usually radiates to the ear. High fever, malaise, anorexia, eating difficulties, muffled speech, trismus, drooling, and fetid breath. Redness and bulging of the tonsillar area include the anterior faucial pillar and soft palate. The uvula is pushed toward the unaffected side.

Other symptoms and special features: The head is tilted toward the affected side. Swollen cervical lymph nodes. It is not unusual for the inflammatory peritonsillar infiltration to commence after a symptom-free interval of several days following a sore throat. Respiratory impairment may occur (due to obstruction of the faucial isthmus, especially with *bilateral* abscesses). Peak occurrence is in the 2nd–4th decades. Symptoms may be minimal in older patients.

Causes: Inflammatory infiltration and abscess formation in the peritonsillar tissues.

Diagnosis:
● Mirror examination shows typical findings.
● Blood count (left shift) and elevated ESR.
● Other options: needle aspiration of the abscess, abscess tonsillectomy.

Differentiation is required from Quincke edema, malignant diphtheria, agranulocytosis, tonsillar neoplasms (malignant lymphoma, anaplastic carcinoma), leukosis, internal carotid aneurysm ("hard, throbbing" pulsation), and dentogenic abscess.

Retropharyngeal Abscess in Children
See p. 265.

Retropharyngeal Abscess in Adults
See p. 266.

Abscess of the Tongue (Base) and Oral Floor

Main symptoms: Severe to excruciating rest pain that is aggravated by swallowing and phonation. Speech impairment ranges from muffled speech to complete aphonia. The tongue is swollen and difficult to move, and the oral floor is bulging, indurated, and tender to pressure. There is severe to very severe malaise. Progression to cellulitis of the oral floor ("Ludovici angina") can occur (see p. 390).

Other symptoms and special features: Patient has difficulty eating and may be entirely unable to ingest solids or liquids. Increased salivation, oral fetor, occasional dyspnea. Trismus.

Causes: Infection of the musculature of the tongue and/or oral floor with rapid spread in the fascial compartments.

Diagnosis:
- Typical history; typical indirect and palpable findings.
- With signs of liquefaction, diagnosis is established by needle aspiration.

Differentiation is required from hematoma, malignant tumor, actinomycosis, and gumma of tertiary syphilis.

Epiglottitis
See p. 316.

Stylalgia (Elongated Styloid Process Syndrome, Eagle Syndrome)

Main symptoms: Long history of pain on swallowing, yawning, or after prolonged, loud speech. Usually unilateral. Neuralgiform "gnawing" and episodic pain that is maximal in the tonsillar area or behind the mandibular angle and may radiate to the ear and temple. Symptoms can be reproduced by palpation of the tonsillar cleft. Intraoral inspection offers unremarkable findings. May follow tonsillectomy.

Causes: Elongated styloid process causing mechanical irritation of the adjacent cranial nerves (IX, X, XI, or XII) or of the internal or external carotid artery.

Diagnosis:
- Typical history; typical tenderness in the tonsillar cleft area.
- Radiographic visualization of the styloid process. May be supplemented by internal or external carotid angiography.

Differentiation is required from trigeminal neuralgia, glossopharyngeal neuralgia, vagus neuralgia, and cervical spondylosis.

Stylokeratohyoid Syndrome

Results from persistence of the embryonic hyoid chain (*very rare*). Symptoms are similar to those of stylalgia but may include transient vertigo or disturbance of consciousness induced by certain head and neck movements. There may be associated dysfunction of the recurrent nerve, facial nerve, and phrenic nerve. Diagnosis is established by radiography.

Differentiation is required from neuralgias of cranial nerves IX and X, cervical rib syndrome (see p. 394), subclavian steal syndrome (see p. 396), and stenosis of the carotid artery (see p. 395) or vertebral artery.

Carotidynia
See p. 167.

Acute Pharyngitis

Main symptoms: Sore throat and odynophagia that may radiate to the ear; raw, dry, burning sensation in the throat. Frequent throat clearing. On inspection the pharyngeal mucosa appears red, thickened, and very dry. Occasionally it may be coated with a mucous or purulent exudate that is succeeded by hard, varnish-like crusts. The tonsils and surrounding tissues are usually involved.

Other symptoms and special features: Acute pharyngitis in *children* is usually associated with fever (systemic infection) and frequently with anterior and posterior cervical lymphadenopathy. The blood count often shows a relative lymphocytosis. *Adult* cases generally run a milder course with little malaise but significant throat pain or discomfort. Frequent concomitant involvement of the nose, larynx, trachea, and bronchi (cough, sputum, temporary hoarseness).

Causes: Usual cause is a primary viral infection followed by bacterial superinfection (e.g., with streptococci). Causative agents include influenzal and parainfluenzal viruses, myxoviruses, adenoviruses, enteroviruses, rhinoviruses, and many others. RS (respiratory syncytial) viruses are common in small children. Acute pharyngitis can also result from mechanical injury (indwelling tube, foreign body).

Chronic form: See p. 264.

Diagnosis:
● Typical history and local findings.
● Protracted cases should be evaluated by bacteriologic and mycologic smears and possibly by serologic testing.

Differentiation is required from prodromal signs of acute exanthemas. Exclude burn injury or intoxication. Exclude oropharyngeal manifestation of a generalized mucosal disease (see Table 4.**16**).

Trauma (Including Burns, Caustic Lesions, and Foreign Bodies)

Main symptoms: Severe sore throat and dysphagia correlating with an exogenous insult (foreign body; ingestion of toxic, scalding, and/or caustic substance). There may be concomitant bleeding from the mouth or blood-tinged saliva (see p. 273). Small foreign objects (fish bones, bone fragments, etc.) tend to lodge in the lingual tonsil or a palatine tonsil.

Diagnosis:
● History, indirect examination, possibly endoscopy.
● Suspected fish bones and similar objects can be recognized by digital palpation of the oropharynx and hypopharynx (base of tongue, tonsils, lateral pharyngeal wall).
● If a foreign body is suspected, biplane radiographs should be taken of the pharynx, perhaps using contrast swallow, *before* endoscopy is performed.

Neoplasms

Main symptoms: Often the only initial symptom of an oropharyngeal malignancy is pain, which may be constant, or provoked by swallowing or chewing. The tumor itself may be very small or in an obscure location and detectable only by careful, repeated searches. Meanwhile, large malignancies that are easily detected may cause no pain or only minimal discomfort for some time. Unexplained pain of long duration, especially in older patients, requires a systematic workup using all available means until a diagnosis is established and malignancy has been confirmed or excluded. See p. 267 for further details.

Oral Pain and Dysesthesia

This relatively general symptom is produced by a multitude of disorders. Pain or dysesthesia may assume the status of a *cardinal symptom* in some disorders, but usually they are combined with other marked symptoms that allow for at least a crude differential diagnosis. Most disorders belonging to this group are discussed elsewhere in greater detail (see page references).

Cheilitis
See p. 240.

Stomatitis
See p. 243.

Other Inflammatory Mucosal Diseases
See p. 252 ff.

Burning Tongue (Glossalgia, Glossopyrosis, Glossodynia)

Burning of the tongue is a common symptom that occurs predominantly in middle-aged and elderly women. Table 4.**3** lists the potential causes, which often must be painstakingly and systematically pursued in the course of differential diagnosis.

Diseases of the Dental System

Main symptoms: Pain in the diseased tooth or its immediate surroundings triggered or aggravated by mechanical loading of the affected tooth (chewing, eating, percussion) and by exposure to heat or cold. The pain may radiate to the ear.

Dental and periodontal diseases that can cause oral pain are shown schematically in Figure 4.1a,b. The accurate diagnosis of these disorders generally requires dental consultation, so a detailed discussion is not presented in this context.

Osteitis and Osteomyelitis of the Jaws
See pp. 141, 144.

Table 4.**3**   Causes of burning tongue

Local irritation
- Glossitis (and/or stomatitis)
- Fissured tongue, geographic tongue, exfoliatio linguae areata (wandering plaques)
- External irritants, e.g., chemicals, topical medications (mouthwashes), electrogalvanic potential difference between metals and alloys used in the mouth, denture plastics (contact allergy), microtrauma (carious teeth, faulty bite, traumatic cleaning, poorly fitting denture), chronic inflammatory foci in the oropharynx (tonsils, pharynx, periodontal pockets, etc.). Radiation mucositis. Candidiasis. Food allergy

Dermatologic causes
- Systemic mucosal diseases such as erosive lichen ruber planus, scleroderma, epidermolysis bullosa, tertiary syphilitis glossitis, etc., see Table 4.**7**

Toxic mucositis
- Caused, for example, by gold, bismuth, lead, mercury, nitrogen mustard; see Tables 4.**8** and 4.**9**

Drug side effects, see Table 4.**8**

Metabolic disorders
- Vitamin deficiency: B complex vitamins and vitamin C
- Iron deficiency anemia (Plummer–Vinson syndrome)
- Latent tetany*
- Diabetes mellitus*
- Gout*

Hematologic disorders
- Pernicious anemia with Möller–Hunter glossitis (vitamin B_{12} deficiency)
- Lymphogranulomatosis, see p. 407

Gastrointestinal disorders
Achylia or hypoacidity of the gastric juice
- Gastritis, ulcerative colitis; dyspepsia and other gastrointestinal disorders including tumors
- Liver and biliary tract infections

Neurologic disorders
- Organic brain disease (cerebral atrophic syndrome)
- Autonomic–neurotic disorders
- Glossopharyngeal neuralgia, intermedius neuralgia, lingual neuralgia
- Progressive paralysis and tabes dorsalis
- Zoster neuralgia

Endocrine disorders
- Menopause
- Glossopyrosis (senile lingual pruritus)

Vascular disorders
- Arteriosclerosis
- Arteritis

Miscellaneous causes
- Sjögren syndrome and preliminary stages, see p. 303
- Cystic fibrosis, see p. 189
- Decompensated cardiac defects
- Malaria
- Chronic alcoholism
- Sublingual varices
- Lingual myalgia, myofacial pain syndrome
- Psychogenic glossodynia
- Latent depression (?)
- Carcinophobia

* No further commentary

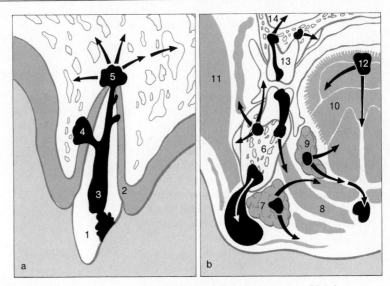

Fig. 4.**1 a,b**   Inflammatory processes involving the teeth and mouth (from Becker, Naumann, Pfaltz)

a Inflammation in and around the tooth
b Inflammation in the oral region
  1 Carious incisor tooth
  2 Periodontium
  3 Pulpitis
  4 Periapical abscess
  5 Apical granuloma
  6 Mandible (teeth, osteomyelitis)
  7 Submandibular gland (inflammation, salivary stone, etc.)
  8 Oral floor musculature
  9 Sublingual gland (inflammation, retention, etc.)
10 Lingual musculature
11 Buccal musculature
12 Abscess formation spreading into the lingual musculature
13 Apical granuloma of a maxillary tooth spreading to the maxillary sinus
14 Lumen of maxillary sinus

Oral Pain Due to Salivary Gland Disease
See Table 5.**1**.

Trauma (Scalds, Caustic Injuries, Foreign Bodies)
See p. 235.

Neoplasms
See pp. 235, 267.

Paroxysmal Pain in the Oropharyngeal Region

This can result from neuralgia of the trigeminal nerve and its branches (see p. 159), the nervus intermedius (see p. 16), the glossopharyngeal nerve (see p. 162), or the vagus nerve (see p. 163).

Dysphagia and Odynophagia
See pp. 279, 380, Table 4.**25**, and Table 8.**8**.

Symptom   **Mucosal Lesions of the Lips**

(Inflammation, deposits, discoloration, ulceration, circumscribed hyperplasia, and other phenomena)

The disorders that must be considered in the differential diagnosis of this symptom are too numerous to be fully explored in the present context, so we shall confine our attention to the more common mucosal diseases that have special significance in otorhinolaryngology (Table 4.4). For convenience, the disorders are arranged according to their preferred sites of occurrence. It should be noted, however, that many of these mucosal diseases do not respect topographic boundaries, and classification according to involvement of the *lips, oral cavity, tongue*, and *lymphoepithelial organs* is artificial and done purely for convenience. The following brief commentaries are limited to a few salient points, because this group of diseases is generally diagnosed from typical local findings while doubtful cases are referred for dermatologic evaluation.

Pyodermas

Impetigo Contagiosa

Main symptoms: Smear infection contracted mainly by children and chiefly involving the lips and the area around the mouth and nose. Superficial skin infection is marked by the presence of small and large vesicles and honey-yellow crusts.

Causes: Hemolytic streptococci, occasionally staphylococci.

Differentiation is required from herpes simplex and secondary syphilis.

Furuncles and Carbuncles of the (Upper) Lip
See p. 208.

Chronic Staphylogenic Folliculitis

Main symptoms: Very refractory abscess-formation occurring predominantly on the upper lip and less commonly on the lower lip due to staphylogenic folliculitis. A relatively common sequel to purulent rhinitis or sinusitis.

Differentiation is required from furunculosis, fungal infection, chancriform pyoderma (especially on the lower lip), and primary syphilis.

Other Bacterial Diseases

Erysipelas
See p. 173.

Tuberculosis
See p. 247.

Leprosy
See p. 248.

Syphilis

See p. 247. All three stages of syphilis may be manifested in the *lip region. Primary stage*: Chancre and swollen regional lymph nodes. *Secondary stage* (about 9 weeks later): Patchy enanthema of the lip mucosa (and possibly all the oral mucosa), generalized syphilids on the skin about the mouth, and regional lymph node enlargement. *Tertiary stage* (starting 3–5 years after the early stage): Tuberoserpiginous syphilids and/or gummata on the mucosal aspect of the lip (usually the upper lip).

Differentiation in *stage I* is required from herpes simplex, furunculosis of the lip, and carcinoma of the lip; in *stage II* from aphthosis, herpes simplex, lichen ruber, and leukoplakia; in *stage III* from cheilitis granulomatosa (Melkersson–Rosenthal disease) and macrocheilia due to other causes (see Table 4.6).

Table 4.**4** *Symptom* Cutaneous and mucosal lesions of the lips (selected according to otolaryngologic criteria)

Synopsis	
Pyodermas	**Dermatoses that commonly involve the lips**
Impetigo contagiosa	Hereditary hemorrhagic teleangiectasis (Osler–Rendu disease)
Furuncles and carbuncles of the (upper) lip, see p. 208	Lentigo simplex and lentiginosis, see p. 150
Chronic staphylogenic folliculitis	Nevi*
	Psoriasis*
Other bacterial diseases	Contact eczema*
Erysipelas, see p. 173	Progressive systematic scleroderma, see p. 255
Tuberculosis, see p. 247	Dermatomyositis, see p. 255
Leprosy, see p. 248	Lupus erythematosus, see pp. 210, 255
Syphilis	Keratoacanthoma (pseudocarcinomatous molluscum)*
Viral diseases	
Herpes simplex labialis	**Macrocheilia**
Verruca vulgaris	See Table 4.**6**
Various forms of cheilitis	**Precancerous lesions**
Cheilitis simplex	Abrasive precancerous cheilitis, see p. 241
Angular cheilitis (perlèche), see also Table 4.**5**	Leukoplakia, see p. 256
Actinic cheilitis	Bowen disease (erythroplasia), see p. 257
Chronic actinitic cheilitis	
Cheilitis glandularis	**Tumors of the lips**
Cheilitis granulomatosa	Benign neoplasms
	Malignant neoplasms (basal cell carcinoma, see p. 148; carcinoma, see p. 148)
Dystrophies and malformations of the lips	
Various cheilopathies	
Angioneurotic (Quincke) edema, see p. 143	
Melkersson–Rosenthal syndrome, see p. 153	
Hypersensitivity reactions, see p. 249	

* No further commentary

Viral Diseases

Herpes Simplex Labialis

Main symptoms: Usually recurrent, episodic eruptions of vesicles with clear contents on the upper and/or lower lip or in the nasal vestibule at the mucocutaneous junction. Itching, tension, or neuralgiform complaints can occur as prodromes. An episode is often brought on by factors such as sun exposure, fever, menstruation, or mechanical skin irritation.

Causes: Primary infection with type I HSV (generally asymptomatic), usually contracted in childhood. Endemic prevalence is very high (about 30% of the population are believed to carry the virus, but only some manifest clinically overt HSV symptoms).

Diagnosis: Isolation of the virus from the vesicular contents on the rabbit cornea. Immunofluorescent detection. Cytopathic effects in cell culture. Epidermal giant cells in the Tzanck test. The organisms are demonstrable by electron microscopy.

Table 4.**5** Causes of angular cheilitis (perlèche)

Infections

- Strepto- or staphyloderma (most common in children)
- Fungal infection (e. g., *Candida albicans*) (most common in adults)
- Syphilis (primary, secondary, very rarely tertiary, congenital syphilis)
- Pyogenic granuloma

Genetic factors

- Endogenous eczema
- Atopic eczema
- Congenital fistulae at the oral commissures
- Acanthosis nigricans

Neoplasms

- Squamous cell carcinoma
- Keratoacanthoma (pseudocarcinomatous molluscum, molluscum sebaceum)

Other causes

- Hypersalivation
- Prognathism, dental misalignment, ill-fitting dentures
- Hypochromic (iron deficiency) anemia (Plummer–Vinson syndrome)
- Hypovitaminoses (e. g., vitamin B_2 deficiency)
- Diabetes mellitus (predisposing factor for candidiasis)
- Malnutrition
- Achylia
- Pernicious anemia
- Cheilitis granulomatosa (Melkersson–Rosenthal syndrome)

Differentiation is required from varicella, chronic recurrent aphthosis, acute infectious exanthemas, herpetic or aphthous gingivostomatitis, Pospischill–Feyrter aphthoid, and impetigo contagiosa.

Verruca Vulgaris

Main symptoms: Common warts occurring singly or in clusters on skin and mucosal surfaces about the lips (and on the tongue!). Isolated mucosal warts = mucosal papillomas. Children and adolescents are mainly affected.

Causes: Various types of karyotropic DNA wart virus (HPV = human papillomavirus). Detectable by electron microscopy ("negative contrast").

Differentiation is required from keratoacanthoma, spindle cell carcinoma, and Bowen disease.

Various Forms of Cheilitis

Cheilitis Simplex (Cheilitis Sicca)

Main symptoms: Lip mucosa is rough, dry, fissured, sometimes reddened, and scaling or covered with flat crusts. Itching or burning. "Cracked lips."

Causes: Exogenous damage by weather, solar radiation, drying (fever), and occasionally by cosmetics or local medications ("contact cheilitis"). Often only the lower lip is affected.

Differentiation is required from contact eczemas and leukoplakia.

Angular Cheilitis (Perlèche, Commissural Rhagades)

Main symptoms: Redness and rhagade formation, usually bilateral, at the corners of the mouth. Later crusting and induration of the commissural tissue.

Causes: Potentially diverse (Table 4.**5**).

Diagnosis: Bacteriologic and mycologic (*Candida albicans*) smears. Exclude or establish one of the causes listed in Table 4.**5**.

Differentiation is required from early carcinoma, congenital syphilis, secondary syphilis, congenital commissural fistulae, and atopic eczema.

Actinic Cheilitis (Solar Cheilosis)

Main symptoms: Edematous swelling, redness, scaling, and vesiculation of the lower lip following intense exposure to sunlight. Progression to chronic actinitic cheilitis (= abrasive precancerous cheilitis) can occur after years of exposure to actinic radiation (most common in persons working outdoors; see below).

Chronic Actinic (Abrasive Precancerous) Cheilitis

Main symptoms: Crusted, erosive lesions of the lower lip with no signs of significant inflammation but with whitish, plaque-like epithelial thickenings and atrophic areas in the red of the lips. Most common in older males (farmers, road workers, construction workers, seamen, etc.). End result of recurrent actinitic cheilitis. A definite *precancerous lesion*!

Differentiation from early carcinoma (in which submucous tissue is already indurated and infiltrated) is accomplished by biopsy.

Cheilitis Glandularis

Main symptoms: Enlarged lip with raised, pinhead-sized purple or glazed macules (gland ostia) on the mucosa that extrude a slightly viscous, colorless fluid when compressed. The lip has a gritty, nodular texture ("bag of shot") on palpation. Onset is in adolescence with about a 2:1 preponderance of males. May progress to *cheilitis glandularis apostematosa* (Volkmann disease), marked by suppuration of the lip glands.

Differentiation is required from Osler disease and other forms of macrocheilia (see Table 4.6).

Granulomatous Cheilitis

Main symptoms: Chronic swelling of the lip with granulomatous inflammation in Melkersson–Rosenthal syndrome (see p. 153). Chiefly affects the upper lip ("tapir mouth") and occasionally the tissue of the cheek (parietitis granulomatosa).

Cause: Unknown.

Diagnosis: Check for Melkersson–Rosenthal triad (transient episodes of facial paralysis, fissured tongue, cheilitis granulomatosa). *But:* all symptoms are not *always* present at the onset of the disease!

Differentiation is required from herpes simplex, cheilitis glandularis, lichen ruber, drug rash, syphilis, mucous granulomas, other forms of macrocheilia (see Table 4.6), and malignant disease.

Dystopias and Malformations Involving the Lip

It is relatively common to find *ectopic sebaceous glands* on the inner surface of the lip and occasionally on the buccal mucosa. Less common are *congenital fistulae*, which represent true malformations and may involve the paramedian or lateral portion of the lower lip. Other easily diagnosed lesions are *mucous cysts* and *mucous granulomas*, which present infrequently in the upper lip as globular, moderately displaceable masses of variable size. *True dermoid cysts* and *epidermoid cysts* are rare in this area.

A *"double lip"* (usually the upper lip) may be congenital or acquired, e.g., as a symptom of the *Ascher syndrome* (blepharochalasis, double lip, juvenile goiter). This condition is not a true malformation but results from the formation of a furrow parallel to the border of the lip. The white lesions known as "lip calluses" (seen in trumpet players and other wind instrument players, also in glassblowers) may convey the impression of a horizontal division of the lips. They represent sites of gradually developing hyperkeratosis of leukoplakia incited by constant mechanical pressure.

Lip Clefts
See p. 271.

Miscellaneous Cheilopathies

Angioneurotic Edema (Quincke Edema)
See p. 143.

Melkersson–Rosenthal Syndrome
See pp. 153, 241.

Table 4.**6**   Causes of macrocheilia

Genetic
- Ascher syndrome ("double lip")
- Familial macrocheilia
- Sturge–Weber syndrome
- Quincke edema (hereditary form)
- Melkersson–Rosenthal syndrome
- Hemangioma
- Lymphangioma

Infectious
- Recurrent herpes simplex
- Recurrent erysipelas
- Cheilitis glandularis
- Acute or chronic inflammatory macrocheilia (lip furuncle, insect sting, Quincke edema, leprosy, leishmaniasis, granulomatous blastomycosis, candidiasis, benign cutaneous lymphadenosis, syphilis, tuberculosis)

Neoplastic
- Neurofibromatosis, neurofibroma
- Mycosis fungoides
- Sarcoma
- Basal cell epithelioma
- Carcinoma

Other causes
- Posttraumatic
- Sarcoidosis
- Acromegaly
- Myxedema
- Storage diseases

○ Lentigo simplex and lentiginosis, see p. 150
○ Nevi
○ Psoriasis
○ Contact eczema
○ Progressive systemic scleroderma, see p. 255
○ Dermatomyositis, see p. 255
○ Lupus erythematosus, see pp. 210, 255
○ Keratoacanthoma (pseudocarcinomatous molluscum, molluscum sebaceum)

Macrocheilia

This descriptive term encompasses a variety of diseases and causes, the most important of which are listed in Table 4.**6**.

Precancerous Lesions

Chronic Actinic Cheilitis
See p. 241.

Leukoplakia
See p. 256.

Bowen Disease
See p. 257.

Tumors of the Lip

The more common *benign neoplasms* of the lip (e.g., fibromas, hemangiomas, lymphangiomas, neurofibromas, granular cell tumors, papillomas, and warts) pose no exceptional problems of differential diagnosis. Biopsy confirms the diagnosis in doubtful cases.

Malignant Tumors

Basal cell epithelioma and carcinoma of the lip are the most important entities in this clinical group.

Basal cell epithelioma of the lip, see p. 148.
Carcinoma of the lip, see p. 149.

Hypersensitivity Reactions

Exaggerated reactions of the lips to certain foods, drugs, and synthetic materials generally affect the oral cavity as well and are discussed on p. 249ff.

Other Skin Diseases that Commonly Involve the Lips

○ Hereditary hemorrhagic teleangiectasis (Rendu–Osler disease), see p. 198

The number and potential manifestations of diseases affecting the mucosae of the mouth and pharynx are quite large. Oral or pharyngeal symptoms may predominate, depending on the location of the disease. Some diseases produce accompanying cutaneous manifestations, raising interdisciplinary issues of differential diagnosis that may necessitate mutual dermatologic and otorhinolaryngologic consultation. In Table 4.7 an attempt is made to group the many relevant disorders into a manageable scheme. This classification is based not just on etiologic criteria but, for convenience of differential diagnosis, on symptomatic criteria as well. Diseases that often cause predominantly *pharyngeal* symptoms are also noted in Table 4.**15**.

Given the large number of diseases listed in Table 4.**7** and the fact that many of the diseases are not the exclusive province of otorhinolaryngology but overlap with other specialties such as dermatology, internal medicine, and pediatrics, the following brief commentaries are limited to some essential key words for diseases that cannot be considered "ENT specific." Diseases in the synopsis that are rarely encountered in ENT practice or fall mainly within the province of other specialties are not included in the brief commentaries that follow.

Viral Diseases

Papillomas

Main symptoms: Single or multiple, soft, grayish-white or reddish neoplasms with an irregular ("villous", "raspberry-like" (surface, attached to the mucosa by a broad or pedunculated base. Sites of predilection are the uvula, cheek, faucial pillars, tongue, and red of the lips. See also p. 325.

Causes: A true viral etiology (human papillomavirus) is assumed. Closely related to cutaneous warts.

Diagnosis: Complete excisional biopsy and histologic examination.

Differentiation is required from papillary carcinoma, Bowen disease, fungal infection, and pemphigus vegetans.

Herpetic Gingivostomatitis (Aphthous Stomatitis)

Main symptoms: Appearance of multiple, yellowish, approximately lentil-sized erosions and/or vesicles ("aphthae") with red halos on the oral mucosa. The lips may be spared. Chiefly affects infants and small children. Onset marked by high fever and oral pain and burning. Feeding difficulties, drooling, oral fetor. Regional lymph nodes are tender and swollen.

Other symptoms and special features: Lesions are mainly localized to the anterior oral cavity and gums. There are recurrent crops of new lesions with no apparent pattern of clustering. Lesions persist for $1-2$ weeks and heal without scarring.

Causes: Primary infection with herpes simplex virus. Droplet infection.

Diagnosis: Very typical location. Isolation of virus from the vesicle contents (inoculated onto rabbit cornea) may be tried.

Differentiation is required from herpes zoster, recurrent (habitual) aphthae, varicella, acute infectious enanthemas (exanthemas), herpangina (see Table 4.**2**), foot-and-mouth disease ("aphthous fever"), Behçet disease, pemphigus, and fungal infections.

Pospischill—Feyrter Aphthoid

Main symptoms: Sequel to whooping cough, measles, scarlet fever, rubella, mumps, or varicella in sick, weak infants and small children. Very severe form of herpetic gingivostomatitis (see above). Also occurs in immunocompromised adults (tumor patients). Infection tends to spread peripherally from the oral cavity and may involve the pharynx, esophagus, face, or limbs. Ulceration can occur. A rare form of herpes simplex infection.

Table 4.**7** *Symptom* Lesions of the oral mucosa (selected according to otolaryngologic criteria)

Synopsis

Viral diseases

Papillomas

Herpetic gingivostomatitis (aphthous stomatitis)

Pospischill–Feyrter aphthoid

Zoster

Herpangina, see p. 231

Epidemic stomatitis (foot-and-mouth disease)

AIDS (acquired immune deficiency syndrome)

Sporadic viropathies (varicella, influenza, measles, mononucleosis)

Bacterial diseases

Ulceromembranous stomatitis

Mucosal tuberculosis

Tonsillar tuberculosis

Mucosal lupus

Syphilis

Diphtheria, see p. 233

Gonorrhea

Rhinoscleroma

Leprosy

Protozoal infections and zoonotic diseases

Leishmaniasis, see Table 4.**28**

Malleus, see Table 4.**28** and p. 248

Listeriosis, see Table 4.**28** and p. 248

Tularemia, see Table 4.**28** and p. 248

Brucelloses, see Table 4.**28** and p. 248

Fungal infections (mycoses)

Candidiasis

Actinomycosis, see p. 397

Blastomycoses, see Table 4.**28**

Histoplasmosis, see Table 4.**28**

Sporotrichosis, see Table 4.**28**

Toxic exanthemas (stomatitis medicamentosa)

Drug-related stomatitis

Allergic and pseudoallergic reactions

Tissue injury

Acute edema within the oral cavity

Quincke edema

Insect sting

Aphthous mucosal diseases

Recurrent aphthae

Solitary aphthae

Behçet aphthosis

Aphthous stomatitis (herpetic gingivostomatitis), see p. 243

Pospischill–Feyrter aphthoid

Zoster

Herpangina, see p. 231

Epidemic stomatitis, see p. 245

Various common lesions of the oral and dental mucosae

Gingivitis

Periodontitis (periodontosis)

Gingival hyperplasia (macrogingivae)

Epulis

Bullous dermatoses that may involve the oropharyngeal mucosae

Pemphigus vulgaris

Dermatitis herpetiformis

Bullous pemphigoid

Benign mucous membrane pemphigoid ("ocular pemphigoid")

Epidermolysis bullosa (dystrophic forms)

Erythema multiforme (including Stevens–Johnson syndrome)

Lyell syndrome

Other dermatoses occasionally manifested in the mouth or pharynx

Lichen ruber planus

Progressive systemic scleroderma

Dermatomyositis

Lupus erythematosus

Granulating diseases of the oropharyngeal mucosae

Sarcoidosis

Melkersson–Rosenthal syndrome, see p. 153

Foreign body granuloma

Specific granulomas (tuberculosis, syphilis, fungal infections), see pp. 247, 248, 249

Histiocytosis X and eosinophilic granuloma

Wegener granulomatosis

Midline granuloma

Continuation Table 4.**7**

Synopsis	
Hypovitaminoses Especially vitamin B₁, B₂, B₆, B₁₂, niacinamide, vitamin C, an occasionally vitamin A	**Benign and malignant neoplasms of the oral and pharyngeal mucosae** See Table 4.**18**
Manifestations of hemorrhagic diathesis in the mouth and pharynx See Table 3.**9**	**Mucosal lesions of the tongue** See Table 4.**12**
Precancerous lesions of the oral and pharyngeal mucosae Leukoplakia Chronic lichen ruber mucosae Bowen disease	**Superficial discoloration of the tongue** See Table 4.**12** **Xerostomia** See pp. 301, 303, and Table 5.**7**

Zoster (Herpes Zoster, Shingles)

Main symptoms: Segmental distribution pattern, generally unilateral. Lesions consist of firm, flat vesicles that all erupt simultaneously, have red halos, and whose contents turn a dull yellowish color after a few days. The vesicles dry (after about 1 week) leaving brownish-yellow crusts that persist for an additional 8 days. No high fever, but significant malaise and burning pain in the affected area (often the second and/or third division of the trigeminal nerve; tongue, cheek, palate).

Other symptoms and special features: Prodromal symptoms may be absent. Chiefly affects elderly patients with impaired host defenses (e.g., due to chemotherapy, radiotherapy, etc.). Severe neuralgiform pain often accompanies the eruptions or persists after they have healed.

Causes: Neurotropic reinfection with varicella zoster virus.

Diagnosis:
- Typical local findings (vesicles all at the same stage, segmental distribution).
- Infecting organism may be isolated from vesicle contents.

Differentiation is required from herpes simplex and recurrent aphthosis.

Herpangina
See p. 231.

Epidemic Stomatitis (Foot-and-Mouth Disease, Aphthous Fever)

Main symptoms: Dry, burning sensation in the mouth, significant malaise with fever and headache. In 1−2 days "primary aphthae" (painful, lentil- to bean-sized vesicles with perifocal redness) erupt within the oral cavity and especially on the hands and feet! Lesions persist for about 2 weeks. A very rare disease in the oral region.

Causes: Infection with a rhinovirus (picorna group). May be transmitted by cattle or raw milk.

Diagnosis: Recovery of organism from vesicle contents, blood, saliva, or urine. Also complement binding reaction (CBR).

Differentiation is required from herpetic gingivostomatitis.

AIDS (Acquired Immunodeficiency Syndrome, HIV Infection)

AIDS is a disease that, while affecting the whole organism, produces relatively frequent (about 40%) and early head and neck manifestations. The symptoms are very diverse and mostly nonspecific. HIV-related symptoms tend to resemble those of other common diseases. Features that may distinguish HIV symptoms include an *atypical location* and *atypical efflorescence*, an *atypical course*, and an *atypical age of onset* for the symptoms observed.

○ *Typical HIV-associated lesions:*

  a) *Disseminated Kaposi sarcoma:* Reddish, brown, or purple macules on the skin and/or mucous membranes that increasingly assume the form of raised, nodular, ulcerating lesions. Initial lesions usually appear on the upper trunk. A classic Kaposi sarcoma occurs on the lower extremities, but its primary manifestation may be in the head and neck region. A Kaposi sarcoma in patients < 60 years of age is raises a strong suspicion of HIV infection. Diagnosis is established by biopsy or HIV serology.

  b) *Hairy leukoplakia* on the tongue: White, hairy patches seen most commonly on the lateral border of the tongue. Generally signifies an advanced stage of AIDS. Lesions may become secondarily infected with *Candida albicans.*

○ *Conditions preferentially associated with underlying HIV infection:*

  – Lymphadenopathy
  – Candidiasis (mouth, nose, pharynx, larynx, tracheobronchial tree, esophagus)
  – Zoster (also generalized)
  – Herpes simplex
  – Mononucleosis
  – Rare infections (e.g., disseminated coccidioidomycosis, disseminated histoplasmosis)
  – Non-Hodgkin lymphoma of B-cell type
  – Toxoplasmosis.

○ *Other potential "nonspecific" manifestations:*

Sinusitis, tonsillitis, herpangina, gingivitis, periodontitis, pharyngitis, esophagitis, tracheitis, bronchitis, sudden deafness, facial paralysis, neuralgias of the face or head.

○ *General associated symptoms*

Fever, anorexia, headache, muscular and/or joint pain, transient or persistent lymph node enlargement, diarrhea, weight loss (> 10 kg).

Causes: Infection with human immunodeficiency retrovirus (serotypes HIV 1 and HIV 2).

Diagnosis: *Screening test* for HIV antibodies in the serum, such as ELISA, and a *confirmatory test* such as the Western blot test. Highly specific HIV detection methods can also be applied.

Systemic viral diseases commonly associated with lesions of the oral mucosa are:

○ *Varicella* (chickenpox): Enanthema and exanthema, most common in children.
○ *Influenza:* Edema of the soft palate and pharynx, sparing the hard palate. Rarely with petechial mucosal hemorrhages; see also p. 183.
○ *Measles:* Koplik spots appear in the prodromal stage (2nd–3rd day of the disease): White spots appearing on the buccal mucosa, succeeded by enanthemous red spots on the oropharyngeal mucosa and then by the typical skin eruption.
○ *Mononucleosis* (see p. 231), which can produce oral mucosal lesions similar to those of aphthous stomatitis, even *without* the typical tonsillitis.

Diseases Caused by Bacteria and Protozoa

Ulceromembranous (Ulcerative) Stomatitis

Main symptoms: Redness, swelling, and tenderness, usually commencing at the gingival margin. Dirty-gray fibrinous exudate or sharply marginated mucosal ulcerations with *severe* pain, often directly adjacent to the tooth. Oral fetor, sialorrhea, bad taste in the mouth, eating difficulties. Onset is usually associated with high fever and malaise.

Other symptoms and special features: Lesions may involve a broad area including the buccal mucosa and/or tongue. Ulcerations may be deep with a red margin and a pink base that bleeds easily. The fibrinous deposits are easily wiped away. See also p. 260.

Causes: Infection with fusiform rods and spirochetes. Poor oral hygiene is a predisposing factor.

Diagnosis: Identification of the organism in smears: *Fusobacterium nucleatum plauti* and spirilla (*Borrelia vincenti*).

Differentiation is required from aphthous stomatitis (usually *not* directly adjacent to the teeth), fungal infection of the mucosa (smear), viral infection of the mucosa, syphilis, tuberculosis, AIDS, and blood diseases (agranulocytosis, leukemia).

Noma (cancrum oris) is an extreme form occurring in debilitated or malnourished patients and characterized by rapidly progressive necrosis and destruction of facial and oral soft tissues.

The following *specific infections* have become rare but can still occur sporadically:

Tuberculosis of the Oral Mucosa (Exudative, Ulcerative Mucosal Tuberculosis)

Main symptoms: Flat, painful mucosal ulcerations with undermined borders, a greasy coating, and swelling and redness of the surrounding mucosa. Eating difficulties. Tuberculoma formation (e.g., on the uvula) is less common.

Other symptoms and special features: Usually secondary to tuberculosis of an internal organ (lung, alimentary tract, etc.). Peak occurrence is in middle-aged males. Morphologic manifestations are highly variable (primary complex or postprimary mucosal disease).

Causes: Usually due to hematogenous or intracanalicular spread from a primary visceral focus (usually the lung).

Diagnosis:
- Smear from an ulcer (Ziehl−Neelsen stain).
- Culture and animal test.
- Biopsy.
- Exclusion of organ tuberculosis (pulmonologic consultation).

Differentiation is required from tertiary syphilis (absence of tubercle bacillus with very similar local findings; serum tests), aphthosis, fungal infection, and mucosal carcinoma.

Special Forms:

Tonsillar Tuberculosis

Main symptoms: Painless swelling of a palatine tonsil with peritonsillar edema. Flat ulcerations or deep tissue defects in the tonsillar area, coated with a greasy material. Regional cervical lymphadenopathy: Lymph nodes are enlarged but not painful. Tumor-like enlarge-

ment of the tonsil is uncommon. Analogous infection can involve the adenoid.

Cause: See above.

Diagnosis: Identification of the causative organism, biopsy.

Differentiation is required from syphilis, carcinoma, and fungal infection.

Mucosal Lupus

Main symptoms: Clusters of round nodules in the mucosa (diascopy pressure demonstrates yellow-brown macules in the oral mucosa). The mucosal lesions are painless and progress very slowly, with or without ulceration. Heavy mucosal scarring. May coexist with lupus of the nose, marked by characteristic cutaneous and cartilaginous lesions in the anterior nasal soft tissues. Has become a *very* rare tuberculous manifestation!

Diagnosis: Identification of the causative organism in culture and/or experimental animals. Biopsy.

Differentiation is required from tertiary syphilis, precancerous disease, and early malignancy.

Syphilis of the Oral Mucosa

Main symptoms: All three stages of acquired syphilis may be manifested in the oral cavity.

Stage I (primary lesion): After about 3 weeks' incubation, a dark red erythema appears, which is succeeded by a hard, painless, reddish-brown ulcer (sites of predilection: lips, tonsils, soft palate, anterior third of tongue, oral commissure, cheek). Followed somewhat later by nonpainful swelling and induration of regional lymph nodes. Chancre resolves in 3−6 weeks. Serum reaction is not positive until 3−4 weeks after the onset of stage I!.

Stage II (secondary): Appears 8−10 weeks after infection, marked by generalized cutaneous and organ manifestations and patchy lesions of the oral mucosa (beefy red, lentil-sized macules that tend to coalesce). Mucosal signs are of variable degree (formation of dark red papules and/or plaques, patchy loss of papillae on the tongue, syphilitic sore throat [see p. 261], involvement of pharyngeal mucosa).

Increasing induration of regional lymph nodes. The mucosal lesions resolve in weeks or months.

Stage III (tertiary): Gumma formation occurring an average of 3–15 years after infection. Tongue involvement manifests as interstitial glossitis. Gummas are generally painless and occur chiefly on the hard palate, tongue, tonsils, lips, oropharynx, and hypopharynx. They are prone to ulcerative degeneration with punched-out ulcer margins and subsequent, very characteristic radial scar formation. Perforation from the oral to the nasal cavity is a relatively common sequel.

Cause: Infection with *Treponema pallidum.*

Diagnosis:
- Endoscopy and general inspection.
- Identification of the causative organism (smear, dark-field examination) in stage I or II.
- Serologic test is positive after 4 weeks (FTA test = fluorescent treponema antibody test). Nelson test is not positive until the 9th week and is rarely performed. The TPHA and VDRL tests are more important.
- Stage III: Serologic tests, biopsy.

Differentiation is required from the following: In stage I: neoplasms, tuberculosis, fungal infections, herpes; in stage II: tuberculosis; in stage III: malignant tumor, leukosis.

Congenital Syphilis

Main symptoms: *Early congenital syphilis* produces a neonatal syphilitic coryza commencing in the first months of life (see p. 184) with subsequent oral rhagade formation and radial lip scarring as the disease progresses. *Late congenital syphilis* begins at age 3–16 with partial or complete Hutchinson triad (parenchymatous keratitis, barrel teeth, sensorineural hearing loss).

Diphtheria

See pp. 233, 316. Involvement of the oral cavity is rare.

Other Rare Bacterial Infections

Involvement of the oral cavity and pharynx may accompany the following bacterial infections:

- *Gonorrhea* occurring as an oral infection with erosive or aphthous stomatitis and burning pain. Tendency to recur. Diagnosed by identification of the causative organism (smear).
- *Rhinoscleroma* presenting as a granulomatous outgrowth spreading from the nose to involve the palate, alveolar processes, or tongue and culminating in very severe cicatricial adhesions and stenoses (see Table 4.**28**).
- *Leprosy* producing infiltration of the mucous membranes of the tongue, palate, lips, and pharynx with gradual ulceration and subsequent scarring of the defects (see Table 4.**28**).

Protozoal Infections and Zoonotic Diseases

This rare group of oropharyngeal infections includes:

- *Leishmaniasis* (see Table 4.**28**).
- *Malleus* can spread from the nose to the oropharyngeal region (palate, lips, gums) leading to granulations, degenerative infiltrations of a livid color, ulcers with degenerating borders, and cicatricial adhesions. Diagnosed by identification of the causative organism (see Table 4.**28**).
- *Listeriosis* can produce rhinitis and conjunctivitis in addition to tonsillitis with white coatings. Tonsillar ulcers, peritonsillar inflammatory infiltration, and severe ulcerative stomatitis and/or pharyngitis are also observed. Diagnosed by identification of the causative organism (see Table 4.**28**).
- *Tularemia* (rabbit fever) can produce areas of rapidly degenerating infiltration and necrosis (primary lesions) or other, nonspecific mucosal lesions in the oral cavity (tonsil, tongue, palate, pharynx, gums). Involvement of regional lymph nodes! For diagnosis see Table 4.**28**.
- The group of *brucelloses* (e.g., Malta fever, Bang disease) can also cause intraoral mucosal lesions (aphthae, ulcers, degenerative infiltrate). For diagnosis see Table 4.**28**.

Fungal Infections (Mycoses)

Candidiasis (Thrush, Moniliasis)

Main symptoms: Stippled chalk-white deposits that can be wiped away; they may be plaque-like or encompass large areas of the mucosa. Intraoral sites of predilection: in the cheek, at folds, and on the tongue (borders and inferior surface). Also common at the corners of the mouth. Stripping away the fungal plaques leaves an erythematous mucosal surface. "Granulating" mycoses are uncommon.

Other symptoms and special features: Thrush occurs in newborns (in about the first week of life) and infants but can affect anyone as a result of impaired host factors or deficient oral hygiene. Especially in the elderly, thrush can develop intercurrently when predisposing factors are present (marasmus, underlying wasting disease, prolonged use of antibiotics or corticosteroids, antineoplastic therapy, endocrine alterations [pregnancy], contraceptives, diabetes, leukoses, etc.). Thrush occurs opportunistically in AIDS patients (see p. 245).

Cause: Infection with the yeast fungus *Candida albicans. But:* Colonization with candida does not always produce clinical symptoms!

Diagnosis:
- Typical local findings.
- Identification of the fungus in fresh smears or culture.
- Exclusion of (consumptive) underlying disease (see above).

Differentiation is required from leukoplakia and lichen ruber (in which the deposits *cannot* be wiped away); also from other erosive mucosal diseases and HIV infection.

Other Fungal Species that May Infect the Oral Cavity

- *Actinomycosis* (see p. 397).
- *Blastomycoses* (extremely rare in Europe; almost always associated with cutaneous or organ manifestations). See Table 4.**28**.
- *Histoplasmosis:* Relatively common granulomatous infection of the oral mucosa including the tongue, pharynx, and larynx with ulcerations and extensive areas of deep necrosis. For diagnosis see Table 4.**28**. Differential diagnosis includes leishmaniasis, tertiary syphilis, and yaws.
- *Sporotrichosis:* Gummous infiltrations and ulcerations. For diagnosis see Table 4.**28**. Differential diagnosis includes carcinoma, tertiary syphilis, and tuberculosis.

Other Causes of Mucosal Lesions

Toxic Enanthemas (Stomatitis Medicamentosa, Toxic Stomatitis)

Mucosal symptoms: Besides causing polysymptomatic skin reactions, certain drugs (and other substances) can incite aphthoid, lichenoid, erosive and/or ulcerative reactions in the oral mucosa. *Stomatitis medicamentosa* is marked by the sudden appearance of these reactions following the use of newly prescribed drugs (see also Table 3.**15**). The variable and sometimes dramatic subjective complaints range from a mild burning or itching to severe pain and fullness, restiveness, and a feeling of suffocation. The mucosa may be severely erythematous and/or edematous. The symptoms subside following withdrawal of the offending agent.

Diagnosis:
- Directed history.
- Elimination trial. Exposure tests: intradermal, epicutaneous.
- Laboratory tests; RAST; possibly lymphocyte transformation test and detection of precipitated immunoglobulin.

The principal medications that can cause stomatitis by various mechanisms are listed in Table 4.**8**.

Allergic and Pseudoallergic Reactions

These oropharyngeal reactions do not differ significantly from those involving the nose and may be manifested concomitantly in both regions (see Table 3.**15**). The local symptoms differ, however, in accordance with the different anatomic and histologic substrates. The oral cavity is involved less often by *inhalation allergies* and more often by *food allergies*. It can also be affected by specific *contact allergies*

Tabel 4.**8**   Common drugs that can incite stomatitis (after Bork, Hoede, and Korting; Schuermann, Greither, and Hornstein)

Manifestations	Precipitating drug groups
Macular enanthemas, erosive and ulcerative stomatitis	Analgesics of the pyrazolone group; barbiturates; benzodiazepines; chloramphenicol (+ blood changes!); chlorpromazine; glucocorticoids (long-term therapy); gold compounds; hydantoin and derivatives; immunosupressive drugs; indomethacin; ipecac; penicillin and derivatives; phenacetin; phenolphthalein; phenylbutazone; pyrazolone and derivatives; mercury; salicylates; streptomycin; sulfonamides; cytostatics, etc.
Mucosal edema	Analgesics; anticonvulsants; local anesthetics; penicillin (especially ampicillin); sulfonamides, etc.
Lichenoid reactions	Antimalarial drugs; beta-receptor blocking drugs; gold compounds; sulfonylurea and derivatives; tetracycline, etc.
Purpura (nonallergic form)	Acetylsalicylic acid; anticoagulants; cytostatics
Allergic reactions	See p. 249
Drug enanthemas	Analgesics; antibiotics (especially tetracycline); atabrine; barbiturates; quinidine; quinine; eucalyptus oil; fungicides; gold compounds; ofloxacin (Tarivid); phenolphthalein; pyrazolone derivatives; mercury compounds; salicylates; sulfonamides; bismuth compounds, etc.
Pigmentation	Contraceptives; antimalarial agents; gold, silver, bismuth, lead; phenothiazines (chlorpromazine); cytostatics, etc.
Black tongue	Chlorhexidine; iron preparations; corticosteroids; mouthwashes containing sodium perborate or hydrogen peroxide; penicillins; tetracycline
Tooth discoloration	Chlorhexidine; ferric ammonium chloride; fluorine and its compounds; tetracycline
Gingival hyperplasia	Hydantoin and derivatives; estrogens; progesterone; phenobarbital; cyclosporin A, see p. 253
Sialopenia	See Table 5.**7**
Sialorrhea	See Table 5.**6**

evoked by mouthwashes, dental materials (plastics and metal alloys), dental pharmaceuticals, toothpastes, etc. Intravenously administered diagnostic agents (radiographic contrast media) and therapeutic agents (plasma expanders, plasma protein solutions, etc.) can also elicit these reactions.

Occupational Injuries

The injurious effects of occupational agents in the oropharyngeal region are basically caused by the same agents that can damage the nasal tissues (see Table 3.**16**). Additionally there are some special disease symptoms listed in Table 4.**9**. The immediate and occupational history can provide clues important for differential diagnosis.

Table 4.9   Tissue injury involving the oral mucosa or teeth

Acute injury

Accidental scalding or caustic injury by vaporous emissions, acids, lyes, gases, fog, smoke, or dust

Aspiration of acids, lyes, etc.

Chronic injury

Teeth
Acid vapors
"Confectioner's caries"

Caustic dusts
Fluorine overdose (with ulcerative gingivitis)

Discoloration of the teeth or gums
Lead (bluish-black)
Cadmium and cadmium–sulfur compounds (yellow)
Copper (greenish)
Picric acid (yellow)

Mercury and its compounds (grayish-blue)
Silver (ashen gray, "argyria")
Vanadium (grayish-green)
Tin (brownish-black)

Stomatogingivitis

Antimony	Acrolein
Arsenic dust	Benzene and derivatives
Lead dust	Dimethylsulfate
Bromine vapor	Organic dyes
Chlorine (hydrochloric acid, chlorosulfonic acid)	Pyridine
Chromic acid (chromium salts)	Carbon tetrachloride
Fluorine (gas, fluorite, FH)	Trichloroethylene
Iodine	Trinitrotoluene
Calcium (oxide, cyanamide)	Etching agents
Copper dust	Plastics and synthetic resins
Manganese dust	Enamels
Nickel sulfate	Mineral oils
Mercury compounds	Tabacco dust
Hydrogen sulfide, sulfuric acid	Tarry substances
Sulfur dioxide, sulfur hexafluoride	Terpentine
Thallium compounds	Sawdust
Vanadium dust	Hops
Hydrogen peroxide	Insecticides
Bismuth	Jute
	Wool dust

Occupational groups at risk

Mechanical injury	Glassblowers, saddlers, shoemakers, paperhangers, grinders, etc.
Thermal injury	Glassblowers, machinists, blast furnace operators, stokers, cooks, etc.
Infectious diseases	Physicians, nurses, veterinarians
Other	Glassblowers (atrophy of the buccal muscles and skin, dilatation of the parotid excretory duct system)

Acute Edema Within the Oral Cavity

Acute circumscribed edema of the oral tissues including the lips,, palate, uvula, tongue, oropharynx, hypopharynx, and larynx can cause alarming symptoms and can be acutely life-threatening when it involves the tongue, pharynx, or larynx.

Main symptoms: Massive, paroxysmal edematous swelling of the oral mucosa (and tongue) that may involve the lips ("trunk mouth") and portions of the face. Burning pain or occasional itching may precede the edema. The boundaries of the edematous areas are ill-defined, but the areas are circumscribed and are more pale than red. The mucosa appears glazed. An edematous episode may last for hours or even days, may show a strong propensity for recurrence, and may "skip" at intervals ranging from days to years.

Other symptoms and special features: Temperature elevation in children. Peak incidence is in the 3rd and 4th decades, with a 2:1 female preponderance, but acute intraoral edema can occur at any age. An hereditary predisposition (irregular dominance) has been confirmed in some patients.

Causes: Very numerous: Both physical (cold) and psychological factors can precipitate edema formation in predisposed individuals. Allergic mechanisms are apparently involved in many cases but cannot always be demonstrated. Inhalation and food allergens (eggs, fish, chocolate, nuts, milk, yeast, etc.), food additives (dyes and preservatives), other chemical substances, and drugs have been implicated (see Table 4.**8**). Attacks can also be triggered by nonallergic factors such as infectious diseases, insect stings, or "pseudoallergic" mechanisms (intolerance or ideosyncratic reactions). Acute edema not associated with a demonstrable allergen is generally characterized as a "pseudoallergic reaction" (see also p. 249).

Diagnosis:
• History, clinical findings.
• Allergy screening tests and serum IgE determination (PRIST and RAST). Exclusion of intolerance reaction. Oral provocative testing (inpatient!).
• Some cases may require biopsy.

Differentiation is required from erysipelas (fever, high ESR, leukocytosis), the Melkersson−Rosenthal syndrome, insect venom, macrocheilia, macroglossia, herpes simplex, zoster, and chronic persistent lymphedema.

Special Situation:

Insect Sting in the Oropharyngeal Region

Main symptoms: Very intense pain of sudden onset, usually experienced during eating, followed within an hour by severe edematous swelling of the tongue base, epiglottis, and/or pharynx. The laryngeal inlet (arytenoid area, arytenoepiglottic folds) may also be affected. Odynophagia, increasing dyspnea with stridor (in some cases), possible hoarseness. Increasing agitation.

Other symptoms and special features: Mild to very severe systemic reactions can occur, depending on the degree of sensitization to bee or wasp venom. Reactions range from nausea, urticaria, vertigo, and daze to shock with cyanosis, collapse, and loss of consciousness.

Causes: Sting from a "swallowed" bee, wasp, or other venomous insect.

Diagnosis:
• Indirect and/or endoscopic findings in conjunction with the history.
• Immediate administration of high-dose corticosteroids (diagnostic *and* therapeutic).

Aphthous Mucosal Diseases

Recurrent Aphthae (Habitual, "Noninfectious" Aphthae)

Symptoms: Reddened, raised, millet-seed- to pea-size infiltrations, ulcerated at the center and covered by a yellowish-white fibrinous exudate. Generally there are no more than one to three eruptions occurring at mucosal folds, on the oral floor (near the frenulum), on the border or base of the tongue, on the soft palate, or in the pharynx. Regional lymph nodes are usually painful and enlarged. *No* fetor, sialorrhea, or stomatitis. The aphthae are very tender when touched. Long history.

"Solitary aphthae" and solitary "giant aphthae" probably have the same pathogenesis.

Causes: Unknown. Apparently not a viral infection but a "trophoneurotic" disturbance in older children and young adults who are autonomically labile. An autoimmune pathogenesis has also been suggested.

Diagnosis: Typical local findings; history of numerous recurrences. *Absence* of sialorrhea and oral fetor.

Differentiation is required from herpes simplex (fetor, fever, many aphthae arranged in clusters) and epidemic stomatitis.

Behçet Disease (Behçet Aphthosis)

Mucosal symptoms: Chronic syndrome with periodic eruptions of oral aphthae. The aphthae are very painful, ulcerate, and are subject to deep necrosis. The lesions can occur anywhere within the oral cavity, pharynx, or larynx. Sialorrhea and oral fetor are present. Swelling of regional lymph nodes (in some patients). Acute episodes manifest temperature elevation, joint and muscle pain, and severe systemic signs and malaise. Cochleovestibular dysfunction can occur. Ocular symptoms are characteristic (hypopyon iritis, uveitis, papilledema, possible blindness). Involvement of genital skin and renal involvement are very common! Men are affected five times more frequently than women. Common in eastern Mediterranean countries, rare in Central Europe. The *symptom triad* of oral aphthae, aphthous genital ulcers, and hypopyon iritis is typical.

Cause: Unknown. May relate to an autoimmune disorder, a viral infection, or both.

Diagnosis:
● Typical clinical and endoscopic findings.
● A specific HLA pattern (HLA B_5, B_{12}, or B_{27}) can often be demonstrated.

Differentiation is required from recurrent aphthae.

Aphthous Stomatitis (Herpetic Gingivostomatitis)
See p. 243.

Various Common Lesions of the Oral and Dental Mucosae

Isolated inflammation of the gum (*gingivitis*) generally presents no problems of differential diagnosis. It basically represents a *stomatitis* confined to the gingival tissue, with its various associated clinical manifestations.

Inflammatory processes are a particular threat to the gingival margin (*marginal gingivitis*) in desiccated states associated, for example, with Sjögren disease or the use of certain medications (atropine, scopolamine, morphine, analgesics, psychotropic drugs, antibiotics, etc.).

Other potential sources of gingivitis are acute and chronic diseases of the periodontium (periodontitis, periodontosis) and/or of the teeth themselves (see p. 237 and Fig. 4.**1**) as well as poor oral and dental hygiene. Dental consultation is indicated!

Differential diagnosis should include early malignant disease and HIV infection.

Circumscribed *gingival hyperplasia* (usually with dark red discoloration) is alternately known as *macrogingivae* or *gingival fibromatosis*. A *variety of causes* should be considered for these patients in differential diagnosis:

○ Subacute or chronic gingivitis
○ Hereditary factors
○ Endocrine factors with coexisting gingivitis (pregnancy, menopause)
○ Leukoses (monocytic leukemia), hemoblastoses, see p. 408
○ Storage diseases (lipoidproteinosis)
○ Melkersson–Rosenthal syndrome, see p. 153
○ Scurvy (vitamin C hypovitaminosis)
○ Hydantoin medication
○ Contraceptive use
○ Cyclosporin A

Epulis is a collective term for various tumors and tumor-like masses arising from the gingiva (e.g., epulis fibromatosa, giant cell epulis, etc.). The diagnosis is established by biopsy. Differentiation is required from specific granulomas and malignancies.

Bullous Dermatoses that May Involve the Oropharyngeal Mucosae

Pemphigus Vulgaris

Main mucosal symptoms: The mucosal symptoms of pemphigus vulgaris are often the earliest signs of disease, consisting of tense or flaccid, rapidly erupting bullae with no significant redness of surrounding tissue. Rupture of the bullae typically leaves a red base surrounded by a thin, ragged epithelial border. Occasionally the eroded surface is covered by a fibrinous exudate. Lesions in the lip area may form hemorrhagic crusts. All portions of the oral cavity may be involved to variable extents, including the pharynx and esophagus. Affected mucosal surfaces are very delicate and easily traumatized ("like tissue paper"). Eroded areas are extremely painful, and eating becomes difficult. The *granulating form* features tissue proliferation in the eroded areas with mucosal swelling, severe pain, and profuse salivation.

Diagnosis:
● Typical local findings; oral lesions are similar to cutaneous lesions.
● Dermatologic consultation.
● Histologic findings and immunohistologic detection of antibodies against antigenic structures on desmosomes.

Differentiation is required from other bullous mucosal diseases such as drug rash, erythema multiforme (the Stevens–Johnson syndrome), epidermolysis bullosa, bullous pemphigoid, etc.

Dermatitis Herpetiformis

Mucosal symptoms: Oral involvement is less common than with pemphigus. Transient bullae are succeeded by slightly raised erythematous lesions 1–3 cm in diameter that bleed easily. Aphthae and/or ulcerations can also occur. Sites of predilection are the palate, cheek, and tongue. Almost *always* preceded by cutaneous manifestations!

Bullous Pemphigoid

Mucosal symptoms: Intraoral vesiculation with subsequent scarring in patients with corresponding cutaneous manifestations of the disease. The mucosal lesions erupt some time *after* the skin lesions appear.

Benign Mucous Membrane Pemphigoid

Main symptoms: Predilection for women over 50 years of age. Lesions may involve the mucous membranes of the mouth, pharynx, nose, larynx, or esophagus. Cutaneous involvement is unusual. *Small* bullae with erosions and ulcerations are succeeded by heavy scarring and stricture formation. No pain. Sites of predilection: lip and buccal mucosa, palate, tongue, pharynx (posterior wall). Concomitant conjunctival involvement is the rule *("ocular pemphigoid").*

Epidermolysis Bullosa

Mucosal symptoms: Very rare! The oral mucosa (tongue, palate, cheek) is most commonly affected in this autosomal dominant disease. Analogous lesions can occur in the pharynx, larynx, and esophagus. Bullae usually rupture quickly, leaving erosions and/or ulcers. Coexisting dental anomalies are common (hereditary disposition). The bullous mucosal lesions appear immediately after birth!

Erythema Multiforme (Including Stevens–Johnson Syndrome)

Mucosal symptoms: Painful erythema, edema, target-like maculopapules and vesicles chiefly affecting the cheek, soft palate, tongue, and vermilion border of the lower lip. Very foul breath odor, sialorrhea. Speech and eating are impaired. Regional lymph nodes are enlarged, soft, and painful. Peak occurrence is in children and young men. Blood count may demonstrate monocytosis. The Stevens–Johnson syndrome = severe form that may involve the pharynx, larynx, and trachea. Presumably has an allergic pathogenesis based on various causes. Differential diagnosis includes drug exanthema, pemphigus vulgaris, Behçet disease, diphtheria, secondary syphilis, epidemic stomatitis, and the Lyell syndrome.

Lyell Syndrome (Bullous Drug Exanthema)

Generalized form of erythema multiforme (see above). Mucosal involvement is marked by bulla formation with cleavage of mucosal tissues ("scalded skin and mucous membranes"). Many (not all) patients have a history of drug use, especially barbiturates, pyrazolone derivatives, sulfonamides, and hydantoins (see Table 4.**8**). Diagnostic options are reviewed on

p. 252. Differentiation is required from the staphylogenic Lyell syndrome (in children), erythema multiforme, and pemphigus.

Other Dermatoses that Occasionally Involve the Mouth or Pharynx

Lichen Ruber Planus

Mucosal symptoms: Lesions may present as milky-white dots that cannot be wiped away, or they may be arranged in a reticular, annular, lacy, or spiderweb pattern or as long, fine striae with adjacent normal-appearing mucosa. Sites of predilection: buccal mucosa, oral commissures, tongue, vermilion border, palate, gingiva. Subjective complaints are mild or absent. Bullous erosive lichen planus is considered a potentially *precancerous lesion!*

Differentiation is required from leukoplakia, chronic lupus erythematosus, secondary syphilis, and thrush.

Progressive Systemic Scleroderma

Mucosal symptoms: A rare disease that mainly affects older women. Mucosal lesions consist of variable-sized areas of atrophy and sclerosis with loss of papillae on the tongue, sclerosis of the oral commissures (patient cannot whistle), microcheilia and microstomia ("purse-string mouth"). Tongue mobility is reduced (frenulum is shortened and hardened). Dry mouth. Frequent esophageal involvement with dysphagia and reflux (see pp. 374, 380). Autoimmune disorder (collagen disease), see Table 4.**29**.

Diagnosis:
● Typical local findings (face, frenulum).
● Detection of antinuclear antibodies. Biopsy.
● Involvement of other body regions.

Differentiation is required from incipient dermatomyositis and lupus erythematosus.

Dermatomyositis

Mucosal symptoms: Dark red to purple erythematous areas with associated edematous swelling mainly affecting the gingiva, tongue, and lips. Also telangiectasias, bullae, superficial erosions, and epithelial opacities. Pain, especially in the tongue. Dry mouth. Autoimmune disorder (collagen disease).

Diagnosis: Skin and muscle biopsy.
● Also: Increased creatine excretion in the urine.
● Electromyography and serologic enzyme tests (CPK, GOT, aldolase, LDH).
● Exclude underlying malignant disease!

Differentiation is required from lupus erythematosus, progressive scleroderma, and periarteritis nodosa.

Lupus Erythematosus

Mucosal symptoms: Involvement of the oral mucosa is common in this generalized autoimmune disease, which chiefly affects younger women. The *systemic or visceral* form is marked initially be erythematous areas that tend to become ulcerated, causing pain. This form most commonly affects the hard palate and buccal mucosa, less commonly the tongue and gingiva. The *discoid* form is marked by livid red erythematous lesions, often sharply demarcated, with raised borders and teleangiectasias on the vermilion border or buccal mucosa and occasionally on the tongue or palate. Lesions are often bilateral and may progress to painful ulcers. See also pp. 210, 291.

Diagnosis: See p. 210.

Differentiation is required from leukoplakia, lichen ruber planus, secondary and tertiary syphilis, erythema multiforme, lupus vulgaris, and systemic scleroderma.

Granulating Diseases of the Oropharyngeal Mucosae

Sarcoidosis (Besnier−Boeck−Schaumann syndrome)

Mucosal symptoms: Pinhead- to hazelnut-sized, prominent, blue to bluish-red granulating areas with a smooth or nodulated surface. Firm consistency. No pain. Very slow growth. The nodules are not prone to ulceration. Concomitant manifestations are common in the

Table 4.**10**   Precancerous oral lesions

Leukoplakias
– Homogeneous (simple) leukoplakia
– Verrucous leukoplakia
– Erosive (speckled, nodular) leukoplakia
– Erythroleukoplakia
Rare:
– Leukoplakia in congenital dyskeratosis
– Leukoplakia in Touraine polykeratosis
– Florid oral papillomatosis
Abrasive precancerous cheilitis, see p. 241
Bowen disease (and erythroplasia or erythroplakia)

skin, eye, salivary glands, lymph nodes, lung, liver, spleen, etc.

Causes: Unknown. A possible relationship to tuberculosis and immune pathology have been suggested.

Diagnosis:
- Typical local findings.
- Biopsy from the infiltrate.
- Intradermal Kveim test. Tuberculin sensitivity test (decreased reaction). Other options: macrophage migration inhibition test, ACE.
- Chest radiographs.
- Examination by an internist (to exclude additional foci).
- Dermatologic consultation.

Differentiation is required from lupus (negative probe sign, i.e., a probe does not penetrate to the soft granulation tissue as in lupus vulgaris), juvenile melanoma, syphilis, fungal infection, foreign body reaction, and lymphoma.

Other Granulomatous Neoplasms

Oral granulomatous neoplasms similar to those of sarcoidosis can occur in:

○ *Melkersson–Rosenthal syndrome* (see p. 153).
○ *Foreign body granuloma.*
○ *Eosinophilic granuloma* (see p. 217).
○ *Wegener granulomatosis* (see p. 192) and *midline granuloma* (see p. 192) should also

be in the differential diagnosis. Wegener granulomatosis typically originates in the nose, paranasal sinuses, or nasopharynx and involves the mouth and the rest of the pharynx secondarily, whereas *midline granuloma* can involve the oral region primarily. These granulomas are diagnosed from biopsy and clinical findings.

Manifestations of Hemorrhagic Diatheses in the Mouth and Pharynx

See Table 3.9

Precancerous Lesions of the Oral and Pharyngeal Mucosa

Leukoplakia

Not all leukoplakias are not precancers! The mucosal lesions of leukoplakia are reviewed in Table 4.**10**. It is believed that the great majority of *all* leukoplakic manifestations are benign and remain so. Nevertheless, *every* leukoplakic mucosal lesion should be scrupulously diagnosed and followed, possibly within the framework of dermatologic consultation.

Distinctions between the various forms of leukoplakia that have differential diagnostic importance are noted below:

Main symptoms: *Simple leukoplakia* (approximately 50% of cases) is a protean entity that may present as velvety or slightly nodulated, usually sharply circumscribed areas of epithelial overgrowth (hyperkeratosis), as a patchy epithelial opacity, or as a with patch of mucosa that cannot be wiped away. Sites of predilection are the buccal mucosa, oral floor, lips, tongue, and palate. Men are affected with much greater frequency than women, with a peak incidence in the 4th–7th decades. Lesions are painless and take a very indolent course (may be present from birth).

Verrucous leukoplakia (approximately 30% of cases), exhibiting an irregular, furrowed, grayish-red surface, *may* be precancerous or become so. "*Denture-rim leukoplakia*" belongs to this group.

Erosive leukoplakia (speckled leukoplakia, nodular leukoplakia) (~ 20%) features small, irregular patches of erythematous leukoplakia that present an "unsettled," nodulated surface. There is an estimated *40% incidence* of malignant transformation in this erosive form. It is closely related to Bowen disease (see below).

Causes: Multifactorial: Hereditary (constitutional) abnormalities. Endogenous irritative reactions (e.g., lichen planus mucosae, granulomatous mycoses, syphilis, lupus erythematosus, lupus vulgaris). Exogenous insults (by physical or chemical agents, e.g., actinic cheilitis, denture-associated leukoplakia, tobacco leukoplakia, etc.). Also "idiopathic."

Diagnosis:
● Typical local findings and history (often an incidental finding!).
● Biopsy (may be a complete excisional biopsy). Malignant transformation depends on the degree of epithelial dysplasia (Table 4.**11**). Leukoplakias on the border or inferior surface of the tongue and on the oral floor are thought to pose a greater cancer risk than lesions on the hard palate, cheek, or alveolar process.

Differentiation is required from ulcerative stomatitis, white spongy nevus, smoker's palate, and migratory glossitis. Also median rhomboid glossitis, AIDS, fungal infection, lichen planus, and pemphigus.

Abrasive Precancerous Cheilitis
See p. 241.

Bowen Disease

Main symptoms: Sharply marginated, deep red foci of variable size presenting either a smooth surface or leukoplakic features (see above). Very slow progression. Sites of predilection: cheek, tongue, gingiva. Years may

Table 4.**11** Terms designating grades of dysplasia (after O. Kleinsasser)

Grade I: Simple squamous hyperplasia, simple dysplasia, atypical epithelium
Grade II: Epithelial hyperplasia with isolated atypias, moderate dysplasia, atypical epithelium
Grade III: Carcinoma in situ, premalignant epithelium, severe or high-grade dysplasia; increased atypical epithelium; intraepithelial carcinoma; stage 0 carcinoma

pass before lesions undergo malignant change. Predilection for males in the 4th–7th decades.

Causes: Manifestation of carcinoma in situ with all potential associated carcinogenic factors. Closely related (if not identical) to erythroplasia or erythroplakia.

Diagnosis: Typical local findings. Long history. Biopsy.

Differentiation is required from lupus erythematosus, leukoplakia, vegetative papillomatosis, and squamous cell carcinoma.

Circumscribed Precancerous Melanosis (Lentigo Maligna)

Involvement of the oral mucosa appears as a small brown macule, which gradually turns slate-colored to bluish-black and may degenerate to malignant melanoma. See p. 150 for further details.

Benign and Malignant Neoplasms of the Oral and Pharyngeal Mucosae
See p. 267.

Symptom   **Mucosal Lesions of the Tongue**

Many of the mucosal diseases of the mouth and pharynx described in the previous section (see Table 4.**7**) can arise in the tongue or spread from their primary focus to involve the tongue. The present section focuses on mucosal lesions that affect the tongue with some frequency.

Coated Tongue (Table 4.**12**)

Table 4.**12**   Mucosal lesions of the tongue (drawn in part from Schuermann, Greither, and Hornstein)

Coated tongue	– Nonspecific oral infections (whitish coat)
	– Chronic gastrointestinal disorders, hyperacidic gastritis, gastric ulcer (whitish coat)
	– Oral thrush (candidiasis) (whitish, membrane-like plaques with red borders, difficult to wipe away)
	– Febrile diseases (whitish coat)
	– Scarlet fever (dirty white coat with marked redness of the tip and borders of the tongue)
	– Hypovitaminosis (e. g., vitamin B_2, B_6)
	– Prolonged liquid diet (white coat)
	– Smoking (grayish-white coat)
Superficial changes	– Fissured tongue (lingua plicata)
	– Geographic tongue (exfoliatio areata linguae)
	– Median rhomboid glossitis
	– Black hairy tongue
	– Various forms of glossitis
Change in the size of the tongue	– Macroglossia, see Table 4.**15**
	– Microglossia, see Table 4.**15**
Smooth gray tongue	– Vitamin A deficiency (whitish mucosal opacities)
	– Previous local radiotherapy
	– Lichen ruber planus
	– Glossitis in tertiary syphilis
	– Progressive systemic scleroderma
	– Epidermolysis hereditaria dystrophicans
Smooth red tongue	– Sjögren disease
	– Scarlet fever (strawberry tongue)
	– Median rhomboid glossitis
	– Hepatic cirrhosis (glossy, dry red tongue)
	– Pernicious anemia (Möller–Hunter glossitis)
	– Iron deficiency anemia (Plummer–Vinson syndrome)
	– Malnutrition, dystrophy (red, glossy, "mirror smooth")
	– Vascular congestion (purple, swollen tongue)
	– Hypertension (pink to crimson)
	– Allergy (strawberry or raspberry red, edema)
	– Pellagra ("checkerboard tongue") (hypovitaminosis due to deficiency of niacinamide and other B-group vitamins)
	– Right heart failure ("congestive tongue" with increased volume and venous markings)
	– Left-sided cardiac decompensation (pink–crimson–bluish)
	– Respiratory insufficiency (ashen gray–red–bluish)
	– Asthma
	– Antibiotics and other drugs, see Table 4.**8**
Neoplasms	– Benign tumors, see Table 4.**18**
	– Malignant tumors, see Table 4.**18**
	– Pseudotumors and dysgenesis, see Table 4.**18**

Superficial Lesions of the Tongue

○ *Fissured tongue (lingua plicata):* Increased furrowing of the dorsal surface of the tongue and sometimes the lateral borders, most pronounced in the anterior two-thirds of the tongue. *Differential diagnosis* includes the Melkersson–Rosenthal syndrome (granulomatous glossitis, see pp. 153, 241); syphilitic, tuberculous, and fungal infections; acromegaly; myxedema; and the Sjögren syndrome.

○ *Exfolatio areata linguae (mappy tongue, geographic tongue):* Red, map-like areas on the tongue that change patterns rapidly ("migratory glossitis") and tend to coalesce.

Table 4.**13**   Macroglossia and microglossia (drawn in part from Schuermann, Greither, and Hornstein)

Macroglossia	
Inflammatory	– Mucosal erysipelas
	– Tongue abscess
	– Wasp or bee sting
	– Contact glossitis
	– Actinomycosis
	– Granulomatous glossitis (Melkersson–Rosenthal)
	– Glossitis in tertiary syphilis (deep interstitial syphilitic glossitis)
	– Gumma
	– Candidiasis
	– Sarcoidosis
	– Leprosy
	– Rhinoscleroma
Genetic	– Marfan syndrome
	– Bruck–de Lange syndrome
	– Peters–Hövels syndrome
	– Mongolism (Down syndrome)
	– Von Pfaundler–Hurler syndrome (gargoylism)
	– Congenital macroglossia (facial hemihypertrophy, [hemi]macroprosopia)
	– Neurofibromatosis and other phakomatoses
	– Fissured tongue
	– Lingual goiter
Angiomatous	– Cavernous hemangioma
	– Lymphangioma
	– Venectasias ("caviar tongue")
Other causes	– Acromegaly
	– Myxedema
	– Lingual goiter
	– Ranula
	– Glycogen storage disease
	– Musculocutaneous amyloidosis (paramyloidosis)
	– Mucocutaneous hyalinosis (Urbach–Wiethe glycoproteinosis)
	– Acanthosis nigricans
	– Hemophilia (organized hemorrhages)
	– Right-sided heart failure
	– Benign and malignant neoplasms
Transient macroglossia	– Angioneurotic (Quincke) edema
	– Hereditary angioedema
Microglossia	– Progressive systemic scleroderma
	– Previous infarction of the tongue
	– Previous trauma or surgery

The red plaques may show conspicuous pale or yellowish outlines that are most prominent centrally. *Differential diagnosis* includes Hunter–Möller glossitis (pernicious anemia), lichen ruber, secondary syphilis, AIDS, Reiter disease, and drug rash.

○ *Median rhomboid glossitis:* Oval or rhomboid, smooth, indurated area of mucosa, devoid of papillae, surrounding the foramen cecum (developmental abnormality?). The affected area may be slightly prominent or depressed below the lingual surface. *Differential diagnosis* includes leukoplakia, early malignancy (biopsy!), and candidiasis.

○ *Black hairy tongue (lingua villosa nigra):* Dark brown to blackish coating on the median portion of the central and posterior dorsal surface of the tongue with the filiform papillae forming long, hyperkeratotic processes. Affects males almost exclusively. *Differentiation* is required from acanthosis nigricans, Darier disease, and stomatitis medicamentosa (see Table 4.**8**).

○ *Glossitis:* Inflammation of the mucosa and/ or body of the tongue. Inflammatory Conditions of the lingual mucosa are like those that involve the oral mucosa (see Table 4.**7**).

Particularly severe forms are *Hunter–Möller glossitis* in pernicious anemia (megaloblastic anemia) with burning tongue, severe redness of the mucosa, which looks smooth and slick ("like raw meat"), and later caramel-colored patches and striations; and *glossitis sicca* in Sjögren disease (see p. 303), featuring extreme dryness of the tongue, atrophy of the papillae, redness, fissuring, and rhagades. The *differential diagnosis* of glossitis sicca includes diabetic tongue, progressive systemic scleroderma, dermatomyositis, drug effects, and sialopenic syndrome (see Table 5.**7**).

Change in the Size of the Tongue

Macroglossia and microglossia, see Table 4.**13**.

Superficial Discoloration of the Tongue (Smooth Gray or Red Tongue)
See Table 4.**12**.

Benign and Malignant Neoplasms of the Tongue
See Table 4.**18**.

Symptom   Disease of the Lymphoepithelial Organs of the Waldeyer Ring

Many of the mucosal diseases occurring in the oropharyngeal region involve the lymphoepithelial structures of the Waldeyer ring. At the same time, tonsils and solitary nodules integrated into the mucosa can form a nidus for disease that later spreads to involve the oral cavity and pharynx. Because diseased tonsillar structures often present a distinctive symptomatology, it is reasonable to consider them separately in terms of differential diagnosis.

Various forms of acute inflammation of the tonsils were discussed previously in the section on Throat Pain (see p. 229). Corresponding page references are given in the Synopsis (Table 4.**14**).

Ulceromembraneous Tonsillitis (Plaut–Vincent Angina)

Main symptoms: Whitish tonsillar membrane, easily wiped away, with potentially deep ulceration of the tonsillar parenchyma, usually affecting one side. Swelling of ipsilateral cervical lymph nodes. Systemic effects are usually mild and contrast with the severity of local findings. No fever. Moderate or slight throat pain with little pain on swallowing; often there is only a foreign-body sensation in the throat. Breath is fetid. Adolescents are predominantly affected.

Other symptoms and special features: The tonsillar membrane may spread onto the palate and buccal mucosa. Concomitant *bilateral* tonsillar symptoms can occur.

Causes: Involvement of spirochetes and fusiform rods in the infection is characteristic. Infection is transmitted by droplets, contaminated eating utensils, etc.

Diagnosis: Mirror examination of the tonsils. Smear analysis confirms fusospirochetal infection.

Differentiation is required from diphtheria, infectious mononucleosis, agranulocytosis, syphilis, tuberculosis, and leukemia.

Syphilitic Tonsillitis (Secondary Syphilis)

Swelling and deep-red discoloration of the tonsils developing about 8–10 weeks after infection. Lentil-sized areas of dark red enanthema are later accompanied by papules and/or opaline plaques on the soft palate, buccal mucosa, gingiva, and tongue, sparing the hard palate. Induration of cervical lymph nodes. Positive serologic test. See p. 274 for further details.

Chronic Tonsillitis (of the Palatine Tonsils)

Main symptoms: History of frequent sore throats or nonspecific symptoms involving *mild* throat complaints ("scratchy throat"). Oral fetor is often but not invariably present. Cervical lymph nodes are frequently enlarged. Local findings: peritonsillar redness, poor "displaceability" of the tonsils; pressure with a tongue depressor extrudes a purulent fluid from the crypts. Tonsillar surface is often "fissured." Tonsillar size is *not* pathologically significant!

Causes: Chronic inflammation or microabscess formation in the tonsillar crypts or tonsillar parenchyma, especially involving group A β-hemolytic streptococci.

Diagnosis:
- Chronic tonsillitis often cannot be diagnosed from local findings alone.
- If clinical suspicion exists, the diagnosis can be supported by determining the antistreptolysin titer (values > 400 are pathologic) and examining a tonsillar smear (group A β-hemolytic streptococci support the diagnosis).

Table 4.**14** *Symptom* Disease of the lymphoepithelial organs of the Waldeyer ring

Synopsis

Inflammatory conditions

Acute tonsillitis, see p. 229

Acute lateral [sic] tonsillitis, see p. 231

Acute adenoiditis (retronasal tonsillitis), see p. 231

Infectious mononucleosis, see p. 231

Tonsillitis in:
- Agranulocytosis, see p. 232
- Syphilis, see p. 247
- Diphtheria, see p. 233
- Scarlet fever, see p. 232
- Listeriosis, see Table 4.**28**

Ulceromembranous tonsillitis

Tubercular tonsillitis, see p. 247

Fungal infection of the tonsils

Peritonsillar abscess, see p. 233

Chronic palatine tonsillitis

Other diseases

Tonsillar hyperkeratosis

Tonsillar hyperplasia in children and adolescents

Tonsillar involvement in hemopathies

Tonsillogenic complications (Fig. 4.2)
- Complication during and after tonsillitis, see p. 262
- Peritonsillar abscess, see p. 233
- Tonsillogenic sepsis
- Tonsillogenic cervical cellulitis
- Tonsillogenic cavernous sinus thrombosis
- Tonsillogenic erosive hemorrhage

Tonsilar neoplasms
○ Epithelial
  - Papilloma, see p. 243
  - Adenoma*
  - Squamous cell carcinoma, see p. 268
  - Anaplastic carcinoma, see p. 220

○ Mesenchymal*
  - Angioma
  - Fibroma
  - Lymphoma
  - Lymphosarcoma
  - Sarcomas

* No further commentary

- An elevated ESR and left shift in the white blood count are also suggestive of chronic tonsillitis.
- Accompanying symptoms may suggest a focal infection.

Differentiation is required from tonsillar hyperkeratosis and fungal infection.

Tonsillar Hyperkeratosis

Symptoms: Yellowish-white dots on the (palatine) tonsils that do not wipe away and exhibit no changes over time. No subjective complaints.

Cause: Innocuous keratinization of the tonsillar epithelium and particularly the crypt epithelium.

Tonsillar Hyperplasia (in Children and Adolescents)

Main symptoms: Marked increase in the volume of the palatine and/or pharyngeal tonsils. Mouth breathing due to nasal airway obstruction. Enlarged palatine tonsils can cause eating difficulties. Snoring, hyponasal speech. No pain. Possible predisposition to tonsillitis. Cervical lymph nodes are usually enlarged.

Other symptoms and special features: Mechanical obstruction predisposes to concomitant disease of the ears, nose, paranasal sinuses, masticatory apparatus, and lower airways. Full-blown obstructive sleep apnea syndrome may be present (see Tables 3.**11** and 3.**12**).

Causes: Excessive reactive proliferation of immunocompetent lymphoepithelial tissue.

Diagnosis: Typical local findings in the oropharynx or nasopharynx.

Differentiation is required from choanal atresia, intranasal foreign bodies, nasopharyngeal fibroma, choanal polyp, and nasopharyngeal or oropharyngeal malignancies.

Tonsillar Involvement in Hemopathies

This ist most commonly seen in *agranulocytosis*, *panmyelophthisis*, *acute* and *chronic leukemia*, and *megaloblastosis*.

Symptoms of Tonsillogenic Complications

Complications During and After Tonsillitis
See below.

Peritonsillar Abscess
See p. 233.

Tonsillogenic Septis (via Thrombophlebitis of the Internal Jugular Vein)

Main symptoms: Chills, septic fever. Tenderness along the internal jugular vein at the anterior border of the sternocleidomastoid muscle. Tendeness and swelling of the lymph nodes. Cervical lymphadenopathy. Possible redness and swelling of the tonsillar area. ESR greatly increased, blood count consistent with inflammation. Severe systemic illness. With progression of disease, splenomegaly ensues and metastatic abscesses may form in the lung, skin, liver, or brain. A "masked" course is also possible (due to antibiotic masking).

Causes: Bacterial seeding into the bloodstream from a primary tonsillar focus (Fig. 4.**2a,b**).

Diagnosis:
- Frequently a prior history of tonsillitis (with or without an asymptomatic interval).
- Mirror examination of the offending tonsil does not always show clear evidence of disease! But adjacent tissues are usually tender, and tenderness is noted along the internal jugular vein (protective muscular defense) and in the ipsilateral cervical nodes.
- Hematologic findings and other laboratory values that are consistent with sepsis.
- Causative organism can be isolated from blood drawn while chills are present. Temperature should be taken at 3-h intervals.

Differentiation is required from sepsis due to other causes.

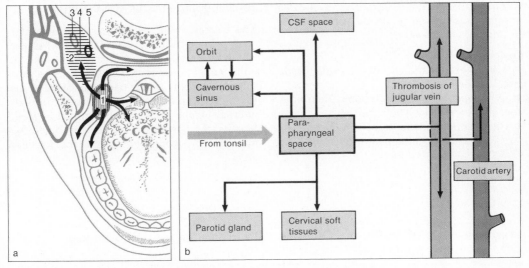

Fig. 4.**2 a,b** Tonsillogenic complications (from Becker, Naumann, Pfaltz)

a Spread from the tonsil to adjacent tissues
  1 Palatine tonsil
  2 Parapharyngeal space
  3 Internal jugular vein

  4 Vagus nerve
  5 Internal carotid artery
b Other routes for spread of tonsillogenic infection

Tonsillogenic Cervical Cellulitis (Malignant Angina)

Main symptoms: Rapidly progressive swelling of the peritonsillar tissue, usually during or after a bout of tonsillitis, spreading to the soft tissues of the lateral pharynx and invading the deep fascial compartments of the neck (parapharyngeal space, see Fig. 4.2). Bull neck. The affected side of the neck is extremely tender, and the head is held in a guarded position. Dysphagia, possibly accompanied by progressive dyspnea. Mediastinal involvement may occur (see p. 386). Rapid spread and rapid physical debilitation with persistent high fever and even septic temperatures once the organisms have entered the circulation.

Causes: Deficient host resistance to the spread of a tonsillar infection, and/or high virulence of the infecting organisms. "*Descending*" inflammation.

Diagnosis:
● Mirror examination shows a tonsillitis.

● Localization of the abscess by CT or MR imaging of the cervical soft tissues.
● Hematologic and other laboratory findings indicate a highly acute, severe inflammatory process.
● Identification of the causative organism in smears (or aspirate) and antibiotic sensitivity testing.

Differentiation is required from cellulitic processes due to other causes (e.g., dentogenic, tongue base, foreign body, traumatic perforation, etc.).

Tonsillogenic Cavernous Sinus Thrombosis

Main Symptoms: Development of symptoms typical of cavernous sinus thrombosis during or after a bout of tonsilitis: ipsilateral proptosis, chemosis, edema of the upper and lower eyelids, decreased ocular mobility, septic temperatures (see p. 214 for further details).

Causes: Inflammation "ascending" to the cavernous sinus via the pterygoid venous plexus or internal jugular vein.

Diagnosis:
● Mirror examination shows a florid or decreasing tonsillitis.
● Ophthalmologic consultation. Neurologic consultation may also be required.
● Blood count and laboratory findings consistent with an acute inflammatory process.

Tonsillogenic Erosive Hemorrhage

This usually occurs as an *arterial* hemorrhage from a branch of the external carotid artery (often the ascending pharyngeal artery) due to inflammatory erosion caused by a tonsillogenic cellulitic process in the parapharyngeal space (Fig. 4.**2**). Rarely the internal carotid artery or internal jugular vein may be eroded as well. Massive hemorrhage is often preceded by multiple "prodromal bleeds" in the tonsillar area.

Symptom   **Inflammatory Disease with Predominantly Pharyngeal Symptoms**

Many of the mucosal diseases discussed in the section on the oral cavity can also be manifested in the pharynx, the site of involvement determining whether the symptoms are predominantly oral, predominantly pharyngeal, or mixed. The principal disorders in which *pharyngeal* symptoms tend to overshadow other signs are listed in Table 4.**15**.

Acute Pharyngitis
See p. 234.

Chronic Pharyngitis

Main symptoms: Three forms are recognized, all with a peak incidence after 40 years of age:

a) *Simple chronic pharyngitis.* Local findings: The posterior pharyngeal wall may show varying degrees of inflammatory irritation or may appear normal. Habitual throat clearing, chronic phlegm congestion, proneness to infections. Full or subdued coughing. Viscous, usually colorless secretions. Globus sensation in the throat. Symptoms are variable, but there is no fever and no significant malaise.

b) *Chronic granular (hyperplastic) pharyngitis.* Local findings: The posterior pharyngeal mucosa is thickened and coarsened, pink to grayish-red in color, and presents a "granu-lating" surface studded with prominent granules or lymph follicles. There is excessive production of a very viscous, usually colorless secretion. Chronic, very troublesome phlegm congestion. Frequent throat clearing, swallowing, and coughing with possible gagging or nausea. A continuum exists from (a) to (b).

c) *Chronic pharyngitis sicca (chronic atrophic pharyngitis).* Pharyngeal mucosa is dry and glossy and may be coated with tough, glue-like, yellow-gray or yellow-brown crusted secretions. The mucosa may be pink and delicate or red and thickened. Marked general discomfort is produced by a foreign-body sensation in the pharynx, habitual throat clearing, and occasional mild pain. Crusting and dryness may cause sleep disturbance and a suffocating sensation at night. Other mucosal areas (nasal, laryngeal, etc.) often exhibit similar symptoms.

Causes: Weakened host defenses, acquired or constitutionally determined, and chronic mucosal infection with a gradual alteration of tissue structure by very diverse exogenous and/or endogenous factors (Table 4.**16**).

Diagnosis:
● Typical local findings; intermittent course, usually lasting for years.
● Bacteriologic and mycologic smears. Search and identify causative factors (Table 4.**16**).

Table 4.**15** *Symptom* Inflammatory disease in which pharyngeal symptoms predominate

Synopsis
Acute pharyngitis, see p. 234
Pharyngitis secondary to trauma (e. g., indwelling tube, foreign body, decubital necrosis)

Chronic pharyngitis
  – Simple
  – Granular
  – Sicca

Ulceromembranous pharyngitis, see pp. 264, 260
Diphtheric pharyngitis, see p. 233
Retropharyngeal abscess in small children
Retropharyngeal abscess in adults
Hypopharyngeal abscess

Associated symptoms
  – With pharyngoesophageal (Zenker) diverticulum, see p. 279
  – With reflux disease, see p. 374
  – With other esophageal diseases, see Table 8.**2**
  – With gastric diseases*

Pharyngoesophagitis (Plummer–Vinson)
Specific pharyngeal diseases (tuberculosis, syphilis, leprosy), see p. 247 ff.
Sarcoidosis of the pharynx, see p. 255
Candidiasis (moniliasis, thrush) of the pharynx, see p. 249
Tularemia of the pharynx, see p. 248 and Table 4.**28**
Pharyngeal bursitis (Tornwaldt)
Other nasopharyngeal diseases, see Table 3.**11**
Tonsillar diseases, see Table 4.**14**

* No further commentary

Table 4.**16**   Causes of chronic pharyngitis (selection)

Congenital or acquired functional weakness of the mucosa
Sjögren disease (sicca syndrome), see Table 5.**7** and p. 303
Specific and nonspecific infections, see Table 4.**15**
Compulsory mouth breathing (nasal airway obstruction), see Table 3.**12**

Chronic inflammatory conditions of adjacent organs
  – Rhinosinusitis
  – Tonsillitis
  – Hypopharyngeal diverticulum
  – Esophagitis
  – Laryngotracheitis

Exogenous injury caused by
  – Alcohol
  – Smoking (active and passive)
  – Physical injury, e. g., due to a hot or dusty work environment
    – Improperly climatized working and living spaces
    – Pronounced, frequent changes in temperature and humidity
  – Chemical injury, see Table 4.**9**
  – Toxic, allergic, or pseudoallergic drug effects, see Table 4.**8**
  – Mucosal allergy to inhalation or food allergens, see Table 3.**16**

Radiation mucositis
Faulty vocal and breathing techniques

Vitamin deficiency states
  – Vitamin A
  – B group vitamins
  – Vitamin C

Endocrine causes
  – Menopause
  – Hypothyroidism
  – Diabetes mellitus

Internal underlying diseases
  – Bronchopulmonary disease
  – Cardiovascular disease
  – Renal disease
  – Gastrointestinal disease
  – Intoxication

Differentiation is required from the Sjögren syndrome, the Plummer–Vinson syndrome, rhinosinusitis, chronic tonsillitis, specific pharyngitis (tuberculosis, syphilis, HIV), immunodeficiency diseases (electrophoresis), pharyngeal bursitis, spondylosis deformans, and psychoneurosis.

Retropharyngeal Abscess in Small Children

Main symptoms: Most common in children under 2 years of age. Balloon-like swelling and redness of the posterior pharyngeal wall, which is soft or fluctuant on palpation. Muffled speech, pain, dysphagia, and eating difficulties (with nasal regurgitation of food).

Other symptoms and special features: Fever. Guarded head position. Occasional nasal airway obstruction. Frequent croup-like cough. Risk of asphyxiation from accompanying laryngeal edema.

Causes: Acute lymphadenitis with liquefaction of the retropharyngeal lymph nodes.

Diagnosis:
• Endoscopy shows a bulging posterior pharyngeal wall, which has a water-cushion consistency on palpation.
• Differential blood count (acute inflammation) and ESR (increased).
• Puncture (with head dependent due to risk of aspiration). Smear from abscess pus with sensitivity testing.
• Lateral head and neck radiograph (demonstrating the cervical vertebrae and adjacent soft tissues).

Differentiation is required from torticollis and from benign and malignant prevertebral tumors.

Retropharyngeal Abscess in Adults

Main symptoms: Chronic course. Globus or pressure sensation in the throat, dysphagia, dry cough. Endoscopy reveals diffuse bulging of the posterior pharyngeal wall, which often shows *no* significant redness. Guarded head carriage but little or no pain.

Causes: Usually a prevertebral "cold" gravitation abscess originating from tuberculous caries of a cervical vertebra or an osteitic abscess gravitating to the pharynx from a focus of petrositis, mastoiditis, or malignant otitis externa.

Diagnosis:
• Endoscopic findings.
• Radiographic views of the cervical spine and skull base including tomograms and/or CT scans. Chest films also may be helpful.
• Needle aspiration, bacteriologic smear.

Differentiation is required from spondylosis deformans (palpable findings, radiographs of cervical spine), benign and malignant prevertebral tumors, retrovisceral goiter, and cervical lymphoma. Needle aspiration or biopsy.

Hypopharyngeal Abscess

Main symptoms: Lower and more laterally situated than retropharyngeal abscess, usually produces more severe symptoms (odynophagia and dysphagia). The lateral wall of the hypopharynx is protuberant, the piriform sinus effaced. There is unilateral edema of the laryngeal inlet, with or without involvement of the epiglottis. Generally speech is preserved despite the edematous laryngeal inlet.

Causes: Foreign body injuries are most common in older patients. Can also result from iatrogenic trauma (e.g., misdirected intubation or endoscopy).

Diagnosis:
• The occult location of the lesion makes diagnosis difficult. Indirect laryngoscopy is not sufficient.
• *Rigid*, "classic" endoscopy is most informative.
• Plain or contrast-enhanced tomography. MRI.

Differentiation is required from laryngeal perichondritis, abscess of the tongue base, collateral edema from a peritonsillar abscess, foreign bodies, and hypopharyngeal malignancy.

Pharyngoesophagitis (Plummer—Vinson Disease, Paterson—Brown—Kelly Disease, Chronic Hypopharyngitis, etc.)

Main symptoms: Affects women almost exclusively. Patients experience moderate to severe dysphagia and may be able to swallow only small bites. Burning tongue. Mucosal surfaces of the tongue and pharynx appear atrophic and dry on indirect inspection. Angular rhagades.

Other symptoms and special features: Most common in persons over 40 years of age. Characteristic features include pale, shriveled, dry skin, koilonychia (spoon nails), and dry, shaggy hair. Occasional precursor of esophageal carcinoma!

Causes: Iron deficiency is probably the underlying cause ("sideropenic dysphagia").

Diagnosis:
• Typical mirror findings with dry, atrophic

mucosa and typical general impression. Fingernails (see above).

● Blood count shows hypochronic anemia with anisocytosis and microcytosis. Extremely low serum iron levels (normal values: $50-150$ µg/100 mL or $9-27$ mol/L).

● Contrast radiographs show spasm of the upper esophageal sphincter with an indentation at the level of the cricoid cartilage and may show a mucosal web at the level of the esophageal inlet.

● *Rigid* esophagoscopy.

Differentiation is required from postcricoid carcinoma, hypopharyngeal carcinoma, cicatricial stricture due to corrosive injury, and functional dysphagia (see Tables 4.**25** and 8.**8**).

Hypopharyngeal Diverticulum (Zenker Diverticulum, Pharyngoesophageal Diverticulum)

This is not a primary inflammatory disease in itself but may incite pharyngitic symptoms. Details on p. 279.

Pharyngeal Bursitis (Tornwaldt Disease)

Main symptoms: Foul-smelling discharge from the nasopharynx, which the patient perceives as a bad taste in the mouth, especially in the morning. Mirror examination and/or endoscopy shows redness and a slight circumscribed bulging of the posterior wall of the nasopharynx. Secondary inflammatory signs may be noted in the upper pharynx, with associated symptoms of chronic pharyngitis. A *rare* disease.

Causes: Attributed to persistence of the central groove of the adenoid with the formation of a pouch, or to an anatomic malformation.

Diagnosis: Postrhinoscopic and endoscopic examination (with velotraction and perhaps general anesthesia). A viscous, yellow-brown, malodorous fluid can be extruded from the pouch. Cyst formation is occasionally observed.

Differentiation is required from chronic sinusitis (especially of the posterior paranasal sinuses) and nasopharyngeal malignancy.

Symptom   **Morphologic Change in the Oropharyngeal Region (Swelling, Tumor)**

Morphologic changes in the mouth and pharynx usually lead rapidly to *functional disturbances* (of eating, mastication, respiration, speech), which can then determine the initial cardinal symptoms. Soft-tissue swellings of inflammatory origin are not always readily distinguishable from neoplasms, especially since inflammation and neoplasia may coexist. The history and associated symptoms usually provide important clues for differential diagnosis, but the definitive diagnosis is established by *biopsy*. The principal swellings and neoplasias affecting the mouth and pharynx are listed in Table 4.**17** along with page references to brief commentaries. This synopsis is intended purely as a guideline to facilitate differential diagnosis.

Malignant tumors of the oropharyngeal region are relatively common compared with benign neoplasms, and their incidence is rising (smokers, alcoholics). Because many of the malignant tumors listed in Table 4.**18** show marked clinical differences from one another and from malignancies at other sites, their symptomatology is briefly discussed below as it relates to the mouth and pharynx.

Carcinoma

Carcinoma of the Oral Floor

Main symptoms: The lesion ulcerates early, presenting raised borders around a surface that bleeds easily. Usually there is rapid super-

Table 4.**17** *Symptom* Morphologic change (swelling, tumor) in the mouth and pharynx

Synopsis
Swelling
Specific and nonspecific inflammatory conditions
– of the lips, see p. 238ff.
– of the oral cavity, see p. 229ff.
– of the nasopharynx, see Table 3.**11**
– of the oropharynx and hypopharynx, see pp. 260, 264, 267
Edema formation, see pp. 143, 153
Granulomas and granulomatoses, see pp. 192, 217
Hyperplasias, see pp. 253, 262
Cysts and celes, see pp. 142, 180
Tumors
See also Table 4.**18**
Benign tumors
– of the lips, see Tables 2.**5**, 4.**4**
– of the mouth, see Table 4.**7**
– of the nasopharynx, see Table 3.**22**
– of the oropharynx, see Table 4.**18**
– of the hypopharynx, see Table 4.**18**
Malignant tumors
– Epithelial malignancies
– of the lips, see Tables 2.**5**, 4.**4**
– of the mouth and oropharynx, see Table 4.**7**
– Second tumors, see p. 249
– of the nasopharynx, see p. 181 and Table 3.**22**
– of the hypopharynx, see p. 270
– Mesenchymal malignancies, see Table 4.**18**
– Malignant melanoma, see pp. 150, 270
"Pseudo"tumors, see Table 4.**18**
Ectopic tissue
– Lingual goiter of the tongue base, see p. 410

ficial growth and deep infiltration with involvement of adjacent bone. Early lesions cause little or no pain, but involvement of sensory nerves or periosteum usually causes constant, severe pain (accompanying inflammation). Most oral carcinomas occur in the gutter between the alveolar ridge and the lateral border of the tongue (75%), often near the sublingual caruncle. The breath is fetid. Usually the tumor is easily detected by mirror examination. The base of the lesion feels indu-

rated on palpation. Any ulcer that does not heal promptly and any hyperkeratotic or leukoplakic area is guggestive of an early malignancy!

Other symptoms and special features: Males predominate by 9:1. Lesions manifest most commonly in the 6th–7th decades, but younger age groups are increasingly affected. Regional lymph node involvement occurs relatively early and is often bilateral! As tumor growth progresses, pain increases and may radiate to the ear and neck. There is gradual impairment of eating and speech and increasing physical debilitation.

Carcinoma of the Tongue

Main symptoms: Most cancers of the tongue involve the anterior portion, showing a predilection for the lateral surfaces and middle third. The base of the tongue is less commonly involved. Lesions of the *lateral tongue* produce marked induration of the tongue in the area of tumor growth with associated impediment of eating and speech. Increasing pain often radiates to the ear. The breath is fetid, and salivation may be increased. Mirror examination shows circumscribed thickening of the tongue, usually with heaped-up ulcer margins and rarely with a slightly indrawn center. There is early, potentially bilateral metastasis to regional lymph nodes, often accompanied by hematogenous spread (to lung, bone, and liver). Lesions of the *tongue base* cause early pain that is often restricted to one side initially. There is early onset of muffled speech and early eating difficulties leading to weight loss and physical debilitation. Again, there is early metastasis to regional nodes. Primary or secondary involvement of at least *one* palatine tonsil is common!

Carcinoma of the Tonsil

Main symptoms: Similar to carcinoma of the tongue base, but generally more pronounced on one side. May involve *both* tonsils, however, especially if the carcinoma has spread from the tongue base. Mirror examination generally shows a size discrepancy between the healthy and cancerous tonsils. Marked induration is noted on palpation of the involved tonsil, which may already be fixed to underlying tis-

Table 4.**18**   Common tumors of the mouth and pharynx (excluding the salivary glands and lips) (selection)

Benign	Malignant
Papilloma	Squamous cell carcinoma
Adenoma	Anaplastic carcinoma (lymphoepithelial tumor,
Pleomorphic adenoma	Schmincke tumor)
Keratoacanthoma	Adenoid cystic carcinoma
Fibroma	Adenocarcinoma
Lipoma	Mucoepidermoid tumors
Histiocytoma	Various sarcomas
Leiomyoma and rhabdomyoma	Malignant lymphoma, see p. 408
Myxoma	Melanoma, see pp. 150, 270
Hemangioma and lymphangioma	Plasmocytoma (extramedullary), see p. 218
Neuroma (neurilemmoma, schwannoma)	Malignant chordoma, see p. 219
Neurofibroma	Ewing sarcoma, see Table 3.**22**
Granular cell tumor	
Chondroma	**Precancerous lesions,** see Table 4.**10**
Osteoma	
Giant cell tumor (osteoclastoma) (approximately	**Tonsillar tumors,** see p. 268
10% malignant)	
Myoblastic myoma (Abrikossoff tumor)	**"Pseudotumors"**
Tumors arising from jaw bone:	Fibrous dysplasia, see p. 141
– Osteoma	Ossifying fibroma, see p. 142
– Osteoblastoma	Cysts:
– Chondroma	– Dermoid cyst and epidermoid
– Chondroblastoma	– Dentogenic cyst, see p. 142
– Osteochondroma	– Tornwaldt cyst, see p. 267
– Myxoma	– Salivary gland cyst, see p. 302
	Hamartoma
Dentogenic tumors:	Lingual goiter (heterotopia)
– Adamantinoma (5% malignant)	Foreign-body granuloma
– Ameloblastoma	Plasma-cell granuloma
– Odontoma	Pyogenic granuloma
– Dentinoma	Epulis
– Odontogenic fibroma	Giant-cell granuloma
– Cementoma, etc.	Brown tumor (hyperparathyroidism)
	Xanthogranuloma
Occurring only in the nasopharynx:	Gouty tophi
	Sarcoidosis
Craniopharyngioma (Erdheim tumor)	Wegener granulomatosis
Juvenile nasopharyngeal fibroma (angiofibroma)	Midline granuloma
Lymphoepithelioma	Exostosis
	Torus palatinus
	Paget disease

sues. Early involvement of regional lymph nodes. Distant metastasis is not uncommon (lung, skeleton, liver).

Anaplastic Carcinoma (Schmincke Tumor)

See p. 220.

Second Tumors (Multiple Tumors)

Neoplasms that follow upon a tumor in the *oral cavity* but are *not* recurrent, residual, or metastatic to the original tumor are relatively common (incidence 8–12%). Sites of predilection are the hypopharynx and larynx. The average interval to manifestation of the second tumor is 4–5 years.

Carcinoma of the Nasopharynx

See p. 220.

Carcinoma of the Hypopharynx

Main symptoms: Dysphagia, pain (sometimes radiating to the ear). Early ulceration of the mucosa. Not infrequently, the *initial warning sign and cardinal symptom* of hypopharyngeal carcinoma is enlargement and induration of the lymph nodes below the mandibular angle and below the sternocleidomastoid muscle (often bilateral!). Respiration is unaffected initially, but increasing mechanical airway obstruction develops in advanced cases. Sites of predilection (in descending order of frequency) are the piriform sinus (lateral wall), postcricoid region, and posterior pharyngeal wall. Rigid endoscopy is generally required for visual identification, especially in early stages. A second carcinoma (e.g., of the esophagus) is not uncommon.

Aspects Common to Carcinomas of the Oral Floor, Tongue, Tonsil, Nasopharynx, and Hypopharynx

Causes: As with all carcinomas, the causes remain largely speculative. Smoking, alcohol abuse, and certain textiles and tar products have been statistically established as carcinogens for the oropharyngeal region. The tumors may develop from precancerous lesions (see p. 256) or may arise without discernible cause.

Diagnosis:
- Mirror and palpable findings, depending on tumor site (includes bilateral examination of regional lymph nodes!).
- Lesions not accessible to mirror examination or palpation (tongue base, nasopharynx, hypopharynx) can be visualized with a magnifying endoscope and/or hypopharyngoscope (use a *rigid*, large-caliber endoscope for this region!).
- Tumor extent can be defined with imaging techniques such as contrast radiography, tomography, or preferably CT and MRI. B-mode sonographic imaging can also be of value.

Differentiation is required from tertiary syphilis, tuberculosis, ulceromembranous stomatitis, agranulocytosis, sarcoma, malignant lymphoma (especially with tonsillar involvement), and metastases from extraoral tumors (e.g., hypernephroma, breast carcinoma, gastric carcinoma, melanoma).

Sarcoma and Malignant Lymphoma

Connective-tissue tumors, unlike carcinomas, are rare in the oropharyngeal region. The most common are *spindle-cell sarcomas, myxosarcomas, plasmocytomas, malignant giant-cell tumors, rhabdomyosarcomas, Kaposi sarcomas, hemangioendotheliomas,* and *malignant lymphomas* (see p. 408). These mesenchymal neoplasms have far less tendency than carcinomas to undergo ulceration, so an intact mucosal lining combined with suspect tissue proliferation is more likely to signify a sarcomatous tumor or possibly a distant metastasis of carcinoma.

Diagnosis: See above.

Melanoma

Melanomas occur rarely in the oropharyngeal region (accounting for less than 1% of all melanomas and about one-third of melanoblastomas of the upper aerodigestive tract). Most occur in the maxillary region, followed by the hard and soft palate, alveolar ridge, cheek, and lip (in declining order of frequency). These mucosal melanomas differ from skin melanomas (see p. 150) in that they usually start as a flat macule with an intact mucosal covering whose melanin content is highly variable, usually ranging from a pale grayish-brown to reddish-gray color. Metastatis is rapid!

Symptom   **Malformation Involving the Mouth or Pharynx**

Table 4.**19**   *Symptom*   Malformation of the mouth or pharynx

Synopsis

Mouth

Cleft anomalies (dysraphias)

- (Lateral) cleft of the upper lip (cheiloschisis, harelip)
- (Lateral) cleft of the alveolus (gnathoschisis)
- (Lateral) palatal cleft (palatoschisis, uranoschisis)
- Combinations of the above clefts (see Fig. 4.**3**)
- Bilateral clefts
- Median cleft of the upper lip (usually as part of a linguofacial dysplasia)
- Bifid uvula
- Oblique facial cleft (meloschisis)
- Transverse facial or malar cleft

Paramedian (lateral) or commissural (angular) *lower lip fistula,* a relatively common dysraphia of the embryonic *mandible*

Hypo- and hyperplasias of the lips, tongue, maxilla, and mandible

Heterotopias

- Lingual goiter, see p. 410
- Cheilitis glandularis, see p. 241
- Fordyce disease (heterotopic sebaceous glands)*
- Dermoid cyst, see p. 241

Other anomalies

- Palatolingual atresia*
- Ankyloglossia (shortening of the frenulum)* Fissured tongue, see p. 258 Median rhomboid glossitis, see p. 260
- Epithelial pearls and/or fistulae in the palatal region*
- Cysts (nasopalatal, oronasal, nasoalveolar) (fissural embryonic remnants)*
- Pigmentary anomalies (e.g., melanosis of oral mucosa)*
- Lateral and midline cervical cysts, see p. 402 ff.

Pharynx

- Choanal atresia, see. p. 206
- Persistent craniopharyngeal canal
- Nasopharyngeal meningoencephalocele, see p. 139
- Pharyngeal bursa (Tornwaldt disease), see p. 267
- Nasopharyngeal cysts
- Teratoma, see p. 218
- Dermoid cysts, see p. 241 and Table 3.**23**
- Branchiogenic anomalies, see p. 402

- Anomalies of the thyroglossal duct, see p. 403
- Ectopic thyroid, parathyroid, and/or thymic tissue in the oropharynx or hypopharynx (e. g., lingual goiter)

Multiple anomalies, see Table 4.**26**

See also Table 3.**23** (facial anomalies) and Table 3.**24** (respiratory and swallowing difficulties due to dysontogenic causes)

* No further commentary

Most of these morphologic abnormalities and associated functional disturbances are easy to recognize, but it can be difficult to assign them to a particular class of anomalies or a specific syndrome, especially since many of these oropharyngeal malformations are rare. The more common anomalies of this group are reviewed in Table 4.**19**. It is relatively common, moreover, for these anomalies to coexist with malformations in other body regions (see Tables 2.**13** and 4.**26**).

Clefts

A fully developed *(lateral) cleft* of the maxillary anlage in all its variations presents few problems of differential diagnosis (Fig. 4.**3a–f**). It should be emphasized, however, that maxillary clefts:

○ Generally imply severe functional disturbances involving the ear, nose, and paranasal sinuses

○ Cause varying degrees of speech and eating

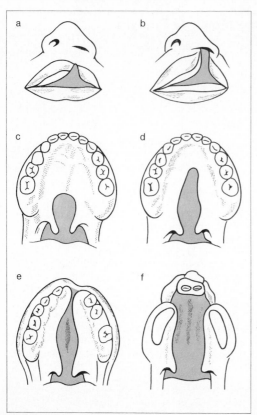

◁ Fig. 4.**3a–f**   Typical cleft anomalies

a   Unilateral cleft lip
b   Unilateral cleft lip and alveolus
c   Partial cleft palate
d   Complete cleft palate
e   Cleft (lip), alveolus, and palate
f   Bilateral cleft lip, alveolus, and palate

impairment and thus require surgical correction at the earliest opportunity
○ Frequently coexist with other anomalies
○ Of the *submucous* type are easily missed and simulate an intact palate, but can still cause the functional deficits noted above.

With submucous clefts, the bony palatal shelf is not closed. This can be recognized by palpating the hard palate or by CT imaging.

These facts should always be carefully considered in the otorhinolaryngologic differential diagnosis of a suspected maxillary dysraphia!

Symptom   **Oral Fetor**

Oral fetor ("bad breath") is a symptom that, while produced by many diverse causes, is often not perceived by the patient. The principal causes are listed in Table 4.**20**. There are also cases in which the patient fears having bad breath in the absence of demonstrable fetor. This phobia can so handicap interpersonal contacts that psychiatric consultation is advised.

Table 4.**20** *Symptom* Oral fetor (causes)

Synopsis			
Site of origin	Disease	Site of origin	Disease
Oral cavity	Stomatitis	Respiratory tract (upper section)	Ozena
	Abscess of tongue and oral floor		(Chronic) sinusitis
	Ulcerated tumor		Dentogenic sinusitis
	Pemphigus		Choanal atresia
	Behçet disease, see p. 253		Tornwaldt disease
	Erythema multiforme	(Halitosis)	Purulent bronchitis
	Other erosive mucosal diseases		Bronchiectasis
	Gingivitis		Tracheal and bronchial foreign bodies
	Dental caries		Pneumonia
	Pyorrhea		Lung abscess
	Periodontal disease		Pulmonary gangrene
	Neglected dentures		Ulcerating or degenerating tumors of the respiratory system
Oropharynx	Prolonged fasting		
	Acute tonsillitis	Digestive tract	Hypopharyngeal or esophageal diverticulum
	Ulceromembranous tonsilitis (Plaut–Vincent angina)		Hiatal hernia
	Infectious mononucleosis		Esophagitis
	Pharyngeal and tonsillar diphtheria		Diseases of the stomach and duodenum
	Chronic tonsillitis		Ulcerating or degenerating tumors of the pharynx, esophagus, or stomach
	Tonsillar plugs		
	Pharyngitis		
	Xerostomia	Other causes	Diabetes mellitus
	Foreign body		Comatose and precomatose states (diabetes, liver, kidney)
	Peritonsillar abscess		
	Retropharyngeal abscess		Vitamin B$_1$ preparations
	Tertiary syphilis		Arsenic, phosphorus, sodium tellurate, dimethyl sulfoxide

---

Symptom   **Blood in the Sputum**

Various terms are applied to the expectoration of blood from the mouth:

1. *Hemoptysis,* in which the varying amounts of blood are present in the sputum, and the bleeding site is generally located in the respiratory tract. With severe grades of hemoptysis, the oral discharge consists largely or entirely of blood.

2. *Hematemesis,* usually characterized by massive bleeding from the mouth originating from a site in the lower digestive tract.

3. The above conditions are distinguished from *"ENT hemorrhage,"* which also can be life-threatening depending on the source of the bleeding.

Table 4.**21**   *Symptom*   Blood in the sputum (causes)

Synopsis

"ENT hemorrhage"

Foreign-body hemorrhage in the oropharyngeal region

Variceal bleeding from the tongue

Postoperative hemorrhage

Trauma

Fracture of the cranium, skull base, larynx, or trachea, see pp. 37, 135ff., 177, 316ff., 363

Rendu–Osler disease, see p. 198

Bleeding hemangioma

Hemorrhagic diathesis, see p. 195 and Tables 3.**8**, 3.**9**, and 3.**10**

Gingival bleeding

Epistaxis discharging through the nasopharynx

Erosive hemorrhage due to ENT malignancies

Erosive hemorrhage due to abscess, cellulitis, or chronic inflammatory infiltration and necrosis

Bleeding tendency in influenza and other infectious diseases

Acute pharyngitis

Acute tracheitis

Intubation trauma

Vigorous retching and vomiting

Bleeding hypopharyngeal diverticulum

Pharmacologic causes (anticoagulants, cyto-statics, etc.)

"True hemoptysis" (bleeding from the respiratory tract)

Acute or chronic bronchitis

Pulmonary infarction

Pneumonia

Bronchiectasis

Aspirated foreign body

Trauma

Fungal infection (aspergillus mycetoma)

Parasitic infection (echinococci, ascarids, hydatid cyst)

Pulmonary abscess

Pulmonary embolism

Pulmonary edema

Congested lung

Bronchopulmonary tumor (e. g., bronchial adenoma, bronchial carcinoma, carcinoid)

Pulmonary endometriosis

Pulmonary tuberculosis

Wegener granulomatosis

Mitral stenosis

Left heart failure

Ruptured aortic aneurysm

Thoracic trauma

Bronchial rupture

Unusually severe cough

Pneumoconiosis, sarcoidosis, honeycomb lung

Hemorrhagic diathesis

Anticoagulant therapy

Hematemesis

Esophageal varices

Esophageal malignancy

Trauma, foreign body, corrosion

Esophagitis

Bleeding esophageal diverticulum

Duodenal ulcer

Erosive gastritis

Gastric peptic ulcer

Gastric carcinoma

Anastomotic ulcers (postresection)

Whenever blood is found in the sputum (aside from gingival bleeding), the patient should be assumed to have a potentially life-threatening condition. The following special features are useful for *gross differentiation:*

a) ENT hemorrhage, especially when massive (e.g., erosive hemorrhage caused by neoplastic or inflammatory erosion of a carotid artery branch [tonsillogenic erosive hemorrhage]), is manifested by profuse, bright red blood or by a large volume of dark red blood due, for example, to inflammatory or neoplastic venous damage and erosion. Smaller oozing hemorrhages and paroxysmal bleeding can result from venous stasis and venous rupture. An important differen-

Table 4.**22**   Procedure for the otorhinolaryngologic differential diagnosis of blood in the sputum

With an acute, severe hemorrhage:	*With slight or intermittent hemorrhage:*

Gross differentiation:
– ENT hemorrhage
– Hemoptysis
– Hematemesis, see p. 385
 	
If possible, make a (presumptive) diagnosis as to:
– The urgency of the condition
– The cause of the bleeding
– The location of the bleeding source
 	
Immediate institution of appropriate emergency treatment by a competent specialty
	1. ENT evaluation:
	  – Detailed history, including parallel diseases, current medications, etc.
	  – Examination of the blood-tinged sputum
	  – Mirror examination of the nose, mouth, pharynx, and larynx
	  – Blood pressure, blood status, ESR
	  – Endoscopy including bronchoscopy and esophagoscopy
	  – Chest radiographs and any special views that are required
	
	2. If all findings are negative, refer for internal medical evaluation and/or surgical evaluation of the chest and abdomen

tiating sign: In contrast to hemoptysis from the lower respiratory tract, *ENT hemorrhage generally does not begin with an initial cough* but with the ejection of blood-tinged sputum and a stale taste of blood in the mouth. Coughing occurs only after blood has been secondarily aspirated into the larynx and trachea.

b) An ENT hemorrhage usually does *not* produce prodromal signs. By contrast, hemoptysis from the lung commonly produces *prodromes* such as a sensation of retrosternal warmth or pressure, a trickling sensation in the chest, and possibly chest pain and severe cough followed by the expectoration of a predominantly bright red, often foamy sputum.

c) *Hemoptysis* in persons under age 40 frequently originates from bronchiectasis or open pulmonary tuberculosis, while significant hemoptysis in older patients is more apt to signify chronic bronchitis or bronchial carcinoma. Small recurrent hemorrhages suggest a tumor, while hemoptysis with copious bright red blood is suggestive of tuberculosis or aspergilloma. A fetid odor suggests a lung abscess.

d) In *hematemesis*, blood is *vomited* with a typical *emetic reflex*. The vomited blood is usually dark red to black, clotted ("coffee grounds"), often has an acidic smell, and is mixed with food residues. Generally there is a history of gastric or hepatic disease.

The more common causes of blood in the sputum are reviewed in Table 4.**21**, and the steps that are important for otorhinolaryngologic differential diagnosis are listed in Table 4.**22**.

Symptom   **Disturbance of Salivation**

See p. 309 and Tables 5.**6** and 5.**7**.

Symptom   **Paralysis Involving the Mouth and/or Pharynx (Sensory, Motor)**

Table 4.**23** *Symptom* Disturbance of the motor and/ or sensory innervation of the mouth and pharynx (common causes)

Synopsis
Peripheral
Interruption (trauma, destruction, etc.) of cranial nerves V, VII, IX, X, or XII
Interruption of the sympathetic and/or parasympathetic trunk
Central and/or spinal
Craniocerebral trauma
Cerebral and/or cerebellar ischemia
Multiple sclerosis
Bulbar paralysis
Pseudobulbar paralysis
Meningitis
Encephalitis
Brain and brain stem tumors
Bulbar poliomyelitis
Amyotrophic lateral sclerosis
Polyneuritis
Syringomyelia
Diabetic neuropathy
Alcoholic neuropathy
Toxic neuropathy (e. g., lead)
Vertebrobasilar insufficiency
Hyperkalemia
Botulism
Myasthenia gravis
Toxic diphtheria
Polyradiculitis (Landry–Guillain–Barré syndrome)
Foramen jugulare syndrome (cranial nerves IX, X, and XII), see Table 1.**18**
Tapia syndrome, see Table 1.**18**
Wallenberg syndrome, see Table 10.**16** and p. 106

Disturbances of Taste Sensation

See p. 291.

Disturbances of Innervation in the Mouth and Pharynx

The mouth derives its sensory innervation from the third division of the trigeminal nerve (= the mandibular nerve), the pharynx from the glossopharyngeal nerve and vagus nerve (see Fig. 3.**1**).

Isolated *sensory* disturbances of the trigeminal nerve present as a *trigeminal neuralgia* or *neuropathy* (see p. 159), while pharyngeal sensory disturbances are manifested as *glossopharyngeal or vagus neuralgia* (see pp. 162, 163).

Besides typical neuralgic symptoms, functional disturbances of these three cranial nerves may be manifested as *motor* deficits or *mixed* palsies, for the trigeminal, glossopharyngeal, and vagus nerves transmit a combination of motor, secretory, sensory, and autonomic fibers. Accordingly, lesions of the glossopharyngeal and vagus nerves, and to a lesser degree of the trigeminal nerve, tend to produce mixed neurologic symptoms depending on the cause and location of the lesion.

Neurologic consultation is essential in the differential diagnostic workup of these symptom complexes, in which a focal lesion, a systemic disease, a peripheral injury, or multiple pathologic foci may have causal significance.

The routine otorhinolaryngologic examination very often provides obvious clues to neurologic deficits in the oropharyngeal region. Some common *cardinal symptoms* of these (principally motor) deficits are outlined below:

○ *Paralysis of the lesser (motor) portion of the trigeminal nerve.* Distribution: masticatory muscles, tensor veli palatini and tympani muscles, mylohyoid muscle, and the anterior belly of the digastric. Paralysis of the masseter muscle is detectable by palpation; also, the masseter reflex may be absent. Functional effects: masticatory problems, deviation of the mandible toward the paralyzed side, dysphagia.

○ *Paralysis of the facial nerve.* Symptoms chiefly affecting the mouth: motor palsy of the lips, mouth, and cheek (flaccid cheek, sagging mouth angle); damage to the nerve supply of the soft palate; disturbance of salivation and taste affecting the anterior two-thirds of the tongue (see p. 150ff).

○ *Paralysis of the glossopharyngeal nerve.* Motor: Paralysis of the inferior and middle constrictor muscles of the pharnyx, the levator muscle of the pharynx, and the soft palate. Dysphagia, usually on one side. Absent or diminished palatal and gag reflex: The soft palate is displaced toward the healthy side with a positive "backdrop sign" (posterior pharyngeal wall is drawn toward the healthy side). The initial phase of swallowing is impaired, with aspiration. Taste disturbance affects the posterior two-thirds of the tongue. Impaired pharyngeal sensation (test!). Disturbance of salivation and mucous gland secretion (particularly affecting the parotid gland).

○ *Paralysis of the vagus nerve.* (Laryngeal innervation is disregarded in this context; for details see p. 350 and Fig. 6.2). Motor: Paralysis of the inferior pharyngeal constrictor (responsible for the hypopharynx and upper esophagus) and of the palate. Cranial nerves V, VII, IX, and X contribute to the motor innervation of the palate! Palatal reflex is absent (pharyngeal sensory impairment).

○ *Paralysis of the hypoglossal nerve.* Paralysis of the tongue with atrophy, fibrillations, and fasciculations. The tongue deviates toward the healthy side. Speech and eating are impaired; possible traumatic malocclusion and bite injury.

The more common causes of innervation disturbances of the mouth and pharynx are listed in Table 4.23.

Symptom   **Trismus**

Various *grades of trismus* are recognized according to the distance between the upper and lower incisors when the jaw is fully open: 2.5−4 cm is classified as *grade 1*, 1−2.5 cm as *grade 2*, and <1 cm as *grade 3*. In *total* trismus (extremely rare), the patient cannot move the jaw to any degree.

The causal mechanism of trismus may be *reflex, spastic, inflammatory, cicatricial,* or *bony* in nature. Trismus also may be characterized etiologically as *myogenic, arthrogenic, dermatogenic, neurogenic,* or *psychogenic.*

The functional counterpart of trismus is *lockjaw,* like that occurring with TMJ dislocation (abnormal position of the mandibular condyle, palpable and demonstrable by radiography).

With a unilateral dislocation, the mouth is half open while the mandible deviates toward the unaffected side. The jaw cannot be closed and offers a springy resistance to passive closure. An important sign differentiating inflammatory trismus from tetanic trismus is that the latter is abolished by general anesthesia, while inflammatory trismus is not.

The principal causes of trismus are outlined in Table 4.24.

The differential diagnostic workup includes a detailed history, assessment of the grade of trismus, palpation of the jaw and TMJ, and a thorough ENT examination. Some cases will additionally require consultation with an oral surgeon or internist.

Table 4.**24** *Symptom* Trismus (causes) (from W. Becker, H. H. Naumann, C. R. Pfaltz: Ear, Nose, and Throat Diseases. Thieme, Stuttgart 1989)

Synopsis	
Group	Individual cause
Inflammation of the teeth or mandible	Unerupted dentition
	Stomatitis
	Pulpitis
	Osteomyelitis (maxilla and mandible)
	Peri- and submandibular abscess
	TMJ arthritis
	Osteoarthritis
	Manifestation of chronic rheumatoid arthritis
Acute inflammation in the TMJ region	Peritonsillitis and peritonsillar abscess
	Sialadenitis and sialolithiasis (affecting the parotid and submandibular glands)
	Otitis externa and furunculosis of the external auditory canal
	Malignant otitis externa
	Parapharyngeal soft-tissue abscess
Trauma	TMJ fracture
	Fracture of the zygoma and zygomatic arch
	Mandibular fracture
	TMJ dislocation
	Posttraumatic scars and adhesions
Muscle spasm	Epilepsy
	Spasticity due to CNS lesions (brain tumor)
	Meningitis
	Tetanus
	Tetany
	Psychogenic spasticity
Tumors	Benign tumor involving the TMJ
	Malignant tumor involving the TMJ
	Previous tumor resection
	Postirradiation scarring
Miscellaneous	Congenital ankylosis of the TMJ

Symptom   Dysphagia

"Dysphagia" is a vaguely defined, "catch-all" term for a symptom that can have numerous causes based or located in a variety of organs and structures. It encompasses *pain on swallowing* (odynophagia) as well as functional or physical *difficulty swallowing*. Ordinarily the following subgroups of dysphagia are recognized:

1. *Odynophagia,* i.e., pain precipitated by swallowing that disturbs and hampers at least the oral phase of deglutition. In *esophageal* odynophagia, pain is initiated during the esophageal phase of swallowing.
2. *Oropharyngeal dysphagia,* in which movement of the food bolus is hampered by incoordination of the oral and/or pharyngeal phase of swallowing.
3. *Pharyngeal or esophageal (mechanical) dysphagia,* in which there are one or more physical obstructions to passage of the bolus in the pharynx or esophagus.
4. *Functional ("hysterical") dysphagia,* in which the chief complaint is a foreign body sensation of variable degree, usually paroxysmal, with no demonstrable organic dysphagia or neurologic impairment ("globus nervosus or hystericus"). It is considered to represent a dysfunction in the setting of a psychoneurotic disturbance (see p. 383).

The *diagnostic workup of dysphagia* consists of an otorhinolaryngologic examination that includes plain radiographs of the paranasal sinuses, endoscopy and esophagoscopy, and contrast radiographs. Optional studies include cinefluoroscopy of the upper digestive tract from the mouth to the stomach, tomography, MRI, chest radiographs, and esophageal manometry (using three-point, pull-through or radiomanometric technique). Exclusion of a neurologic cause may be required (Table 4.**25**).

Hypopharyngeal Diverticulum (Pulsion Diverticulum, Zenker Diverticulum, Pharyngoesophageal Diverticulum)

Main symptoms: Foreign-body sensation, scratchiness, or fullness during and after eating. Habitual throat clearing. Larger diverticula cause constant fullness and a sensation of food "sticking in the throat." They also cause frothy saliva, oral fetor, cough, and regurgitation of undigested food that may have been eated several days before. Middle-aged and elderly individuals are most commonly affected.

Other symptoms and special features: As the sac enlarges, it may cause sustained esophageal obstruction leading to dehydration, electrolyte disturbances, and malnutrition.

Causes: Outpouching of the hypopharynx at the Killian triangle immediately above below the upper esophageal sphincter, presumably based on an incoordination of esophageal motility.

Diagnosis:
● Typical history.
● Radiographic studies: Barium swallow.
● Hypopharyngoscopy, esophagoscopy (using a rigid scope!).

Differentiation is required from globus hystericus; posttraumatic strictures; malignant tumor of the hypopharynx, esophagus, or stomach; hiatal hernia; achalasia; the Plummer—Vinson syndrome; and true esophageal diverticula (see p. 378).

Table 4.**25** *Symptom* Dysphagia (causes)

Synopsis

Type I: Oropharyngolaryngeal dysphagia

Inflammatory or traumatic

- Glossitis, see p. 258
- Abscess of the tongue (base) and oral floor, see p. 234
- Stomatitis, see p. 243 ff.
- Tonsillitis, see pp. 229, 262 and Tables 4.**1** and 4.**14**
- Pharyngitis due to various causes, see pp. 234, 266
- Peritonsillar abscess, see p. 233
- Ludwig angina, see p. 390
- Angioneurotic (Quincke) edema, see p. 143
- Epiglottitis, see p. 316
- Laryngitis, see p. 315
- Laryngeal perichondritis, see p. 317
- Laryngeal tuberculosis, see p. 323
- Thermal burns and caustic injury, see pp. 317, 376
- Internal and/or external injury to the bone and soft tissues, see p. 316
- Posttraumatic state
- Postoperative state
- Foreign bodies, see pp. 235, 317

Noninflammatory

- Zenker diverticulum
- Pharyngeal stricture
- Benign and malignant tumors of the mouth, pharynx, or larynx, see pp. 218, 267, 326
- Carotid body tumor, see p. 405
- Macroglossia, see Table 4.**13**
- Cleft anomalies, see p. 271
- Lingual goiter, see p. 410
- Acromegaly, see p. 138
- Pharyngeal cysts
- Cervical cysts, see p. 402
- Anomalies of the hyoid bone, see p. 392
- Ranula, see p. 302
- Laryngocele, see p. 328
- Xerostomia, see Table 5.**7**
- Sicca syndrome, see p. 303 and Table 5.**8**
- Previous radiotherapy

Neurologic

- Palsy of the soft palate in diphtheria, see p. 233
- Glossopharyngeal or vagus nerve lesion, see p. 277
- Hypoglossal nerve lesion (especially bilateral), see p. 277
- Mandibular nerve lesion
- Superior laryngeal nerve lesion, see p. 350 ff.
- Stylalgia, see p. 234
- Upper (cricopharyngeal) achalasia, see p. 382
- Central nervous diseases such as bulbar paralysis, botulism, toxic diphtheria, multiple sclerosis, amyotrophic lateral sclerosis, brain tumor, cerebral ischemia, pseudobulbar paralysis, polyneuritis, poliomyelitis, syringomyelia, etc.
- Other relationships with neurologic syndromes, bulbar disturbances, or central nervous disorders, see Table 1.**18**

Muscular

- Diseases affecting the pharyngeal musculature, e. g., myasthenia gravis, myotonic dystrophy, dermatomyositis, thyrotoxic myopathy

Neurotic or psychogenic

- Autonomic ("functional") dysphagia, globus hystericus, see pp. 279, 383

Cervical spine

- Osteoarthritis, spondylosis deformans
- Hyperostitic spondylosis (Forestier disease)
- Whiplash injury, see p. 392
- Dislocation
- Fracture
- Herniated disk
- Spondylolisthesis
- Cervical rib, see p. 394
- "Cervical vertebragenic" dysphagia

General diseases

- Botulism, pernicious anemia, agranulocytosis, tetany, tetanus, goiter, hypokalemia, leukoses, vitamin deficiency (A, B_2), mitral valve disease, aortic aneurysm, thyrotoxicosis, collagen diseases, etc.

Dermatologic diseases

- Scleroderma, lupus erythematosus, erythema multiforme, pemphigus, zoster, herpes simplex, recurrent aphthosis, hereditary epidermolysis bullosa, dermatomyositis, etc.

Type II: Esophageal dysphagia, see Table 8.**8**

Symptom   Airway Obstruction in the Mouth and Pharynx

The first lesions to be considered under this heading are *benign and malignant neoplasms in the nasopharynx* (see p. 218), *oropharynx* and *hypopharynx* (see p. 270 ff.), and tumors of the *oral cavity* (see p. 267). In patients with a brief history, the differential diagnosis should include *inflammatory processes and abscesses* in the *mouth*, on the *tongue*, in the *faucial isthmus*, and *anywhere within the pharynx*. Pain in these cases usually significantly *precedes* the onset of airway obstruction.

Angioneurotic edema can cause acute airway obstruction without pain. Airway obstruction in *children* is most commonly a result of *adenoid and/or tonsillar hyperplasia*. Other potential causes are listed in Table 3.24.

Symptom   Disturbance of Speech

See p. 353 ff.

Syndromes Involving the Mouth and Pharynx

The more common *dysgenetic syndromes* involving the oropharyngeal region are summarized in Table 4.26. Other common syndromes are listed in Table 4.27.

Table 4.26   Congenital syndromes involving the mouth, pharynx, and neck (modified from Leiber and Olbrich)

Syndrome	Classification	Typical ENT deficits	Other symptoms
Ascher syndrome	Combination of double lip, blepharochalasis, and goiter, probably transmitted as an autosomal recessive trait	Double lip (upper lip), recurrent or persistent edematous swelling of the lip	Swelling of the upper eyelid with blepharochalasis. Onset in puberty. Goiter
Bonnevie–Ullrich syndrome	Webbed neck combined with multiple dysplasias	Skull abnormalities with hypertelorism, mandibular hypoplasia, auricular dysplasia, and dystopia. Possible cranial neuropathies (facial nerve, eye muscles, eyelids)	Edema of the hands and feet, limb malformations, joint pathology. Possible mental retardation
Down syndrome	See Table 2.13		
Gardner–Turner syndrome (see also Table 2.13)	Bilateral acoustic neuroma, autosomal dominant mode of inheritance	Manifestations do not appear until 2nd–3rd decade. Typical, gradually progressive symptoms; see pp. 29, 78, and Table 1.8	Additional cranial nerve deficits and cerebral compression symptoms due to the acoustic neuromas

Table 4.**26**   (cont.)

Syndrome	Classification	Typical ENT deficits	Other symptoms
Edwards syndrome (trisomy 18 syndrome)	Autosomal trisomy of group E chromosomes with multiple deformities	Dysplasia of the external ear, conductive hearing impairment, short neck, microgenia, possible cleft lip and palate, high palate. Possible choanal atresia	Mental retardation, ocular dysplasias. Multiple malformations of the limbs and/or internal organs
Franceschetti–Zwahlen syndrome	See Table 2.**13**		
Goeminne syndrome	Cervicodermorenogenial dysplasia	Congenital wryneck, craniofacial asymmetry	Keloids on the chest and arms. Renal dysplasia. Cryptorchidism
Grob syndrome	See Table 2.**13**		
Goldenhar syndrome	See Table 2.**13**		
Klippel–Feil syndrome	Multiple derformities of the vertebral column combined with other anomalies. Autosomal dominant transmission is presumed	Short ("frog") neck with decreased mobility of the vertebral column. Elevated scapula. Possible low-set ears, microtia, atresia of the external auditory canal, cleft palate, dysmelias	Numerous skeletal anomalies, barrel chest, etc.
Moebius syndrome	Congenital paralysis of various (cranial) nerves	Facial paralysis, paralytic dysphagia, lingual paralysis and ocular muscle paralysis in various combinations. Ear deformity, atresia of the ear canal, hearing impairment, and vestibular neuropathy also occur	Symptoms are highly variable depending on the affected nerves
Naffziger syndrome (cervical rib syndrome)	See p. 394		
Papillon–Léage–Psaume syndrome	Orofacial–digital dysostosis	Hypertelorism, narrow nose, short upper lip. Cleft palate. Fixation of tongue and/or upper lip. Dental dysplasias. Possible conductive hearing loss	Skeletal anomalies involving the skull and extremities

Table 4.26 (cont.)

Syndrome	Classification	Typical ENT deficits	Other symptoms
Patau syndrome (trisomy 13–15 syndrome)	Autosomal trisomy of group D chromosomes with multiple deformities	Varying degrees of craniocephalic dysplasia. Cleft lip, alveolus, and palate. Deafness. Possible hypoplasia or aplasia of the nasal bones. Possible dysplasia of the external ear	Ocular dysplasias. Microphthalmia. Possible multiple malformations of internal viscera
Pendred syndrome	Enzymopathy (defective iodine utilization in goiter) combined with sensorineural hearing loss; hereditary etiology	Bilateral progressive sensorineural hearing loss, possibly with vestibular dysfunction. Goiter, initially euthyroid, develops during the first 2 decades	
Peutz–Jeghers syndrome	Pigmentary anomalies and intestinal polyposis; hereditary etiology	Multiform melanin spots on the oral mucosa, face, and lips	Associated pigmented lesions on the extremities; extensive polyposis in the gastrointestinal tract. Secondary anemia
Von Pfaundler–Hurler syndrome	See Table 2.13		
Robin syndrome	See Table 2.13		
Schimmelpenning–Feuerstein–Mims syndrome	Neuroectodermal syndrome	Multiple sebaceous gland nevi on the face, neck, head, and in the oral cavity	Ocular dysplasias, possible internal hydrocephalus
Sturge–Weber syndrome	See Table 2.13		
Turner syndrome	See Table 1.43		
Urbach–Wiethe syndrome	Disturbance of protein and lipoid metabolism with lipoprotein storage in the skin and mucosa (mouth); hereditary etiology	Firm, whitish inclusions in the mucosae of the mouth, pharynx, larynx, and esophagus. Possible macrocheilia and macroglossia. Hoarseness	Dysproteinemia, dyslipoidemia. Possible epileptiform seizures and intellectual retardation

Table 4.**27**   Other common syndromes involving the mouth and pharynx

Syndrome	Classification	Typical ENT deficits	Other symptoms
Immunodeficiency diseases	Collective term for congenital or acquired disturbances of the cellular and humoral immune system, e. g., absent or deficient IgA or IgM	Greatly increased susceptibility to respiratory infections and/or proneness to viral, bacterial, and fungal infections. The respiratory tract is particularly affected	The digestive tract may also be affected (malabsorption syndrome); possible disturbances of hematopoiesis
Angioneurotic syndrome (Quincke edema)	Paroxysmal (pseudo-)allergic angioneurotic edema; hereditary etiology	See p. 143	May also be manifested in the genitals or extremities. Abdominal pain and vomiting can also occur
Apnea syndrome	Obstructive form of sleep apnea	Apnea syndrome due to ENT disease (Table 3.**11**), generally combined with loud, irregular snoring. At least 10 apneic episodes per hour lasting 10 s or more	See Table 3.**12**
Eagle syndrome	Stylalgia	See p. 234	
Hutchinson syndrome	Symptom complex typical of congenital syphilis	Triad of barrel-shaped central upper incisors, sensorineural hearing loss, and interstitial keratitis	Positive syphilis tests; possible syphilitic arthritis and nephritis
Lyell syndrome	Severe form of erythema multiforme, generally occurring as a drug reaction	Manifestations may include severe mucosal lesions in the mouth and pharynx	Very severe, febrile systemic illness with multiform epidermolysis, see p. 254
Melkersson–Rosenthal syndrome	Circumscribed orofacial soft-tissue swelling with transient facial paralysis	See pp. 153, 241	Ophthalmic symptoms may occur
Plummer–Vinson syndrome (Paterson–Brown–Kelly syndrome, sideropenic syndrome)	Iron deficiency dysphagia	See p. 266	
Reiter syndrome	Infection, probably coupled with abnormal immune responses	Erosive, inflammatory mucosal lesions involving the mouth, pharynx, and lips. Chronic course with exacerbations	Arthritis, conjunctivitis, urethritis. Possible iritis, keratitis, iridocyclitis. Inflammatory skin conditions. Balanitis
Sjögren syndrome (sicca syndrome)	Systemic disease with exocrine gland dysfunction	See p. 303	

Rare Infections and Their Causative Organisms

Infections relevant to otorhinolaryngology are
reviewed in Table 4.**28**.

Table 4.**28**   Rare infectious otorhinolaryngologic diseases

Name	ENT symptoms	Causative organisms	Diagnosis	Epidemiology	Remarks
AIDS (acquired immunodeficiency syndrome, HIV syndrome)	Kaposi sarcoma. Oral symptoms (hairy leukoplakia of the tongue, etc.). Cervical lymphadenopathy, many other nonspecific ENT manifestations	Human immunodeficiency virus (HIV)	Antibody detection (ELISA) and confirmatory test (e. g., Western blot test)	Worldwide distribution Human to human transmission	See p. 245
Blastomycosis					
a) European blastomycosis (Busse–Buschke disease) (cryptococcosis; torulosis)	Soft outgrowths, prone to necrosis, occurring on the oral mucosa, tongue, tonsils, and lips. Also ulcerating bluish-red nodules in the oral and pharyngeal mucosa; ulcers and fistulae	*Cryptococcus neoformans* (yeast fungus)	Biopsy, culture	Worldwide distribution, very common in the United States. Farm works particularly affected	Chiefly involves the internal organs (lung, heart); also CNS and bone
b) South American blastomycosis (Lutz–Spendore–de Almeida disease) (paracoccidioidomycosis)	Infection often starts on the oral mucosa (gingiva) and may spread to the entire mouth, pharynx, lips, and perioral region; grayish-white to reddish mucosal granulations. Mulberry-like glossitis, diffuse stomatitis. Enlarged regional lymph nodes. Nasal and laryngeal mucosa may also be affected	*Paracoccidioides brasilensis* (yeast fungus)	Biopsy, isolation of organism from lymph node aspirate or smear, culture	Distributed throughout South America, occurs sporadically in Central America	Most commonly affects agricultural workers. Clinical picture similar to lymphogranulomatosis
c) North American blastomycosis (Gilchrist disease, Chicago disease)	Microabscesses on the lips and the nasal vestibule, usually spreading from infected skin areas. Granulating mucosal ulcers, draining nodules; may also involve the oral commissures, auricle, and larynx	*Blastomyces dermatidis* (yeast fungus)	Organism can be identified in pus or discharge, culture; serologic: CBR	Apparently confined to North American continent and Central America. Also endemic to areas in South America	Chiefly lung involvement, followed by hematogenous spread

(cont. on next page)

Table 4.**28**   (cont.)

Name	ENT symptoms	Causative organisms	Diagnosis	Epidemiology	Remarks
Brucellosis (Bang disease, Malta fever, sheep and swine brucellosis)	Generalized lymph node swelling, rarely affects the oral mucosa; nonspecific aphthosis; also enanthemas, gingival bleeding, ulcers	*Brucella abortus, B. melitensis, B. suis,* and *B. ovis*	Can sometimes be cultured from blood; serology: CBR; rapid agglutination test; cutaneous test	Transmitted by animals (cattle, goats, house pets)	Veterinarians, animal keepers, and meat processors are at highest risk. Generalization with involvement of liver, spleen, and heart
Yaws (frambesia, bouba, parangi, pian)	Stage III features rhinopharyngeal involvement with destructive lesions of the nose, pharynx, and maxilla. "Rhinopharyngitis mutilans." Enlarged lymph nodes (also in the preceding stages). Facial pseudotumors. Coryza with bloody, purulent discharge. Occasional hypertrophic osteitis ("goundou")	*Treponema pertenue* (nonvenereal treponematosis)	Organism can be isolated from tissue fluid. Indistinguishable from syphilis by serologic testing	Africa, South America; Southern Asia; Pacific Islands	Lesions are usually manifested first on the legs; later the infection may become generalized. Disease may be present for years before reaching tertiary stage!
Histoplasmosis	Airway saprophytes. Infection distinguished by regional lymph node involvement. Nonspecific nasopharyngeal symptoms	*Histoplasma capsulatum* (yeast fungus)	Organisms can be identified in culture. Biopsy. Serology: CBR. Intradermal test	Worldwide distribution with greatest prevalence in North, Central, and South America and the Far East. Rare in Europe	Children affected more often than adults. Symptoms similar to those of tuberculosis (lung!)
Cat scratch fever (viral scratch lymphadenitis)	Granulating mucosal lesions may appear initially in the mouth and pharynx. Picture is dominated by lymphadenitis with liquefaction (and a draining fistula with purulent discharge)	*Chlamydia*	Intradermal test, CBR	No geographic predilection. Transmitted by cats or stinging insects	Children are principally affected. Course is usually self-limiting

Table 4.**28**   (cont.)

Name	ENT symptoms	Causative organisms	Diagnosis	Epidemiology	Remarks
Coccidioido-mycosis (California disease, "desert rheumatism")	Involvement of nose, lips, oral cavity, tongue, and larynx. Nodular, degenerating protuberances on the face and nose (first involving the soft tissues and later the bone). Concomitant paranasal sinus involvement can occur. Swelling and subsequent necrosis	*Coccidioides immitis* (yeast fungus)	Organism can be identified in pus or expectorate. Animal test. Biopsy. Intradermal test	Southwestern United States, Mexico, South America, also Africa	Lesions may be manifested anywhere on the body. "Pulmonary" and "cutaneous" forms. Joint involvement is also possible
Leishmaniasis. Various forms: a) Kala-azar, mucocutaneous (American) espundia	Involvement of lips and oral cavity; possible involvement of pharynx, tonsils, and larynx. Dark-red papules on pale oral mucosa with mucosal bleeding. Post-kala-azar leishmaniasis: Also can involve mouth and pharynx, producing plaque-like or ulcerating lesions of the pharyngeal mucosa. Lymph node swelling	*Leishmania donovani* (flagellate protozoa)	Organisms can be isolated from blood or lymph nodes	Mediterranean countries and many other warm regions (India, Africa, South and Central America)	Transmitted by phlebotomine sandflies
b) South American leishmaniasis (espundia)	Involvement of the nasal, oral, pharyngeal, and laryngeal mucosae: Granulomas, severe mucosal ulcerations, papillomatous outgrowths. Possible auricular involvement. Typical nasal lesions consist of granulomas and ulcers on the septum and turbinates with crusting. Lesions also form on the palate and oropharynx. Succeeded by constricting scars and mucosal atrophy. Septal perforation	*Leishmania brazilensis* (flagellate protozoa)	Intradermal Montenegro test. Organism can be identified by culturing curetted material on blood agar. Biopsy. Smear	Central and South America	Transmitted by lutzomyian sandflies

(cont. on next page)

Table 4.**28**   (cont.)

Name	ENT symptoms	Causative organisms	Diagnosis	Epidemiology	Remarks
c) Cutaneous leishmaniasis (oriental boil)	Facial cutaneous lesions may spread to nasal or oral cavity, resulting in severe tissue defects	*Leishmania tropica*	See above	Central American countries, Africa, Middle East, India, Northern China, Southern Russia	Transmitted by sandflies
Leprosy Three different forms (tuberculoid; lepromatous; borderline, indeterminate leprosy)	Chronic coryza with sticky, viscous discharge, epistaxis, mucosal atrophy. Intranasal nodule formation may be accompanied by nodules in the mouth, pharynx, and larynx, which ulcerate and produce a fetid discharge. Subsequent scarring with synechiae and stenoses (leonine facies). Neurologic symptoms! Hyposmia or anosmia	*Mycobacterium leprae*	Intradermal lepromin test, biopsy; organism can be identified in tissue scrapings	Tropical and subtropical countries (Africa, Asia, South America). Sporadic occurrence in Southern Europe	Human-to-human transmission. See pp. 191 and 248 for further details
Listeriosis	Diverse symptomatology: Rhinitis, tonsillitis, flu-like infections, stomatitis, pharyngitis. Possible mucosal ulcerations. Multiple necrotizing granulomas on the posterior pharyngeal wall. The parotid gland and esophagus also may be involved. Regional lymphadenopathy	*Listeria monocytogenes* (flagellated bacterium; zoonosis)	Microbiologic detection of the causative organism; possibly CBR	Worldwide distribution	See p. 248 for further details
Malleus	Extensive necrotizing ulcers involving the external nose, cheek, lips, nasal cavity, hard and soft palates. Nasal mucosa is swollen with nodulation, ulcerative degeneration, and a bloody, purulent discharge. Lesions may spread to the pharynx and larynx. Crusted necrotic areas and extensive tissue defects are succeeded by heavy mucosal and facial scarring	*Actinobacillus mallei* (zoonosis)	Bacteriologic identification of the causative organism. Serologic options: CBR and agglutination test	Has become very rare. Still occurs in areas of Eastern Europe, Southeastern Europe, and apparently in North America	Mainly transmitted by solipeds (horses, donkeys, mules). Keepers, veterinarians, and farmers are at highest risk. See pp. 191 and 248 for further details

Table 4.**28**   (cont.)

Name	ENT symptoms	Causative organisms	Diagnosis	Epidemiology	Remarks
Rhinoscleroma	Nasal symptoms usually appear first: Atrophic rhinitis followed by mucosal nodules in the central and posterior parts of the nasal cavity. Nasal obstruction by granulation tissue. Epistaxis. Granulomas may spread to the pharynx, larynx, and trachea; are succeeded by hard scars that constrict the airways	*Klebsiella rhinoscleromatis*	Organism can be identified in culture. Biospy	Chiefly in Eastern Europe (Galicia, Poland, Hungary, Black Sea, Italy). Also Asia, Africa, North America, Central America, South America	
Rhinosporidiosis	Granulations and polyposis in the anterior nose. Epistaxis. Slow-growing, soft, reddish, papilloma-like outgrowths causing nasal airway obstruction. The oral cavity, pharynx, larynx, trachea, and paranasal sinuses may also be involved. Granulation polyps may undergo ulcerative degeneration, resulting in large mucosal defects. Chronic relapsing course	*Rhinosporidium seeberi* (Phycomycetes)	Biopsy	India, Ceylon, also Africa and America	
Mold stomatopathies (e.g., aspergillosis)	Ear, sinuses, and upper lip are involved in patients with weakened host defenses	At least 5 different *Aspergillus* species	Mycologic detection in sputum and discharges. Identifiable in culture. Serology: precipitation test	Widespread distribution in the United States	May present as mycetogenic asthma (farmers, poultry breeders, climatized spaces). Acquired by inhalation of contaminated dust. Pulmonary or gastrointestinal symptoms are usually predominant. Common in leukemia patients

(cont. on next page)

Table 4.**28**   (cont.)

Name	ENT symptoms	Causative organisms	Diagnosis	Epidemiology	Remarks
Mucor-mycosis	Especially common in person with diabetes or chronic debilitating disease: Bloody nasal discharge with grayish-red granulations on the mucosa; lesions may spread to the sinuses, with a potential for "rhinocerebral" progression. The ear may also be involved	*Phycomyce-tes mucor* or *Thizopus* or *Absidia*	Organism can be identified in sputum or washings. Culture		
Sporotricho-sis	Primary manifestation is an ulcerating, flat infiltrate in the nasal and/or oral cavity. Larynx and esophagus also may be involved. Cutaneous lesions usually predominate: Papules, pustules, and ulcers showing necrotic degeneration. Lymph nodes are swollen but nonpainful	*Sporotrix schenckii*	Organism can be identified by culture. Biopsy; immunofluorescent detection. Sporotrichin skin test	Worldwide distribution with predilection for warm, moist subtropical or tropical climates	Minimal systemic complaints. Men are affected 10 times more frequently than women
Toxoplasmo-sis	Nonspecific intraoral symptoms. Mild pharyngitic complaints. Isolated cervical or nuchal regional lymphadenitis (Pirringer–Kutchinka). Congenital and postnasal forms. Possible sensorineural hearing loss	*Toxoplasma gondii* (protozoan)	Organism can be identified by animal tests or biopsy. Serology involves detecting humoral antibodies by the immunofluorescent antibody test (IFAT); CBR; hemagglutination test	Worldwide distribution	Mainly transmitted in raw meat. Principal host: cat
Tularemia (rabbit fever) Diverse forms	Painful primary lesion may occur in the oral cavity (aphthous mucositis, tonsillitis). Crater-like ulcers in the oral or pharyngeal mucos are typical. Subsequent lymph node swelling is usually very painful	*Francisella tularensis* (zoonosis)	Organism can be identified in pus. Intradermal tularin test. Agglutination test, CBR	Only in the northern hemisphere, especially Russia, Japan, and North America	Hunters are at highest risk. Infection may become generalized

Collagen Diseases (Autoimmune Diseases)

This term is applied to diseases ranging from rheumatic and pararheumatic disorders to the vasculitides that are based on an immune disturbance and must be classified separately from other known entities. Given the lack of definite knowledge about the etiologies of these diseases, their definitions remain somewhat unclear, and their clinical delineation is correspondingly obscure and in some cases even speculative, making differential diagnosis difficult. The relatively few autoimmune diseases that are presently of clinical interest in otorhinolaryngology are reviewed in Table 4.**29**. The differential diagnostic evaluation of the laboratory features of these disorders requires appropriate consultation with an internist and pathologist.

Table 4.**29**   Common collagen diseases in the ENT region

Wegener granulomatosis, see p. 192

Myoepithelial sialadenitis (Sjögren disease), see p. 303

Progressive systemic scleroderma, see p. 255

Temporal arteritis, see p. 167

Systemic lupus erythematosus, especially discoid lupus (DLE) confined to the skin and mucosae, see pp. 210, 255

Dermatomyositis, see p. 255

Suggestive laboratory findings (characteristic of the various collagen disorders in varying degrees):

ESR:	Greatly increased
Blood count:	Usually anemia, possible leukopenia or leukocytosis
Serum iron:	Decreased
Total protein:	Usually increased
Electrophoresis:	α and β fractions increased, hypergammaglobulinemia
Urinary sediment:	Pathologic
Antinuclear antibodies:	Demonstrable
Rheumatoid factors:	Latex, Waaler–Rose test (positive in approximately 20% of cases)
Antistreptolysin titers:	Frequently >200 I.U./mL
Biopsy:	Typical immunohistologic findings

Symptom   **Disturbance of Taste**

H. Scherer

Taste is a complex chemosensory process mediated by impulses transmitted to the CNS by at least four distinct afferent pathways. Within the CNS the neuronal information is processed in a complex interactive network involving the olfactory, somatic, autonomic, and other sensory systems. Because of these interconnections, disturbances of taste are always linked with olfactory disturbances and vice versa, while sensory disturbances of the tongue are usually combined with gustatory dysfunction. This accounts for the diversity of sensations that are associated with taste disturbances and for the diagnostic problems that can arise — compounded by a lack of precise and objective neurophysiologic methods of examination. Aspects relating to the symptom of taste disturbance are outlined in Table 4.**30**.

Basic Anatomic Principles

Taste receptors are distributed over the entire surface of the tongue, the posterior pharyngeal wall, the epiglottis, and the soft palate. They are the remnants of a much larger taste-sensitive area that in childhood extends well into the esophagus, the trachea, and the epipharynx. Some of the taste buds in this area are superficial, but most lie within the sulci of the vallate, foliate, and fungiform papillae. Serous salivary glands open into these sulci to wash out the substances that are tasted.

As in olfaction, contact of the flavored substance with the sensory cell is established stereochemically, with water solubility of the substance as a necessary criterion. Different zones of the lingual mucosa are sensitive to the four taste qualities of *sweet, sour, salty*, and *bitter*. This "gustatory map" and the different modes of afferent transmission of gustatory signals play an important role in the investigation and differential diagnosis of taste disturbances.

○ *Gustatory map:* The distribution of specialized receptors for the four taste qualities is mapped in Figure 4.**4**. It can be seen that the receptors for sweet are concentrated at the tip of the tongue, while those for bitter are located at the base of the tongue.
○ *Afferent flow of impulses:* The neuronal information is transmitted to the CNS by at least four different pathways (Fig. 4.**4**). These pathways are located so far apart that a very severe trauma causing massive parapharyngeal disruption would be needed to damage all of the afferent nerves (a fact to be considered in compensation evaluations).

1. Information from the *tip* and *anterior two-thirds* of the tongue is relayed to the CNS first by the *lingual nerve*, then via the *chorda tympani* and the *facial nerve*.
2. Information from the *posterior third* of the tongue and the *mesopharynx* is transmitted by the *glossopharyngeal nerve*. The fibers leave this nerve in the inferior ganglion and pass via the tympanic nerve to the lesser petrosal nerve, which relays the information to the CNS. (For simplicity, the pathway via the tympanic nerve is not shown in Figure 4.**4**.)
3. Information from the *hypopharynx* and *laryngeal inlet* is carried to the CNS by the vagus nerve.
4. Information from the *palate* passes with the lesser palatine nerves to the *pterygopalatine ganglion*, thence to the *greater petrosal nerve* and then the *nervus intermedius* (of cranial nerve VII).

○ *Central connections:* The four afferent nerves terminate in the solitary tract nucleus (Fig. 4.**4**). From there secondary fibers are distributed to the medial lemniscus of the opposite side, to the ventrocaudal nucleus of the thalamus, and to the hypothalamus, where they are linked with other sensory systems. The tertiary neuron terminates in the area of the parietal cortex where taste perception occurs. A gustatory reflex pathway projects from the solitary tract nucleus to the salivatory nucleus. Certain taste stimuli can evoke an increase in salivation via this reflex pathway. Another reflex tract stimulating the production of gastric juices passes to the dorsal part of the nucleus of the vagus nerve.

Diagnostic Options

The sense of taste is evaluated by using *test solutions* of varying concentrations and by *electrical stimulation* (electrogustometry). In each case the examiner relies on subjective responses reported by the patient. Objective studies using evoked potentials have been developed but have not been successfully adapted for clinical use.

○ *Filter paper test:* Small pieces of filter paper are immersed in graded concentrations of test solution and are applied to appropriate sites on the tongue. Glucose solutions, sodium chloride solutions, and citric acid solutions are used in concentrations of 0.1, 1, and 10%; bitter quinine solution is applied in concentrations of 0.001, 0.01, and 0.1% (Rollin 1978). Herberhold uses five concentrations for each solution:
Sodium chloride: 0.3, 1.5, 2.5, 5, and 15%
Citric acid: 0.035, 0.5, 1, 7.5, and 15%
Quinine sulfate: 0.001, 0.005, 0.01, 0.05, and 0.2%
Cane sugar: 0.5, 2, 4, 10, and 40%

○ *Electrogustometry:* An electrode probe is used first to apply a suprathreshold direct-current stimulus of 50–100 microamperes (μA) to produce a metallic, acidic taste. The counterelectrode is held in the hand. The current is then reduced in stages to the threshold level. At each level the probe should touch the tongue for no more than 2 s to avoid threshold migration. The *normal threshold* in the tip area is *5–20 μA*. In a positive test, a discrepancy is noted between the right and left sides of the tongue. This difference is not measured on the absolute microamperage scale but on a logarithmic scale (Table 4.**31**). A right–left discrepancy *greater than 4–5 dB* is considered *pathologic*. Complete ageusia of the tested area is present if current levels up to 300 μA fail to evoke a taste sensation. Current levels higher than 350 μA are sufficient to stimulate sensory nerve endings of the trigeminal nerve in the tongue.

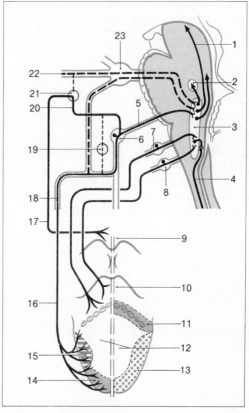

Fig. 4.**4** Gustatory apparatus and pathways

1 Central gustatory pathway
2 Salivatory nucleus
3 Solitary tract nucleus
4 Reflex pathway via the vagus nerve
5 Facial nerve
6 Geniculate ganglion of the facial nerve
7 Glossopharyngeal nerve
8 Vagus nerve
9 Faucial pillars and oropharynx
10 Epiglottis and hypopharynx
11 Base of tongue (sensitive to bitter taste)
12 Dorsum of tongue
13 Lateral border of tongue (sensitive to salty taste)
14 Tip of tongue (sensitive to sweet taste)
15 Side of tongue (sensitive to sour taste)
16 Chorda tympani
17 Lesser palatine nerves
18 Lingual nerve
19 Otic ganglion
20 Greater petrosal nerve
21 Pterygopalatine ganglion
22 Maxillary nerve
23 Semilunar (gasserian) ganglion

Table 4.**31** Unit-of-measure equivalents in electrogustometry. Comparison of dB scale, electrogust units (EGUs), and the corresponding microamperage values (μA) (after Rollin)

dB	8	4	0	4	8	12	16	20	24	28	32
μA	3.18	5.05	8	12.7	20.1	31.9	50.5	80	127	201	318
EGU	–	–	4	8	12	17	21	25	29	33	37

○ *Test for feigning:* Since all the tests are based on subjective responses, a feigning test should be added to all examinations for disability assessment and compensation. It is based on "rhinogenic" taste testing. Much as in the gustatory olfaction test of Güttlich, a flavored substance such as chloroform (sweet) or pyridine (bitter) is presented to the patient to "smell." If a gustatory component of the stimulus is recognized, ageusia cannot be present.

Definitions

Fikentscher, in a survey work on the definition of taste disturbances, attempted to coordinate the terminology with that used for olfactory dysfunction:

○ *Normogeusia:* Ability to recognize a test substance within the limits of the normal taste threshold. This threshold is quite difficult to define when test solutions are used. Rollin, using the three concentration levels noted above, found that approximately 10% of normal subjects could recognize the lowest concentration, while 50% could recognize the second level, and 90% could detect the highest level. In electrogustometry, the threshold is between 2 and 7 μA for young adults and may be as high as 20 μA in older adults.
○ *Dysgeusias:*
  – *Quantitative dysgeusias:* Analogous to olfactory disturbances, taste disturbances are classified by degree as ageusia, hypogeusia, or hypergeusia. Hypergeusia (increased taste sensitivity) can result from drug use and psychiatric disorders.
  – *Qualitative dysgeusias:* Parageusia, pseudogeusia, and phantogeusia are defined as they were for olfactory disturbances (see p. 225).

Diseases and Causes

Epithelial and Receptor Dysgeusias

As with olfaction, epithelial and neural pathology overlap in the region of the sensory cells. Diphtheria, for example, leads both to mucosal damage and to diphtheritic neuritis.

○ *Dysgeusia due to disturbances of mucus production:* Mucus secretion by the salivary glands is decreased by *irradiation*, leading to receptor dysfunction. The different taste qualities are affected differently: Sweet is affected first, followed by salty, bitter, and finally sour. Partial recovery usually ensues in the months following the termination of radiotherapy. Marked dysgeusia for the salty, bitter, and sour qualities also occurs in *Sjögren syndrome*. Decreased mucus production is a very common *side effect of certain drugs* such as antivertiginous drugs, psychotropic drugs, some cardiac medications, and atropine (see Table 4.**32**).
○ *Dysgeusia due to mucosal atrophy:* Mucosal atrophy with pronounced dysgeusia results from acute and chronic caustic injuries, lichen ruber planus, irradiation, and from vitamin B_2, vitamin B_{12} and zinc deficiencies. Differentiation is required from involution of aging, which leads to a marked decrease in the number of papillae (the circumvallate papillae decrease from about 250 in children to about 90 in old age). Complete dysgeusia is a feature of *familial dysautonomia*, a congenital anomaly involving the nervous system, skin, and mucous membranes. The atrophic mucosa of the oropharynx is devoid of gustatory sensory cells. Other symptoms of this disease are decreased temperature and pain sensation, resulting in constant lip biting, and absent or deficient lacrimation, which can lead to keratitis.

Table 4.**32**   Drugs that can cause taste disturbances (after Rollin)

Drug	Indications	Incidence of taste disturbance
d-Penicillamine	Chronic rheumatoid arthritis	25–30%
Niridazole	Helminths	30%
l-Dopa	Parkinsonism	4.5–22%
Carbamizol	Trigeminal neuralgia, epilepsy	10%
Biguanidine	Diabetes mellitus	3%
Phenylbutazone	Rheumatic diseases	Rare
Oxyfedrine	Coronary insufficiency	Rare
Gold	Chronic rheumatoid arthritis	?
Methylthiouracil	Hyperthyroidism	Rare
Phenindione	Anticoagulation	?
Bamifylline	Chronic bronchitis	Frequent
Metronidazole	Protozoal and bacterial infections	?
Griseofulvin	Fungal infections	?
Lincomycin	Bacterial infections	?
Acetylsalicylic acid	Pain, thrombosis	?
Ethambutol	Tuberculosis	Frequent

Another congenital disorder is a specific *blindness* for the *bitter taste quality* produced by PTC (phenylthiocarbamide) and other substances with an $N-C=S$ group. It is transmitted as a recessive homozygous trait. The remaining taste qualities are perceived normally. This disorder is encountered in all parts of the world but has a variable distribution. There are "tasters" and "nontasters." Nontasters have been found in 2% of American Indians and Eskimos, 7% of Japanese, 10% of Chinese, and 25–30% of Europeans. The prevalence of nontasters among Greenland Eskimos is as high as 50%. This disorders has a high association with trisomy, athyreotic cretinism, and duodenal ulcers.

o *Dysgeusia due to receptor damage by exogenous toxins:* Some of the many industrial toxins that cause gustatory dysfunction are listed in Table 4.**33**. Heavy *smoking* leads acutely to dysgeusia in all receptor fields and chronically to isolated impairment of bitter taste sensation. *Toothpastes* that contain the foaming and cleansing agent sodium

Table 4.**33**   Substances that can cause dysgeusia when chronically inhaled

Tetrachloroethane
Tobacco smoke
Hydrazine
Benzene
Gasoline
Aniline and derivatives
Lacquers and their solvents
Rubber dust
Chromates
Cobalt

laurylsulfate or other tensides can impair taste sensation for up to 2 h in some persons. *Oral antiseptics* produce a similar effect. Many *drugs* (see Table 4.**32**) have a toxic effect on taste receptors, leading to parageusia (metallic taste) and impaired sensitivity to sweet and other qualities.

Table 4.**34**   Local causes of peripheral gustatory nerve lesions

Trauma	Temporal bone fracture
	TMJ fracture
	Fracture of the sphenoid wing
Iatrogenic lesions	Middle ear surgery
	Surgery in the internal acoustic meatus
	Surgery in the posterior cranial fossa
	Tonsillectomy
	Injury by dental instruments
Compression	Glomus jugulare tumor
	Hourglass tumor in the foramen ovale (e. g., glossopharyngeal neuroma)
	Pleomorphic adenoma of the soft palate
	Meningioma of the posterior cranial fossa, etc.
Destruction	Middle-ear cholesteatoma
	Carcinoma of the middle ear and external auditory canal
	Nasopharyngeal malignancy
Polyneuritis	
Pterygopalatine ganglion syndrome (Sluder syndrome)	See p. 162

○ *Dysgeusia due to hormonal disorders:* Taste disturbances are known to accompany diabetes and hypothyroidism.

○ *Dysgeusia due to receptor damage caused by infections:* Gustatory receptors have a remarkable regenerative capacity, so damage caused by viral, bacterial, and fungal infections is generally transient.

Neural Dysgeusias

These result from damage to the peripheral nerves of the gustatory system. The widely distributed nerves are inherently susceptible to injury.

○ *Infectious diseases:* Afferent nerve damage can result from influenza, zoster, diphtheria, and typhus.

○ *Local damage to peripheral nerves:* These disorders go unnoticed if they develop *slowly*, first because taste information reaches the CNS by many different pathways, so that local damage only affects discrete por-

tions of taste sensation, and second because disturbances of gradual onset can be centrally compensated. *Rapidly* developing lesions are generally perceived, although there are patients who, for example, do not report taste impairment following section of the chorda tympani, even though the loss is verifiable by electrogustometry. Section of the chorda tympani in many patients produces a parageusia (metallic taste) that gradually subsides. The mechanism of this parageusia remains unexplained. Potential causes of peripheral lesions of gustatory nerve fibers are listed in Table 4.**34**.

Central Dysgeusias

Abnormalities of taste sensation can occur as a symptom of central nervous disease but often are less important clinically than other associated neurologic symptoms. Taste disturbances can be important, however, for site-of-lesion determinations.

○ *Lesions of the medulla oblongata* cause ipsilateral hypogeusias or ageusias. Some or all taste sensations may be affected depending on the extent of pathology in the solitary tract nucleus. The most frequent cause is multiple sclerosis.

○ *Lesions of the thalamus* cause contralateral hypogeusias and ageusias. Hypergeusias and parageusias also occur.

○ *Lesions of the gustatory cortex* (operculum, postcentral and precentral gyri) cause hypogeusias, hypergeusias, and parageusias affecting all taste sensations. As in other sensory systems, handedness is a factor. For example, the left-sided gustatory center is thought to be dominant in right-handed individuals. Lesions of the gustatory cortex are frequently combined with sensory disturbances of the perioral region and hand (especially the thumb and index finger) and with motor aphasia (parietal operculum syndrome).

Dysgeusia Combined with Dysosmia

Concomitant disturbances of taste and smell can occur peripherally only if there has been massive trauma causing damage to multiple cranial nerves. Trauma of this magnitude is rarely survived. Extensive central lesions may, however, be associated with combined olfactory and gustatory dysfunction, which will invariably be accompanied by other neurologic symptoms. The following list covers symptom complexes of the kind reported in the literature:

○ Bilateral ageusia and anosmia combined with small zones of sensory impairment in the oronasal region.

○ Unilateral ageusia and anosmia combined with ipsilateral hemihypoesthesia and various autonomic symptoms.

○ Unilateral hypogeusia and hyposmia combined with disturbances of proprioception and exteroception, impairment of gnostic association, increased susceptibility to affective disturbance, decreased intentional spontaneity, and a hyperkinetic symptom pattern (Head–Holmes syndrome).

○ Episodic hypogeusia and hyposmia occurring as "uncinate attacks" in the setting of temporal lobe epilepsy.

5. Salivary Glands

The Symptoms

○ Pain (and dysesthesia), p. 299

○ Morphologic change (swelling, tumor), p. 302

○ Malformation, p. 309

○ Disturbance of salivary production, p. 309

○ Common syndromes, p. 312

Principal Diagnostic Methods

○ A careful *history* is particularly helpful in the evaluation of salivary gland diseases and will often suggest a presumptive diagnosis. The *duration of the disease*, the *description of symptoms*, and the patient's *age* are as rewarding as:

○ *Inspection* and *palpation*. The healthy *parotid gland*, located in front of the auricle, blends harmonioulsy with the facial contours on visual inspection, as do the *submandibular gland*, located in the submandibular trigone, and the *sublingual gland* lying between the tongue and oral floor musculature. Most diseases of these three salivary glands are associated with visible swelling. *Inspection* and *bimanual palpation* will generally quickly disclose an *increase in size* or *consistency, tenderness* to pressure, and *mobility* relative to the surrounding soft tissues. If enlargement of a parotid gland is marginal or questionable, it can be compared with the opposite parotid by viewing *both* glands from the posterior aspect.

○ *Sonography:* Ultrasound is frequently used to screen for salivary gland disease owing to its convenience, wide availability, and low cost. The two-dimensinal B-mode scan is particularly useful for evaluating the parotid and other salivary glands.

○ *Radiographic studies*
Sialography: Contrast radiography of the glandular duct system, perhaps utilizing the subtraction technique, can sometimes contribute to differential diagnosis. Combining sialography with
Computed tomography can be particularly effective for the delineation of tumors.
Radionuclide scanning is most helpful for determining organ size, detecting inflammatory intraglandular processes, and defining the relationships between glandular and neoplastic tissue.

○ *Magnetic resonance imaging (MRI)* is very rewarding in the diagnosis of salivary gland diseases.

○ *Determination of salivary flow rate (sialometry)* yields information on salivary production and thus on the function of the affected gland. The results depend strongly, however, on interindividual, circadian, and peristatic influences, and physiologic variations are substantial.

○ *Biochemical analysis of the saliva (salivary chemistry):* this type of study is still reserved for specialized laboratories. The parameters of diagnostic interest are listed in Table 5.5.

○ *Punch biopsy:* This method of tissue sampling for morphologic study is useful in experienced hands and more reliable than *fine-needle aspiration cytology*. Both methods are *less reliable* and *less informative* for salivary gland investigations than

○ *Incisional biopsy*, for which the major salivary glands are readily accessible, and which establishes a tissue diagnosis. If desired, benign lesions can be removed by a complete *excisional biopsy* combined with frozen-section confirmation and routine histology.

Symptom   **Pain (and Dysesthesia)**

Pain is generally a conspicuous feature of *acute* salivary gland diseases, *stasis* of salivary secretions (ductal obstruction), and *malignant tumors* of the major salivary glands. Pain is less pronounced in chronic inflammatory conditions.

The synopsis in Table 5.**1** lists significant diseases that can affect the parotid, submandibular, and sublingual glands in varying degrees.

Trauma and Sequelae

Injuries of the parotid gland are relatively common, injuries of the submandibular and sublingual glands less so. The cause is obvious with a gunshot wound, stab injury, blunt trauma, or surgical trauma, and the differential diagnosis must establish whether there is concomitant injury to the glandular capsule, major blood vessels, large salivary ducts, or important nerves (facial nerves, lingual nerves, hypoglossal nerve). The consequences of inadequate surgical repair can range from severe nerve deficits, painful stasis and other disturbances of the ductal system, possibly with fistula formation, to complete degeneration of the involved salivary gland.

Acute Bacterial Sialadenitis

Main symptoms: The parotid gland is most commonly affected. Pain is very severe and may occur in waves. The gland is hard and swollen, and the overlying skin is warm and erythematous. The earlobe is protuberant on the affected side. A discharge—purulent, cloudy/viscous, sometimes gelatinous—can be expressed from the punctum of the gland. Salivary flow is absent or diminished (hyposialosis).

Other symptoms and special features: Fever is often present. With liquefaction, the gland becomes fluctuant, and pus may erupt from a fistula over the gland. The orifice of the Stensen duct (opposite the second upper molar in the buccal mucosa) is reddened. Trismus may be present. Inflammation of the submandibular

Table 5.**1**   *Symptom*   Pain (and dysesthesia)

Synopsis
Trauma and sequelae
Acute bacterial sialadenitis
Chronic recurrent parotitis
Chronic sialadenitis of the submandibular gland, see p. 302
Viral sialadenitis
– Epidemic parotitis (mumps)
– Cytomegaly parotitis, see p. 302
– Coxsackie parotitis, see p. 302
Sialolithiasis
Electrolyte sialadenitis
Drug-related salivary gland pain
Auriculotemporal neuralgia, see p. 16
Sialadenitis of the minor salivary glands (granulomatous cheilitis), see p. 241
Radiation sialadenitis
Malignant tumors

gland and, rarely, the sublingual gland present analogous manifestations.

Causes: Ductogenic or hematogenous infection. Streptococci or staphylococci are commonly identified as pathogens. Individuals with a deficient metabolic status (diabetes, renal failure) or lowered general host resistance (e.g., after surgery) are predisposed.

Diagnosis:
● Typical history, typical local and palpable findings.
● Bacteriologic examination and sensitivity testing of material expressed from the affected gland.
● Internal medical consultation may be indicated (metabolism).

Differentiation in *parotid gland* disease is required from dentogenic buccal abscess, mumps, lymphadenitis (e.g., with furunculosis of the external auditory canal), infected atheroma, otogenic zygomaticitis, and TMJ arthritis. With disease of the *submandibular gland*, differentiation is required from abscess of the tongue (base and oral floor and from dentogenic abscess formation. See also p. 237 and Table 2.**10**.

Chronic Recurrent Parotitis

Main symptoms: Inflammation is usually unilateral and most common in children and adolescents. Generally runs a painful course of 3–8 days with marked glandular swelling. Active phases, marked by hyposalosis with a milky, granular, or purulent discharge, alternate with asymptomatic periods lasting weeks to years.

Other symptoms and special features: Cases may resolve spontaneously during puberty.* Adult cases have a less favorable prognosis (atrophy of the glandular parenchyma culminating in a chronic sialectatic parotid gland with absent or diminished salivation).

Causes: Not fully understood. Based on disturbances in the production and transport of glandular secretions. Viral disease, immunopathologic processes, and congenital ductal ectasia have been postulated.

Diagnosis:
- Typical history with characteristic local and palpable findings in the active phase. During quiescent periods the gland usually appears normal or may be slightly indurated.
- Sialography shows a "tree-in-leaf" figure with ectatic ducts forming a string-of-beads or cluster-of-grapes pattern.
- Some cases may require biopsy.
- Laboratory tests show leukocytosis with a left shift, an elevated ESR, and a rise of serum amylases.

Differentiation is required from sialolithiasis, a slow-growing tumor, fungal infection, tuberculosis, actinomycosis, and allergic sialadenitis.

Chronic Sialadenitis of the Submandibular Gland
See p. 302.

Epidemic Parotitis (Mumps)

Main symptoms: Painful, doughy swelling of the parotid gland, chiefly affecting children. Involvement is bilateral in 75% ("hamster cheeks"). Fever need not be present! *Non*purulent discharge from the Stensen duct.

Other symptoms and special features: The other major salivary glands may also be involved. Potential involvement of the gonads, pancreas, CNS, and inner ear (see p. 65). Peak occurrence is from 2 to 14 years of age.

Cause: Paramyxoma viruses transmitted by droplet infection.

Diagnosis:
- Direct detection of the causative virus (possible only in the early stage)
- Initial leukopenia with relative lymphocytosis.
- Serologic testing (complement binding reaction and/or hemagglutination inhibition test). Fourfold rise of antibody titer (within about 3 weeks) confirms mumps infection.
- Transient elevation of amylase and diastase in the serum and urine.

Differentiation is required from true (bacterial) parotitis, chronic recurrent parotitis, sialolithiasis, dentogenic infection, coxsackievirus infection (serologic titer assay), cytomegalovirus infection in infants and newborns, and parotid tumors.

Cytomegalovirus and Coxsackievirus Parotitis
See p. 302.

Sialolithiasis

Main symptoms: Marked, usually painful swelling of the affected salivary gland ("tension pain") brought on by eating. The overwhelming site of predilection is the submandibular gland (85%). In long-standing cases the gland remains swollen between meals. Calculi in the parotid gland account for only about 10% of cases.

Other symptoms and special features: Males are affected twice as frequently as females. The stone may be detectable in the gland or its excretory duct by bimanual palpation. If the stone is located near the duct orifice, a grating sound may be heard and a rough surface felt when a probe is passed into the duct. It is not uncommon to encounter multiple stones in one gland.

Causes: Calculus formation (calcium phosphate or calcium carbonate) in the excretory duct of the salivary gland secondary to electrolyte sialadenitis (=abnormal salivary composition; see Table 5.5) or the presence of a foreign body (nidus for crystalization) in the duct.

Diagnosis:
● Typical history; often positive findings on palpation or probing.
● Stones may be identified by radiographic examination or sialography (filling defect).

Differentiation is required from an intraglandular tumor, calcified tuberculous lymph node, and chronic sclerosing sialadenitis of the submandibular gland (a Küttner tumor).

Electrolyte Sialadenitis

Main symptoms: Transient swelling of the submandibular gland during and after eating, usually with tension pain, which may be very severe. The glandular discharge is milky or purulent, usually with increased viscosity. Electrolyte sialadenitis is on a continuum with sialolithiasis.

Causes: Changes in the composition of the salivary electrolytes ("dyschylia") with ductal inflammation and the formation of organic stenoses and microliths.

Diagnosis:
● Sialometry and determination of biochemical salivary parameters.
● Sialography may be informative.
● Some cases require biopsy, preferably done as a complete excisional biopsy.

Differential diagnosis is the same as for sialolithiasis.

Drug-Related Salivary Gland Pain

Patients taking antihypertensive medication (e.g., clonidine, a-methyldopa, guanethidine derivatives) or psychotropic drugs may experience pain, especially in the parotid region, which may be transient (most pronounced at the start of mastication) or prolonged and very bothersome. Local findings are negative, though oral dryness may be present. A correct diagnosis can be made empirically by questioning the patient about current medications and, if necessary, by trial withdrawal and replacement of the suspect agent. See also Table 5.7.

Auriculotemporal Neuralgia
See p. 16.

Sialadenitis of the Minor Salivary Glands
(e.g., granulomatous cheilitis)
See p. 241.

Radiation Sialadenitis

Main symptoms: Increasing, burning pain and dry mouth ("xerostomia"), which may be transient or permanent depending on the radiation dose. Hypogeusia or ageusia (see p. 294).

Cause: Damage of the salivary gland parenchyma by ionizing radiation.

Diagnosis:
● Typical history and symptomatology.
● Sialometry and salivary chemistry are seldom indicated.

Differentiation is required from drug side effects, dehydration in a debilitated patient, and hematologic disease.

Tumors

Many malignant tumors of the salivary glands cause significant pain at a relatively early stage or at least a troublesome sensation of tension and pressure. The gradual, unilateral enlargement of a gland combined with pain should always raise suspicion of malignant disease.

Symptom   **Morphologic Change (Swelling, Tumor)**

This section deals with salivary gland diseases whose cardinal symptom is swelling or alteration of shape. Pain is either absent or is overshadowed by the morphologic change.

This disorders listed in Table 5.2 were not classified as inflammatory versus noninflammatory due to persisting discrepancies of nomenclature.

Cytomegalovirus Sialadenitis

Main symptoms: Most common in children under 2 years of age. Swelling of the parotid glands; the other major salivary glands are less commonly affected. Occasional features: jaundice, hepatosplenomegaly, anemia, hemorrhagic diathesis.

Other symptoms and special features: The course in small children is variable; pediatric management is required. Symptoms in adult cases are highly variable and nonspecific.

Causes: Viral infection acquired transplacentally or postnatally (DNA virus of the herpes group).

Diagnosis:
● Serologic antibody testing (> 1:64). Increased complement binding reaction.
● Cytodiagnostic or histologic diagnosis may be required.
● Pathogenic organism can be grown from saliva and urine in human tissue culture.

Differentiation is required from other infectious salivary gland diseases. Exclusion of rhesus incompatibility may be required.

Coxsackievirus Sialadenitis

Main symptoms: Parotid swelling and/or swelling of minor salivary glands, gingivitis. Some cases commence with herpangina (see p. 231).

Diagnosis: Serologic titer determination.

Chronic Sialadenitis of the Submandibular Gland ("Küttner Tumor")

Main symptoms: Enlargement and induration of the submandibular gland. Possible feeling of pressure but no pain. Inspissated saliva. Gradual conversion to sclerosing fibrosis of the glandular parenchyma ("salivary gland cirrhosis").

Cause: Apparently secondary to electrolyte sialadenitis (see p. 301). An autoimmune pathogenesis has been suggested.

Diagnosis:
● Typical local and palpable findings.
● Diagnosis may be aided by analysis of salivary chemistry.
● Excisional biopsy of the affected gland.

Differentiation is required from a salivary gland malignancy, tuberculosis, Sjögren disease, fungal infection, calcified submandibular lymph nodes, etc.

Cystic Lesions

Main symptoms: Tense, spherical, nonpainful masses in the (parotid) gland body, which enlarge very slowly and usually are poorly displaceable on palpation. Other cysts are extraglandular and present as a soft, boggy, submucous mass (e.g., *sublingual ranula*). Cysts of the salivary glands are relatively common, accounting for approximately 7% of all salivary gland diseases.

Causes: Salivary gland cysts are classified etiologically as follows:

○ Primary (true dysgenetic) cysts
○ Secondary cysts resulting from ductal obstruction and stasis (calculi, ductal angulation, trauma)
○ Pseudocysts that lack an epithelial lining
○ Cysts forming in neoplasms
○ Mucoceles ("mucous granulomas") in the minor salivary glands (especially of the lower lip), the most common type of secondary cyst

Special features: Most cystic lesions of the *parotid gland* are secondary *salivary duct cysts.* Peak occurrence is in the 6th−7th decades with a predilection for males. Dysgenetic cysts based on congenital sialectasis and a cystic parotid gland are very rare. *Ranulas* are relatively common in the *sublingual gland*; presumably they can have both a dysgenetic and a secondary monocystic or polycystic pathogenesis. Most common around puberty, ranulas of sufficient size can cause impairment of swallowing and/or speech.

Diagnosis:
● Typical local and palpable findings.
● Some cases may require sialography or needle biopsy.
● Complete excisional biopsy.

Differentiation is required from enlarged intraglandular lymph nodes, (foreign-body) ductal and parenchymal granulomas (e.g., following contrast extravasation from the duct system during sialography), salivary gland neoplasms (mostly benign), and occupational *"pneumatocele"* in glassblowers and musicians (stretching of the glandular duct system by the constant action of high air pressures).

Allergic and Pseudoallergic Sialadenitis

Main symptoms: Transient but recurrent, usually bilateral swelling, chiefly affecting the parotid gland, in response to allergen exposure (medications such as nitrofurantoin or phenylbutazone, certain foods). *Diagnosis* of this rare disorder is by exclusion or possibly by histologic examination. See also Tables 3.**5** and 4.**8** and p. 249.

Myoepithelial Sialadenitis (Sjögren Disease)

Main symptoms: Swelling of the parotid gland and occasionally the submandibular gland with gradual enlargement, usually bilateral. No pain. Increasing xerostomia with atrophy of the lingual mucosa and replacement of the glandular tissue by fatty or connective tissue. Xerophthalmia with involvement of the lacrimal glands.

Other symptoms and special features: Women are affected almost exclusively (during meno-

Table 5.**2** *Symptom* Morphologic change (swelling, tumor)

Synopsis
Acute course
Intracapsular hemorrhage, see p. 299
Cytomegalovirus sialadenitis
Coxsackievirus sialadenitis
Sialolithiasis, see p. 300
Chronic course
Chronic sialadenitis of the submandibular gland (Küttner tumor)
Cystic lesions, ranulae
Allergic sialadenitis
Myoepithelial sialadenitis (Sjögren disease)
Epitheloid cell sialadenitis (sarcoidosis, Heerfordt syndrome, uveoparotid fever)
Sialadenoses
Specific inflammatory conditions (tuberculosis, syphilis)
Inflammation of the paraglandular and/or intraglandular lymph nodes
Other rare salivary gland diseases (fungal infection, actinomycosis, lipomatosis)
Tumors of the salivary glands (sialomas), see Table 5.**3**

pause). Common accompanying manifestations are pharyngitis and laryngotracheitis sicca, rheumatoid arthropathies, purpura rheumatica, and periarteritis nodosa. The disease does not always manifest in a fully developed form.

Causes: Presumably autoimmune (collagen disease, "autoimmune exocrinopathy").

Diagnosis:
● Typical local findings of salivary gland swelling, and sometimes combined with augmentation of the lacrimal glands, sicca symptoms.
● Decreased lacrimal production in the Schirmer test.
● Sialography shows ductal ectasia and, in later stages, a "tree-in-leaf" pattern. Sialochemistry (usually difficult to analyze due to paucity of saliva) shows increased levels of sodium, chlorine, lactoferrin, albumin, and immunoglobulin A, G, and especially M with reduced phosphate levels.

• Greatly increased ESR, hypochromic anemia, elevated serum gamma globulins. Rheumatoid factors can be demonstrated. Immunofluorescent detection of antibodies against salivary ductal antigen and antinuclear factors.
• Biopsy from the glandular parenchyma or lip mucosa (immunohistology).

Differentiation is required from chronic sialadenitis, drug side effects, actinomycosis, adenolymphoma, malignant lymphoma, and other malignancies.

Epitheloid-cell Sialadenitis (Sarcoidosis, Heerfordt Syndrome, Unveoparotid Fever)

Main symptoms: Symmetrical parotid swelling is common, but unilateral symptoms can occur. Gland has a moderately firm consistency and may present a humped surface. Possible reduction of salivary flow. Pain is unusual. An undulant fever pattern may be observed.

Other symptoms and special features: Possible lacrimal gland involvement and uveitis. Women are affected more frequently than men. Other concomitant organ manifestations of sarcoidosis may occur.

Causes: Extrapulmonary manifestation of Besnier–Boeck–Schaumann disease (see p. 255).

Diagnosis:
• Local findings.
• Positive Kveim test; tuberculin test is generally negative.
• Elevated serum levels of angiotensinase I.
• Diagnosis is proven by biopsy.
• Search for possible additional organ manifestations (lung, bones, etc.).

Differentiation is required from Sjögren disease, glandular tuberculosis, sialadenosis, and neoplasia.

Sialadenosis

Main symptoms: Usually painless but occasionally painful swelling of *both* parotid glands, which may be intermittent or persist for just a few days. "Hamster cheeks." The saliva may be normal in quantity and consistency, or salivary viscosity may be increased leading to dry mouth.

Other symptoms and special features: Prolonged use of sympathicomimetic drugs (asthma therapy) can also lead to bilateral parotid swelling and oral dryness.

Causes: Endocrine and metabolic disorders (e.g., in diabetes, pregnancy, menopause, adrenocortical dysfunction, vitamin deficiency, protein deficiency, alcoholism, starvation dystrophy) and neurogenic causes are known.

Diagnosis:
• Typical local findings; painless fluctuant swelling is suggestive of sialadenosis.
• Sialography shows a "leafless tree" pattern signifying a very narrow ductal system.
• Biopsy.
• Head and neck examination is followed by an endocrinologic workup to establish the cause. If a pharmacologic cause is suspected, trial withdrawal of the suspect drug is indicated.

Differentiation is required from chronic parotitis and Sjögren disease.

Specific Diseases of the Salivary Glands

Tuberculosis of the salivary glands is the most clinically important disease of this group. It can affect any of the major salivary glands, is generally unilateral, and produces a virtually painless swelling of the gland that may culminate in a draining fistula with purulent discharge. Primary involvement is very rare, and most cases represent a postprimary infection of the gland or lymph nodes by the hematogenous route. The affected gland presents an irregular, indurated surface on palpation. Sialography may show pooling of contrast medium in intraglandular degenerative foci. Biopsy confirms the diagnosis.

Other Rare Glandular Diseases

Fungal Infection

Fungal infection of the salivary glands is extremely rare. It most commonly affects the submandibular gland or one of the minor salivary glands occurring throughout the oral cavity, possibly in conjunction with a mucosal fungal infection.

Lipomatosis

This diffuse proliferation of fatty tissue in the parotid gland ("pseudohypertrophy") occasionally occurs in children and is also observed in diabetes, obesity, hypertension, or as a sequel to a coxsackievirus infection ("lipomatosis parotid atrophy").

Tumors of the Salivary Glands (Sialomas)

Benign Sialomas

The more common *epithelial neoplasms* of the salivary glands are listed in Table 5.**3**. The problem of differential diagnosis in this group is that, while the history, length of illness, local findings, and other symptoms may suggest a benign neoplasm with a very high index of probability, histologic examination is necessary to reach a definitive diagnosis. The consequences of mistaking a malignancy for a benign tumor are so potentially grave that the slightest doubt regarding tumor nature warrants excisional biopsy (removing the entire lesion with clear margins confirmed by frozen sections)!

Seifert reports that 90% of salivary gland tumors are epithelial in origin. Approximately 25% of these tumors are malignant. Only about 20% of epithelial tumors of the *parotid gland* are malignant, as opposed to 45% for the *submandibular gland*, 90% for the *sublingual gland*, and 45% for the *minor salivary glands!*

Pleomorphic Adenoma

Main symptoms: Smooth, round or nodular, painless mass with a tense consistency ("tennis ball") and very slow growth (often >5 years). There is no fixation of the overlying skin.

Other findings and special features: Peak occurrence is in the 4th and 5th decades with a slight preponderance of females. Even with very large tumors, the facial nerve remains functional for a remarkably long time.

Diagnosis:
● Long history and typical findings on palpation.

● Sialography shows displacement of the ductal system (basket-like ductal pattern). May be supplemented by CT. Salivary production and chemistry are normal.
● Complete excisional biopsy. It is best *not* to precede the excision by an incisional or punch biopsy (risk of tumor cell dissemination).

Differentiation is required from other parotid tumors, including malignancies, parotid cysts, and sialolithiasis.

Special Form

A *"dumbbell"* or *"iceberg" tumor* results from the extension of a pleomorphic adenonma toward the pharynx. Inspection in these cases reveals a firm, poorly displaceable, mucosa-covered neoplasm with a round or humped surface located, for example, *behind the palatine tonsil* in the pharynx. Larger growths cause speech impairment and dysphagia.

Cystadenolymphoma (Warthin Tumor)

Main symptoms: Soft, mobile, painless, slow-growing, frequently bilateral mass most commonly occurring in the parotid gland.

Other symptoms and special features: Chiefly affects males between 50 and 60 years of age.

Diagnosis:
● Typical long history, typical palpable presentation of a soft, mobile mass. Frequently bilateral.
● Biopsy, preferably by complete excision.

Differentiation is required from monomorphic adenoma, hemangioma, cyst, and enlarged lymph nodes.

Monomorphic Adenoma

This tumor belongs to the same group of sialomas as cystadenolymphoma.

Main symptoms: Usually arising in the parotid gland, the tumor produces a painless swelling that has much the same clinical presentation as pleomorphic adenoma and cystadenolymphoma. The tumor is rare and generally unilateral.

Diagnosis:
● Palpable findings.

- Sialography may show displacement of the ductal system.
- Incisional or complete excisional biopsy.

Malignant Salivary Gland Tumors

Even more so than with benign sialomas, the differential diagnosis of malignant salivary gland tumors *always* requires biopsy. The present section, then, centers on clinical features that are specific for certain tumor types.

Acinous Cell Tumor (Acinous Cell Carcinoma)

Main symptoms: Spherical mass with a somewhat firm consistency, usually located in the parotid gland and rarely in the submandibular gland. Clinical behavior is relatively "benign," and pain is not typical. Peak incidence is between 30 and 60 years of age, and males predominate by 3:1.

Diagnosis and prognosis rely on biopsy. Lymphogenous metastases are rare, hematogenous very rare.

Differentiation is mainly required from adenocarcinoma.

Mucoepidermoid Tumor (Mucoepidermoid Carcinoma)

Main symptoms: Most tumors affect the parotid gland (65%), with one-third occurring in the minor salivary glands. Two grades of malignancy are recognized: *Low-grade tumors* (about 75% of cases) present as a slow-growing, painless, circumscribed nodule having a variable (usually rubbery) consistency. *High-grade tumors* (about 25%) present as a fast-growing, painful, poorly displaceable mass with occasional associated facial paralysis (25%) and regional lymphogenous spread (50%). Most cases occur in the 4th–5th decades, with a 3:1 predominance of females.

Differential diagnosis requires biopsy.

Carcinoma of the Salivary Glands

Adenoid Cystic Carcinoma

Main symptoms: This tumor very often involves the minor salivary glands (in the palate, cheek, etc.) as well as the sublingual gland, submandibular gland, and parotid. Palpation reveals a hard, often nodulated mass that is fixed or poorly displaceable. Growth is generally very slow initially (5 years or more) and is often associated with severe pain or paresthesia, especially in later stages. The tumor tends to track along nerves and vessels, and facial paralysis is relatively common (25%). Other cranial neuropathies (V–VII, IX–XII) are common in later stages. There is about a 15% incidence of regional lymphogenous spread. Distant hematogenous spread (to lung, brain, bones, liver, etc.) is relatively common (15–20%), especially in advanced cases.

Diagnosis:
- Typical symptoms.
- Sialography (filling defects in the ductal system, possible diffuse contrast extravasation). CT. Sonography may also be useful.
- Diagnosis and prognosis rely on biopsy.

Adenocarcinoma

See Table 5.3 for prevalence. The parotid gland is the site of predilection in more than 70% of cases. Peak incidence is from 60 to 70 years of age. Palpation discloses a hard mass that is fixed or poorly mobile. Fixation of the overlying skin is common. There is usually severe pain. Early facial paralysis occurs in 40% of cases with parotid involvement, but lymphogenous and hematogenous metastasis are relatively late events. Diagnosis is the same as for adenoid cystic carcinoma.

Squamous Cell Carcinoma

See Table 5.3 for prevalence. The tumor presents as a firm, poorly circumscribed mass, fixed or poorly mobile, in the parotid or other major salivary glands. Pain is usually severe. Preoperative facial paralysis develops in more than half of cases. Tumor may metastasize to the parotid gland from distant sites or may in-

Table 5.**3**   Histologic classification of salivary gland tumors (after G. Seifert, A. Miehlke, J. Haubrich, R. Chilla: Speicheldrüsenkrankheiten. Thieme, Stuttgart 1984)

Adenomas		**65.5%**
Pleomorphic adenomas		47.5%
(approx. 85% of which are in the parotid)		
Monomorphic adenomas		18 %
Cystadenolymphoma	73%	
Salivary duct adenoma	19%	
Others (e.g., basal cell adenoma, oncocytic adenoma,		
sebaceous adenoma, clear cell adenoma)	8%	
	100%	
Malignant epithelial tumors		**22.5%**
Acinous cell tumors		2 %
Mucoepidermoid tumors		4.5%
Carcinomas		16 %
Adenoid cystic carcinoma	23%	
Adenocarcinoma	14%	
Squamous cell carcinoma	11%	
Carcinoma in pleomorphic adenoma	31%	
Salivary duct carcinoma	5%	
Undifferentiated carcinoma	8%	
Other carcinomas	8%	
	100%	
Nonepithelial tumors		**4.5%**
Angiomas		
Lipomas		
Neuromas		
Neurofibromas		
Chondromas, etc.		
Various sarcomas		
Periglandular tumors and metastases		**7.5%**
		100 %

(n = approximately 3000; some of the above numbers were rounded)

vade the gland from contiguous structures, and vice versa. Superficial cancers cause relatively early fixation of the overlying skin, which later ulcerates in the tumor area. There is early lymphogenous spread to cervical lymph noses. The diagnostic steps are the same as for adenoid cystic carcinoma.

Carcinoma in Pleomorphic Adenoma

See Table 5.**3** for prevalence. Malignant transformation of a known, long-standing pleomorphic adenoma may be signaled by sudden rapid growth, pain, or increasing facial paralysis.

Peak incidence is in the 6th–7th decades. Suspicion of malignancy warrants immediate biopsy, preferably a complete excision with frozen-section confirmation of margins.

Nonepithelial Sialomas

Nonepithelial sialomas are salivary gland tumors and neoplasms that do not arise from the salivary gland tissue itself but from tissues accompanying the gland. Aside from hemangioma, lipoma, and neuroma, these are rare or very rare neoplasms involving the salivary glands.

Special Tumors

Hemangioma and Lymphangioma

These relatively common benign tumors account for some 1% of all salivary gland neoplasms. Seventy-five percent are congenital, and 90% are manifested before 1 year of age. Eighty percent occur in the parotid gland, 18% in the submandibular gland, and the rest in the remaining salivary glands. See pp. 146 and 405 for further details.

Neural Tumors (Neuromas, Neurofibromas, Components of Neuofibromatosis), Lipomas, Fibromas, and Granular Cell Tumors

All of these are rare. Diagnosis is established by biopsy.

Sarcomas

Various types of sarcoma occur in all age groups but *rarely* involve the salivary glands. Diagnosis necessitates biopsy.

Malignant Lymphomas

More than one-third of malignant lymphomas in the head and neck region are located in the salivary glands (parotid, submandibular gland, minor glands of the palate and oropharynx). The majority are non-Hodgkin lymphomas, which may be associated with Sjögren disease. Peak incidence is from age 60 to 70 (versus 20 to 30 for Hodgkin lymphoma), but children may be affected. Biopsy is essential for differential diagnosis.

Other malignant diseases that can involve the major salivary glands and especially the parotid are *leukemia* and *melanoma*, in which swelling is the cardinal symptom. Virtually all of these cases are secondary manifestations, however.

Symptom   **Malformation**

Malformations and anomalies of the salivary glands are of little clinical importance and play a very minor role in differential diagnosis. The most important are listed in Table 5.**4**.

Table 5.**4**   *Symptom*   Malformation or anomaly of the salivary glands (after Seifert)

Synopsis	
Disease	Cardinal symptom or distinctive clinical feature
Glandular aplasia and ductal atresia	If complete, extreme xerostomia; since most cases are partial and unilateral, dysfunction is not severe. Other coexisting anomalies are not uncommon. Parotid is chiefly affected
Dystopic and accessory glands	Glands are generally functional but have a misplaced ductal orifice (oral commissure, palate, etc.). Parotid is most commonly affected
Aberrant glands	These glands are nonfunctional because they lack an excretory duct (secondary salivary fistula may occur). Located in the lateral neck, pharynx, middle ear; pituitary

Cysts and sialectasias
– Dysgenetic (sialocele)
  – Cystic parotid gland
  – Sialectasia (parotid)
  – Salivary duct diverticulum
  – Sublingual gland ranula
  – Branchiogenic cyst
– Acquired
	See p. 302
	
	See p. 302
	See pp. 27, 402

Salivary fistulae – Congenital – Acquired	Depends on site and nature of causative trauma

Symptom   **Disturbance of Salivary Production**

Disturbances of salivary production are manifested either by an *abnormal quantity of secretion* (sialorrhea, hypersialia, hypersalivation versus sialopenia, hyposialia, asialia, hyposalivation) or by an *abnormal composition of the secretion* (dyschylia). Congenital factors and/or acquired functional disturbances may have causal significance. Exogenous factors (drugs, toxic effects, etc.) should also be included in the differential diagnosis. Normal values for salivary production and chemistry are summarized in Table 5.**5**.

A causal distinction is drawn between *primary dyschylia* (caused by metabolic and neurohormonal influences) and *secondary dyschylia* (e.g., due to sialadenitis or a salivary gland tumor). *Proteodyschylia* is distinguished from

Table 5.**5**   Parotid secretion (biochemical values)

Biochemical salivary values fluctuate interindividually and with time of day, season, nutritional state, gender, etc. They can also vary markedly among the glands of an individual subject, and significant discrepancies appear in the values reported by different investigators. The figures below represent approximations, therefore.			
Criterion	At rest		After stimulation
Flow rate	up to 1 mL/10 min		2–15 mL/10 min
Sodium (mEq)	up to 10		20–80
Potassium (mEq)	15–35		20–40
Total protein (mg/mL)	2–10		2–10
Lysozyme (µg/mL)	16–520		8–60
Amylase (U/mL)	150–600		100–700
Immunoglobulin A (mg/mL)	0.03–0.3		0.01–0.1
Protease inhibitor (U/mL)	5–18		0.5–10
	Flow rate	Lysozyme	Protein	IgA
Sialadenosis	Normal to slightly increased	Decreased	Decreased	Decreased
Sialadenitis	Decreased	(Strongly) increased	Strongly increased (especially albumin)	(Strongly) increased

mucodyschylia and *hydrodyschylia* according to the pathologic change in the *biochemical composition* of the secretion. While these abnormalities of salivary composition are of substantial clinical interest, their biochemical detection has not yet become a routine diagnostic procedure. Thus, the data currently available in this area and their discriminating ability are not yet adequate to provide a reliable basis for differential diagnosis.

For the present, then, the quantity of saliva and its variations provide the best index for purposes of differential diagnosis. The synopsis in Table 5.**6** lists diseases and states that are characterized by *excessive salivation (sialorrhea)*. Potential causes of *deficient salivation (sialopenia)* are listed in Table 5.**7**. The extreme case is *asialia*, which is associated with the clinical picture of *xerostomia* (see pp. 301, 303 and Table 5.**7**).

Table 5.**6** *Symptom* Sialorrhea (hypersalivation, hypersialia) (causes)

Synopsis

Physiologic states
Acidic foods (fruit, vinegar, etc.)
Pregnancy (ptyalism)
Appetite stimulants
States of excitation
Nausea and vomiting

Diseases
Stomatitis, diseases of the mouth and tongue
Foreign body in the pharynx
Head injury
Diabetes insipidus
Parkinson disease
Cerebral palsy, hemiplegia
Encephalitis
Brain tumors
Paralysis
Sluder neuralgia
Erythroprosopalgia (Bing–Horton)
Myasthenia gravis
Wilson disease
Rabies
Botulism
Pellagra
Mongolism (Down syndrome)
Schizophrenia
Manic–depressive psychoses

Toxicity
Metal poisonings (mercury compounds)

Pharmacologic agents
Acetylcholine
Alkylphosphates (parathion)
Amanita muscaria
Ammonium chloride
Apomorphine

Beta-receptor blocking drugs
Quinine
Chloroform
Clonazepam
Cocaine
Caffeine
Cyclopropane
Digitalis
Ethionamide, prothionamide (tuberculostatics)
Fluorions
Halogen compounds
Cardiac glycosides
Ipecac
Methacholine
Morphine
Neostigmine
Nicotine in small doses
Nitrazepam
Peppermint
Picrotoxin
Pilocarpine
Physostigmine
Prostigmin
Reserpine
Strychnine
Sympathicomimetic drugs (e. g., atropine)
Theophylline
Veratrum alkaloids (veratrin)
Citric acid
Parasympathicomimetic drugs, cholinergic agents, anticholinesterases
Sympathicolytic drugs (e. g., α-dibenamine, β-propranolol)
Direct action on salivary glands (e. g., physalaemin, eledoisin, nitrogen mustard)
Ganglion-blocking drugs (e. g., hexamethonium)

Table 5.**7** *Symptom* Sialopenia (hyposalivation, hyposialia, asialia, sicca syndrome) (causes)

Synopsis	
Physiologic states	Anticholinergic agents
Hot work environment	Antiparkinson drugs
Dusty work environment	Antihistamines
	Antihypertensive drugs (reserpine, clonidine,
Diseases	guanethidine group, α-methyldopa)
Acute inflammation of the mouth and pharynx	Atropine
Febrile infections	Barbiturates
Epitheloid cell sialadenitis (Sjögren disease)	Belladonna
Electrolyte sialadenitis	β-Receptor blocking drugs (e. g., propranolol)
Radiation sialadenitis (dose > 10 Gy)	Broad-spectrum antibiotics (some)
Alcoholism	Cannabinol and derivatives
Vitamin A deficiency	Chlorothiazides
Hyperthyroidism, Basedow disease	Cocaine
Hypertension	Decongestants
Diabetes mellitus	Dinitrophenol
Pernicious anemia	Ganglioplegics
Iron deficiency anemia (Plummer–Vinson)	LSD
Gastric achylia	Mescaline
Dehydration (diarrhea, vomiting)	Methadone
Central nervous disorders (pituitary, trauma)	MAO inhibitors
Uremia	Nicotine in *large* doses
Other comatose or precomatose states	Oligomycin
Cachexia and marasmus	Pethidine
Endogenous depression	Psychotropic drugs (antidepressants, tricyclic
	thymoleptics)
Toxicity	Scopolamine
See Tables 4.**8** and 4.**9**	Spasmolytics
	Tolbutamide (Rastinon)
Pharmacologic agents	Xylocaine
Aldosterone antagonists (e. g., Aldactone)	
α-Receptor blocking drugs (e. g., phenylephrine)	

Syndromes Associated with Salivary Gland Disorders

See Table 5.**8**.

Table 5.8 Syndromes associated with salivary gland disorders

Syndrome	Classification	Typical ENT deficits	Remarks
AOP syndrome (obesity–hyperthermia–oligomenorrhea–parotid syndrome)	Diencephalic dysfunction of unknown cause	Painful, recurrent parotid enlargement in women	Additional features: obesity (Froelich type), oligo- or dysmenorrhea. Symptoms are not always fully developed
Frey syndrome (auriculotemporal syndrome, gustatory, sweating)	Increased sweating due to disturbance of auriculotemporal innervation	Skin redness and hyperhidrosis over the parotid region stimulated by eating (especially of acidic, bitter, hard, or hot foods) or emotional stress, usually following parotidectomy (after an asymptomatic interval > 10 months) or parotitis	Presumably identical to salivosudoriparous (Dupuy) syndrome. May be combined with auriculotemporal neuralgia
Heerfordt syndrome (subchronic uveoparotid fever)	Manifestation of Bresnier–Boeck–Schaumann disease in the parotid gland, lacrimal glands, and eye	See p. 304	
Mikulicz syndrome	Oculosalivary syndrome that may develop in various systemic diseases	Slowly increasing, painless swelling of the lacrimal and salivary glands (sometimes only partial). Xerostomia, hypolacrimia	Retention of this disease name is problematic because it is not based on a consistent etiology or uniform morphologic substrate (occurs, for example, in sarcoidosis and Hodgkin disease)
Sjögren syndrome (sicca syndrome)	Systemic disease with secretory insufficiency of the eccrine glands. Autoimmune disease of the rheumatoid group	See p. 303	Xerostomia

6. Larynx

General Clinical Aspects

The Symptoms

○ Pain (and dysesthesia), p. 315

○ Habitual throat clearing, p. 318

○ Cough, p. 318

○ Morphologic change (swelling, tumor), p. 320

○ Malformation, p. 327

○ Hoarseness, p. 329

○ Hemoptysis, p. 273

○ Dyspnea, p. 365

○ Stridor, p. 329

Principal Diagnostic Methods

The larynx performs a combination of vital and communicative functions (respiration, protection of the lower airway, phonation). Consequently, different diagnostic methods will be applied depending on the nature of the differential diagnostic inquiry. Some of the same methods are used in investigations of the *trachea*.

Besides the *history*, the following primary and adjunctive procedures are available for *routine evaluations* of the larynx:

○ *External palpation* of the larynx and surrounding soft tissues. This can be especially rewarding in traumatologic and oncologic investigations (displacements of the cartilage skeleton, abnormal mobility, swelling, fixation, status of the large cervical vessels and reginal lymph nodes, etc.).

○ Classic *indirect laryngoscopy* with a mirror. This precedes any instrumental exploration of the larynx, at least as a pilot examination.

○ The *magnifying laryngoscope* also employs an indirect light path but offers the option of optical magnification and photographic documentation of the interior of the larynx.

○ A very rewarding procedure is *direct laryngoscopy* in the form of *microlaryngoscopy*. This combines use of a self-retaining laryngoscope with the operating microscope, permitting the examination of structures at varying magnifications, selective tissue sampling, and other endolaryngeal manipulations. It allows for photographic, video, and cinematographic documentation and follow-ups at least as far as the upper trachea. The necessity of general anesthesia limits the indications for direct laryngoscoopy.

○ If a self-retaining laryngoscope cannot be used, *endoscopic biopsy* can still be performed "indirectly" with appropriate instruments using the laryngeal mirror as a guide.

○ *"Transconioscopy"* (Euler and Mårtensson) involves the introduction of a rod-lens telescope from the outside through a portal in the conical ligament (cricothyroid membrane). This procedure can assist differential diagnosis in very rare cases, e.g., for subglottic evaluation in patients with glottic stenosis.

○ *Biopsy.*

○ *Microbiologic smears.*

○ *Cytodiagnosis* (very rarely indicated).

○ *Diagnostic imaging:*
  − *Conventional radiography:* Soft-tissue radiographs of the larynx and/or trachea in the sagittal and lateral projections.
  − *Xeroradiography,* a special contrast-enhancing technique that can be useful for studying the larynx.

- *Tomography* in its various technical modifications is still the most widely used method for radiographic evaluation of the larynx and trachea in many places. One modification, *laryngography*, provides enhanced contour definition by coating mucosal surfaces with contrast material.
- *Computed tomography* (CT), with or without contrast enhancement, is increasingly supplanting "conventional" tomography of the larynx, trachea, and surroundings owing to its superior diagnostic information content and higher yield.
- *Radionuclide imaging* can be useful for selected investigations of the cricoarytenoid joint, thyroid gland, and lymph nodes.
- *Angiography*, especially using the digital subtraction technique.
- *Magnetic resonance imaging* (MRI) can provide detailed images of the larynx and trachea and offers a strong alternative to CT.
- *Sonography* plays a very minor role in evaluations of the larynx and trachea.
○ *Stroboscopy* with video recording permits detailed observation, analysis, and documentation of vocal cord vibration and movement (see p. 336).
○ Various *special phoniatric tests* are also available (see p. 336).

Symptom   Pain (and Dysesthesia)

There is considerable diversity in the subjective perception of pain and especially "dysesthesia" in the laryngeal region as symptoms of disease. Some degree of discomfort is present in almost all laryngeal disorders. The present section deals only with diseases in which pain or dysesthesia is generally reported as a *main symptom* (Table 6.**1**).

Acute Laryngitis

Main symptoms: Pain or a disturbing "rough" feeling and dryness in the larynx. Dry cough and/or habitual throat clearing and tickling. Increasing hoarseness ranging to painful aphonia. Laryngoscopy: Vocal cords appear red and sometimes swollen, and cord adduction may be incomplete.

Causes: Ascending or descending mucosal infection—usually a primary viral infection with risk of bacterial superinfection. Exogenous noninfectious insults; dry, dusty air; gases and caustic vapors. Attacks of coughing. Damage by physical, thermal, or chemical agents is also common. Systemic diseases can be predisposing (diabetes, dystrophy).

Diagnosis:
● History, giving special attention to the duration of complaints and any underlying diseases or contact with injurious agents.
● Laryngoscopic findings.

Differentiation is required from chronic laryngitis, vocal cord pachyderma, specific laryngitis (typically causing monocorditis with *unilateral* cord redness and swelling, see p. 323), and neoplasms (see p. 325). "Acute laryngitis" persisting for more than 2–3 weeks requires very careful evaluation!

Special Forms
Associated with Pain or Discomfort

○ *Acute vocal abuse ("fatigue catarrh")*. Even in the *absence* of an infectious inflammatory cause, poor vocal habits or misuse of the voice can produce laryngitis-like symptoms of irritation with pain (see also pp. 339, 349).
○ *Fibrinous laryngitis*, marked by fibrinous membranes coating the laryngeal mucosa.
○ *Ulceromembranous laryngitis*, marked by a greasy coating and mucosal ulcerations on

Table 6.1 *Symptom* Pain and dysesthesia

Synopsis
Acute "simple" laryngitis and special forms
– Acute vocal abuse
– Fibrinous laryngitis
– Ulceromembranous laryngitis
– Diphtheric laryngitis
– Acute stenosing laryngotracheitis in children (pseudocroup), see p. 332 and Table 6.**11**
Cricoarytenoid arthritis
Acute and hyperacute epiglottitis
Laryngeal trauma (caustic injury, blunt and sharp trauma)
– Sharp and blunt external or internal trauma
– Injurious physical and chemical agents
– Foreign bodies
– Iatrogenic trauma
Laryngeal perichondritis
Laryngeal abscess and cellulitis
Superior laryngeal neuralgia
Chronic laryngitis, see p. 320
Contact ulcer, see p. 350
Specific laryngitis, see p. 323
Benign and malignant tumors, see p. 325

the inside of the larynx and the epiglottis, usually coexisting with Plaut–Vincent angina.

○ *Diphtheric laryngitis*, marked by patchy and later confluent, dirty white, firmly adherent mucosal deposits (see p. 233).

Acute (Stenosing) Laryngotracheitis in Children (Pseudocroup)

See p. 332 and Table 6.**11**.

Cricoarytenoid Arthritis

Main symptoms: Pain and a feeling of pressure during speech and swallowing. Hoarseness or other vocal dysfunction. Laryngoscopy shows redness and edema about the cricoarytenoid joint with variable fixation of the arytenoid cartilage.

Causes: Partial manifestation of rheumatoid arthritis, trauma to the cricoarytenoid joint, or

involvement of the joint by cellulitic or neoplastic disease in the laryngeal area.

Diagnosis:
● Mirror laryngoscopy.
● Direct laryngoscopy (with a self-retaining instrument).
● Biopsy in doubtful cases.

Differentiation is required from recurrent nerve palsy, specific inflammatory condition (tuberculosis), trauma, postcricoid tumor, and gout.

Acute Epiglottitis

Main symptoms: Most common in children under 10 years of age, very rare in adults. Severe pain (on swallowing). Fulminating course. Muffled speech. Severe systemic signs with fever and rapid deterioration. Some patients develop increasing dyspnea (stridor) and must sit upright in bed. There is *no* cough, and there may be *little or no* change in voice (see Table 6.**11**). Mirror laryngoscopy demonstrates a markedly swollen, cherry-red epiglottis.

Causes: Usually bacterial infection with abscess formation, possibly following "microtrauma" of the mucosa or a previous viral infection.

Diagnosis:
● Very short history.
● Typical alarming symptoms, typical indirect findings in the oropharynx.
● Resuscitative facilities should be available during the examination (reflex cardiac arrest!).

Differentiation is required from acute subglottic stenosing laryngitis in children (see Table 6.**11**) and peritonsillar abscess.

Laryngeal Trauma

The larynx may be unjured by external trauma (accident, gunshot, stab injury, sports-related injury, etc.) or by damage to its internal surface (caustic substance, foreign body, physical or chemical agents, iatrogenic injury). The history is usually clear-cut, and *pain and hoarseness are cardinal symptoms*.

The primary *diagnostic measures* in the absence of life-threatening symptoms are as follows:

- History followed by inspection, palpation, and laryngoscopy.
- Findings or suspicion may also warrant radiography (CT) or MRI.
- Specific attention is given to the condition of the cartilage skeleton (fracture of the thyroid or cricoid cartilage, dislocation of an arytenoid cartilage), soft-tissue lesions, edema and hematoma formation, and the danger of stricture or stenosis formation.
- The innervation and function of the endolaryngeal muscles are assessed.

Endolaryngeal Foreign Body

Main symptoms: Generally there is a typical history, but this may be absent in small children! Major symptoms are pain, severe cough, and a foreign-body sensation deep in the throat. There is variable hoarseness, which may alternate with a clear voice. Dyspnea depends on the type and location of the foreign body. Severe unrest. Increasing airway obstruction by reactive endolaryngeal swelling. Patient repeatedly grasps at the larynx.

Diagnosis:
- Laryngoscopy, which may be supplemented by radiographic evaluation and documentation.
- Direct laryngoscopy with a self-retaining instrument for extraction of the foreign body.

Iatrogenic Trauma

Variable soft-tissue injuries or even the dislocation of an arytenoid cartilage can occur during intubation or instrumental endoscopy of the larynx due to lack of manual experience or anatomic obstacles within the larynx. Prompt recognition and documentation of the trauma is essential. The presence of fresh or even bleeding mucosal lesions and complaints of pain and laryngeal dysfunction shortly following an endoscopic procedure make differential diagnosis an easy matter.

Laryngeal Perichondritis

Main symptoms: Severe pain in the laryngeal region, usually radiating to the ears, and severe dysphagia. The larynx is tender to exter-nal palpation. Hoarseness; possible dyspnea and fever. Laryngoscopy shows endolaryngeal swelling, redness, and restricted movement.

Other symptoms and special features: The symptoms of *acute perichondritis* and rapidly become threatening (stridor, severe pain, fever and chills). In *perichondritis* due to *chronic* specific inflammation, radiation, or tumor-associated inflammation, the symptoms are more insidious and nonspecific. Endolaryngeal swelling with dysesthesia is the main symptom.

Causes: Perichondrial damage due to injury, irradition, tumor infiltration, or as a postoperative complication. Hematogenous infection is very rare.

Diagnosis:
- Clues from the history.
- Laryngoscopic findings. Sites of predilection for swelling: arytenoid cartilage, posterior laryngeal wall, ventricular folds (false vocal cords), epiglottis. Exposed cartilage may be visible inside the larynx.
- Sequestrated cartilage is sometimes demonstrable by radiography.
- Biopsy may also be considered.

Differentiation is required from abscess formation in the endolaryngeal soft tissues and from neoplasia. It is particularly difficult to distinguish between radiation perichondritis and recurrent tumor (biopsy!).

Laryngeal Abscess and Laryngeal Cellulitis

Main symptoms: Rapidly progressive symptoms of acute onset: severe pain radiating to the ear, dysphagia, hoarseness, stridor, fever, and severe systemic illness. Laryngoscopy shows swelling, redness, and possible liquefaction or fistula formation (common during the first week).

Causes: Bacterial infection of endolaryngeal soft tissues. May coexist with epiglottitis and/or laryngeal perichondritis.

Diagnosis:
- Typical local findings on laryngoscopy.
- Bacteriologic smear and sensitivity testing.
- Laboratory findings consistent with highly acute inflammation.

Differentiation is required from laryngeal edema, laryngeal perichondritis, and neoplasia.

Superior Laryngeal Neuralgia

Main symptoms: Most cases present with unilateral, paroxysmal, stabbing pain in the region of the larynx, radiating to the side of the neck, upward to the ear, and sometimes downward as far as the clavicle. Typical findings: The entry site of the superior laryngeal nerve in the thyrohyoid membrane is very tender to pressure, which may occasionally precipitate a neuralgic attack. Additional trigger zones are in the piriform sinus (during swallowing and speech). Peak occurrence is between 40 and 60 years of age.

For further details, see Vagus Neuralgia, p. 163.

Chronic Laryngitis
See p. 320.

Contact Ulcer
See p. 350.

Specific Laryngitis
See p. 323.

Laryngeal Tumors

Pain and discomfort generally are *not* an early major or cardinal symptom of laryngeal tumors. Possible exceptions are laryngeal malignancies that involve either the epiglottis (free margin or petiole) or the aryepiglottic fold. See p. 325 for further details. Pain can also be an early cardinal symptom of "extrinsic" laryngeal cancer (hypopharyngeal carcinoma; see p. 270).

Symptom   **Habitual Throat Clearing**

This symptom may occur with almost any *endolaryngeal disorder*. It can also occur with diseases of the *pharynx* and especially the *hypopharynx* (e.g., hypopharyngeal diverticulum), the *upper esophagus*, and the *upper trachea*. Under no circumstances should *functional voice disorders* (p. 339) be omitted from the differential diagnosis of this symptom!

Symptom   **Cough**

Cough is a very common warning sign of disease in many portions of the respiratory tract. A cough may be classified as *dry* or *productive* (with raising of secretions). *Hemoptysis* is the coughing of blood (see Table 4.**20**).

The *laryngotracheal cough* is of primary interest to the otorhinolaryngologist. Most patients describe the cough as "high" and point spontaneously to the neck area. This cough is predominantly *dry* and is interpreted as a reflex response of the sensory innervation of the mucosa to numerous laryngotracheal diseases. A *productive* laryngotracheal cough is less common and serves to clear the laryngeal and tracheal lumen of secretions, contaminants, and small foreign bodies, which occasionally may ascend to the larynx from lower portions of the respiratory tract.

ENT differential diagnosis must identify an organic or functional cause in the larynx, tra-

Table 6.2 *Symptom* Cough (causes)

Synopsis

Dry cough

- Respiratory tract infection; in children, early measles, whooping cough (initial stage), etc.

Otolaryngologic

- Various forms of acute pharyngitis, laryngitis, and tracheitis
- Chronic laryngotracheitis and possibly bronchitis
  - Simple chronic form
  - Hyperplastic chronic form
  - Atrophic chronic form ("sicca")
  - Chondro-osteoplastic tracheopathy
- Mouth breathing (due to nasal airway obstruction)
- Vocal cord hematoma
- Foreign body
- Smoking (active and passive)
- Environmental and/or occupational influences (inhalation allergens, dusty or hot work environment, gaseous irritants)
- Fungal infection of the larynx or trachea
- Malformation of the larynx or trachea
  - Megatrachea
  - Tracheal diverticulum
- Endolaryngotracheal goiter
- Laryngocele
- Tracheal compression (bitonal cough)
- Recurrent nerve palsy
- Vagus nerve irritation (e. g., styloid syndrome)
- Superior laryngeal neuralgia
- Neoplasm involving the larynx and/or trachea
- Nervous cough

Pneumologic

- Incipient bronchial asthma
- Various forms of pneumonia
- Middle lobe syndrome
- Bronchial stenosis due to various causes
- Pleuritic cough

- Vagus nerve irritation (mediastinal disease)
- Sarcoidosis
- Bronchopulmonary neoplasms

Cardiologic

- Stasis in the pulmonary circulation (mitral stenosis, left heart failure)

Miscellaneous causes

- Mediastinal tumors
- Aortic aneurysm
- Goiter
- Gastroesophageal reflux
- CNS diseases with dysphagia

Wet cough

Otolaryngologic

- Sinusitis
- Laryngotracheitis (and bronchitis) in later stages
- Aspiration tracheobronchitis
- Tracheoesophageal fistula, see p. 380

Pneumologic

- Cystic fibrosis
- Bronchitis
- Bronchiectasis
- Whooping cough (later stage)
- Pneumonias and other parenchymatous lung diseases
- Tuberculosis
- Aspiration pneumonia
- Pulmonary abscess
- Hemoptysis, see Table 4.21

chea, or pharynx or reliably exclude an organic or functional disease. "Nervous" or "psychogenic" cough should always be included in the differential diagnosis.

Some characteristic *differentiating features* of cough:

○ "Exaggerated," forced coughing and throat clearing: pharyngeal cough.
○ Dry, hoarse cough: irritation of the epiglottis and glottis.
○ Whooping cough: staccato-like attacks of a cough that is initially dry and later becomes

wet, a long-drawn inspiration marking the end of the attack. Most common in children (pharyngeal smear, serology).
○ Croupy cough: hoarse, resonant, barking.
○ Nocturnal cough: may signify congestive heart failure.
○ Morning cough: may signify bronchiectasis.
○ Cough during or after meals: hypopharyngeal diverticulum, hiatal hernia, neurogenic dysphagia.
○ Cough relieved by sleep or distraction: "nervous" or psychogenic cough.
○ Cough during fluid ingestion: suggestive of tracheoesophageal fistula.

○ Hemoptysis: See causes in Table 4.**21**.

Generally, the patient's description of the site of the irritation is useful when the cause of the cough is laryngotracheal, although an intrathoracic cause may sufficiently involve the glottis to incite a secondary laryngeal cough.

Differential diagnosis should include diseases of the bronchi, lung parenchyma, heart, mediastinum, pleura, and external auditory canal (auricular branch of vagus nerve!) (Table 6.**2**).

Symptom   **Morphologic Change (Swelling, Tumor)**

The symptoms of "morphologic change" and "hoarseness" are very common but do not always coexist. For this reason and for reasons of differential diagnostic convenience, each of these two symptoms is covered in a separate section with its own synopsis. Accordingly, there is some overlap between Tables 6.**3** and 6.**7**, but page references are furnished to avoid repetition.

External Swelling of the Larynx

By palpating through the relaxed (!) cervical soft tissues, the examiner can detect any deviations in the normal contours of the cartilaginous framework and any abnormal fixation of the larynx. In some diseases, palpation will elicit tenderness; other diseases are painless or are associated with constant pain. *Causes* of external laryngeal swelling include *inflammatory processes* (e.g., perichondritis of the thyroid or cricoid cartilage), sequestration, a pointing abscess, *posttraumatic states*, and bony and soft-tissue changes, especially those caused by *malignant neoplasms* (e.g., tumor invasion through the thyroid cartilage into the extralaryngeal soft tissues). The causes of these palpable swellings are generally established by the history, endoscopic findings, imaging procedures (CT, MRI), and biopsy.

Chronic Laryngitis

The cardinal symptom of "simple" chronic laryngitis is generally hoarseness, which is caused by morphologic changes within the larynx. The term "chronic laryngitis" encompasses various entities:

○ *Simple chronic (catarrhal) laryngitis:* The vocal cords are markedly thickened and pale red, and the ventricular folds are often thickened and coarse. Viscous mucus. Variable hoarseness. Foreign-body sensation, frequent throat clearing, possible cough. Phoniatric aspects, see p. 349. *Causes:* Recurrent and/or chronic infections of the upper or lower airways with canalicular distribution. Chronic irritative laryngitis (vocal abuse; exogenous noxious agents: thermal, mechanical, chemical; smoking, dusty work environment, mouth breathing; alcoholism).
○ *Chronic hyperplastic laryngitis:* Lobular or pad-like hyperplasia of the vocal cords, ventricular folds, or ventricular mucosa ("ventricular prolapse"), either circumscribed or diffusely involving the intralaryngeal soft tissues. Foci of epithelial metaplasia and thickening (*pachyderma*) are common, especially on the vocal cords and/or the ventricular folds. Hoarseness is variable and

Table 6.**3** *Symptom*   Morphologic change (swelling, tumor)

Synopsis	

External swelling of the larynx
– Inflammatory
– Posttraumatic
– Neoplastic
Chronic laryngitis
– Simple chronic (catarrhal) laryngitis
– Chronic hyperplastic laryngitis
– Reinke edema
– Laryngitis sicca (atrophic laryngitis)
Fungal infections
Contact ulcer and contact pachyderma, see p. 350
Vocal polyps
Vocal nodules, see p. 350
Endolaryngeal cyst
Laryngeal edema
Laryngeal abscess, cellulitis, perichondritis,
  see p. 317
Arthritis of the cricoarytenoid joint, see. p. 316
Specific inflammatory conditions
– Tuberculosis
– Sarcoidosis
– Syphilis
	– Leprosy, see p. 324
	– Leishmaniasis, see p. 324
	– (Rhino)scleroma, see p. 324 and Table 4.**28**
	– Malleus, see p. 324 and Table 4.**28**
	– Granulomatoses, see pp. 192, 324
	Various dermatoses such as
	– Herpes simplex, see p. 239
	– Herpes zoster, see p. 245
	– Pemphigus, see p. 253
	– Erythema multiforme, see p. 254
	Storage disease and other rare disorders
	Laryngeal trauma
	Intubation granuloma
	Cicatricial stenosis, see p. 329
	Deformity of the laryngeal skeleton
	Neurogenic morphologic changes,
	  see p. 350
	Benign tumors
	– Laryngeal papillomas
	Precancerous lesions
	Malignant tumors

usually severe. Habitual throat clearing, scant viscous mucus. "False-vocal-cord voice." *Causes* are similar to those of chronic catarrhal laryngitis. Predisposing occupations (bartenders, butchers, construction workers; salesmen, teachers, other speaking professions), and chronic vocal abuse.

○ *Reinke edema:* Polypoid edema strictly confined to one or both vocal cords. The affected cord(s) may present as a glazed, yellowish, edematous "bulla" projecting a variable distance into the glottic space, causing hoarseness or even aphonia. Dyspnea can occur. Inflammatory processes and vocal abuse are thought to have causal significance (see p. 341).

○ *Chronic laryngitis due to noise exposure* (see p. 349).

Diagnosis:

● Detailed history, with special emphasis on exposure to potential irritants.

● Typical indirect findings may be supplemented by endoscopy, especially with hyperplastic laryngitis and pachyderma, and by biopsy (to exclude malignancy).

● Stroboscopy can be used to assess phonation and vocal cord function.

● Phoniatric functional analysis. See also p. 336.

Differentiation is required from specific and allergic laryngitis and neoplasms. Reinke edema requires differentiation from monocorditis and vocal polyps.

Laryngitis Sicca (Atrophic Laryngitis)

Main symptoms: Habitual throat clearing, possibly accompanied by a dry, barking cough. Variable hoarseness. Stridor may be present. On laryngoscopy the vocal cords are seen to be narrow, reddened, and may be covered with dry crusts or lacquer-like secretions. Dyspnea occurs if the crusts produce glottic obstruction.

Usually there are associated sicca symptoms in the pharynx, oral cavity, and/or nose (see pp. 301, 303, and Table 5.**7**).

Causes: Multifactorial. Atrophic condition of the respiratory mucosa due to environmental and/or occupational insult, endocrine factors (laryngopathy of pregnancy), or metabolic influences (e.g., nephrosis). Autoimmune factors can be important in the setting of Sjögren disease.

Diagnosis: Laryngoscopy. Attempt to identify endogenous and/or exogenous causes (see Table. 4.**16**).

Fungal Infection

Main symptoms: *Very rare* in the larynx and usually combined with a fungal infection of the mucosa at a different site (mouth, pharynx, bronchi). Fungi form whitish deposits on the laryngeal mucosa that can be wiped away. The mucosa appears red and thickened. Infiltrates and ulcerations also occur. See p. 249 for further details.

Causes: *Candida albicans* is the usual pathogen. Other fungal infections occasionally encountered in the larynx (and trachea) are blastomycosis, histoplasmosis, actinomycosis, coccidiomycosis (in North and South America), and sporotrichosis (see Table 4.**28**).

Diagnosis: Identification of the causative organism and biopsy.

Differentiation is required from specific inflammation and neoplasia.

Contact Ulcer and Contact Pachyderma
See p. 350.

Vocal Polyp

Main symptoms: Spherical, smooth-walled, soft, red to grayish-red mass, pinhead- to pea-sized, usually attached to the anterior half of the vocal cord by a sessile or pedunculated base. The lesion is painless and slow-growing. Pedunculated polyps may drop into the glottic space during inspiration, causing hoarseness, but coughing can temporarily restore a clear voice by raising the polyp above the glottic plane. This intermittent hoarseness is typical of a floating vocal polyp. There is habitual throat clearing and a paroxysmal cough. Large polyps can occlude the glottis and cause dyspnea! See p. 350 for further details.

Vocal Nodules
See p. 350.

Endolaryngeal Cyst

Main symptoms: Tense, globular, mucosa-covered bulge of variable size with no associated pain or inflammation. Sites of predilection are the vocal cords, the ventricular folds, the epiglottis, and the aryepiglottic folds. Cysts may have a milky, yellow, or bluish coloration. There may be associated hoarseness or aphonia, depending on the site of the lesion.

Causes: Two types are recognized: retention cysts (relatively common) and congenital cysts (less common).

Diagnosis:
● Typical laryngoscopic findings.
● Some cases may require CT or MRI.
● Needle aspiration or incisional biopsy.

Differentiation is required from laryngocele, vocal polyp, and neoplasm (especially with a cyst deep in the soft tissues of the ventricular folds).

Laryngeal Edema

Main symptoms: Edematous swellings in the larynx may be *circumscribed* (e.g., Reinke edema) or *diffuse* (e.g., Quincke edema). The *symptoms* depend on location, extent, and rate of development and include hoarseness to aphonia, occasional dyspnea, a foreign-body or pressure sensation in the laryngeal area, frequent throat clearing, and cough. There is no pain. Laryngoscopy shows a circumscribed glassy edema or general swelling of endolaryngeal soft tissues including the epiglottis, with associated mechanical motion restriction of endolaryngeal structures.

Causes: a) *Inflammatory* edema (most common form) collateral to usually deep-seated endolaryngeal inflammatory processes (e.g., perichondritis) or abscess formation in proximity to the larynx (peritonsillar, oral floor, pharyngeal wall, etc.); also after trauma, caustic injury, scalding, foreign-body aspiration, or during and after radiotherapy. b) *Noninflammatory* edema like that associated with *cardiac, renal*, or *hepatic insufficiency*; myxedema; lymphatic obstruction; *intubation*; or *drug intolerance*. c) *"Angioneurotic"* (Quincke) edema (see p. 143), which is recurrent! d) *Allergic* edema.

Diagnosis: Typical findings on mirror laryngoscopy. Sites of predilection for edema formation are the epiglottis, arytenoid cartilage, aryepiglottic folds, and vocal cords (Reinke edema). Subglottic edema occurs in children (see p. 332). Edema can also cause variable obstruction of the piriform sinus.

Differentiation is required from allergy and pharmacologic pseudoallergy, insect sting, foreign body, and any of the other various causes of laryngeal edema (see above).

Laryngeal Abscess, Laryngeal Cellulitis, Laryngeal Perichondritis
See p. 317.

Arthritis of the Cricoarytenoid Joint
See p. 316.

Specific Inflammatory Diseases

Tuberculous Laryngitis

Main symptoms: This has become a *very rare* disease. Intralaryngeal manifestations are diverse, but almost all cases show hoarseness and cough that increase over a period of months. Pain eventually supervenes and may radiate to the ears. *Laryngoscopic* findings depend on the form of the infection.

a) *Infiltrating mucosal tuberculosis:* Reddish-brown submucous nodules that coalesce. Often only *one* vocal cord is affected initially (*monocorditis*). It is not unusual for disease foci to remain on one side of the larynx. Sites of predilection: vocal cord, posterior laryngeal wall, ventricular fold, the Morgagni ventricle ("ventricular prolapse"), occasinally the epiglottis.

b) *Ulcerating mucosal tuberculosis:* The most common form. Shallow mucosal ulcers with undermined borders are succeeded by deep crater-like soft-tissue ulcers with gradual involvement of the cartilaginous framework of the larynx (necrosis, perichondritis) and cricoarytenoid joints. Greasy coating. Hoarseness, increasing pain that may be severe. Dysphagia.

c) *Tuberculoma ("tuberculous laryngeal tumor").* Very rare. Sessile or pedunculated granular mass with a smooth or nodular surface. Hoarseness, occasional respiratory impairment. Little pain.

d) *Mucosal lupus,* also very rare, can spread from the pharynx to involve the larynx (usually the epiglottis).

Other symptoms and special features: Males predominate by about 2:1, with a peak occurrence in the 3rd−5th decades. Most patients have coexisting tuberculosis of the lung or other organs.

Causes: Secondary infection of the larynx from the lung or by the hematogenous route.

Diagnosis:
● Laryngoscopic findings. Use a self-retaining laryngoscope to obtain a smear for bacteriologic study.
● Biopsy.
● Internal medical consultation to identify the primary focus (lung or other organ). Laryngeal findings may be positive *before* pulmonary findings!
● Identification of the causative organism in culture and/or animal test.

Differentiation is required from "vasomotor monocorditis" (see p. 349), syphilis, and malignant tumor.

Sarcoidosis (Besnier−Boeck−Schaumann Disease)

Main laryngeal symptoms: A *very rare* site of involvement. Lesions consist mostly of small, firm nodules and infiltrates in the laryngeal mucosa with associated dysphonia and a feeling of cervical fullness. Diagnosis is established by biopsy. Look for pulmonary or other manifestations of Boeck disease. See p. 255 for further details.

Syphilis

Main laryngeal symptoms: *Secondary* syphilis produces syphilitic eruptions in the larynx accompanied by corresponding changes in the oropharyngeal mucosae (see p. 247). *Tertiary* cases are marked by endolaryngeal gummata with pseudotumor formation, ulceration, and destruction of the laryngeal skeleton. Dark red swellings are succeeded by ulcers with punched-out borders in the larynx. Hoarseness to aphonia is the rule. Pain and dysfunction may be absent for some time. Ulceration is marked by oral fetor, and perichondrial involvement is marked by severe pain, dysphagia, and possible dyspnea depending on the extent of disease.

Diagnosis: See p. 248.
Secondary syphilis requires *differentiation* from pachyderma, papilloma, pemphigus (see p. 253), and tuberculosis; *tertiary* syphilis from tuberculosis and malignancy.

Other Rare Diseases

The rare diseases of *leprosy, leishmaniasis, scleroma* and *malleus* are never manifested primarily or exclusively in the larynx, so the differential diagnosis is guided by symptoms in the nose and pharynx and by the typical geographic distribution of these diseases (see Table 4.**28**).

A thorough differential diagnosis should include consideration of the extremely rare *endolaryngeal manifestations* of *lipoidosis, lipoid granulomatosis* (Hand−Schüller−Christian disease), *xanthomas, amyloidosis,* and *gout.* The diagnosis is established by biopsy.

Laryngeal Trauma

See the discussion on p. 316, 317. With regard to the symptom of morphologic change, it should be noted that *blunt* and *sharp external laryngeal injuries* can produce all conceivable variants of such change. The differential diagnosis of *acute* trauma should be guided by the patient's immediate vital status: In patients with acutely life-threatening hemorrhage or respiratory distress, life-saving operative measures also serve a diagnostic and differential diagnostic function. In posttraumatic states *beyond the acute stage*, the differential diagnosis of functional disturbances such as hoarseness, aphonia, dysphagia, stridor, pain, etc., relies on the use of all available endoscopic and radiologic techniques in addition to phoniatric analysis.

Circumscribed Endolaryngeal Injuries

See the discussion on p. 316. The lesions of greatest interest in terms of morphologic change are *intubation granulomas, cicatricial stenosis*, and permanent *deformities of the laryngeal skeleton.*

Intubation Granuloma

Main symptoms: Foreign-body sensation in the larynx, usually arising several weeks after intubation (general anesthesia), with variable hoarseness that tends to increase over time. Dyspnea may be present. Laryngoscopy reveals a spherical, grayish-red mass in the posterior third of the true vocal cord (usually at the attachment of the free vocal fold to the vocal process of the arytenoid cartilage). Bilateral occurrence is possible.

Causes: Damage to the mucosal lining by previous intubation, inciting the formation of granulation tissue at mechanically traumatized sites on the vocal cords.

Diagnosis:
● Typical history and laryngoscopic findings.
● Complete excisional biopsy.

Differentiation is required from contact ulcer (see p. 350) and malignancy.

Cicatricial Stenosis
See p. 367.

Deformity of the Laryngeal Skeleton
See p. 329.

Neurogenic Morphologic Changes

These include angulation of the arytenoid cartilage, deformation of the endolaryngeal contours, etc. See p. 350 ff.

Laryngeal Tumors

Benign Tumors

The *benign laryngeal neoplasms* of greatest clinical importance are listed in Table 6.**4**. These tumors produce a uniform symptom complex consisting of a foreign-body sensation, habitual throat clearing, cough, occasional hoarseness to aphonia, and possible dyspnea depending on tumor size and location.

The **differential diagnosis** utilizes endoscopic and radiologic findings (tomography, CT, MRI) but is definitively established by incisional or excisional biopsy.

One benign epithelial tumor is described in somewhat greater detail owing to its frequency and clinical importance:

Laryngeal Papilloma (Papillomatosis)

Main symptoms: Solitary or mutliple, yellowish to red, soft, wart-like lesions, sessile or pedunculated, occurring predominantly on the vocal cords but also on the ventricular folds or at any endolaryngeal site. Papillomatosis is marked by an extensive papillomatous "lawn" covering the endolaryngeal, tracheal, and/or pharyngeal surfaces. Laryngeal papillomas are painless. Patients with vocal cord involvement present with hoarseness to aphonia. Glottic obstruction causes dyspnea with danger of asphyxia. Peak occurrence is from 2 to 4 years of age. *"Juvenile red papillomas"* are the most common form and occasionally affect adults (principally in the 3rd decade).

Solitary *adult papillomas* are hard, *grayish-white* lesions that occur infrequently in persons (chiefly males) over 60 years of age. Adult papilloma is considered a precursor of carcinoma!

Causes: Juvenile papilloma is assumed to have a viral etiology (papovavirus, a type of DNA virus). The cause of adult papilloma is still under discussion.

Diagnosis:
● Typical laryngoscopic findings.
● If possible, papillomatosis in children should be biopsied through a self-retaining laryngoscope.

Table 6.**4**   Benign laryngeal tumors (selection)

Pseudotumors
– Laryngocele
– Primary (congenital) and secondary (rentention) cysts
– Amyloid tumor
– Gouty tophi
– Dysplasias and hyperplasias (pachyderma, leukoplakia, etc.)
– Intralaryngeal goiter

Epithelial
– Papilloma
– Oxyphilic adenoma (oncocytoma)
– Adenoma
– Pleomorphic adenoma (rare)

Mesenchymal
– Fibroma
– Giant cell tumor
– Leiomyoma
– Rhabdomyoma
– Lipoma
– Hemangioma and lymphangioma
– Chondroma

Neuroectodermal
– Granular cell tumor (myoblastoma)
– Neuroma
– Neurofibroma
– Chemodectoma

● With a solitary adult papilloma, at least an incisional biopsy specimen should be taken from the base of the papilloma (using self-retaining microlaryngoscopy) to exclude malignant disease.

Precancerous Lesions

These include:

○ Leukoplakia
   (white pachyderma, hyperkeratosis)
○ Adult papilloma
○ Erythroplakia
   (erythroplasia, red pachyderma)
○ Carcinoma in situ

Main symptoms: Whitish or reddish, flat or nodular deposits on the vocal cord, often involving both the superior and inferior surfaces of the cord. Occasionally both cords are involved. Extraglottic occurrence is uncommon. Hoarseness or cough may be present. Habitual

Table 6.5   Malignant laryngeal tumors (selection)

Precancerous lesions
- Leukoplakia and pachyderma
- (Solitary) adult papilloma
- Erythroplasia (or erythroplakia)
- Carcinoma in situ

Epithelial
- Squamous cell carcinoma
  (>90%, various grades)
- Verrucous carcinoma
- Adenocarcinoma
- Adenoid cystic carcinoma
- Undifferentiated small-cell ("oat-cell")
  carcinoma
- Mucoepidermoid tumor
- Carcinoid

Mesenchymal
- Fibrosarcoma and other sarcomas
- Rhabdomyosarcoma
- Chondrosarcoma

Lymphoreticular system
- Malignant lymphoma
- Plasmacytoma

Neuroectodermal
- Melanoma
- Chemodectoma

Tumors of adjacent structures and metastatic tumors such as:
- Hypopharyngeal carcinoma
- Esophageal carcinoma
- Thyroid carcinoma
- Hypernephroma

throat clearing is typical. Peak occurrence is in the 6th–8th decades, with males predominating by a 9:1 ratio.

Diagnosis:
- Typical vocal cord findings.
- Complete excisional biopsy is indicated so that *all* portions of the growth can be evaluated. Grades of dysplasia are reviewed in Table 4.**11**.

Differentiation is required from carcinoma and chronic hyperplastic laryngitis.

Malignant Tumors

Malignant tumors of the larynx continue to represent the largest group of head and neck malignancies, followed closely by oropharyngeal cancers. The more common types are listed in Table 6.**5**.

It is imperative for prognostic and therapeutic reasons that laryngeal malignancies be given a very thorough and precise workup (including classification, grading, and staging). It would exceed our scope to explore all the clinical details and contrasting symptomatologies of the different tumor types. Here we shall simply outline the symptoms and differential diagnostic steps that characterize the large group of laryngeal carcinomas (which account for more than 90% of laryngeal malignancies). For clinical reasons, hypopharyngeal malignancies are also considered in this context.

Laryngeal Carcinoma

Main symptoms: The most common *warning signs* in order of frequency are: hoarseness, habitual throat clearing, cough, hemoptysis, dyspnea, pain, and dysphagia. Pain is generally a relatively late symptom signifying perichondritis. Depending on tumor location, metastasis to lymph nodes may occur early (with supraglottic and subglottic laryngeal carcinoma and with hypopharyngeal carcinoma), late, or not at all (with carcinoma of the vocal cords).

Other symptoms and special features: *Intralaryngeal carcinoma* is ten times more prevalent in males than females, with a peak occurrence between 55 and 65 years of age. *Hypopharyngeal carcinoma* is most common between 40 and 60 years of age, with about a 6:1 preponderance of males. The following *differentiating symptoms* should be noted for laryngeal carcinomas occurring at different sites:

○ *Carcinoma of the vocal cords:* Early hoarseness and habitual throat clearing. Often there is a history of chronic laryngitis. Carcinoma of the vocal folds is the most common manifestation of laryngeal carcinoma in Central Europe. It usually develops in the anterior half of the vocal cord (including the anterior commissure). Lymph node metastasis is absent or delayed.

○ *Supraglottic carcinoma:* Supraglottic lesions tend to remain asymptomatic for some time. Hoarseness develops as a late feature, especially with tumors arising in the epiglottis. But there is relatively early peritumoral swelling in the area of the ventricular folds and/or aryepiglottic folds. Dysphagia, globus sensation. Early lymph node metastases. Speaking causes throat pain that may radiate to the ear. Epiglottic involvement leads to a rigid epiglottis. Tumors located in the area of the petiole can be *very difficult* to detect.

○ *Subglottic carcinoma:* Often there is an initial paucity of symptoms. Hoarseness is a late feature, and stridorous respiration signifies advanced disease (encroachment on the already narrow subglottic airway). Early lymph node metastases occur along the tracheobronchial tract.

○ *Transglottic or ventricular carcinoma:* Detection is very difficult initially and often requires unfolding of the Morgagni ventricle. Early hoarseness.

○ *Peripheral laryngeal carcinomas* (epiglottic border, aryepiglottic fold, apex of arytenoid cartilage): Hoarseness is a very late sign. Dysphagia may be the initial symptom. Lymph node metastasis is variable, occurring late with tumors at the free epiglottic margin and early with tumors on the aryepiglottic fold.

○ *Hypopharyngeal carcinoma:* The earliest symptom is often a palpable lymph node metastasis at the side of the neck (deep jugular chain) and/or at the mandibular angle. Sometimes symptoms commence with dysphagia and pain radiating to the ear. Hoarseness is absent or delayed until the arytenoid cartilage becomes involved.

○ *Postcricoid carcinoma:* Restricted movement of the arytenoid cartilage can cause early hoarseness. Otherwise the initial symptom is dysphagia, at times accompanied by early lymph node metastases.

Causes: Predisposition by precancerous disease, chronic hyperplastic laryngitis, smoking, alcoholism, chronic inhalation of noxious gases, or ionizing radiation. Some patients are genetically predisposed.

Diagnosis:
● Laryngoscopy. Suspicious findings or symptoms warrant microlaryngoscopy (with a self-retaining rigid laryngoscope) including hypopharyngoscopy.
● Biopsy.
● Various imaging procedures can be used to define the extent of a laryngeal tumor and its relationship to neighboring structures (see p. 314). Tomography and especially CT provide the most detailed information. The procedures of choice for detecting and documenting regional lymph node metastases are CT, MRI, and also B-mode sonography.

Differentiation is required from tuberculosis, secondary or tertiary syphilis, benign true tumors and granulation tumors, chronic hyperplastic laryngitis, and other laryngeal malignancies.

Second Tumors (Multiple Tumors)

The statistical incidence of neoplasms coexisting with laryngeal tumors in 5–15%. Most occur in the bronchial region or oral cavity. The asymptomatic interval is 4 years or more.

Symptom   **Malformation**

Congenital malformations of the larynx are uncommon. Some play a role in differential diagnosis, and most can be diagnosed endoscopically. Table 6.6 lists the conditions that are significant in terms of differential diagnosis.

Laryngomalacia (Congenital Stridor)
See p. 338.

Congenital Webs
See p. 337.

Table 6.**6** *Symptom* Laryngeal malformation (arranged in order of clinical importance)

Synopsis
Laryngomalacia (congenital stridor), see p. 338
Congenital webs (connective-tissue membranes), see p. 337
Congenital stenosis of the cricoid cartilage, see p. 338
Congenital neurogenic disturbances (recurrent nerve), see p. 351
Cysts
Laryngoceles
Hemangiomas and lymphangiomas, see p. 337
Epiglottic anomalies (cleft, curled, absent)*
Thyroid cartilage anomalies (failure of fusion of the alae, asymmetry, absence of the horns or prominence, elongation of the horn to the hyoid bone)*
Cricoid cartilage anomalies (subglottic stenosis, part of the cartilage ring missing or replaced by connective tissue, laryngotracheoesophageal cleft)*

* No further commentary

Congenital Neurogenic Disorders

These are based on unilateral or bilateral recurrent nerve palsy (see p. 351).

Cysts

"Secondary" (retention) cysts are discussed on p. 322.

Primary (congenital) cysts of the larynx are rare. Most are solitary and tend to occur in the region of the Morgagni ventricle (between the true and false vocal cords), though some have an epiglottic or subglottic location. The diagnosis is made endoscopically. The differential diagnosis should include retention cysts, laryngoceles, and neoplasms, especially in adults.

Laryngoceles

Laryngoceles may be classified as *internal* (located within the confines of the larynx), *external*, or *mixed*.

Main symptoms: *Internal* laryngocele presents as a rounded, soft, compressible bulge of the intralaryngeal soft tissues (ventricular fold, aryepiglottic fold, piriform sinus) with associated hoarseness or even dyspnea, depending on the site. Bilateral occurrence is possible! Men are affected more commonly than women, with a peak incidence at 50−60 years of age, but lesions may occur in children and produce ominous symptoms (breathing and eating difficulties). *External* laryngocele presents as a soft protrusion usually situated laterally between the superior border of the thyroid cartilage and the hyoid bone in the area of the hyothyroid membrane. A valvular mechanism causes gradual enlargement of the sac. There is no pain. Mixed laryngoceles are relatively common.

Causes: Persistence of the embryonic laryngeal saccule with herniation of the laryngeal mucosa. A traumatic etiology (acquired laryngocele) has been postulated for cases originating in adulthood.

Diagnosis:
● Laryngoscopy and microlaryngoscopy.
● Palpable findings with external laryngocele: soft, mobile, balloon-like mass at the level of the hyothyroid membrane.
● Radiographs (AP tomograms) show a spherical cavity that may be distorted into bizarre shapes by adjacent structures. The contents consist of air and less commonly of mucus. A mucus-filled sac may exhibit poor radiographic contrast.

Internal laryngoceles mainly require *differentiation* from primary or secondary cysts; *external* laryngoceles from lipomas and lateral or midline cervical cysts.

Hemangioma and Lymphangioma
See p. 337.

Symptom   Hoarseness

Aside from habitual throat clearing, hoarseness is the most common symptom of laryngeal disease and is considered a form of *dysphonia* (see p. 339ff. and Tables 6.**12** and 6.**13**). It occurs in most endolaryngeal diseases to some degree (from slight vocal harshness to aphonia). The underlying decrease in vocal cord mobility may be caused by a lesion of the vocal cords and arytenoid cartilages or by a lesion of the ventricular folds or other parts of the endolarynx. Hoarseness should not be confused with "muffled" speech like that occurring in epiglottitis and hypopharyngeal diseases.

For conciseness, only *groups of diseases* are listed in the synopsis below (Table 6.**7**). The page references will direct the reader to more detailed information (brief commentaries and associated symptoms).

Table 6.**7**   *Symptom*   Hoarseness (causes)

Synopsis
Malformations and anomalies, see p. 327ff.
Congenital dysphonia, see Table 6.**12**
Acquired dysphonia, see Table 6.**13**
Functional disturbances due to organic causes, see pp. 337, 350
Injuries, see pp. 316, 324
Exogenous agents, see Table 6.**1**
Foreign bodies, see p. 317
Acute inflammatory conditions, see p. 315ff.
Chronic nonspecific inflammatory conditions, see p. 320ff.
Chronic specific inflammatory conditions, see p. 323ff.
Metabolic disorders, see p. 324
Circulatory disorders
Pseudotumors, see Table 6.**4**
Benign tumors, see Table 6.**4**
Precancerous lesions, see p. 325
Malignant tumors, see Table 6.**5**
See also Tables 6.**12** and 6.**13**

Symptom   Hemoptysis

See p. 273.

Symptom   Dyspnea

See p. 365 and Figure 6.**1**.

Symptom   Stridor (Obstructive Respiratory Insufficiency)

Airway obstruction, especially when occurring in the pharynx, larynx, or tracheobronchial system, causes a stenotic respiration whose cardinal symptom is *stridor*. Its pathophysiology is based on an *obstructive respiratory insufficiency*, which can be fatal given sufficient

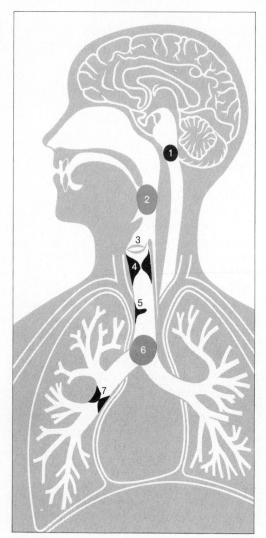

Fig. 6.**1**   Causes of acute and/or chronic obstructive respiratory insufficiency (after Matthys)

1 Lesion of the respiratory center
2 Intrapharyngeal foreign body or swelling
3 Obstruction of the glottis (foreign body, inflammation, neoplasm)
4 Stenosing scar tissue in the trachea, or tracheomalacia
5 Webs in the trachea
6 Intralaryngeal, intratracheal, or intrabronchial foreign body
7 Bronchial stenosis

duration and severity of the obstruction. *Stridor always constitutes an absolute and urgent emergency situation* requiring *immediate* differential diagnostic evaluation so that appropriate therapeutic measures can be initiated without delay.

A *stenosis* in the *pharynx* or *supraglottic area* generally causes a rattling, sonorous inspiratory stridor. The voice may be normal.

A *glottic stenosis* always produces an inspiratory stridor and often an expiratory stridor. The associated voice disturbance ranges from hoarseness to aphonia.

A *subglottic stenosis* is associated with inspiratory and expiratory stridor that may be interrupted by a barking cough. The voice may be normal (see also Table 7.**3** and Fig. 6.**1**).

Severe obstructive respiratory insufficiency caused by a lesion *above the tracheal bifurcation* is generally marked by retraction at the supraclavicular fossae, sternum, and intercostal spaces in addition to cyanosis. By contrast, an airway obstruction *below the bifurcation* causes thoracic asymmetry, possibly with elevation of the diaphragm. A loud, rattling stridor can be auscultated over the bronchial stenosis, and respiratory sounds past the stenosis may be diminished. Generally an airway obstruction below the tracheal bifurcation does *not* constitute an acute emergency as long as the remaining lung is fully functional (see Fig. 6.**1**).

The principal causes of obstructive respiratory insufficiency are summarized in Table 6.**8**. Because the differential diagnosis of stridor generally is not confined to the *larynx*, the *pharynx*, *trachea*, and *bronchial tree* are included in the synopsis as potential sites of airway obstruction.

The following short commentaries deal with *laryngeal* causes for stridor only. For *pharyngeal* and *tracheobronchial* causes, see the page references in Table 6.**8**.

Congenital Stridor (Laryngomalacia)
See p. 338.

Table 6.**8** *Symptom* Stridor (obstructive respiratory insufficiency) (causes)

Synopsis	
Disease	Cardinal symptoms
In the pharynx	
Diphtheria	Dirty gray membranes, see p. 233
Peritonsillar abscess	(Unilateral) swelling and redness in the Waldemeyer ring, odynophagia, trismus, see p. 229
Mononucleosus	Membranes and swelling of the tonsils and surrounding tissues on both sides, see p. 229
Retropharyngeal abscess	Bulging of the posterior pharyngeal wall, see p. 265 ff.
Quincke edema	Sudden onset, edematous mucosa in the faucial isthmus and/or larynx, see p. 143
Tongue retraction in an unconscious patient	Stertorous breath sounds, open mouth, unresponsiveness
Abscess of the tongue and oral floor	Severe inspiratory stridor, muffled speech, short history, see pp. 233, 234
Lingual goiter	Long history, muffled speech, no pain, see p. 410
Neoplasms (chiefly malignant)	Long history, oral fetor, possible pain, bloody sputum; possible visible neck mass, see pp. 267 ff., 326, 364
In the larynx	
Congenital stridor (laryngomalacia)	In newborns and infants, staccato respiration, see p. 338
Obstructive respiratory distress in newborns and infants	Cyanosis, effortful respiratory excursions, agitation, chest retraction
Acute epiglottitis	Most common in children 4–10 years old, severe pain, fulminating course, muffled speech, no cough or hoarseness, see p. 316
Glottic edema	Endolaryngeal edema, occasional hoarseness, see p. 322
Vocal cord paralysis	Bilateral abductor paralysis, see pp. 337, 350
Laryngeal spasm	Reflex closure of the glottis of abrupt onset, see p. 332
Laryngeal diphtheria, croup	Dirty gray endolaryngeal membranes, hoarseness, see p. 315
Stenosing laryngotracheitis, pseudocroup	Most common in children 1–4 years old, hoarseness, hyperacute symptoms, barking cough, see p. 322
Foreign body	History, pain, cough (bitonal), variable symptoms, see pp. 317, 332
Trauma and sequelae	History, see pp. 317, 324
Benign neoplasms, cysts, laryngoceles	Long history, endoscopic findings, see pp. 322
Malignant tumors	Slowly progressive symptomatology, hoarseness (in many cases), possible pain, see p. 325
In the tracheobronchial tree	
Foreign body	History, cough, varying symptoms, see p. 362
Tracheal injury (sharp, blunt, rupture)	History, emphysema or escape of air from the wound, see p. 363

Table 6.**8** (cont.)

Synopsis	
Disease	**Cardinal symptoms**
Stenosing (laryngo)tracheobronchitis	History of infection, prior intubation, endoscopic surgery, tracheotomy, see p. 332
External compression (e.g., goiter, mediastinal neoplasm)	Slowly progressive stridor, also regional symptoms, see pp. 366, 387
Tracheomalacia	Scabbard trachea after trauma, surgery, or with goiter, see p. 366
Cicatricial stenosis	History of trauma or surgery, see p. 367
Intratracheal or intrabronchial neoplasm	Slowly increasing stridor with audible maximum over the trachea, see p. 367. Intrabronchial tumors, see Table 7.**5**
Complication in tracheostomy patients or after removal of the tracheostomy tube	Stridor while tracheal tube is in place or after its removal, see p. 370

See also Tables 7.**3** and 7.**5**

Table 6.**9** Congenital causes of obstructive airways distress in newborns and infants

Craniofacial anomaly, see p. 221 and Table 2.**13**

Micrognathia and retrognathia

Microgenia (Franceschetti–Zwahlen syndrome), see Tables 1.**43** and 2.**13** Glossoptosis

Pierre-Robin syndrome, see Table 2.**13**

Crouzon syndrome, see Tables 1.**43** and 2.**13**

Apert syndrome, see Table 2.**13**

Macroglossia, see Table 4.**13**

Klippel–Feil syndrome, see Table 4.**26**

Bilateral choanal atresia, see p. 206

Transitory edema, obstruction of both nasal cavities

Cleft lip and palate, see p. 271

Space-occupying lesion in the nasopharynx (e.g., encephalocele), see pp. 139, 217ff.

Lingual goiter, see p. 410

Laryngomalacia, see p. 338

Congenital stenosis of the cricoid cartilage, see p. 337

Congenital webs in the larynx or trachea, see p. 337ff.

Laryngocele, see p. 328

Tracheal malformation

Tracheoesophageal fistula, see p. 365

Bronchial malformation

Esophageal malformation, see Table 8.**7**

Obstructive Respiratory Distress in Newborns and Infants

Stridorous respiration in newborns and infants can pose special problems of differential diagnosis due to the high position of the larynx and the inability to rely on auxiliary oral breathing. The diagnostic problems are compounded by the small size of the anatomic structures. The high-risk *period of obligate nasal breathing* lasts for about 3 months postpartum; thereafter, an adequate capacity for oral breathing is available if required. When significant glossoptosis is present, the danger of asphyxiation will be greatly reduced by about 6 months of age owing to natural growth of the mandible.

Main symptoms of an "upper" airway obstruction in this age group are very effortful and to a degree ineffectual respiratory movements and cyanosis, with or without stridor. Supraclavicular, sternal, and intercostal retraction during inspiration. Severe restlessness. Refusal of feed.

The more common dysgenetic causes of mechanical airway obstruction in newborn and infants are listed in Table 6.**9**.

Diagnosis: See Table 6.**10**.

Acute Epiglottitis
See p. 316.

Table 6.**10**   Diagnostic evaluation of obstructive respiratory distress in newborns and infants

1. *Gross etiologic differentiation* of cyanosis and dyspnea:
   - Mechanical airway obstruction
     (Very effortful respiratory excursions with inspiratory chest retraction. "Struggle for air,"
     with or without stridor)
   - Cardiovascular cause
     (Shunt or cardiac decompensation)
     (*No* "struggle for air," cyanosis, slowed reactions)
   - Central respiratory disturbance
     (Congenital or due to birth injury)
     (Deficient, arrhythmic spontaneous respiration, "cerebral" type of respiratory dysfunction with
     asymptomatic intervals. Infant is limp and unresponsive)
   - "Paradoxical" cyanosis
     (Cyanosis is present when the infant lies supine with the mouth closed and is absent
     when the infant cries)
     (E. g., following thoracic trauma with rib fractures)

   Appropriate consultation should be sought for all presumed cases of cardiovascular, central,
   or "paradoxical" respiratory dysfunction!

2. Presumed mechanical (obstructive) respiratory distress:
   Presumptive site-of-lesion determination
   - Cause in the thorax?
   - Cause in the neck (trachea, larynx, hypopharynx)?
   - Cause in the mouth or oropharynx?
   - Cause in the nose or nasopharynx?

3. If dramatic symptoms are absent but spontaneous respiratory function is precarious:
   - Precede a thorough evaluation by *bridging measures* such as:
     – Insertion of a Guedel tube or similar measure for transoral or transnasal airway maintenance
     – Feeding tube insertion
     – Ventilatory support as required

4. If spontaneous respiratory function is satisfactory:
   - Conduct a *detailed evaluation* in the following sequence:
     – Fix the tongue forward
     – Support the patient in an upright position
     – Suction the airway
     – Palpate all areas of the oropharynx and nasopharynx accessible to the finger
       (e. g., for lingual goiter, encephalocele, etc.)
     – Probe the choanae with a soft catheter or a thin fiberoptic endoscope. If the probing instrument
       can be advanced >35 mm past the nostril, the choana is assumed to be patent. Exclude bilat-
       eral choanal atresia, anterior or central nasal atresia, and midfacial hypoplasia (Crouzon or
       Apert syndrome)
     – Perform laryngoscopy with a thin fiberoptic endoscope or if necessary with an intubation spatu-
       la (to exclude laryngomalacia, vocal cord paralysis, tracheomalacia, tracheoesophageal fistula,
       tracheal stenosis, diaphragmatic hernia, esophageal atresia, etc.).
     – If necessary, intubate the trachea and esophagus
     – Radiographs: chest (possibly multiplanar views), nasopharynx skull, neck. Constrast radio-
       graphs of the esophagus and possibly the nose (to exclude choanal atresia)
     – MRI

Glottic Edema

This term, though in clinical usage, is misleading because the edema does not affect the glottic opening. Glottic edema is a collective term for endolaryngeal manifestations of edema that may involve the epiglottis, the ventricular folds, or any other sites in the larynx. Reinke edema and subglottic edema ordinarily are not considered forms of glottic edema. See also p. 322.

Vocal Cord Paralysis

Main symptoms: By far the most common cause of stridor in vocal cord paralysis is bilateral abductor paralysis or "recurrent nerve palsy," in which *both* vocal cords are fixed in a paramedian position. It is remarkable how well some patients can adapt over time to breathing adequately through a tiny glottic chink. In this situation, however, even minor reactive swelling of the vocal folds can lead acutely to severe dyspnea with risk of asphyxiation. Inspiratory stridor is provoked by the slightest physical effort and even occurs at night in the sleeping position. The voice is weak, the cough impulse feeble and breathy. Stridor can also occur with *unilateral* recurrent nerve palsy if the previously healthy side undergoes edematous, inflammatory, or neoplastic change. See p. 350 for details.

Laryngeal Spasm

Main symptoms: A sudden reflex closure of the glottis following violent coughing, aspiration of a foreign body, or extubation after general anesthesia. Immediate effects range from choking to loss of consciousness, during which the spasm generally subsides. Many patients have a prior history of proneness to glottic spasm.

Cause: Presumably a very low threshold of the endolaryngeal protective reflexes.

Diagnosis: If the patient has suffered previous attacks, the situation, though alarming, is generally not life-threatening. The diagnostic procedure of choice is rigid endoscopy to exclude an obstructing foreign body, followed by ventilation through the endoscope. Reintubation may be required.

Laryngeal Diphtheria (Laryngeal Croup)

See p. 316.

Stenosing Laryngotracheitis ([Hyper]acute Subglottic Laryngotracheitis, Pseudocroup in Children)

Main symptoms: Symptoms begin in early childhood (1–5 years) without prodromes or with "catarrh": Dry, barking, "subglottic" cough with increasing dyspnea for several hours, followed by an inspiratory (and often expiratory) stridor and increasing respiratory distress. Agitation and apprehension. Thoracic retraction. Cyanosis. Climatic and seasonal influences: Predisposed individuals appear to be at particularly high risk on damp fall and winter days.

Causes: Virogenic infection (parainfluenzal virus 1–3). Apparently, bacterial pathogens are also common (group B *Haemophilus influenzae*). Noxious environmental agents and allergic factors have also been suggested.

Diagnosis:
● History often demonstrates a predisposition.
● Very characteristic symptoms. Laryngoscopy shows predominantly *subglottic* edema and inflammatory swelling, sometimes with a viscous secretion succeeded by crusts. See Table 6.**11**.

Differentiation is required from acute epiglottitis in children (see p. 316), foreign-body aspiration, and diphtheria. See also Tables 6.**10**, 6.**11**, and 7.**3**.

Endolaryngeal Foreign Bodies

Main symptoms: Symptoms are usually quite dramatic with sudden aphonia, a voiceless cough, stridor, and possible reflex respiratory arrest. Severe unrest. Danger of asphyxiation, with a critical stenosis causing loss of consciousness.

Diagnosis:
● History.
● If the situation permits, indirect laryngoscopy. Radiographic localization of the foreign body is also an option.

Table 6.**11**   Differentiating features of stenosing laryngotracheitis (pseudocroup) and acute epiglottitis (after Truckenbrodt and Richter)

Feature	Stenosing laryngotracheitis (pseudocroup)	Acute epiglottis
Location	Subglottic	Supraglottic
Peak occurrence	Age 1–3 years	Age 2–7 years
Pathogen	Viruses (often parainfluenzal viruses) with possible bacterial superinfection	Usually *Haemophilus influenzae* (group B)
Incidence	Approximately 90%	Approximately 10%
Onset	Often follows an infection, with dyspnea increasing over a period of hours	Fluminating; very severe dyspnea often develops within 1–2 h
Stridor	Inspiratory; independent of body position	Inspiratory (if present), often stertorous; expiratory rattle, gurgle; exacerbated by recumbent position
Voice	Harsh, hoarse to aphonic	Clear, soft, muffled, slurred; not hoarse
Cough	Barking, dry	Often absent
Deglutition	Normal with no excessive salivation	Painful dysphagia with excessive salivation
Local findings	Redness of the vocal cords and subglottic swelling	Massive swelling of the epiglottis; larynx cannot be visualized
General condition	Satisfactory	Severe systemic toxicity
Fever	$<39\,°C$	$>39\,°C$

● Otherwise: immediate endoscopy under emergent conditions (ventilation, preparations for tracheotomy, general anesthesia, *rigid tube!*).
● Extraction.

Differentiation is required from endotracheal or endobronchial foreign bodies (see p. 362) and acute stenosis due to other causes (see Table 6.**8**).

Trauma and Posttraumatic States
See pp. 316, 324.

Benign Neoplasms, Cysts, and Laryngoceles
See pp. 325 ff., 328, and Table 6.**4**.

Malignant Tumors
See p. 326, also Tables 6.**5** and 7.**5**.

Other Causes of Respiratory Distress

Causes of dyspnea that are *not* located in the pharynx, larynx, or tracheobronchial system are reviewed in Table 7.**3**.

Voice and Speech Disorders

F. Martin

Principal Diagnostic Methods

- General and specific *history*.
- ENT *mirror examination.*
- *Logopedic evaluation.*
- *Audiologic evaluation.*
- *Examination of the larynx* includes *external inspection and palpation, indirect laryngoscopy, magnification laryngoscopy,* and *microlaryngoscopy. Direct laryngeal microscopy* is useful for defining diagnostic and therapeutic tasks. *Magnification stroboscopy* and *microstroboscopy* are among the routine diagnostic procedures of the phoniatrician. *Electromyography* is reserved for special inquiries.
- *Vocal function* is assessed perceptually by determining the habitual pitch of the speaking voice and the pitch range, vocal usage (soft, hard, breathy), loudness range, maximum duration of phonation, and vocal quality. The most important electroacoustic study is the frequency/intensity profile (phonetogram). Vocal quality analyses and hoarseness analyses can be performed for specific inquiries. Vocal capacity can be evaluated by voice stress tests and fitness studies.
- The *respiratory examination* covers various types of respiration and is concerned with maximum phonatory duration, vital capacity, and pneumography. Aerodynamic measurements are too costly for routine clinical use.
- Assessment of *phonatory function* includes examination of the articulatory areas (inspection, palpation, orofacial motor function, velopharyngeal function), sound testing, nasality testing, testing of phonematic discrimination, speech comprehension, vocabulary, grammatical ability, reading/writing ability, fluency, and prosody.
- An important component is the *documentation of findings* by means of recording tape (for auditory data) and photographic or video documentation (for visual data).
- Some patients require psychologic evaluation, which may include intelligence testing as well as neurologic, neuropediatric, genetic, endocrinologic, general medical, (adolescent) psychiatric, and special pedagogic studies.
- Imaging studies are discussed on p. 314.

Symptom   **Congenital Dysphonia**

This refers to congenital alterations of vocal quality, which are either associated with organic abnormalities in the larynx or perceived abnormalities of the infant cry that suggest central or peripheral disease. In some congenital anomalies of the larynx (dysplasias), vocal fatigue may be the only prominent symptom that is noted (Table 6.**12**).

Congenital Organic Malformations of the Larynx

Laryngeal Web

Main symptoms: Hoarse to aphonic cry from birth, possibly accompanied by inspiratory and expiratory stridor, depending on the degree of webbing between the vocal folds.

Cause: Congenital reduction deformity.

Diagnosis: Direct laryngoscopy shows a web-like membrane spanning the ligamentous portions of the vocal cords. With pronounced synechia, the vocal cords cannot always be identified. Webbing can also occur at the supraglottic (rare) or subglottic level (more common).

Differentiation is required from congenital synechia of the vocal processes or stenosis of the cricoid cartilage (main symptom: stridor).

Hemangioma

Main symptoms: Increasing stridor during initial postnatal weeks due to progressive enlargement of a capillary hemangioma. Hoarseness and dyspnea may occur, depending on the site of the lesion.

Causes: Disseminated congenital hemangiomatosis with involvement of the trachea and subglottic space.

Diagnosis:
● Direct laryngotracheoscopy under general anesthesia shows a reddish-blue, cavernous mass in the trachea and/or subglottic space with a variable residual lumen. Tracheotomy is occasionally required.

Table 6.**12** *Symptom*   Congenital dysphonia

Synopsis
Laryngeal web
Hemangioma
Vocal cord paralysis
Laryngomalacia
Laryngeal clefts
Anomalies of laryngeal shape
Pathologic infant cry:
Intracranial hemorrhage
Brain tumor
Meningitis
Hydrocephalus
Hyperbilirubinemia
Asphyxia
Congenital hypothyroidism
Langdon–Down disease (mongolism)
Chromosome abnormalities (e. g., cri-du-chat)
Myasthenia gravis
Congenital amyotonia (Oppenheim disease)

● CT to evaluate extent and monitor progression.

Differentiation is required from subglottic hypoplastic cricoid stenosis or subglottic soft hyperplastic connective-tissue stenosis.

Vocal Cord Paralysis

Main symptoms: Feeble infant cry. Stridor and dyspnea occur with bilateral paralysis.

Causes: Most cases are familial, hereditary, and congenital. Birth trauma is a less common etiology.

Diagnosis:
● Direct laryngoscopy shows respiratory vocal cord arrest in a median or paramedian position.
● Evaluate vocal cord mobility under light general anesthesia (spontaneous respiration). Attempt careful mobilization of the arytenoid cartilages.

● If the vocal cords are immobile, evaluate the vocalis muscle by electromyography.

Differentiation is required from congenital ankylosis of the cricoarytenoid joint (EMG) and perinatal subluxation of the arytenoid cartilages by intubation (history).

Laryngomalacia

Main symptoms: Inspiratory stridor. Generally the voice is normal. A weak, quiet voice signifies obstruction of the laryngeal inlet by exceptionally soft cartilage.

Causes: Most common congenital laryngeal anomaly, based on extreme softness of the laryngeal skeleton (maturation defect) with a folded or curled epiglottis.

Diagnosis:
● Typical history of stridorous respiration in the supine position or during forceful inspiration or crying. Stridor is better at rest and in the prone or lateral position.
● Endoscopic examination with a flexible nasopharyngoscope or direct laryngoscopy under light general anesthesia with spontaneous respiration. Soft laryngeal cartilage with curled epiglottic halves that collapse and vibrate on inspiration. Concomitant indrawing of the flaccid mucosa of the aryepiglottic folds and arytenoid cartilage. "Choking fits" are harmless.

Differentiation is required from organic stenoses of the larynx and trachea.

Laryngeal Clefts

Main symptoms: An anterior laryngeal cleft produces congenital aphonia. A posterior or laryngoesophageal cleft produces dysphagia, aspiration, and possible inspiratory stridor.

Causes: Congenital failure of fusion of the thyroid cartilage laminae or cricoid plate.

Diagnosis:
● Palpation of the anterior border of the thyroid cartilage reveals an anterior cleft in the thyroid cartilage with decreased angulation of the laminae.
● Direct laryngotracheoscopy shows increased vocal-cord separation at the anterior commissure with a phonatory anterior glottic cleft. A posterior cleft is marked by a gaping posterior commissure.
● Esophagoscopy.
● Exclude additional anomalies in the upper aerodigestive tract.

Differentiation is mainly required from congenital hypoplasia or aplasia of the vocalis muscle (normal vocal-cord separation at the anterior commissure, bowing of the cords).

Anomalies of Laryngeal Shape

Main symptoms: Symptoms are nonspecific and may include vocal fatigue, especially under stress, and constant hoarseness ("dysplastic dysphonia"). With severe malformations, inspiratory stridor and airway distress predominate.

Causes: Congenital morphologic anomalies or malformations of the larynx. The milder forms are most prevalent.

Diagnosis: Phoniatric and logopedic evaluation. Voice stress test.

Differentiation is required from phonasthenia and from functional, neurogenic, and psychogenic voice disorders.

Abnormal Infant Cry

The abnormal infant cry is characterized by continuous, dominant noise components and/or by constant or repetitive structural changes in the fundamental frequency and overtone structure. Relevant noise manifestations tend to arise from local lesions, while changes in acoustic structure usually signify developmental anomalies, chromosomal, central, or myogenic causes, or neurologic disease. The site of the lesion may correlate with the character of the cry.

Main symptoms: Hoarse or tonally altered voice, or the cry may be stridorous but clear. Cough quality is altered by glottic, subglottic, or tracheal lesions.

Causes: Besides congenital organic laryngeal abnormalities, potential causes include intracranial hemorrhage, brain tumors, meningitis, hydrocephalus, hyperbilirubinemia, asphyxia, congenital hypothyroidism, Langdon–Down disease (mongolism), chromosome abnormalities (e.g., cri-du-chat), myasthenia gravis, and congenital amyotonia (Oppenheim disease).

Diagnosis:
- Endoscopy of the complete aerodigestive tract (microlaryngoscopy, bronchoscopy, esophagoscopy) to exclude organic pathology. The workup should not terminate when a peripheral lesion is found, as there may be coexisting airway disease.
- In the absence of demonstrable organic airway disease, detailed neurologic (EEG, CT, EMG, muscle biopsy) and pediatric investigations (including chromosome studies) are indicated.

- The spectral analysis of vocal pathology is reserved for specially equipped voice laboratories.

Differentiation is required from pharyngeal stridor with posterior displacement of the tongue in patients with bilateral choanal atresia, microgenia, the Robin syndrome, the Cornelia de Lange syndrome, the Hurler syndrome, and mental retardation. Stridorous phonation and pathologic cough occur with tracheal diseases such as congenital goiter, vascular anomalies, mediastinal tumor, functional tracheal narrowing in tracheobronchomalacia, circumscribed malformation of the tracheal cartilage, tracheal dyskinesia, rigid tracheal stenosis, and occasionally congenital tracheoesophageal fistula or esophageal atresia.

Symptom   **Acquired Dysphonia** (Table 6.13)

Functional Voice Disorders

This is a collective term for voice disorders that involve distortions of vocal quality and capacity in the absence of a primary pathologic organic condition. Functional abnormalities in the tonicity of structures that contribute to voice production (respiratory apparatus, larynx, resonator, even the body as a whole) may be in the direction of "too much" (=hyperfunctional dysphonia) or "too little" (=hypofunctional dysphonia).

Causes: Presumably a multifactorial etiology (Table 6.14) involving constitutional, habitual, phonogenic, and psychogenic factors.

Hyperfunctional Dysphonia

Main symptoms: History of vocal failure. Stress-dependent decline in vocal capacity during the day or week with recovery overnight or over the weekend. Following vocal exertion the voice sounds raspy, harsh, grating, strained, and diplophonic. The degree of hoarseness

depends on the degree of vocal strain. Other symptoms are throat discomfort (most common early symptom) such as scratching, burning, a foreign-body sensation, or anterior internal and external neck and throat pain. There is habitual throat clearing and swallowing with a sensation of increased mucus formation. The pharynx feels dry. There is laryngeal tickling with a paroxysmal cough followed briefly by spasmodic aphonia. Characteristic late symptom is a hoarse, strained, grating voice.

Causes: Multifactorial. Besides constitutional factors, a disproportion exists between individual vocal capacity and vocal misuse/abuse, e.g., a protracted increase in vocal pitch and loudness in a noisy environment, when speaking with a hearing-impaired person, or when singing out of range. Other causes are mechanical trauma by coughing and throat clearing. Psychogenic factors include an inability to cope with general life tasks and conflicts, excessive psychosocial demands, and adverse working conditions. Organic factors such as in-

Table 6.**13** *Symptom* Acquired dysphonia

Synopsis	
Functional voice disorders	**Hormonal voice disorders**

Functional voice disorders

Hyperfunctional dysphonia

- Primary hyperfunctional dysphonia
- Secondary hyperfunctional dysphonia
- Juvenile hyperfunctional dysphonia
- Occupational dysphonia
- False-vocal-cord voice
- Hyperfunctional psychogenic aphonia
- Spastic dysphonia

Hypofunctional dysphonia

- Primary hypofunctional dysphonia
- Secondary hypofunctional dysphonia
- Hypofunctional form of occupational dysphonia
- Psychogenic dysphonia/aphonia

Developmental voice disorders

Mutation disorders

- Persistent childlike voice
- Delayed mutation
- Precocious mutation
- Perverse mutation

Dysphonias relating to the female cycle

- Premenstrual dysodia
- Menstrual dysodia
- Laryngopathia gravidarum
- Mutation of pregnancy
- Menopausal dysphonia
- Senile voice

Hormonal voice disorders

Dysphonia induced by androgens
Dysphonia induced by anabolic steroids

Endocrine disorders

Pituitary disorders
- Acromegaly
- Pituitary microsomia and dwarfism
- Anterior pituitary insufficiency

Gonadal disorders
- Male hypogonadism
- Hormone-producing gonadal tumors

Thyroid disorders
- Hyperthyroidism
- Hypothyroidism

Adrenocortical disorders
- Addison disease
- Adrenogenital syndrome
- Androgen-producing tumors of the adrenal cortex

Myogenic voice disorders

Myopathy of the vocalis muscle
Myasthenia gravis pseudoparalytica

Secondary organic voice disorders

Vocal cord hyperemia
Vasomotor monocorditis
Chronic catarrhal laryngitis
Chronic laryngitis due to noise exposure
Vocal polyps
Vocal nodules
Contact pachyderma

Neurogenic voice disorders

flammatory and allergic vocal cord lesions, previous vocal cord surgery, and postintubation states combined with inadequate voice rest can, by altering kinesthetic feedback, affect phonation by inciting a compensatory tone increase in the phonatory muscles.

Diagnosis:
- History, giving special attention to habitual and psychosocial factors.
- Vocal status: increased habitual pitch, vocal abuse.

- Inspection: abnormal speech respiration, abnormal position and tonicity of orofacial and neck muscles and even of the body musculature as a whole. Excessive muscle tension in the tongue is difficult to appreciate when the tongue is extended. Soft palate is stiff during phonation and shows little elevation.
- Abnormal muscle tension hampers laryngeal examination. Tight, cylindrical vocal folds with narrow light reflexes and poor posterior closure. Possible concomitant movement of the false vocal cords.

Table 6.**14** Etiology and pathogenesis of functional dysphonias (after Bauer)

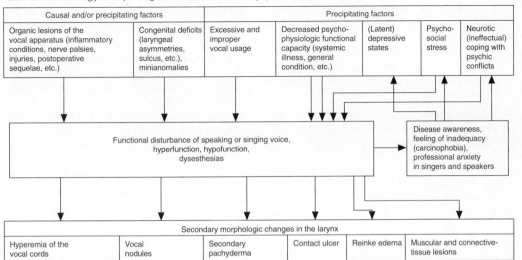

Causal and/or precipitating factors		Precipitating factors				
Organic lesions of the vocal apparatus (inflammatory conditions, nerve palsies, injuries, postoperative sequelae, etc.)	Congenital deficits (laryngeal asymmetries, sulcus, etc.), minianomalies	Excessive and improper vocal usage	Decreased psycho-physiologic functional capacity (systemic illness, general condition, etc.)	(Latent) depressive states	Psycho-social stress	Neurotic (ineffectual) coping with psychic conflicts

Functional disturbance of speaking or singing voice, hyperfunction, hypofunction, dysesthesias

Disease awareness, feeling of inadequacy (carcinophobia), professional anxiety in singers and speakers

Secondary morphologic changes in the larynx					
Hyperemia of the vocal cords	Vocal nodules	Secondary pachyderma	Contact ulcer	Reinke edema	Muscular and connective-tissue lesions

- Stroboscopy shows decreased glottic edge movements of low amplitude that do not increase with loudness level.
- Phonetogram.

Differentiation is required from laryngeal catarrh or (sub)acute laryngitis in which there is redness of the vocal cords or their free edges (maginal corditis) as an expression of stress-related hyperemia. Differential diagnosis includes hormonal voice disorders in hyperthyroidism or hypothyroidism with compensatory hyperfunctional symptoms, and incomplete mutation with an excessively high vocal pitch.

Special Forms:

- *Secondary hyperfunctional dysphonia* occurring as a compensatory stage in primary hypofunctional dysphonia. Approximation of the false vocal cords, depression of the epiglottis, constriction of the supraglottic sphincter. Vocalis gap shows normal amplitudes and marked edge movements. Raising the pitch narrows the vocalis gap and produces a clear voice.
- *Juvenile hyperfunctional dysphonia:* Most common voice disorder in children. Loud, aggressive children (3:1 ratio of boys to girls) of school age or preschool age. Vocal cords are edematous or show fusiform thick-

ening. Predisposition to vocal nodules (see p. 350).

- *Occupational dysphonias:* Occupation-related voice disorders are most often a clinical manifestation of hyperfunctional dysphonia. Professional voice users are predisposed (lecturers, teachers, salesmen, attorneys, persons in noisy work settings; also mothers of several children, relatives of hearing-impaired persons, etc.). Vocal intensity and speaking fundamental frequency are increased. Besides constitutional differences in the capacity and stress tolerance of the phonatory apparatus, potential causes include faulty vocal technique, psychoautonomic factors, conflicts, and unfavorable environmental conditions (noise, dry air, gymnasiums). May lead to development of secondary organic voice disorders (see p. 348). Occupational dysphonias may render the patient unable to continue in the same work setting.
- *False-vocal-cord voice:* Secondary, extreme form of hyperfunctional dysphonia. The voice sounds deep, strained, and harsh. The false vocal cords approximate to the point of medial contact and are often hyperplastic. There is simultaneous constriction of the remaining supraglottic sphincter with posterior displacement of the petiole and epiglottis and narrowing of the laryngeal inlet, so that

the true vocal cords are hidden from view. A compensatory mechanism for glottic insufficiency, e.g., in chronic laryngitis, Reinke edema, vocalis atrophy, and after cordectomy, laryngeal trauma, or paresis of the true vocal folds. A psychogenic "undesired false-cord voice" can develop in patients whose true cords are intact.

Differentiation is required from primary hyperplasias of the false vocal cords due to cystic glandular lesions (dyschylic pseudotumor), internal laryngoceles, prolapse of ventricular mucosa thickened by inflammatory edema, allergic or radiogenic inflammatory thickenings of the ventricular folds with unilateral bulging of the false vocal cords, and especially concealed tumors (intramural, ventricular, or on the laryngeal aryepiglottic surface).

○ *Hyperfunctional psychogenic aphonia:* History of sudden onset brought on by acute psychic trauma (fright, humiliation, despair, or joy), usually after long-standing conflict situations. Also voice guarding after acute laryngitis or decortication of the vocal cords. Discrepancy between severe vocal dysfunction (dysphonia to aphonia) and a normal-appearing larynx. Attempted phonation produces tight glottic closure with no sound emission and constriction of the supraglottic sphincter. Most patients can cough and laugh normally, and speech is normalized by white noise masking through headphones.

Differentiation is required from vocal cord paralysis. Paradoxical adduction: Psychogenic motility disturbance with glottic closure during inspiration with inspiratory stridor.

○ *Spastic dysphonia:* Phonatory glottic spasm during speech (vocal stutter). Spasms of the respiratory and phonatory muscles lead to a very strained, grating, and saccadic vocalization with irregular voice breaks and vocal tremor. The patient has a "strangled" appearance during speech. As speech is continued, the symptoms increase to the point of intermittent vocal failure and complete physical exhaustion. Noncommunicative vocalizations (whispering, singing) are unaffected. Laryngoscopy usually shows hyperemic vocal cords (stress hyperemia) and thickened ventricular folds that approxi-

mate on phonation, partly or completely obscuring the true cords. Intermittent, jerky, ataxic vocal cord movements lead to fleeting glottic closure.

Differentiation is required from tonic stutter, false-cord voice (hoarse singing voice), the hyperfunctional form of psychogenic dysphonia, pseudobulbar dysarthria, spastic cerebral palsy, amyotrophic lateral sclerosis, multiple sclerosis, and tabetic crises.

The **prognosis** is poor, especially in long-standing cases.

Hypofunctional Dysphonia

Main symptoms: Soft, breathy, quiet, easily fatigued voice that cannot be effectively raised to a higher loudness level. Occasional functional flaring of the nares due to deficient activation of the soft palate. Subjective discomfort such as throat dryness and pain.

Causes: Congenital hypotonicity of the laryngeal muscles or the general body musculature.

Diagnosis:
● The tongue is flaccid and easily grasped. Laryngoscopy shows elliptical closure defect (vocalis weakness) and/or triangular posterior gapping (arytenoid weakness).
● Stroboscopy shows increased amplitudes and edge movements with accentuated vertical vibrations. With pronounced hypofunction, there is bowing of the vocal cords in the respiratory position.
● Vocal status.
● Phonetogram.

Differentiation is required from phonasthenia, in which abnormal vocal fatigue is accompanied by normal laryngostroboscopic findings. Hypofunctional form of psychogenic dysphonia. Residuum of vocal cord paralysis. Vocal cord atrophy with bowing secondary to myositis or mechanical stretching by prior intubation.

Special Forms:

○ *Secondary hypofunctional dysphonia:* Decompensated form of primary hyperfunctional dysphonia due to exhaustion. On laryngoscopy, the posterior commissure is seen to extend over the ligamentous area. Marked reduction of the glottal chink and the resumption of edge movements in response to low-pitched phonation are typical of this condition.

○ Hypofunctional forms of *occupational dysphonia* are rare. They are characterized by a contracted vocal range, decreased maximum phonatory duration, and posteriorly displaced, indistinct articulation.

○ Psychogenic dysphonia/aphonia with hypofunctional symptoms: Psychogenic components predominate (stressful situations, vocal anxiety, psychic stresses, depression, neuroses). The gaping glottal chink mimics paresis. Reflex vocal cord mobility is preserved during coughing and laughing.

Developmental Voice Disorders

Mutation Disorders

Persistent Childlike Voice

Main symptom: High-pitched, infantile voice in an individual with physical dimensions appropriate for an adult male.

Causes: Prepubertal castration (history). Primary hypogenitalism due to loss of testicular function (testicular atrophy, malformations, tumors, trauma) leads to an eunuchoid male with an infantile habitus, eunuchoid gigantism or obesity, and a small larynx with a high-pitched, childlike voice. Secondary hypogonadism due to pituitary insufficiency. Lack of gonadotropic hormones.

Diagnosis:
● History. Laryngoscopy and general physical examination: failure of pubertal development (beard growth) after 15 years of age, small larynx, eunuchoid gigantism or obesity. Hypoplastic genitals.
● Endocrine evaluation.
● Gonadotropin assay. Testicular biopsy.

Differentiation is required from pubertas tarda and psychogenic forms.

Delayed Mutation

Main symptoms: Delayed onset of vocal mutation in males over 16 years of age or in females over 14 years of age.

Causes: Constitutional developmental abnormality. Developmental retardation secondary to chronic disease. Testicular insufficiency due to gonadotropin deficiency (secondary hypogonadotropic hypogonadism) or direct testicular damage with normal gonadotropin production (primary hypergonadotropic hypogonadism). The Klinefelter syndrome. Gonadal dysgenesis in girls. Adiposogenital dystrophy.

Diagnosis: Laryngoscopic findings, vocal status, endocrine studies.

Differentiation is required from pituitary microsomia and dwarfism and from forms of growth retardation not associated with deficient gonadotropins.

Precocious Mutation

Main symptom: Deepening of the voice before 8 years of age in both sexes. Accelerated body growth. Enlarged genitals. Age-appropriate mental status.

Causes: Premature sexual maturation (precocious puberty) based on premature activation of the hypothalamic−pituitary−gonadal axis (hypothalamic gonadotropin releasing hormones, pituitary gonadotropin secretion, androgen production). Tumors or inflammatory lesions involving the third ventricle or hypothalamus. The Albright syndrome, pseudopubertas praecox due to peripheral lesions such as neoplasia or hyperplasia (adrenal cortex, testes), ectopic hormone-producing tumors, exogenous hormone administration.

Diagnosis: Laryngoscopy, vocal status, pediatric endocrine studies.

Perverse Mutation in Girls

Main symptoms: Harshness of the voice during puberty with a masculine vocal quality. Menarche may fail to occur.

Causes: Disturbance of the normal hormonal system at the level of the pituitary, ovaries, or adrenal cortex. (A hormonal disturbance cannot always be demonstrated). Psychic factors, mimicry.

Diagnosis is based on endocrine studies, signs of virilization, and masculine dimensions of the female larynx.

Differential diagnosis includes hormonal, exogenous androgenic, psychogenic, and constitutional causes and pregnancy-related vocal change. Exclude organic laryngeal disease.

Dysphonias
Relating to the Female Cycle

Premenstrual Dysodia

Main symptoms: Limitation of subtle voice performance, especially the singing of high notes (dysodia). Voice is dull to hoarse, deepened, harsh, cracked, and easily strained. The speaking voice is not impaired.

Causes: Variable. Emotional lability, progesterone-induced ergotropic–sympathicotonic state. Increased premenstrual water retention with secondary aldosteronism.

Diagnosis: History with emphasis on general physical premenstrual tension and discomfort. The vocal cord mucosae are slightly swollen or edematous and are congested to hyperemic. Circumscribed subepithelial petechiae may be present. Mucus production is increased. Stroboscopy shows a hypofunctional vibratory pattern.

Differentiation is required from functional voice disorders, laryngitis, abuse of the singing voice, and iatrogenic administration of virilizing hormones.

Menstrual Dysodia

Main symptoms: Accentuation of premenstrual complaints, with a lowering of vocal pitch and a contracted upper range. Vocal intensity may be increased.

Causes: Same as for premenstrual dysodia.

Diagnosis: Typical cyclic history. Mild mucosal swelling with accentuated vascular markings and incomplete glottic closure.

Differential diagnosis: same as for premenstrual dysodia.

Laryngopathia Gravidarum

Twenty percent of all pregnant women give a history of laryngopathic complaints starting in about the 5th month of gestation.

Main symptoms: Dryness, pain, and foreign-body sensation in the upper airways; variable hoarseness with a rough, raspy, hoarse to aphonic voice. The vocal pitch drops by from two to three tones. Positive vocal changes may persist after parturition, however (voice is more mature, fuller, warmer, stronger).

Causes: Physiologic changes relating to pregnancy. True preeclampsia–eclampsia. Predisposition for manifesting a latent voice disorder. Nervous etiology.

Diagnosis: The vocal folds are edematous, bulging, and livid on laryngoscopy, with involvement of the arytenoid cartilage region, aryepiglottic folds, and false vocal cords. The mucosae are dry or covered with secretions; crusting is less common. Similar mucosal changes are found on the nasal septum and turbinates. Symptoms are entirely reversible after delivery.

Differentiation is required from functional voice disorders, subacute laryngitis, laryngitis sicca, other causes of edema, mutation of pregnancy, and drug side effects.

Mutation of Pregnancy

Extremely rare.

Main symptoms: Deep, clear, masculine-type voice commencing during pregnancy and persisting afterwards. Possible laryngeal enlargement.

Causes: Presumably a transient hormonal imbalance involving excessive androgen production.

Diagnosis: Endocrine studies are indicated if the voice deepens by a full octave.

Differentiation is required from laryngopathia gravidarum, hormonally or pharmacologically induced vocal virilization, and androglottia (feminine larynx with masculine voice quality).

Menopausal Dysphonia

Main symptoms: Slight deepening of the voice with a contracted upper pitch range. Speaking fundamental frequency is lowered, with significant loss of singing ability and vocal fatigue. Voice is harsh, breathy, and easily strained.

Causes: Estrogen deficiency due to ovarian insufficiency, relative predominance of adrenocortical androgens.

Diagnosis:
- Often there is a history of associated neuroautonomic and psychic symptoms.
- Laryngoscopy shows slight thickening and occasional asymmetry of the vocal cords.
- Stroboscopy shows irregular vibrations of variable amplitude, phase aperiodicities, and glottic hypofunction.

Differentiation is required from iatrogenic hormonal dysphonia (ask about hormone use!) and functional voice disorders.

Senile Voice

Main symptoms: A lower fundamental frequency in women and a higher fundamental frequency in men. Contracted vocal range. The senile voice fatigues easily and has a dull, weak, shallow quality with little volume. Monotonicity and tremor are common. Maximum phonatory duration is shortened. Voice may be breathy and husky with breaks or may be sharp and shrill. There is loss of resiliency in the respiratory organs (decreased thoracic respiratory excursions and vital capacity) and larynx.

Causes: Complex psychophysical involutionary processes that involve morphologic, endocrinologic, biochemical, central nervous, and neuromuscular factors.

Diagnosis:
- Estimate biological (not chronological!) age. Laryngoscopy shows expansion of the (para)laryngeal spaces due to soft-tissue atrophy. The mucosae are dry due to involution of the false-cord glands. Usually there is vocalis weakness and less commonly a transverse arytenoid muscle gap. The vocal cords appear widened due to dilatation of the laryngeal ventricles, and their contours are enhanced due to atrophy.
- Stroboscopy shows irregular vibratory amplitudes.

Differentiation is required from functional voice disorders, hypofunctional symptoms of abrupt onset in severe systemic diseases, consumptive diseases, and postintubation states.

Hormonal Voice Disorders

Dysphonia Induced by Androgens or Anabolic Steroids

Main symptoms: *Early symptoms* are entirely subjective and consist of increased susceptibility to vocal strain and fatigue and a vocal quality that the patient perceives as "strange." Later there are objective, irreversible symptoms of a harsh, cracked voice with loss of singing and shouting ability. The *late symptom* is a low habitual pitch.

Causes: *Androgenic hormones* administered for the treatment of breast or ovarian cancer (Amenose, Famandren, Femovirin, Lylaudrone, Masteril, Primodian, testosterone, Testoviron). *Combination products* containing androgens and estrogens given for menopausal complaints, premenstrual complaints, endometriosis, fibrocystic breast disease, or osteoporosis. *Ovulation inhibitors* in the form of synthetic estrogen−progesteron products. Voice disorders are especially common with nortestosterone derivatives; hydroxyprogesterone derivatives tend to produce laryngitis sicca-type symptoms. Dysphonia also results from *anabolic steroid use* to promote protein synthesis during convalescence from a debilitated condition, underweight, anorexia, exhaustion, chronic hepatic and renal diseases, and growth disturbances (Anadur, Dianabol, Diane, Durabolin, Primobolan, Steronabol, Stromba). Also *hepatic protectants* (Dacomid, Fortabol), *antihypotensive drugs* (Docabolin). Aldosterone antagonists (Aldactone, spironolactone) for diuresis can also cause vocal dysfunction in males. *Hydantoins* in antiepileptics. *Ablactational injections* (Ablactone, Pravidel). Factors predisposing to increased sensitivity to androgens: increased endogenous androgen production, high target-organ sensitivity, laryngeal asymmetry, asthenic male habitus with proness to acne, hirsutism, hypomenorrhea, and deep voice.

Diagnosis: Specific, detailed history of drug use is essential. Laryngologic findings are subtle and nonspecific. Vocal cords are reddened, show marginal edema, and have a porous, spongy appearance. Stroboscopy during deep phonation shows amplitude expansion with decreased edge movements. Glottic gaps form at various sites.

Differentiation in boys is required from true isosexual precocious puberty; in women and girls, from adrenogenital syndrome, androgen-elaborating tumors, and polycystic ovaries with virilization. Differential diagnosis also includes mutation of pregnancy, androglottia, constitutional hirsutism, acromegaly, functional voice disorder, acute laryngitis, and laryngitis sicca.

Endocrine Disorders

Pituitary Disorders

Acromegaly

Main phoniatric symptoms: Hollow, rough, hoarse, strained voice with a dark quality, contracted vocal range, reduced phonatory duration, and muffled, indistinct articulation. General enlargement of the hands and feet.

Causes: Intrasellar eosinophilic pituitary adenoma producing excessive growth hormone after the cessation of longitudinal growth.

Diagnosis: Endocrine evaluation. Indirect ENT examination shows nasal airway obstruction with general nasal enlargement. Macrocheilia, macroglossia, progenia, interdental gap. Later hypersalivation. Resonant cavity is narrowed. There is substantial laryngeal enlargement with long, wide vocal folds. Mucosal thickening is also noted in the arytenoid cartilage area and on the aryepiglottic folds.

Differentiation is required from constitutional acromegalic habitus and reversible acromegaloidism of pregnancy.

Pituitary Microsomia and Dwarfism

Main phoniatric symptoms: Persistent child-like voice in adulthood with small laryngeal dimensions and proportionate microsomia.

Causes: Puberty and vocal mutation fail to occur due to pituitary hypoplasia with growth-hormone deficiency and secondary gonadotropic pituitary dysfunction.

Diagnosis: Endocrine studies can confirm the clinical impression. The larynx is soft due to failure of ossification of the laryngeal cartilages. Microgenia. Gothic-arch-shaped palate.

Differentiation is required from nonpituitary forms of growth deficiency.

Anterior Pituitary Insufficiency

Main symptoms: Phonatory symptoms of hypofunctional dysphonia. Breathy, mono-pitched voice with contracted vocal range.

Causes: Ischemic necrosis of the anterior lobe of the pituitary. Postpartum Sheehan syndrome, infectious or traumatic hemorrhage, primary idiopathic fibrosis, fibrosis secondary to syphilitic or tuberculous granuloma, pituitary neoplasms.

Diagnosis: Endocrine studies. Laryngoscopy shows flaccid vocal cords and a ligamentous glottic gap.

Differentiation is required from primary hypothyroidism, primary adrenocortical insufficiency, hypergonadotropic hypogonadism, anorexia nervosa, chronic consumptive diseases, and amenorrhea due to various causes.

Gonadal Disorders

Male Hypogonadism

Main symptoms: Prepubescent androgen deficiency leads to failure of vocal mutation with lack of development of secondary sex characters.

Causes: Direct, irreversible testicular damage with a reactive inrease in gonadotropin formation (hypergonadotropic hypergonadism) or secondary hypogonadism due to absent or deficient gonadotropin formation (hypogonadotropic hypogonadism).

Diagnosis: Andrologic evaluation.

Differentiation is required from constitutional or psychogenic mutational voice disorders, anterior pituitary insufficiency, the Klinefelter syndrome, and the Kallmann syndrome (hypogonadotropic hypogonadism with anosmia). Female hypogonadism, even with gonadal dysgenesis, is characterized by a persistent child-like voice.

Hormone-producing Gonadal Tumors

Main symptoms: In boys, isosexual pseudopubertas praecox with premature change of voice or signs of feminization, depending on the type of hormone produced. In girls, isosexual or heterosexual pseudopubertas praecox with precocious mutation or postpubescent virilization.

Causes: Testicular tumors with isosexual or heterosexual activity. Ovarian tumors with isosexual activity. Androgen-producing ovarian tumors.

Diagnosis: Gynecologic or andrologic examination.

Differentiation is required from true isosexual precocious puberty, androgenital syndrome, androgen-producing adrenocortical tumors, and iatrogenic administration of androgens or anabolic steroids. In women: polycystic ovaries with virilization (Stein–Leventhal syndrome), mutation of pregnancy, androglottia, constitutional hirsutism. In males with gynecomastia: the Klinefelter syndrome, administration of aldosterone antagonists.

Thyroid Disorders

Hyperthyroidism

Main phoniatric symptoms: Diminished vocal capacity in terms of range, pitch, loudness, and duration. Voice is harsh, jittery, tremulous, and hoarse.

Causes: Hyperfunction of the thyroid gland due to diffuse hyperplasia, hyperthyroid nodular goiter, or toxic adenoma.

Diagnosis: Medical and endocrinologic evaluation. Laryngoscopy shows normal laryngeal findings with hypofunctional or hyperfunctional symptoms; a jittery or tremulous vocal quality; shallow, adynamic phonatory respiration; reduced vital capacity; a weak singing and shouting voice; rapid vocal fatigue; and decreased phonatory duration.

Differentiation is required from functional and psychogenic dysphonias, myopathic dysphonia, and thyrovocal syndrome with reflex laryngeal hyperemia in patients with large goiters.

Hypothyroidism

Main phoniatric symptoms: With *congenital hypothyroidism*, the infant cry is deep, hoarse, harsh, and monopitched. Vocal range is diminished, and phonatory duration is greatly reduced. Developmental speech delay is difficult to treat, especially with regard to sibilant production and nasality.

With *acquired hypothyroidism*, the habitual pitch is deepened and the voice fatigues rapidly. Vocal quality is hoarse, grating, scratchy, and cracked. Articulation is crude and indistinct. Bradylalia. Monotone voice. General physical and mental inertia.

Causes: Congenital etiology, acquired pituitary disease, faulty iodine utilization, radical strumectomy, thyroiditis, thyrostatic drugs, radioiodine therapy.

Diagnosis: Medical and endocrinologic evaluation. Audiography, as 50% of affected children have sensorineural hearing loss (the Pendred syndrome). Laryngoscopy in congenital cases shows a small larynx and gross, bulging, flaccid vocal folds with edematous margins. Acquired cases feature edematous mucosal changes in the nose, pharynx, and larynx with waxy-yellow, edematous infiltration in the arytenoid cartilage area.

Differentiation is required from edematous mucosal changes due to other causes and senile voice changes.

Adrenocortical Disorders

Addison Disease

Main symptoms: Muscular adynamia with weak, breathy voice that fatigues rapidly. Disturbed shouting and singing voice. Decreased vital capacity and phonatory duration. Speech is slow and feeble. Habitual pitch is lowered in women.

Cause: Adrenocortical dysfunction.

Diagnosis: Clinical presentation is predominant. Hormone assays.

Differentiation is required from hypofunctional dysphonias due to other causes and from secondary adrenocortical insufficiency in pituitary diseases.

Adrenogenital Syndrome

Main symptoms: Boys develop isosexual precocious puberty with laryngeal enlargement and a dark vocal timbre after 7 years of age and vocal change after 10 years of age. Girls develop virilization signs after birth consistent with heterosexual pseudopubertas praecox. After 10 years of age they manifest vocal changes like those of normal male mutation.

Causes: Inreased adrenocortical androgen production based on congenital enzyme defects with a recessive mode of inheritance.

Diagnosis: Elevation of urinary 17-ketosteroids. Levels should be determined whenever deepening of the voice occurs in childhood.

Differential diagnosis: Congenital changes require differentiation from true hermaphroditism and feminine pseudohermaphroditism due to nonadrenal causes. Masculine pseudohermaphroditism should be considered in intersexual boys, and true isosexual precocious puberty in male children. Differential diagnosis in females should include virilizing ovarian tumors, Stein–Leventhal syndrome, androglottia, congenital hirsutism, androgen and anabolic steroid use, and androgen-producing tumors of the adrenal cortex.

Androgen-producing Tumors of the Adrenal Cortex

Main phoniatric symptoms: Vocal changes like those occurring in adrenogenital syndrome.

Causes: Androgen-producing carcinomas, less commonly adenomas of the adrenal cortex in children, some of which may be congenital.

Diagnosis: CT, specific steroid hormone analyses, elevated urinary 17-ketosteroid levels.

Differential diagnosis is like that for adrenogenital syndrome and should include pregnancy-related vocal change.

Myogenic Voice Disorders

Myopathy of the Vocalis Muscle

Main symptoms: Hoarse, breathy, weak voice with strained phonation as in secondary hyperfunctional dysphonia.

Cause: Noncompliance with voice rest in acute (interstitial) laryngitis or inflammatory infiltration of vocalis muscle (myositis).

Diagnosis: Laryngoscopy shows an elliptical glottic gap or glottic sulcus. Stroboscopy shows variable amplitudes and discontinuous edge movements. Often there are compensatory hyerfunctional supraglottic adductions.

Differentiation is required from hypofunctional disorders, reflex or psychogenic vocal cord guarding after acute laryngitis, and bilateral cricothyroid muscle paralysis.

Myasthenia Gravis Pseudoparalytica

Main phoniatric symptoms: Rapid decline in vocal capacity with hypernasal speech to aphonia, with spontaneous recovery following brief voice rest.

Causes: Impairment of neuromuscular signal transmission based on acetylcholinesterase deficiency.

Diagnosis:
- Neurologic evaluation.
- Neostigmine test.
- EMG.

Differentiation is required from bulbar lesions.

Secondary Organic Voice Disorders (Due to Vocal Abuse)

Vocal Cord Hyperemia (Noninfectious Laryngitis)

Main symptoms: Hoarseness following vocal exertion, most pronounced in the evening. Frequent throat clearing. Potential development of hyperfunctional dysphonia.

Causes: Aberrant vocal usage in speaking professions or in a noisy environment. Vigorous coughing. Vocal stress or overuse in singers.

Diagnosis: Detailed, specific history. Laryngoscopy shows marginal or diffuse hyperemia of the vocal folds with vascular congestion.

Differentiation is required from the inflammatory form of laryngitis (hoarseness present on waking), psychogenic dysphonia (varying, inconstant symptoms), hormonal dysphonia (constant pattern of dysfunction), and primary hyperfunctional dysphonia. History, clinical presentation, and follow-ups are often necessary for differentiation.

Vasomotor Monocorditis

Main symptoms: Hoarse, diplophonic, rapidly fatiguing voice with a contracted range.

Causes: Unclear. May relate to faulty or excessive vocal usage in the setting of a neuroautonomic and hormonal imbalance. Women are more commonly affected.

Diagnosis:
● Laryngoscopy shows redness and edema of one vocal cord with a normal-appearing opposite cord.
● Stroboscopy shows decreased amplitudes and edge movements and possible phonatory arrest.

Differential diagnosis: If the voice does not improve after a 4-week course of voice rest and anti-inflammatory therapy, a biopsy is taken to exclude a specific inflammatory disease (tuberculosis) or malignancy. With premenstrual hyperemia affecting one vocal cord, stroboscopy demonstrates a normal vibratory pattern.

Chronic Catarrhal Laryngitis

Main symptoms: Hoarseness that is more severe in the morning than in the evening. Pitch range and fundamental frequency are reduced. Habitual throat clearing. Dryness and foreign-body sensation. Also burning, scratching, tickling, and pain in the throat.

Causes: Inadequate voice rest in acute laryngitis. Vocal abuse. Often combined with smoking; the inhalation of caustic vapors; a dry, dusty environment; or mouth breathing. Upper respiratory tract infection, alcohol, allergy.

Diagnosis: Detailed history. Laryngoscopy shows cylindrical thickening and grayish-red discoloration of the vocal folds, which have blunt and rounded edges. Viscous mucous strands. Stroboscopy shows irregular vibratory pattern with abbreviated edge movements or even phonatory arrest.

Differentiation is required from allergic laryngitis (allergy test), smoker's laryngitis, subacute laryngitis, hyperfunctional dysphonia, and hormonal forms of dysphonia. See also p. 320.

Chronic Laryngitis
Due to Noise Exposure

Main symptoms: Hoarseness, frequent throat clearing, strained, raspy voice.

Causes: Chronic vocal abuse with use of high loudness levels and increased conversational volume in a noisy work setting. Hyperfunctional dysphonia is usually secondary. Pathologic vocal changes occur in 50% of speakers past 85 dB(A) and in 90% of speakers past 90 dB(A). Secondary vocal damage occurs by the 3rd to 7th year of employment.

Diagnosis:
● Laryngoscopy may show either a chronic atrophic or chronic hyperplastic form.
● Stroboscopy usually shows a hyperfunctional pattern.

Differentiation is required from chronic laryngitis of other etiology and from carcinoma. See also p. 326.

Vocal Polyps

Main symptoms: Usually there is severe hoarseness with aphonic episodes. With pedunculated lesions, the voice may be essentially normal at low volume. Habitual throat clearing. Feeling of dryness in the throat.

Causes: Phonation trauma (shouting), excessive vocal use in smokers or in the setting of laryngitis. Middle-aged males are predominantly affected.

Diagnosis: Laryngoscopy generally shows a typical unilateral lesion involving the center or anterior third of the ligamentous vocal cord.

The polyp may be sessile or pedunculated and may arise from the upper surface, free margin, or undersurface of the cord. A *teleangiectatic polyp* is red to dark red and richly vascular. A *gelatinous polyp* appears grayish-yellow, glassy, and translucent. Stroboscopy will reveal any associated inflammatory reaction of surrounding tissues (important before microsurgical ablation!).

Differentiation is required from varices, hematoma, cyst, vocal nodules (always bilateral, females). Sessile polyps require differentiation from edema due to vocal abuse, unilateral Reinke edema, vocal cord amyloidosis, and polypous mucosal thickenings (in older patients). See also p. 322.

Vocal Nodules

Main symptoms: Hoarseness, vocal cord disuse, diplophonia, habitual throat clearing, foreign-body sensation. Vocal nodules in singers ("singer's nodes") limit the ability to sing softly or reach higher notes. Increased effort is required for singing, but vocal quality may remain normal. Affects children of both sexes and women.

Causes: Vocal abuse with hyperfunctional symptomatology. Caused by demands that exceed vocal capacity (shouting), vocally abusive singing (e.g., excessively loud or high-pitched voice), or forced vocalization with excessive muscle tension.

Diagnosis:
- Check for history of aberrant vocal usage and infection.
- Laryngoscopy shows bilateral marginal nodules at the center of the ligamentous vocal cords. Lesions in children tend to be broad-based and involve the middle third of the cord. Incipient nodules are most clearly visible in the respiratory phase and disappear during high phonation.
- Stroboscopy shows a hyperfunctional pattern with small amplitudes and decreased edge movements with cylindrical thickening of the true cords. Soft, reversible nodules are associated with intact edge movements. Hard, fibrous nodules are marked by an absence of edge movements at the site of the lesion.

Differentiation is required from vocal polyps, circumscribed Reinke edema, vocal cord cysts, varices, hematomas, polypous mucosal thickening in older patients, and edge thickening during mutation.

Contact Pachyderma and Contact Ulcer

Main symptoms: Hoarseness, hard vocal usage, odynophagia on the affected side. Occasionally there may be some blood in the sputum and a foreign-body sensation in the throat.

Causes: Forceful approximation of the arytenoids with secondary hyperfunctional dysphonia of the masculine voice.

Diagnosis:
- Laryngoscopy shows vocalis muscle weakness, the vocal cords typically appearing markedly long and narrow, and symmetric adduction of the cords with unilateral epithelial thickening above the base of the vocal process and a corresponding hyperkeratotic contact reaction of the epithelial tissue.
- Stroboscopy frequently shows hyperfunctional compensation accompanying the underlying hypofunctional pattern.

Differentiation is required from intubation granulomas, papillomas, pyogenic granuloma, interarytenoid pachyderma, tuberculosis, and carcinoma.

Neurogenic Voice Disorders

Main symptoms: Mild hoarseness to aphonia, depending on the position of the paralyzed vocal cord in relation to the healthy cord. Cord paralysis may be unilateral or bilateral, flaccid or rigid. Dyspnea at rest is strictly a feature of bilateral paralysis. Exertional dyspnea may occur with unilateral paralysis.

Causes: Diverse. Vocal cord paralysis may be called "idiopathic" only after the causes in Table 6.15 have been excluded.

Diagnosis:
- History.
- Laryngoscopic findings: Paralysis is indicated by respiratory and phonatory arrest of one or both vocal cords with loss of inspiratory ab-

Table 6.**15** Causes of neurogenic vocal cord arrest (after Wirth)

Allergic:	Serum prophylaxis, as for tetanus (tetanus antitoxin)
Allergic–toxic:	Following tonsillectomy or dental extraction
Bronchial carcinoma:	Located in upper and middle lung field
Diabetes mellitus:	Diabetic neuropathy
Endotracheal intubation:	Excessive stretching by tube placement or pressure injury by inflated cuff
Hereditary:	Bilateral congenital or developing postnatally (Sipple syndrome). With congenital paralysis, cords are always fixed in a paramedian position
Diseases of the nervous system:	Bulbar paralysis, pseudobulbar paralysis, multiple sclerosis, amyotrophic lateral sclerosis, syringobulbia
Vascular surgery:	Carotid endarterectomy (superior or inferior laryngeal nerve)
Cervical lymph nodes:	Preoperative or following radical neck dissection
Herfordt syndrome:	Swelling of salivary glands, uveitis
Cardiac diseases:	Dilatation of the left atrium in mitral stenosis (Ortner syndrome), pulmonic stenosis, aortic aneuryms, dilatation or displacement of the pulmonary artery in mitral stenosis, pericarditis, primary pulmonary hypertension
Cardiac surgery:	Patent ductus arterious, atrial septal defect
Brain abscesses, brain tumors, surgical repair of hypopharyngeal diverticulum:	Pulsion diverticulum
Toxic–infectious:	Rheumatic processes, influenza, herpes zoster, mononucleosis, diphtheria, streptomycin, quinine, lead, arsenic, poliomyelitis
Pulmonary tuberculosis, mediastinal diseases:	Metastases, lymphogranulomatosis
Malformation of the hyoid chain:	Ossification of the horn of the hyoid bone, stylohyoid ligament, and thyrohyoid ligament
Esophageal carcinoma, esophageal surgery:	Proximal third
Sharp or blunt cervical trauma:	Accident, strangulation, excessive stretching in gymnastics or chiropractic therapy, mediastinoscopy, puncture of the jugular vein
Thyroid diseases:	Malignant goiter, substernal goiter
Thyroid surgery:	Nerve stretch, nerve transection
Tumors of the skull base:	Garcin syndrome
Tumors of the vagus nerve:	Schwannoma
Wallenberg syndrome:	Occlusion of the posterior inferior cerebellar artery
Cytostatic drugs:	Neurotoxic effect of vinblastin and vincristin

duction and by failure of the piriform recess to open with phonation. The position of the vocal cords (median, paramedian, or intermediate) does not necessarily reflect the site of the cranial nerve lesion!

● Stroboscopy in flaccid paralysis shows increased amplitudes with vertical vibration and no edge movements. Stroboscopy in rigid paralysis shows decreased amplitudes with no edge movements. Old palsies demonstrate a

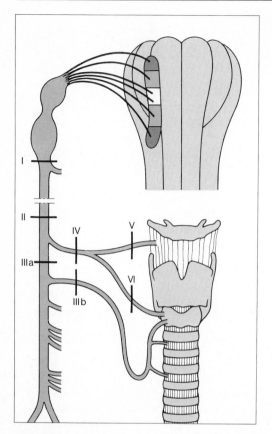

Fig. 6.2 The vagus nerve and its branches, with sites of possible lesions (I–VI) and their effects on the larynx, soft palate, and pharyngeal walls

I = Lesion between the nucleus ambiguus and the origin of the pharyngeal rami below the inferior ganglion: Intermediate position of the ipsilateral vocal cord, ipsilateral paresis of the soft palate and posterior pharyngeal wall (backdrop sign), extinction of gag and palatal reflexes on the affected side, loss of laryngeal sensation

II = Lesion between the pharyngeal rami and superior laryngeal nerve: Intermediate position and sensory loss

III = Vagus nerve lesion below the superior laryngeal nerve (a) or recurrent laryngeal nerve (b): Vocal cord paralysis (recurrent nerve paralysis) in a paramedian position

IV = Lesion of the superior laryngeal nerve: Paresis of the cricothyroid muscle with loss of tone and bowing of the mobile vocal cord. Sensory loss in the ipsilateral supraglottic mucosa

V = Lesion of the internal branch of the superior laryngeal nerve: Sensory loss in the ipsilateral supraglottic mucosa

VI = Lesion of the external branch of the superior laryngeal nerve: Paresis of the cricothyroid muscle

recovery of edge movements through collateral reinnervation of the vocalis muscle.
● Etiologically unclear cases should be evaluated by further neurologic and radiologic studies that include testing of the pharyngeal reflexes, soft palate and tongue mobility, and sensitivity testing of the laryngeal mucosa.
● Palpation of the neck.
● Radiographs of the chest and upper third of the esophagus including cinematography, skull base, thyroid examination. The outstanding feature of *central paralysis* is not vocal cord arrest but motor disturbances such as paradoxical vocal cord movements, rest tremor, intention tremor, impairment of fine coordinated movements, slowing of abduction and adduction, and combined vocal-cord and velopharyngeal nystagmus.

With *lesions involving the medulla oblongata* as far as the origin of the pharyngeal rami, there are associated disturbances with paralysis of the palatal, pharyngeal, and laryngeal musculature (cranial nerves IX–XII), producing a variety of syndromes (e.g., Tapia, Avellis, Schmidt, Vernet, Collet–Siccard, Villanet, Garcin) (see Table 1.18 and Fig. 6.2).

Differential diagnosis of vocal cord arrest includes postintubation, dislocation or fracture of the arytenoid cartilage (history), arthritis, ankylosis,, scarring after prolonged intubation or laryngeal surgery, postirradiation perichondritis, laryngoceles, intramural carcinoma, tetany due to hypoparathyroidism following strumectomy, laryngeal apraxia, and a hyperfunctional form of psychogenic aphonia. EMG and ENG are useful differentiating studies.

Speech and Language Disorders (Table 6.16)

Disorders of *voice* and disturbances of *speech and language* fall within the otolaryngologic specialty of *phoniatrics*. Though only *voice disorders* are caused by diseases of the larynx, the differential diagnosis should include speech and language problems for reasons of practical clinical utility, even though we must depart temporarily from our usual topographic–etiologic format.

Table 6.**16** *Symptom* Speech or language disorder

Synopsis
Developmental speech disorder
Articulation disorder   Dyslalia (stammering)   Dysglossias   Dysarthrias   Dyspraxias
Resonance disorder   Hypernasality   Hyponasality   Mixed nasality
Symbolization disorder   Aphasias
Fluency disorder   Stuttering   Cluttering

Symptom   Developmental Speech Disorder

Main symptoms: Speech production (expressive function), or, less commonly, speech comprehension (receptive function) that is absent, abnormal for age, or is delayed, fragmentary, and defective on various functional levels. Includes disturbances of sensory perception (recognition of auditory and visual symbols), integrative functions (ability to interrelate and utilize auditory or visual symbols), retrieval (ability to reproduce sequences of auditory or visual stimuli after central engramming), and disturbances in the recognition or reproduction of symbol sequences.

Causes: A myriad of anomalies or insults can occur during pre-, peri-, and postnatal development (Fig. 6.**3**). Particular significance is ascribed to hereditary disposition (familial speech deficit), brain damage, intellectual impairment, hearing impairment, environmental insult, and complex insults.

Diagnosis:
● Behavioral observation in the play setting (attentiveness, endurance, stimulability, response to auditory and visual stimuli, vocal utterances). Parent interview, family history. General cause-oriented history.
● ENT mirror examination.
● Logopedic status.
● Pediatric audiometry. Vestibular function testing as indicated.
● Developmental neurologic evaluation may be required (neurologic findings, psychological examination including intelligent tests, testing of motor maturity).

Differential diagnosis is based on etiologic aspects or linguistic principles and includes multiple handicaps, central hearing impairment, acoustic agnosia, mutism, early childhood autism, schizophrenia, dysphasia/aphasia, cerebral dysfunctions, isolated performance deficits, stammering, and dyslexia.

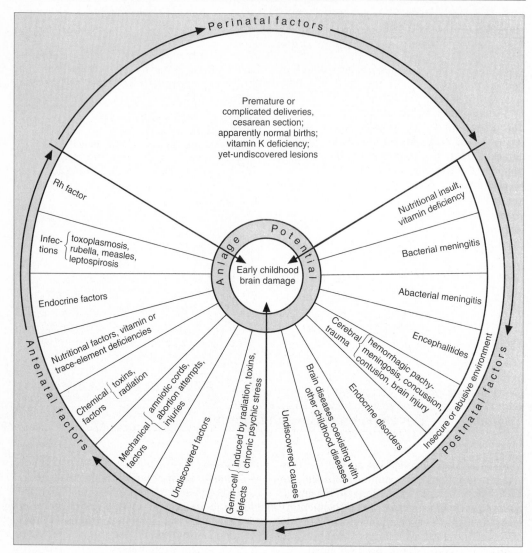

Fig. 6.**3**   Pre-, peri- and postnatal etiologic factors in delayed speech development (after Göllnitz)

Symptom   **Articulation Disorder**

Dyslalias (Stammering) = Developmental Articulation Disorders

Main symptoms: Faulty articulation with an inability to pronounce certain sounds or sound combinations correctly.

Causes: Much the same as in developmental speech disorders: The interaction of disordered sensory functions (especially acoustic, motor, and kinesthetic), a disordered capacity for central phonologic and phonetic–motor pattern formation, anatomic deficiencies and deficient functional capacity of the organs of articulation, impaired intellectual development, and abnormalities of personality structure, emotional profile, and social milieu (Fig. 6.3).

Diagnosis:
● History, organic findings, and auditory testing.
● Sound status with evaluation of phonematic discrimination. Assessment of vocabulary and grammatical abilities. In older children test reading and writing proficiency, rapidity of speech, struggling, pause placement, and prosody.
● Psychological evaluation is indicated in patients with apparent behavioral abnormalities or developmental delays; pathologic findings warrant additional neuropsychiatric studies.

Differentiation is required from audiogenic dyslalia (deaf and hearing-impaired speech is distinguished by distortions of sibilants and fricatives, terminal syllable omissions, misplaced stresses, and an increased, monotone habitual pitch). Differentiation is also required from dysglossia and dysarthria.

Dysglossias
(Peripheral Articulation Disorders)

Main symptoms: Isolated pronunciation errors due to changes in the organs of articulation and/or associated peripheral cranial nerves.

Causes: Congenital cranial neuropathies (facial nerve, hypoglossal nerve) or organic lesions (cleft lip, macroglossia, microglossia, lingual goiter, etc.). Traumatic, postoperative, or paralytic causes.

Diagnosis: History and organic findings are suggestive. Cranial nerve testing, especially of V, VII, IX, X, and XII. Speech should be tested for circumscribed articulation disorders.

Differentiation is required from dyslalias, dysarthrias, dyspraxias, and dysphasias. Multiple defects may coexist following trauma.

Dysarthrias
(Central Articulation Disorders)

Main symptoms: General speech disturbance involving articulation, voice production, and respiratory support with normal language symbolization.

Causes: Lesions of cerebral centers, tracts, and nuclei of the nerves involved in speech. Early childhood brain damage. Birth trauma, injuries, circulatory problems, inflammatory conditions, exposure to toxic substances, tumors, and neurologic diseases (multiple sclerosis, amyotrophic lateral sclerosis, epilepsy, progressive paralysis, alcohol abuse, postconcussional defects).

Diagnosis: Neurologic investigation of the underlying disease and the site of the lesion (pyramidal, extrapyramidal, cerebellar, bulbar, mixed). Logopedic workup with evaluation of articulation, voice, and respiration.

Differentiation is required from dysphasias, dysglossias, dyspraxias, and psychoses.

Dyspraxias

Main symptoms: Inability to perform voluntary, purposeful movements with certain muscle groups in the absence of paralysis. Affective movements are intact.

Causes: Lesions of the dominant hemisphere, especially in the frontal and parietal areas, or involving the nondominant, associative connections. Disordered movement pattern for articulation.

Diagnosis: Special neurologic, phoniatric, and logopedic examinations are required.

Differentiation is required from aphasias and motor dyslalia.

Hypernasality (Rhinophonia Aperta, Hypernasal Speech)

Main symptoms: Production of speech sounds with predominantly nasal resonance due to velopharyngeal incompetence.

Causes: Functional due to nonstructural problems or resting of the soft palate after tonsillectomy or adenoidectomy. Psychogenic or habitual. Congenitally short soft palate. Paralytic conditions of the soft palate. Submucous or open palatal cleft. Postoperative sequelae. Motility of the soft palate may be constrained by tumors or hyperplastic tonsils.

Diagnosis:
● Inspection of the nasal cavities, oral cavity, and nasopharynx. Functional observation of the soft palate.
● Tests of nasality and nasal air flow (I−A test of Gutzmann, fogged mirror test of Czermak, phonendoscopy).
● EMG for suspected paralysis of the soft palate. Head rotation test.
● Exclusion of nasal regurgitation and latent velum incompetence.
● Otologic findings. Auditory testing.

Differentiation is required from hyponasality and mixed nasality, poor speech control in oligophrenia, and hearing impairment (inability to monitor oral−nasal contrast).

Hyponasality (Rhinophonia Clausa, Hyponasal Speech)

Main symptoms: Inability to produce the resonants, m, n, and ng. The voice sounds muffled.

Causes: Organic due to lesions obstructing the nasal airway (mucosal and turbinate swelling due to various causes, nasal polyps, deviated septum, postoperative and posttraumatic sequelae such as synechiae or cicatricial stenosis, choanal atresia, tumors, hyperplastic adenoids, nasopharyngeal fibroma, etc.). See also p. 199. Functional hyponasality (with a clear nasal airway) can result from habitual, sustained contraction of the soft palate.

Diagnosis:
● Examination of the nasal cavities and nasopharynx; may require decongestion of the nasal membranes.
● Nasality tests. Visible elevation of the levator mounds during production of the resonant sounds, as demonstrated by anterior rhinoscopy, suggests functional hyponasality.

Differentiation is required from mixed nasality.

Mixed Nasality (Rhinophonia Mixta)

Main symptoms: Combination of hypernasal and hyponasal components in speech.

Causes: Obstruction of the nasal cavities or nasopharynx with coexisting velopharyngeal incompetence.

Diagnosis: Assessment of velopharyngeal function combined with a search for organ nasal airway obstruction.

Differentiation is required from the pure forms of hypernasal and hyponasal resonance.

Aphasias/Dysphasias

Main symptoms: Central speech disturbances that are caused by circumscribed cerebral lesions, develop after the completion of language acquisition, and are characterized by a disturbance of language−symbol association. Word formation, comprehension, and recall are affected in addition to the symbolization of reading and writing (dysgraphia, dyslexia).

Table 6.**17**   Classification of aphasic syndromes in the Aachen aphasia test

	Amnestic aphasia	Expressive aphasia	Receptive aphasia	Global aphasia
Area of impairment:				
Syntactic structure of spontaneous speech	Not impaired	Severely impaired	Mildly impaired	Severely impaired
Speech comprehension	Mildly impaired	Mildly impaired	Severely impaired	Severely impaired

Causes: The most common cause is cerebrovascular insufficiency. Hemorrhages, mass lesions, and injuries or inflammatory lesions in the distribution of the middle cerebral artery are less common. Left-brain dominance and acute onset are characteristic.

Diagnosis:
● Thorough neurologic evaluation including CT.
● Determination of dominance and handedness.
● Logopedic examination: Aachen aphasia test (AAT) covers spontaneous speech, token test, repetition, written speech, naming, and speech comprehension. Specific forms of aphasia, or aphasic syndromes, can be identified with some consistency about 4−6 weeks after the onset of the acute disease process (Table 6.**17**).

Forms of Aphasia

o *Global aphasia:* Most common form, caused by a general lesion of the speech area secondary to occlusion of the main branch of the middle cerebral artery. Profound impairment of all language functions including speech comprehension, with a predominance of stereotypic (automatic) and neologistic language behaviors. Severe syntactic dysfunction. Relative competence in repeating short phrases. Often there are accompanying dysarthric symptoms such as struggling and poor articulation. Articulatory apraxia.
o *Expressive (Broca) aphasia:* Caused by a circumscribed lesion in the distribution of the prerolandic artery. Severe reduction of syntactic structure in the form of agrammatism, a "telegram" style of speech, struggling, and phonematic paraphrasing. Cortical dysarthria often coexists. Buccofacial apraxia. Writing is altered by agrammatic sentence constructions and phonematic paraphrases.
o *Receptive (Wernicke) aphasia:* Caused by a lesion in the distribution of the posterior temporal artery (the Wernicke center). Cardinal symptom is paragrammatism with severe impairment of speech comprehension, reading,, and writing. Phonematic paraphrasing is common. Fluent speech production, occasional logorrhea; good articulation.
o *Amnestic aphasia:* Not necessarily caused by a circumsribed lesion in a specific vascular area. Cardinal symptom is difficulty in naming, with a tendency to substitute words. Speech comprehension and the syntactic structure of spontaneous speech are largely intact.
o *Conduction aphasia:* Disproportionate difficulty with repetition.
o *Transcortical motor aphasia:* Caused by lesions in the peripheral areas of the speech centers or the supplementary motor area. Initial mutism with rapid recovery of repetition but otherwise severe expressive speech disorder. Favorable prognosis.

Differentiation is required from psychiatric disorders (hysteria, schizophrenia, autism), impairment of consciousness, memory or intelligence deficits, mutism, and dysarthria.

Symptom   **Fluency Disorder**

Stuttering

Main symptoms: Inhibition or interruption of speech fluency that is independent of the will of the stutterer.

o *Clonic stuttering* is characterized by repetitions of words or syllables.

o *Tonic stuttering* is characterized by dysfluent blocks due to straining at the start of a word or sentence.

o *Tonic−clonic stuttering* includes a combination of both components, with associated disturbances of respiration, facial expression, gestures, voice, and vegetative function. Singing is usually not affected.

Causes: *Organic theories:* Occasional hereditary association (usually paternal). Neuropathic family history (e.g., CNS hyperexcitability, migraine, bed wetting, epilepsy). Developmental speech disorder is present in some 30% of cases. Occurs in aphasic settings and after craniocerebral trauma. Early childhood brain damage and minimal cerebral dysfunctions.

Neurosis theories: Spastic coordination neurosis of Kussmaul. Speech neurosis as a constitutionally determined, emotionally triggered overt inhibition of respiration, with a consequent inhibition of sound and speech production. Abusive upbringing in the form of neglect or overprotectiveness.

Learning theories portray stuttering as a learned behavior. Semantic theory of Johnson, frustration theory of van Riper, conflict theory of Sheehan.

Multifactorial theory (currently preferred) postulates a complex etiology that combines hereditary disposition with organic, psychic, and environmental aberrations.

Diagnosis: History. Test speech functions in the play setting. Check for impairment of consciousness. Monitoring of stuttering stages is usually possible only in a therapeutic setting. Evaluation by child and adolescent psychologist. Neurologic examination is indicated if organic brain damage is suspected.

Differentiation is required from cluttering (Table 6.**18**), combined stuttering and cluttering, and aphasic syndromes (especially global aphasia).

Cluttering

Main symptoms: Hurried, muddled speech that has been poorly prepared before utterance and may be difficult to understand due to the omission of sounds, syllables, and words. Speech is often monotonic and nonmusical and is marked by poor concentration, haphazard linkage of thought and speech, and deficient respiratory support. Consciousness is not impaired.

Causes: Unclear. Familial hereditary influences. Expression of a personality disorder.

Diagnosis: Check speech functions. Cluttering improves when the patient's attention is focused on the problem and in conversation with strangers. Symptoms worsen during distraction.

Differentiation is required from stuttering.

Table 6.**18**   Differentiating features of stuttering and cluttering (after Wendler and Seidner)

	Stuttering	Cluttering
Awareness of the problem	Present	Absent
Speaker's attitude toward his speech	Anxious, insecure	Indifferent
Effect of directing speaker's attention to the problem	Aggravates the dysfluency	Improves the dysfluency
Effect of distraction or relaxation	Improves the dysfluency	Aggravates the dysfluency
Important message to be conveyed by the speaker	Aggravates the dysfluency	Improves the dysfluency
Conversation with strangers or authority figures	Aggravates the dysfluency	Improves the dysfluency
Conservation with acquaintances	Improves the dysfluency	Aggravates the dysfluency

7. Trachea and Bronchi

The Symptoms

○ Pain and dysesthesia, p. 361

○ Morphologic change (swelling, tumor, malformation), p. 364

○ Cough, p. 364

○ Dyspnea, p. 365

○ Stridor, p. 329

○ Hemoptysis, p. 273

The trachea is very closely linked to the larynx, as it is to the bronchial system, in its pathology and pathophysiology. For our purposes, however, it is convenient to discuss diseases of the trachea separately from those of the larynx. This is done both to facilitate differential diagnosis and to acknowledge that investigations of the trachea and bronchi often require the use of specialized diagnostic procedures. Significant relationships with the laryngeal region will be noted in this chapter as they arise.

The tracheobronchial region is the domain of various disciplines. Our present emphasis is on aspects of *otorhinolaryngologic* differential diagnosis, but diagnostic procedures and typical findings in neighboring specialities will be noted where appropriate.

Principal Diagnostic Methods

○ *History, external inspection, palpation, laryngoscopy,* and *probing* (where indicated) comprise the minimal diagnostic workup of laryngeal disease. They are supplemented as needed by:

○ *Auscultation* for the gross localization of a low airway stenosis and for the exclusion of,

Table 7.**1** Indications for diagnostic tracheobronchoscopy

With a rigid endoscope
- Aspirated foreign body or suspicion thereof
- Tracheal and bronchial stenoses or suspicion thereof
- Suspected tumor of the trachea or surrounding tissues (assessment of wall elasticity and mobility, etc.)
- Suspected bronchial tumor
- Persistent, unexplained coughing or wheezing
- Hemoptysis of unexplained origin
- Suspected tracheal or bronchial trauma
- Transtracheal or transbronchial aspiration (of a lymph node or central lung tumor)
- Forceps biopsy, especially when there is risk of heavy bleeding
- Examination in children
- Dilatation of stenoses
- Laser application in the trachea, at the bifurcation, or in the main bronchi

With a flexible fiberscope
- Suspected peripheral bronchial tumor (distal to the segmental orifices)
- Parenchymatous lung disease of undetermined nature
- Bronchiectasis; may also be combined with bronchography
- Pleural effusion of unexplained origin
- Pneumonia that is slow to resolve and interstitial pneumopathies
- Middle lobe syndrome
- For bronchoalveolar lavage
- For clearing bronchial secretions (e. g., during intensive care)
- For collecting smears (with a brush, swab, or aspirating catheter)

say, bronchial asthma and other broncho-pulmonary diseases that are the concern of other specialties.

○ *Sputum examination* (microbiologic, microscopic [sputum constituents], rarely cytologic).

○ *Blood gas analysis.*

○ *Diagnostic imaging* with survey radiographs of the cervical and thoracic soft tissues, fluoroscopy (e.g., to screen for a suspected foreign body), and tomography and CT. Contrast medium may be administered to outline the tracheobronchial tree (tracheography, bronchography). Diagnosis can be aided by Müller and Valsalva maneuvers (for tracheal stenosis). MRI is also assuming increasing importance in airway studies. See footnote on p. 1.

○ *Tracheobronchoscopy* using a rigid endoscope or a flexible fiberoptic scope (Table 7.**1**), including:

○ Endoscopic *biopsy* or sometimes *needle aspiration.*

○ *Mediastinoscopy* is occasionally used for investigations of the trachea but more commonly of the bronchi (see p. 386, 389).

○ ENT differential diagnosis may be aided by *spirography* and other respiratory function studies such as *whole-body plethysmography, airway impedance measurement*, etc.

Symptom   **Pain and Dysesthesia**

Tracheobronchial pains is generally retrosternal in location and inspiration-dependent. Pain or discomfort is exacerbated by increasing the depth of inspiration or by breathing poorly conditioned air (temperature, humidity).

The most clinically important diseases associated with tracheobronchial pain are listed in Table 7.**2**.

Acute Catarrhal Tracheobronchitis

Main symptoms: Viral infection that usually begins in the nasopharyngeal area and descends within several days to involve the larynx, trachea, and bronchi. Retrosternal pain, initially dry cough, and moderate fever. Secretions are initially mucous and then purulent with expectoration. Usually there is significant malaise. Occasionally the sequence of infections is ascending, or both may occur in succession. The total course is 1–3 weeks. Childhood cases are common and often take a dramatic course, especially in small children.

Causes: Variable. A highly contagious viral etiology is quite common (influenza, myxovirus, adenovirus, picornavirus, reovirus). There may be secondary infection with pneumococci, streptococci, staphylococci, *Haemophilus influenzae*, etc.

Table 7.**2** *Symptom* Pain and dysesthesia

Synopsis
Acute catarrhal tracheobronchitis
Stenosing laryngotracheitis, see p. 332
Diphtheria of the trachea, see p. 316
Tracheitis sicca
Tracheitis in tracheostomy patients
Specific tracheobronchial infections (tuberculosis, sarcoidosis, syphilis)
Foreign-body aspiration
"Chronic" foreign body
Tracheobronchial injuries – External blunt trauma – External penetrating trauma – Internal injury – Tracheal avulsion – Internal iatrogenic injury – Pressure injury of the tracheal wall
Tumors

Diagnosis:

● Typical clinical presentation, often with an epidemic distribution, especially in the spring and fall.

● Laryngoscopy shows features of acute laryngitis.

● Harsh breath sounds are audible over the trachea, with possible symptoms of acute bronchitis.

Differentiation is required from prodromes of other acute infectious diseases (measles, whooping, cough, chickenpox), spastic bronchiolitis in children, and an aspirated foreign body.

Special Form:

Acute Stenosing Laryngotracheitis (Pseudocroup)
See p. 332.

Diphtheria of the Trachea
See pp. 233, 316.

Tracheitis Sicca

Main symptoms: Chronic relapsing course. "Acute stage" is marked by a painful, barking, gasping cough that concludes with a long-drawn, wheezing inspiration. Coexisting laryngitis and pharyngitis are not uncommon ("sicca syndrome"). Crusts may be raised during coughing attacks.

Causes: Exogenous mucosal damage (physical, chemical, climatic; nicotine or alcohol abuse; drug side effects [see Tables 4.**8** and 5.**7**]; individual disposition [see Tables 3.**14** and 4.**16**]).

Diagnosis: Typical clinical presentation with other manifestations of sicca syndrome (see Table 5.**8**). Tracheoscopy as indicated.

Differentiation is required from an intratracheal tumor, diphtheria, and specific tracheobronchitis.

Special Form:

Tracheitis Sicca in the Tracheostomy Patient

Main symptoms are retrosternal pain and viscous, crusty tracheal secretions, often with interspersed blood. Most prevalent in the spring and fall. There is occasional dyspnea with risk of asphyxiation due to tracheal obstruction by crusts. The *diagnosis* is established by identify-ing the dark brown, viscous crusts in the expectorant or on the tracheostomy tube and by tracheal endoscopy. Bacteriologic and mycologic smears will occasionally disclose "problem organisms" (e.g., *Pseudomonas aeruginosa*) or candidiasis.

Specific Tracheobronchial Diseases

Tuberculosis of the tracheobronchial tract may develop as an intracanalicular infection or may rupture into the airways from an infected lymph node. Sites of predilection are the tracheal bifurcation and posterior tracheal wall. The left bronchus is affected more commonly than the right. Females predominate by a 2:1 ratio. The clinical manifestations resemble those of tubercular laryngitis (see p. 323).

Besnier – Boeck – Schaumann disease is extremely rare as an isolated tracheobronchial disease. Pulmonary involvement generally coexists. See p. 255 for further details.

Involvement of the trachea or bronchi by *syphilis* has become very rare. Tracheobronchial involvement is occasionally observed in the secondary and tertiary stages of syphilis. Isolated cases of primary infection (by instrumental inoculation) have been reported.

Aspirated Endotracheal or Endobronchial Foreign Bodies

Main symptoms: Paroxysmal cough and intermittent or continuous dyspnea with stridor; reflex or mechanical apnea is very uncommon. Retrosternal pain or pressure. Cyanosis, profound unrest. Intermittent or continuous hoarseness is present with laryngeal involvement (see p. 317). Dysphagia can also occur.

Other symptoms and special features: Peak occurrence is in early childhood (<3 years of age). For anatomic reasons, endobronchial foreign bodies in adults tend to lodge in the right main bronchus. Both main bronchi are affected with about equal frequency in small children. Bodies at some sites may remain asymptomatic for days or weeks! With an endobronchial foreign body, percussion often elicits a dull or hypersonorous sound over the lung. Auscultation: hissing, stenotic sound at the level of the foreign body; rhonchi. With bronchial occlusion, respiratory sounds are absent.

Causes: Aspiration of vegetable matter (seeds, beans, peas), metal or plastic objects (toys, bullets, denture parts), biological materials (teeth, sloughed tissue, bone, fishbones), or small organisms (worms, insects, etc.).

Diagnosis:
- Typical history with abrupt onset of symptoms and paroxysmal coughing and pain.
- Radiographic studies: Chest film, lateral neck film, possibly tomograms. Look for overinflated lung areas. The Holzknecht sign: Mediastinal shift on fluoroscopy with bronchial occlusion.
- Tracheobronchoscopy for localization and extraction of the foreign body.

Differentiation is required from diphtheria, pseudocroup, laryngospasm, whooping cough, bronchial asthma, intraluminal tumor, and laryngeal stenosis.

Special Form:

"Chronic" Bronchial Foreign Body and Broncholiths

Forgotten, aspirated foreign bodies in very young or elderly individuals incite a granulating inflammation, stenosis, and abscess formation in dependent lung segments, producing chronic cough and recurrent bouts of pneumonia as the chief symptoms. Differential diagnosis follows the scheme described for "acute" foreign bodies.

Injuries

Tracheobronchial injuries may be external or internal. *Fresh external injuries* usually have an obvious history and pose no problems of differential diagnosis. The effects depend on whether the injury was inflicted by a *blunt* trauma (blow, etc.) or a *penetrating* trauma (cut, stab wound, gunshot):
- A *blunt external injury* generally produces hematoma, edema, and soft-tissue contusions and lacerations. Some injuries may partially or completely sever the trachea or may displace portions of its cartilaginous framework. *Acute symptoms* are pain, dysphagia, dyspnea, and possible stridor. There may be hemoptysis, hoarseness, and occasionally progressive emphysema.
- A *penetrating external injury*, often combined with other injuries (multiple trauma), is generally associated with pain, massive hemoptysis, and a frothy, blood-tinged discharge, at the wound opening during expiration. Accompanying features are cough, dyspnea or apnea, and severe systemic manifestations. The traumatologic differential diagnosis should be oriented toward the general presenting situation and should establish treatment priorities. Very often the differential diagnosis can be completed only after the patient has come to operation.
- *Inhalation injuries* caused by caustic, toxic, or hot gases (occupational injuries, chemical weapons, etc.) are less common. The *main acute symptoms* are pain, cough (sometimes with a sanguinolent discharge), dyspnea, and stridor. Systemic signs can be extremely severe with rapid deterioration.
- *Internal iatrogenic injuries* are more common and can result from intubation, catheterization, probing, or endoscopy. The *main symptoms* are retrosternal pain, cough, hemoptysis, dyspnea, and (rarely) emphysema. Perforation of the tracheobronchial wall during endoscopy is *very* rare when correct technique is employed.

Special Form:

Pressure Injury of the Tracheal Wall

Tracheal wall injury with symptoms of delayed onset — like that caused by excessive cuff pressure during endotracheal anesthesia, a cuffed tracheostomy tube, or mechanical pressure necrosis due to a faulty tube design or endoprosthesis — is of major importance in the clinical setting. Usually several weeks or months elapse before the effects become apparent (see p. 367).

Diagnosis:
- History, inspection, and palpation of the neck.
- Endoscopic evaluation: Indirect laryngoscopy or magnifying laryngoscopy; rigid or flex-

ible endoscopy of the larynx, trachea, bronchi, and esophagus, depending on the type and location of the injury.
• Diagnostic imaging: Radiographic views depend on the type and location of the trauma: Neck films in two planes. Tomograms or CT scans of the larynx and trachea. MRI may also be considered. Other options are contrast radiography of the hypopharynx and esophagus and cervical spine projections, as required.
• Airway impedance measurement as indicated.

• Blood gas analysis as indicated.
• Phoniatric function studies (see p. 336).

Tumors

Pain is most characteristic of the late stages of *malignant tumors*, i.e., various types of carcinoma and, less commonly, mesenchymal malignancies and reticuloses.

Further details are presented in Table 7.**6**.

Symptom   **Morphologic Change (Swelling, Tumor, Malformation)**

Besides *malformations* and *anomalies*, the morphologic changes of greatest clinical interest are *posttraumatic conditions* and *neoplasms*. As a rule, morphologic changes involving the trachea or bronchi can be detected only by endoscopic and/or radiologic examination; so while they are an important finding, they do not constitute a primary cardinal symptom. Dyspnea, hemoptysis, and/or dysphagia are usually predominant and may have a morphologic change as their cause. For this reason "morphologic change" is discussed elsewhere in connection with symptoms that are more clinically prominent.

Symptom   **Cough**

(First review p. 318 and Table 6.**2**). Many diseases provoke coughing but generally produce other symptoms as well that can be utilized for differential diagnosis. There are several tracheobronchial diseases, however, that have cough as their *main symptom* and require endoscopy for definitive diagnosis.

Chronic Tracheobronchitis

As with chronic laryngitis (see p. 320), multiple forms of chronic tracheobronchitis are recognized:

a) *Simple chronic tracheobronchitis*
b) *Chronic hyperplastic tracheobronchitis*
c) *Chronic atrophic tracheobronchitis*
d) *Chondro-osteoplastic tracheopathy*
   (special form, see below)

The mucosal changes in a) through c) are analogous to those of chronic laryngitis (see p. 320) and often affect the larynx and tra-

cheobronchial tree concurrently. In these cases the laryngeal symptoms, especially hoarseness, are predominant. In the absence of laryngeal involvement, the *main symptoms* generally are cough and the expectoration of a thick, mucoid, often colorless sputum. Endoscopy is necessary to localize the cause of the cough to the trachea. Concomitant bronchial involvement can be detected by auscultation. Males are most commonly affected.

Tracheopathia Osteoplastica

Main symptoms: Cough and possible foreign-body sensation in the trachea. Many cases are largely asymptomatic, however.

Causes: Patchy formation of hard bony and cartilaginous deposits in the tracheal wall, usually involving lateral portions of the wall between the tracheal rings.

Diagnosis: Tracheobronchoscopy.

Tracheoesophageal Fistula

See p. 380.

Very *rare* tracheobronchial lesions causing cough include *true* and *false tracheal diverticula* and *megatrachea*. The diagnosis is generally made radiographically and confirmed by endoscopy.

Neoplasms

Both benign and malignant neoplasms of the tracheobronchial system (see Table 7.**6**), if limited, may produce cough as their only symptom. Thus, a cough persisting for several weeks assumes special significance as a potential early cardinal symptom of neoplasia. Endoscopy and radiography should be applied liberally to exclude a neoplasm when this symptom exists.

Special Case:

Endotracheal Goiter

This is not a true neoplasm but a dystopic lesion that is associated with the thyroid gland and is involved by changes in the gland. Peak incidence is between 10 and 30 years of age, with a preponderance of females. The usual site of occurrence is the posterior wall of the upper trachea.

Diagnosis:
● Endoscopy and biopsy.
● Above studies may be preceded by radiologic exploration (tomography, radionuclide scans).

Symptom   **Dyspnea**

Dyspnea is defined by Meakins as "the awareness of the necessity of labored breathing." *Apnea* refers to the cessation of breathing and *asphyxia* to the state of suffocation resulting from prolonged apnea.

Dyspnea and apnea are dramatic symptoms that can be caused by many diverse conditions. The initial step in differential diagnosis is always to determine the *type of dyspnea* that is present. Various causes and cardinal symptoms of *dyspnea* are reviewed in Table 7.**3**, and the *types* of dyspnea are contrasted in Figure 7.**1**.

The type of greatest interest in otorhinolaryngology is *obstructive respiratory insufficiency*, caused by an airway stenosis located between the pharynx and the bronchi. For clarity of differential diagnosis, the more common *causes of dyspnea* located in the pharynx and larynx are discussed in the section on the *Larynx* (symptom: *Stridor*), although the term "dyspnea" is more comprehensive, and dyspnea may occur with or without stridor (see p. 329, Tables 6.**7−9**, and Fig. 6.**1**).

The most common dyspnea-causing lesions of the *trachea* and *bronchi* are listed in Table 7.**4**.

External Compression and Tracheomalacia

Main symptoms: Dyspnea of gradual onset that usually increases over a long period (months) and is eventually accompanied by inspiratory and expiratory stridor.

Causes: Space-occupying lesions adjacent to the trachea (goiter; mediastinal tumors; enlarged paratracheal or parabronchial lymph nodes as in pulmonary tuberculosis, Besnier−Boeck−Schaumann disease, and Hodgkin disease; aneurysms of the great cervical and/or thoracic vessels).

Diagnosis:
● Palpation of the neck.
● Radiographic examination of the neck, trachea, and chest; CT scans. Thyroid isotope scans may also be considered.
● Tracheoscopy. Suspected compression at the bronchial level can be confirmed or excluded by bronchoscopy or CT.

Table 7.**3**   Differential diagnosis of dyspnea (from W. Becker, H.H. Naumann, C.R. Pfaltz: Ear, Nose, and Throat Diseases. Thieme, Stuttgart 1989)

Type	Characteristic symptoms	Examples
Obstructive respiratory insufficiency (stridorous respiration)	Inspiratory stridor; also expiratory stridor if the stenosis is distal to the bifurcation. "Struggle for air." On inspiration: Indrawing of the suprasternal notch, supraclavicular and intercostal retraction. Restlessness and anxiety progressing to disorientation and loss of consciousness. Pulse rate is usually very high. Respiratory rate is usually decreased, with a relatively prolonged inspiratory phase. On auscultation, stridor is loudest over the site of the stenosis. A flopping sound is heard with mobile foreign bodies. Initial skin pallor progressing to cyanosis. Anxious, harried facial expression, increasing exhaustion	Aspirated foreign body; stenosing laryngeal edema; stenosing laryngotracheitis; airway stenosis above the bifurcation caused by tumor, hematoma, or other obstructing lesion or extrinsic compression; blunt or sharp trauma, etc.
Restrictive respiratory insufficiency	Light, shallow, rapid respiration with shortening of the inspiratory *and* expiratory phases. Associated pathologic findings in the lung or pleura. Patient prefers to lie flat	Pneumonia, pneumothorax, atelectasis, bronchial carcinoma, pulmonary fibrosis, pleural effusion, vomiting with aspiration of gastric contents, etc.
Bronchial asthma	Decreased respiratory rate with a typical *expiratory* breath sound (rhoncus and wheeze). Expiration is markedly longer than inspiration. Patient tends to lean on the arms while breathing (to recruit auxiliary muscles of respiration). Typical audible findings over the lung. Dyspnea occurs in paroxysm	Bronchial asthma (endogenous type), asthmoid form of inhalation allergy, occupational asthma, etc.
Cardiac respiratory insufficiency	Increased respiratory rate *without* stridor. Airways clear; skin pale or cyanotic, "blue" lips. Cold sweat on the forehead. Patient favors an upright sitting posture. Frequent nocturnal attacks of dyspnea (cardiac asthma). Associated pathologic findings in the heart and circulation	Left cardiac failure, aortic or mitral valve defect, acute cor pulmonale, acute cardiac pulmonary edema, etc.
Central respiratory insufficiency	Irregular, "gasping, or periodic respiration. Progressive obtundation that may culminate in loss of consciousness. Stridor can occur in this condition if the tongue falls back. Bradypnea combined with apnea	Stroke, cerebral sclerosis, increased intracranial pressure, brain edema, brain tumor, diabetic or uremic coma, drug intoxication, etc.
Psychogenic respiratory insufficieny	Respiratory rate increased. Hyperventilation syndrome. *No* stridor, possible "sighing" respiration. *No* cyanosis; skin and mucosae are well-perfused	Neuroses, psychoses, hysterical reactions

Special Case:

Tracheomalacia (Chondromalacia)

Tracheomalacia is a dystrophic condition of the tracheal cartilages caused by pressure atro-phy, local nutritional deficit, trauma including surgery (prolonged intubation, faulty tracheotomy placement), or local inflammatory disease. (An analogous process can involve the bronchial wall: "bronchial collapse.") A "scabbard trachea" results. The main symptoms and diagnostic procedures are the same as for compression stenoses (radiographic evaluation can be assisted by the Müller and Valsalva maneuvers).

Stenoses

Stenoses may be classified as *acute* or *chronic* and their causes as *extramural, intramural,* or *intraluminal.*

Acute Stenoses

Tracheal trauma (see p. 363), tracheitis (see p. 361), stenosing laryngotracheitis (pseudocroup) (see p. 332).

Chronic Stenoses

Main symptoms: Gradually progressive dyspnea following trauma, surgery, or other mucosal injuries or necrosis (generally with an asymptomatic interval of weeks or months following the trauma). Stridor is mainly inspiratory when the stenosis is at the tracheal level and expiratory when the stenosis involves the bronchi. "Weak voice," hoarse cough. Pallor and possible cyanosis. Typical body and head posture are adopted to maximize the residual lumen (upright body posture with the upper body leaning forward and the chin indrawn). In this situation even slight mucosal irritation or swelling can cause dramatic respiratory distress and asphyxia!

Causes: Scar tissue replacing all (annular stenosis) or part (webbing) of the circumference of the damaged tracheal wall. The causes that most commonly produce this situation are listed in Table 7.**5.**

Diagnosis:
- Radiographic evaluation (neck and chest tomograms, Müller and Valsalva maneuvers, CT scans).
- Tracheoscopy or bronchoscopy, depending on local findings.
- Biopsy.
- With involvement of the bronchial system, consultation should be sought with a pulmonologist or thoracic surgeon.

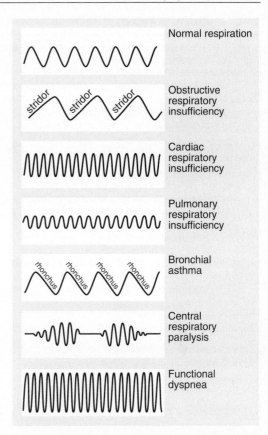

Fig. 7.**1** Various respiratory patterns useful in the differential diagnosis of dyspnea (from H. Feldmann: HNO-Notfälle, 2nd ed. Springer, Berlin 1981)

Table 7.**4** *Symptom* Dyspnea
(causes in the trachea and/or bronchi)

Synopsis
Foreign body, see p. 362
Tracheal injury, see p. 363
Stenosing laryngotracheobronchitis, see p. 332
Spastic bronchiolitis in children*
Asthma, see p. 367
Extrinsic compression of the trachea
Tracheomalacia
Cicatricial stenosis
Intratracheal and intrabronchial neoplasms
Complications in tracheostomy patients
See also Tables 7.**3**, 7.**5**, and 6.**8**
* No further commentary

Table 7.**5** Chronic laryngeal or tracheal stenosis (common causes)

Blunt or penetrating tracheal injury, external or internal, that has not been adequately managed
Exogenous damage to the tracheal muscosa (toxic gases, liquids, etc.)
Infection of the tracheal wall (specific and nonspecific)
Radiation injury (radiotherapy, etc.)

Traumatic intubation
    Mucosal defects caused by pressure or friction: typical intubation granulomas or other endolaryngeal or endotracheal granulations
    Synechiae in the anterior commissure or posterior third of the glottis
    Injury of the cricoarytenoid joint
    Cicatricial stenosis caused by the tube cuff in the trachea

Technically flawed endoscopy or endotracheal surgical manipulation
Improper tracheostomy technique
Faulty surgical technique in the neck region
Intratracheal tumors
Space-occupying lesions adjacent to the trachea (compression)
See also Table 6.**8**

Intratracheal and Intrabronchial Tumors

The overall incidence of intratracheal neoplasms is low. The more common benign and malignant tumors occurring in this area are listed in Table 7.**6**.

Main symptoms: Paroxysmal cough, progressive dyspnea with wheezing and eventual stridor. With a slow-growing tumor, the stenosis may remain clinically silent for some time. Some malignancies produce hemoptysis or blood-tinged sputum, occasionally with increasing retrosternal pain. Bronchial malignancies produce chest pain accompanied by weight loss and physical debilitation.

Diagnosis:
● Detailed history. Percussion and auscultation when thoracic symptoms are present.
● Radiographic evaluation (neck and chest survey films and spot films, possibly CT scans; tracheograms, bronchograms). MRI may also be considered.
● Endoscopy and biopsy. Mediastinoscopy as indicated.
● With bronchial involvement, consultation with a pulmonologist or thoracic surgery is indicated.
● For special inquiries: radionuclide scans (thyroid); MRI; cytologic evaluation of sputum, tracheal secretions, or bronchial secretions; mediastinoscopy.

Table 7.**6** Principal tumors of the trachea and bronchus (selection)

Type of tumor	Special clinical aspects
Benign	
– Fibroma	Most common benign mesenchymal tumor, occurs predominantly in the trachea, rarely in the bronchi. May develop as a neoplasm or from granulation tissue (= pseudofibroma)
– Hemangioma	Rare. Typically occurs near the larynx. Is usually manifested in early childhood. May cause hemoptysis
– Chondroma	Very slow growth with few associated symptoms. Very hard tumor. Most prevalent from 40 to 60 years of age. Tracheopathia osteoplastica is classified as a diffuse chondromatosis. See also p. 364
– Papilloma (solitary or in papillomatosis)	Secondary involvement from laryngeal papillomatosis is relatively common (see p. 325). "Juvenile red" papilloma is most common in the trachea. Males predominate. "Senile" papillomas, see section on Pachyderma and p. 325
Precancerous lesions	Pachyderma, leukoplakia, "senile" papilloma, see p. 325

Table 7.**6**   (cont.)

Type of tumor	Special clinical aspects
"Low-grade malignancy"	
— Bronchial adenoma	Relatively common. Occurs chiefly at the bronchial level (main bronchi near the carina, lower trachea), Clinical parallels with basal cell carcinoma and intestinal carcinoid. Peak occurrence 30–40 years of age, with preponderance of females. Slow growth. Infiltrate growth can occur! Expiratory stridor. Retention of secretions and recurrent bouts of pneumonia. Asthma-like attacks are not uncommon. Cardinal symptom: recurrent hemoptysis
Malignant	
— Carcinoid	Mostly occurs in the central bronchial system, tending to exhibit extrabronchial rather than endobronchial growth. Peak occurrence is 30–60 years of age, with females predominating. About 50% grow invasively, with about a 10% incidence of lymphogenous metastasis and 5% hematogenous. A "cardinoid syndrome" like that occurring with intestinal carcinoids is usually absent with (smaller) bronchial carcinoids. Proneness to hemoptysis, recurrent infections, purulent sputum, and cough
— Squamous cell carcinoma	Rarely primary to the trachea, but primary bronchial involvement is very common. Bronchial carcinoma is second most common form after gastric carcinoma. Peak occurrence is 50–60 years with a 10:1 preponderance of males. Cardinal symptoms: cough progressing to hemoptysis, severe weight loss
— Adenocarcinoma	Far less common than squamous cell cancers. Have the poorest prognosis of all tracheal tumors
— Adenoid cystic carcinoma	Rare. Very slow-growing, is more common in the trachea than in the bronchi. Greater propensity for hematogenous than regional lymphogenous spread
Thyroid carcinoma	Involves the trachea by extension from the thyroid. Most tumors are undifferentiated, a few are well-differentiated
Various sarcomas	Rare in the tracheobronchial tree. Most do not ulcerate, or do so at a very late stage. Overlying mucosa is usually intact
Extraluminal tumors (invade the trachea or produce symptoms by external compression)	Goiter, lymph-node metastases, e. g., from bronchial carcinoma. Malignant lymphomas are very rare in the trachea. Invading esophageal or mediastinal malignancies
Pseudotumors	
— Endotracheal goiter	Intrusion of thyroid tissue into the trachea, usually at the posterior tracheal wall near the inferior border of the cricoid cartilage. The mass communicates with the thyroid gland!
— Mucosal polyp	Granulation tissue or soft, relatively vascular fibroma developing in response to local irritation. Common in the larynx but rare in the trachea and bronchi
— Amyloid tumor	Rare. Subepithelial amyloid deposits. Peak incidence is 20–40 years of age with a 3:1 preponderance of males

Table 7.**7**   Complications in tracheostomy patients

Postoperative bleeding

— Near the stoma:	Thyroid gland, thyroid isthmus
	Mucosal vessels
	Tracheal wall vessels
— Distant from the stoma:	Poor intraoperative management of the wound bed (carotid artery branches, inferior thyroid artery)

Late bleeding:	Decubitus ulcer
	Erosive hemorrhage, e. g., from the brachiocephalic vein (cannula tip)
	Bleeding tumor

Other complications:

Pneumothorax	Infections
Subcutaneous emphysema	— Tracheitis (wet, dry, crusting, etc.)
Mediastinal emphysema	— Granulation formation
Dysphagia and/or spillover	— Bronchitis
Recurrent nerve paralysis	— Pneumonia
Tracheoesophageal fistula	— Lung abscess

Technical deficiencies:

Tube obstruction by crusting	Pharyngeal stenoses
Faulty tube placement (paratracheal)	Intralaryngeal stenoses
Improper tube shape	— Supraglottic
Faulty tube fixation	— Glottic
Poor tube care	— Subglottic
Malposition of the stoma	Intratracheal stenosis
— Cricoid stenosis	— Supraorificial
— Granulation formation about the stoma	— Orificial
Aspiration or spillover in tubes with a phonation valve ("neoglottis")	— Suborificial
	— Low endotracheal
Destabilization, deformation, and collapse of the tracheal wall	Multiple stenoses
Granulation formation at the tube tip with subsequent webbing	
Orificial cicatricial stenosis (after closure of the stoma)	

Differentiation is required from asthma, tracheomalacia, and other mediastinal and pulmonary diseases.

Complications in Tracheostomy Patients

These complications are often challenging in terms of differential diagnosis, because generally they occur at an occult site, are unsuspected, and often pose an acute, significant threat to the patient. The major potential complications are reviewed in Table 7.**7**.

Diagnosis:
● Diagnosis (and treatment) must be carried out by a physician *experienced* in dealing with tracheostomy complications!
● Endoscopic inspection of the tracheostomy and tracheobronchial tree with a rigid endoscope. This is performed under emergency conditions when risk of hemorrhage exists.

8. Esophagus

The Symptoms

- Pain (and dysesthesia), p. 372
- Morphologic change (swelling tumor), p. 377
- Malformation, p. 379
- Esophageal dysphagia, p. 380
- Hematemesis, p. 385

The esophagus is an overlapping area of concern for multiple specialties. The following discussion of differential diagnosis focuses on *otorhinolaryngologic* symptoms and investigations.

Principal Diagnostic Methods

- *Inspection* and *palpation* of the external neck can reveal evidence of disease of the cervical esophagus such as inflammatory redness, swelling, emphysema, tenderness (vascular sheath!), enlarged lymph nodes, etc.
- *Auscultation* over the course of the esophagus (e.g., for stenotic sounds) can assist the localization of esophageal disease.
- A complete *mirror examination of the mouth, pharynx, and larynx* is an essential prelude to the studies that follow.
- The scope of *imaging studies* is determined by the nature of the inquiry. The minimum initial workup includes a *fluoroscopic examination of the neck and chest* (possibly with contrast medium) and *survey radiographs*, which should precede esophagoscopy if at all possible. *Tomograms* and/or *CT scans* have an established role in the investigation of stenoses, foreign bodies, tumors, etc.

- *Cineradiography* is important for analyzing esophageal motion, and *intraluminal scintigraphy* is useful for reflux measurements and other applications.
- *Contrast examination* of the esophageal lumen and mucosa is a widely used, simple, and very informative procedure.
- When combined with a special endoscope, *intraluminal sonography* is an interesting modality for studies of the esophagus.
- *Magnetic resonance imaging* (MRI) offers promising advantages for evaluating the soft tissues of the neck and for locating and delineating tumors in that region (improved contrast resolution and spatial localization).
- The use of *rigid or flexible esophagoscopy*, which may be combined, depends on the specific inquiry and situation. Both methods are complementary (Table 8.**1**). *Pneumatic esophagoscopy* (air insufflation into the esophagus during the examination) can be particularly rewarding for endoesophageal studies.
- *Probing* of the esophageal lumen yields information on the nature and configuration of stenoses and foreign bodies and will facilitate subsequent bougienage.
- *Biopsy* is generally performed during the course of esophagoscopy.
- *Esophageal manometry* (e.g., three-point, pull-through, or radiomanometry), by measuring and recording intraluminal pressures, is useful for assessing the function of the sphincters and thus the overall functional status of the esophagus (normal pressure range of the lower esophageal sphincter: 15−45 mmHg).
- *pH-metry* (normal intraesophageal pH = 4−7) can often yield important diagnostic information.

Table 8.**1**   Applications of rigid and flexible diagnostic esophagoscopy

Rigid telescope with rod-lens optics (classic method)	Endoscopic task	Flexible endoscope, fiberscope
Method of choice	Detailed evaluation of the preesophageal segment (piriform sinus), upper esophageal sphincter, and upper half of the esophagus	Use is often problematic
Well-suited (especially in conjunction with positive intraluminal pressure, "pneumatic" esophagoscope)	Diseases along the full length of the esophagus	Well-suited (especially for screening)
Well-suited	Middle and lower espophagus including the cardia	Well-suited
Method of choice	Foreign bodies (including extraction)	Unsuitable
Well-suited	Diverticula (hypopharynx, esophagus)	Of limited use
Method of choice	Photographic and film documentation	Of limited use
Well-suited	Lumen-restricting lesions and esophagoscopy in small children	Use is often problematic
Unsuitable	Patients with extraesophageal obstructions to esophagoscopy (scoliosis, kyphosis, etc.)	Method of choice
Unsuitable	Observation of functional phenomena (e. g., lower esophageal sphincter)	Well-suited
Unsuitable	Selection for panendoscopy with emphasis on the stomach and duodenum	Method of choice
Method of choice	Selection for diagnostic *and* therapeutic procedures (e. g., hemorrhage, dilatation of cicatricial stenoses, etc.) in the esophagus	

The indications also depend on the personal experience and technical skills of the examiner, on any concomitant therapeutic goals, and on the patient's general condition (ability to tolerate general anesthesia)

Symptom   Pain (and Dysesthesia)

Esophageal pain may be perceived behind the sternum and/or between the scapulae. When caused by disease near the upper esophageal sphincter, the pain may radiate to the hypopharyngeal area, while lesions near the cardia can additionally cause upper abdominal pain. Even "ear pain" (auricular branch of the vagus nerve, see Fig. 1.**1**) can occur with malignant and other esophageal lesions. Conversely, angina pectoris and myocardial infarction may be associated with severe "esophageal" pain!

Pain on swallowing is correctly termed *odynophagia*. The term *dysphagia*, though commonly applied to odynophagia, simply means *difficult swallowing*. The *sensation* of difficult swallowing with no real impairment of deglutition is referred to clinically as *globus* (or globus sensation) (see pp. 279, 383).

Table 8.**2** lists the principal esophageal disorders in which pain or discomfort is generally a prominent symptom. Diseases included in the differential diagnosis of retrosternal pain are listed in Table 8.3.

Idiopathic Diffuse Esophageal Spasm (Spastic Esophagitis, Functional Diverticula)

Main symptoms: Changing, intermittent dysphagia or odynophagia (retrosternal). Transient, painful suspension of bolus progression followed by spontaneous recovery of normal deglutition.

Other symptoms and special features: Average age at onset in 50−60 years; both sexes are affected equally. The intervals between spastic episodes may last days, months, or years. Spasm may be precipitated by stress, hurried eating, poor mastication, or the ingestion of certain foods (dry, hard, granular bolus). The episode lasts from a few minutes to 2 hours or more. In severe cases a total inability to swallow (*aphagia*) may persist for days. Retrosternal pain can be quite severe. Simultaneous cardiac and other autonomic symptoms are not uncommon (cardiac arrhythmias, pallor, faintness, cold sweats, etc.).

Causes: Disturbance of autonomic innervation ("dyschalasia") with an unknown precipitating cause.

Diagnosis:
• Contrast esophagography shows variable, traveling ring-like contractions of the esophageal wall ("rosary bead" figure) with pseudodiverticulum formation. Esophageal findings between episodes are normal!
• *Esophagoscopy* to exclude an organic stenosis or an organic cause of the spasm.
• Esophageal perfusion manometry to detect and analyze proness to spasticity.

Differentiation is required from an ulcer or malignant tumor of the esophagus or stomach, angina pectoris due to myocardial infarction or coronary insufficiency, (hypermotile) achalasia, lower esophageal ring (see below), reflux esophagitis, presbyesophagus, alcoholic polyneuropathy, and diabetic neurogastroenteropathy.

Table 8.**2** *Symptom* Pain (and dysesthesia)

Synopsis
Idiopathic diffuse esophageal spasm (spastic esophagus)
Lower esophageal (Schatzki) ring
Achalasia (cardiospasm), see p. 382
Spasm of the upper esophageal sphincter (cricopharyngeal achalasia), see p. 382
Hypopharyngeal diverticula, see p. 279
Esophageal diverticula, see p. 378
Globus hystericus, see pp. 279, 383
Esophagitis
− Simple acute esophagitis
− Ulcerative esophagitis
− Retention esophagitis
− *Candida* esophagitis
− Reflux esophagitis
− AIDS-related esophagitis
− Sideropenic esophagitis (Plummer−Vinson syndrome), see p. 266
Hiatal hernia
Acquired brachyesophagus (Barrett esophagus)
Esophageal trauma
− Foreign bodies
− Caustic or thermal injury
− Instrumental (iatrogenic)
− Spontaneous rupture (Boerhaave syndrome)
− Mallory−Weiss syndrome
− External injury
Dermatoses
− Herpes simplex, see p. 239
− Epidermolysis bullosa, see p. 254
− Pemphigus, see p. 253
− Pemphigoid, see p. 254
− Lyell syndrome, see p. 254
Collagen diseases
− Progressive systemic scleroderma, see p. 255
− Dermatomyositis, see p. 255
− Periarteritis nodosa, see p. 167
Malignant tumors

Special Form:

Lower Esophageal (Schatzki) Ring

The Schatzki ring is a constant, web-like, concentric narrowing of the distal esophagus, which may coexist with a diaphragmatic hernia. The oral aspect of the ring is covered with squamous epithelium, the aboral aspect with gastric mucosa. The ring is subject to intermittent spastic contractions (intermittent dyspha-

Table 8.**3** Causes of retrosternal pain (from W.E. Hansen: Gastrointestinale Symptome. Springer, Berlin 1984)

Esophageal diseases
- Esophagitis
  (reflux, candidal, caustic injury by acid or lye)
- Functional disorders
  (achalasia, esophageal spasm)
- Neoplasms

Cardiovascular diseases
- Coronary heart disease
  (angina pectoris due to ischemia or infarction)
- Pericarditis
- Aortic aneurysm, aortitis

Other diseases
- Ulcer at the gastric inlet
- Cholelithiasis
- Pleurodynia
- Sternal pathology (e. g., myeloma or leukosis)
- Mediastinitis due to esophageal rupture or pneumothorax
- Bronchial asthma

Table 8.**4** Drugs that can cause ulcerative esophagitis (selection)

Alprenolol (β-receptor blocking drug)

Analgesics and anti-inflammatory agents (especially acetylsalicylic acid, indomethacin, phenacetin, phenylbutazone, etc.)

Antibiotics (tetracyclines, especially older doxycycline products with an HCl component; cephalosporins; clindamycin; erythromycin; lincomycin; penicillins; sulfonamides)

Chlorthalidone (diuretic)

Clomethiazole (psychotherapeutic agent)

Iron preparations

Emepronium (anticholinergic)

Feneterol (β² sympathomimetic, broncholytic)

Fluorouracil (cytostatic)

Glibenclamide (oral hypoglycemic)

Glucocorticoids

Potassium chloride

Mexiletine (antiarrhythmic)

Thioridazine (tranquilizer)

---

gia). *Diagnosis* relies on special radiographic studies ("distention") to demonstrate the ring. Most common in males over 50 years of age.

Globus Hystericus

See pp. 279, 383.

Esophagitis

The differential diagnosis includes various clinical forms:
○ *Simple (acute) esophagitis* is a rare disease with a viral (e.g., HSV) or bacterial etiology (e.g., spread of infection from the rhinopharyngeal mucosa).
○ *Ulcerative esophagitis* is caused by prolonged contact of orally ingested drugs with the esophageal lining (Table 8.**4**), by systemic mucosa-damaging agents such as cytostatics and corticosteroids, or by radiotherapy.
○ *Retention esophagitis* is caused by irritation from foods and other materials that are retained above sites of esophageal stenosis (achalasia, diverticula, presbyesophagus, neoplasms, scleroderma, Crohn disease, the Plummer–Vinson syndrome).
○ *Candida esophagitis* is most common in patients with metabolic abnormalities (diabetes, renal or hepatic failure, hypothyroidism, etc.) or other lower resistance (e.g., after cytostatic or radiation therapy). It also occurs in the setting of HIV infection, reflux esophagitis, achalasia, stenosing esophageal tumors, and broad-spectrum antibiotic therapy.
○ *Reflux esophagitis (peptic esophagitis)*, probably the most common form, occurs when an incompetent lower esophageal sphincter allows regurgitation of acidic gastric contents. The lower third of the esophagus is usually affected. Factors that can cause reflux are listed in Table 8.**5**. Subjective reflux symptoms are typically brought on by bending over or lying flat (horizontal body position); by eating poorly digestible foods; by the use of alcohol, coffee, nicotine, or sweets; and apparently by stress and exertion.
○ *AIDS-related esophagitis* is one of many organ manifestations that can develop in AIDS patients.

Main symptoms: Dysphagia, retrosternal burning ("heartburn"). Occasional epigastric pain is exacerbated by eating acidic foods. Frequent hiccups. Feeling of retrosternal or interscapular pressure.

Diagnosis: The objective diagnostic yield in *simple acute esophagitis* is usually disappointing in relation to the subjective complaints.

In *ulcerative esophagitis*, questioning the patient about drug ingestion at the onset of complaints may identify the cause. Esophagoscopy reveals mucosal erosions and perhaps superficial ulcerations, which will resolve 1−2 weeks after the offending agents has been withdrawn.

Suspected *Candida esophagitis* can be confirmed by esophagoscopy (whitish wall deposits that can be wiped away, coarsened mucosal relief) with the examination of a mycologic smear and biopsy specimen.

Retention esophagitis is diagnosed from a history of dysphagia, radiographic studies (showing an esophageal stenosis or perhaps a gastric ulcer or tumor), esophagoscopic findings, and biopsy. The latter studies also establish the nature of the stenosis.

Reflux esophagitis is the result of reflux disease. Diagnosis is based on the history, esophageal manometry, intraluminal scintigraphy, pH-metry, radiography (e.g., with acidified contrast medium), and especially esophagoscopy (erosive, ulcerative, and cicatricial mucosal lesions and metaplasias chiefly affecting the distal half of the esophagus). Often there are sites of induration and stenosis ("peptic esophageal stenosis"). A sliding hernia frequently coexists.

The local symptoms of *AIDS-related esophagitis* can be quite diverse (whitish membranous deposits, shallow ulcerations, erosions, etc., affecting the esophageal mucosa). Generally there are other, more easily recognized AIDS symptoms in other parts of the body, supported by definitive laboratory findings.

The diagnosis of *sideropenic esophagitis* (Plummer−Vinson syndrome) is discussed on p. 266.

Differentiation from "functional dyspepsia," previous digestive tract surgery, gastric or duodenal ulcer, ulcerative colitis, biliary tract disease, angina pectoris, "pregnancy esophagus," and gastric carcinoma is based on the severity of symptoms and the location of the lesions.

Table 8.**5**   Causes of reflux disease (after W. Rösch)

Primary:
Incompetence of the lower esophageal sphincter
Presbyesophagus
Drug-induced:
anticholinergics, coronary vasodilators
Cyclic contraceptives
Nicotine, alcohol, caffeine
Endocrine factors (e. g., pregnancy)
Constipation
Obesity
Ascites
Psychic factors (stress)
Secondary:
Scleroderma (and other collagen diseases), see Table 4.**29**
Carcinoma of the cardia
Gastrectomy, fundectomy
Antral, pyloric, and duodenal stenosis
Persistent vomiting (hematemesis of pregnancy)
Prolonged immobilization
Indwelling gastric tube
Reflux occurs when the pressure of the lower esophageal sphincter falls to 5 mmHg or less (manometry)

Hiatal Hernia

Main symptoms: Retrosternal and/or epigastric pain. Heartburn, hiccups, regurgitation of food, occasionally reflux symptoms. Proneness to vomiting and bleeding ulcerations with chronic anemia. *But:* Many hiatal hernias, especially the sliding type, produce minimal or *no* complaints (approximately 80%). This depends on the size and location of the hernia.

Other symptoms and special features: Possible effects on the heart and lung (displacement), leading to pain in the cardiac region (aggravated by recumbency) and possible shortness of breath.

Causes: Incompetent esophageal hiatus leading to the development of: a) a *sliding hernia* (approximately 90%), b) *paraesophageal* hernia, or c) *mixed* types. Women are affected more frequently than men. Peak incidence is around 50 years of age, but even children may present with symptomatic hernias ("habitual vomiting"). The paraesophageal type, in particular, tends to become fixed over time; these hernias are no longer reducible and may become incarcerated.

Diagnosis:
● Chest radiographs (may demonstrate retrocardiac shadow), contrast esophagography with the head lowered (typical sliding and paraesophageal hernia formation).
● Esophagoscopy: The transitional zone from squamous epithelium to gastric mucosa is displaced orally above the level of the diaphragm, and a crease is visible in the distal "esophagus" (formed by displaced gastric mucosa). Signs of reflux esophagitis may be noted.

Differentiation is required from congenital brachyesophagus, achalasia, malignant tumor, and gastroesophageal prolapse. Pyloric and duodenal stenosis should additionally be considered in infants.

Special Form:

Acquired Brachyesophagus (Barrett Esophagus, Endobrachyesophagus)

Heterotopic and partially metaplastic columnar epithelium (gastric mucosa) lining mainly the lower portion of the esophagus, which is predisposed to peptic ulceration and stenosis. The *symptoms* closely resemble those of hiatal hernia, which frequently coexists with the Barrett esophagus. The *diagnostic studies* are like those for hiatal hernia. Adenocarcinoma develops in 10% of patients with the Barrett esophagus!

Esophageal Trauma

Foreign Bodies

Main symptoms: Most common in children under 3 years of age and in the elderly (denture wearers). Marked dysphagia is accompanied by odynophagia perceived retrosternally or in the back or neck. Occasional cough. If the foreign body perforates the esophageal wall, ominous mediastinitis-like symptoms arise within

a few days (see p. 386). Mediastinal emphysema also develops in some patients.

Diagnosis:
● Typical history, except in small children.
● Radiographic studies: Fluoroscopic and/or contrast examination depending on the radiopacity of the foreign body. Generally the object will lodge in the upper esophageal sphincter. A perforating foreign body can be demonstrated by tomography of the chest and mediastinum.
● Esophagoscopy
(diagnostic and therapeutic).

Differentiation is required from foreign-body "decubitus" (mucosal lesion left by a foreign body that has traversed the esophagus) and from incipient tumor.

Caustic and Thermal Injuries

Main symptoms: Typical history. Very severe retrosternal pain and dysphagia following the inadvertent or deliberate ingestion of acid, lye, caustic chemicals. Progressive shock symptoms with hypotension, rapid pulse, cyanosis, pallor, and cold sweats. Mucosal "marks" in the mouth and pharynx. This type of injury constitutes an *urgent emergency situation!* The same symptoms may arise after an explosion trauma. See also "Complete Spontaneous Rupture of the Esophagus" below.

Diagnosis:
● Chest radiographs. If local findings and the patient's general condition permit: Contrast radiography of the esophagus and stomach on days 2–6 (with follow-ups at 1 and 2 weeks):
● If the severity of the injury permits, flexible endoscopy should be performed (on day 3–6) to assess the mucosal damage from the mouth at least as far as the stomach ("panendoscopy"). Contraindications are shock and suspicion of perforation. The late effect of the injury is cicatricial stenosis (see p. 380).

Iatrogenic Esophageal Injuries

These are not uncommon and can result from probing, bougienage, dilatation, injection, intubation, or esophagoscopy (even with a fiberscope!). Usually the *cardinal symptom* is *sudden, severe pain* correlating with the procedure. *Sites of predilection* for esophageal perforation are the piriform sinus, the three physiologic esophageal constrictions, and stenoses.

Marking the *diagnosis at the time of injury* is critical in terms of further management.

Complete Spontaneous Rupture of the Esophagus

This condition, known as the *Boerhaave syndrome*, is caused by a sudden rise of intraesophageal pressure due, for example, to severe vomiting. *Typical symptoms* include hematemesis, excruciating retrosternal and interscapular pain, epigastric pain, cervical emphysema, acute abdomen, pneumothorax, dyspnea, and precipitous fall of blood pressure with prostration and risk of rapid deterioration. Predisposing factors are cicatricial stenosis of the esophagus, habitual vomiting, and alcoholism.

Differentiation is required from diaphragmatic rupture, incarcerated hiatal hernia, caustic or thermal injuries, and a perforated gastric or duodenal ulcer.

Mallory–Weiss Syndrome

Main symptoms: Hematemesis with significant retrosternal and/or epigastric pain. Severity of symptoms depends on the severity of the lesion.

Causes: Mucosal lacerations of variable extent and number near the esophagogastric junction. Most common in association with habitual vomiting, sliding hiatal hernia, and alcoholism.

Diagnosis: Esophagoscopy.
Differentiation is required from duodenal or gastric ulcer, hemorrhagic gastritis, esophageal varices, hemorrhagic diathesis, and malignant tumors of the esophagus or stomach.

External Esophageal Injuries

Most are *blunt* injuries sustained in vehicular accidents (steering wheel, motorcycle handlebars) or occupational injuries. *Cardinal symptoms* are cough and retrosternal pain on swallowing (due to a tear in the wall of the esophagus and/or trachea). A tracheoesophageal fistula may not become apparent until several days or even weeks after the injury. Other severe trauma symptoms are found in the region of the chest or neck.

An *open (penetrating) injury* of the esophagus is marked by the discharge of saliva and/or food from the external wound. Causes include vehicular and occupational injuries, gunshot injuries, stab wounds, and suicide attempts. Open injuries generally involve the cervical portion of the esophagus.

The **diagnosis** is made from the history, the posttraumatic symptoms, and the intraoperative findings.

Malignant Tumors

Pain (sometimes radiating to the ear) is usually an early feature of esophageal malignancy. Dysphagia often becomes predominant in later stages, and the terminal stage is typically marked by a return of pain accompanied by physical deterioration.

Further details on esophageal malignancies are given on p. 384.

Symptom   **Morphologic Change (Swelling, Tumor)**

Radiographic procedures or esophagoscopy are needed to verify morphologic changes in the esophagus. The most frequent causes are listed in Table 8.**6**.

All or circumscribed portions of the esophagus may be displaced from their normal position by adjacent mass lesions (benign and malignant tumors of the mediastinum, giant goiter,

Table 8.**6** *Symptom* Morphologic change (swelling, tumor)

Synopsis

Extrinsic displacement or compression of the esophagus
  – Hyporpharyngeal diverticula, see p. 279
  – Mediastinal tumors, see p. 387
Luminal expansion
  – (True) esophageal diverticula
  – Megaesophagus, see pp. 379, 382
  – Esophageal spasms, see pp. 373, 382
Cicatricial stenoses, see p. 376
Hiatal hernia, see p. 375
Esophageal varices
Esophageal fistulae, see p. 380
Benign tumors, see p. 384
Malignant tumors, see pp. 377, 384

Table 8.**7** *Symptom* Malformation (after K. Ungerecht)

Synopsis

Anomalous development of the esophagus itself
 	
Having *no communication* with the respiratory tract:
  – Agenesis*
  – Duplication*
  – Stenoses
  – Atresia*
  – Congenital megaesophagus
  – Diverticula
  – Brachyesophagus
  – Barrett esophagus, see p. 376
  – Ectopic gastric mucosa*
  – Cysts*
 	
Communicating with the respiratory tract:
  – Atresia with a tracheoesophageal or bronchoesophageal fistula*
  – Tracheoesophageal or bronchoesophageal fistula*
  – Laryngeal cleft and/or tracheal cleft, see p. 338

Anomalies adjacent to the esophagus
 	
Vascular malformations
  – Dysphagia lusoria
  – Right-sided aortic arch*
  – Duplication of the aortic arch*
  – Tetralogy of Fallot (cardiac anomaly consisting of pulmonic stenosis, ventricular septal defect, dextroposition of the aorta, and right ventricular hypertrophy)*
  – Visceral transposition*
Congenital cysts*
Congenital hiatal hernias, see p. 375
Cardia–fornix anomaly*

* No further commentary

large lymphomas, etc.), by posttraumatic scar tissue, and by soft-tissue defects and displacements (e.g., after pneumonectomy). Significant esophageal displacement can occur without producing alarming functional problems. On the other hand, even relatively slight compression of a circumscribed portion of the esophagus can lead to dysphagia or at least a feeling of pressure. The *diagnosis* is based on radiographic and endoscopic findings, which may occasionally require biopsy confirmation.

The most clinically important *diverticula* of the upper digestive tract (approximately 70% are the Zenker pulsion diverticula) are *not* esophageal diverticula but *hypopharyngeal diverticula* (see p. 279). Nevertheless, a sufficiently large diverticular sac can exert *extrinsic* compression on the upper esophagus and cause significant dysphasia. This is readily diagnosed by contrast radiography and, if necessary, by endoscopy.

True Esophageal Diverticula

Esophageal diverticula may be *parabronchial* or *thoracic* (approximately 20%), *parahiatal* or *epiphrenic* (approximately 10%). High esophageal protrusions are generally asymptomatic. Lesions near the tracheal bifurcation can occasionally cause mild dyspnea, retrosternal pressure, or even cough. Parahiatal and epigastric diverticula are sited in the distal esophagus (5–10 cm above the sphincter) and frequently cause heartburn, spasms, and epigastric pain. Hiatal hernia coexists in more than 30% of cases. These typically small protrusions are *demonstrated* most clearly by contrast radiography. Esophagoscopy is less rewarding as a solitary study in these cases but is an excellent adjunct for demonstrating local intraesophageal changes.

Esophageal Varices

Main symptoms: Recurrent hematemesis,, usually severe, consisting of *fresh*, (bright) red blood. The absence of acrid-smelling food residues in the vomitus distinguishes this type of hemorrhage from the blackish "coffee ground" appearance of nonvariceal hematemesis. Subsequent tarry stool. Dysphagic complaints and retrosternal pressure are usually mild. Generally the patient is known to have portal hypertension, hepatic cirrhosis, or hepatitis, or a mediastinal tumor is present.

Causes: The varices are part of a collateral circulation evoked by congestion in the portal venous system or superior vena cava.

Diagnosis:
● History (hepatic disease is common!).
● Contrast radiography of the esophageal lumen (varices = coarse longitudinal striations). With occlusion of the portal venous system, the varices are located in the lower half of the esophagus; with stasis in the superior vena cava, they are located in the upper half.
● Esophagoscopy usually provides a better diagnostic yield than radiography.

Differentiation is required from gastric or duodenal ulcer, Mallory–Weiss syndrome, and pulmonary hemorrhage.

Symptom   **Malformation**

Most of the anomalies in Table 8.**7** are very rare. The listing is intended merely to provide a systematic framework for differential diagnosis: Although the otorhinolaryngologist is not the first attending physician in such cases, some of these malformations cause disturbances that call for a differential diagnosis on the part of the ENT specialist. The most important are briefly discussed below.

Congenital Stenoses (Membranes)

These most commonly involve the lower half of the esophagus as well as the physiologic constrictions. Typical *symptoms* of esophageal stenoses, which may develop gradually, are described on p. 380.

Diagnosis: Radiography and esophagoscopy.

Congenital Megaesophagus

This condition is usually manifested several months (or years) postnatally by hiccups, vomiting, the regurgitation of *nonacidic chyme*, and possible hematemesis. Other symptoms are anorexia, failure to thrive, and possibly anemia.

Diagnosis: Radiography and esophagoscopy.

Differentiation is mainly required from achalasia with secondary megaesophagus; also from hiatal hernia, cicatricial stricture, and brachyesophagus.

Congenital Diverticula

These may occur in the extrathoracic or intrathoracic esophagus. They are generally asymptomatic and are discovered incidentally (see also p. 378).

Congenital Brachyesophagus

This results from absence of the lower esophageal segment. *Reflux symptoms* commence in infancy approximately 50% of cases (see p. 374); in the rest they appear at an later age or not at all. Suggestive signs are proneness to vomiting with no organic stenosis, hematemesis, and secondary anemia.

Diagnosis: Typical findings on contrast radiography and esophagoscopy.

Differentiation is required from sliding hiatal hernia with secondary brachyesophagus and from peptic stricture or pylorospasm in small children.

Tracheoesophageal or Bronchoesophageal Fistula ("H Fistula")

Communications between the esophagus and tracheobronchial tree may be congenital or may develop as a result of trauma, infection (tuberculosis, syphilis), or malignant disease. In all cases the *cardinal symptom* is cough precipitated by fluid ingestion. A *congenital* H fistula may remain asymptomatic into adulthood if it possesses a valve mechanism, posing a challenge of differential diagnosis. With an H fistula that is already manifest in infancy, the symptoms are striking and dramatic: Paroxysmal cough with cyanosis and choking precipitated by *fluid* ingestion. Solid foods generally do not evoke respiratory symptoms.

Diagnosis: Contrast radiography using a dilute contrast medium.

Differentiation is required from posttraumatic fistula, a perforated diverticulum, and a malignant tumor.

Dysphagia Lusoria

An anomalous right subclavian artery arising from the aortic arch crosses the midline between the esophagus and vertebral column in about 80% of cases and between the esophagus and trachea in about 15%. Dysphagic symptoms are not generally manifested until middle age or later (loss of vessel wall elasticity, possibly accompanied by blood pressure elevation).

Diagnosis:
- Contrast radiography of the esophagus in at least two planes (fluoroscopy), angiography.
- Esophagoscopy demonstrates an oblique or transverse, pulsating indentation of the esophageal wall.

Symptom   **Esophageal Dysphagia**

Dysphagias can be classified by etiology and clinical presentation as predominantly oropharyngeal (including the larynx and occasionally the trachea) or predominantly esophageal (see also p. 279). The causes of the *oropharyngeal* and rare *laryngotracheal* dysphagias are reviewed in Table 4.**25**, which includes commentaries and appropriate page references.

Suggestive signs useful for the differential diagnosis of *esophageal dysphagia* include marked hypersalivation present *before* swallowing is attempted, slow mastication of food, a tendency to assist swallowing by "chasing" the bolus with fluid, and long pauses between bites.

Table 8.**8** lists the principal disorders associated with *esophageal* dysphagia, and Table 8.**9** reviews the age dependence and relative prevalence of the most common disorders underlying chronic esophageal dysphagia.

Cicatricial Stenosis (Web, Stricture, Ring)

Main symptoms: These depend on the cause, site, and configuration of the stenosis. *Caustic*

scars commonly occur at the physiologic constrictions, especially the second, and tend to cause concentric luminal narrowing. Dysphagia and retrosternal pressure, first variable and then constant and progressive, commence a few weeks following the caustic injury. Larger pieces of food may be retained in the esophagus, and weight loss ensues. *Multiple* successive strictures are not uncommon!

Causes: Necrotizing damage to the esophageal wall with scar formation following a caustic injury, reflux esophagitis, prolonged tube feeding, anastomotic surgery, a neglected foreign body, or mucosal disease such as epidermolysis bullosa.

Diagnosis: Contrast radiography and esophagoscopy.

Differentiation is required from malignancy, achalasia, scleroderma, and peptic stenoses (which tend to involve the distal esophagus).

Progressive Systemic Scleroderma

Main esophageal symptoms: Increasing dysphagia and odynophagia, retrosternal and/or

Table 8.**8**   *Symptom*   Dysphagia

Synopsis

Type II: Esophageal dysphagia

Inflammatory
- Simple esophagitis, see p. 374
- Reflux esophagitis, see p. 374
- Barrett esophagus, see p. 376
- *Candida* esophagitis, see p. 374
- Esophageal ulcer (peptic or pharmacologic), see p. 374
- Sideropenic esophagitis (Plummer–Vinson syndrome), see p. 266
- Inflammatory stenoses
- Cicatricial stenoses, webs, strictures, rings
- Hiatal hernia, see p. 375
- Drug-induced lesions, see p. 374
- Radiation-induced lesions

Traumatic
- Caustic injuries and burns, see p. 376
- Internal and/or external injury, see p. 376
- Posttraumatic states, see p. 380
- Foreign bodies, see p. 376

Motility disturbance
- Idiopathic diffuse esophageal spasm, see p. 373
- Achalasia (cardiospasm)
- High achalasia (cricopharyngeal muscle)
- Muscular dystrophy
- Prior vagus nerve section
- Esophageal varices, see p. 379
- Extrinsic compression and/or displacement (goiter, mediastinal tumor, aortic aneurysm, etc.)
- Presbyesophagus
- Globus hystericus (psychogenic or "functional" dysphagia)

Congenital
- Megaesophagus, see p. 382
- Diverticula, see p. 378
- Stenoses, membranes, rings, see p. 380
- Dysphagia lusoria, see p. 380
- Tracheoesophageal fistula
- Esophageal atresia

Neurologic
See Table 4.**25**

Neoplastic
- Benign neoplasms (esophagus, cardia, stomach)
- Malignant neoplasms (esophagus, cardia, stomach)

Systemic diseases
- Collagen diseases: scleroderma, lupus erythematosus, rheumatoid arthritis, periarteritis nodosa
- Diabetic neuropathy
- Alcoholic neuropathy
- Amyloidosis
- Crohn disease (chronic inflammatory disease of the digestive tract)
- Vitamin A or B_2 deficiency

Dermatologic diseases
- Pemphigus, see p. 253
- Recurrent aphthosis, see p. 252
- Dermatomyositis, see p. 255
- Progressive systemic scleroderma

Neuromuscular disorders from medications
- Antibiotic
- Antiarrhythmic
- Antirheumatic
- Anticonvulsive
- Psychopharmaceuticals

Type I: Oropharyngolaryngeal dysphagia, see Table 4.**25**

pharyngeal burning. Regurgitation. Mucosal lesions in the mouth and pharynx (see pp. 243, 257, 264), cutaneous manifestations. Esophageal dysphagia may be the earliest sign of disease!

Causes: Collagen disorders with neuromotor disturbances affecting the esophagus. Atrophy of the smooth muscle (see Table 4.**29**).

Table 8.**9**   Prevalence by age of selected causes of esophageal dysphagia (after R. Eckhardt, K. H. Mayer zum Büschenfelde in: F. Müller and O. Seifert: Taschenbuch der medizinisch-klinischen Diagnostik. Bergmann, Munich 1985)

Age 15 – 45 years		Age > 45 years
Reflux esophagitis	More common	Carcinoma
Achalasia		Reflux esophagitis
Benign tumors		Achalasia
Extrinsic compression		Diffuse spasm
(vascular anomalies, mediastinal tumors)		Lower esophageal ring
Scleroderma		Extrinsic compression
Carcinoma		(aneurysms, mediastinal tumors)
Lower esophageal ring		Zenker diverticula
Paraesophageal hiatal hernia		Paraesophageal hiatal hernia
Zenker diverticula		Benign tumors
Diffuse spasm	Less common	Scleroderma

Diagnosis:

● Esophageal manometry (using pull-through or three-point technique).

● Cineradiography (aperistalsis, dilatation, retention of air and contrast medium).

● Esophagoscopy may be used to identify secondary changes (esophagitis, ulcers, etc.).

Differentation is required from other collagen diseases such as lupus erythematosus, dermatomyositis, and sicca syndrome.

Achalasia (Cardiospasm)

Main symptoms: Very long history gradually progressive esophageal dysfunction. Sensation of food retention in the esophagus behind the xiphoid process. Tough, solid foods cause more severe dysphagic complaints than liquids, and the patient tends to "chase" solid food with drink. Approximately 60% of patients have retrosternal pain. Dysphasia is initially variable and later constant; it is accompanied by active and position-dependent regurgitation or vomiting of food constituents. Typically the vomitus does *not* have an acrid odor! Gradual weight loss may progress to cachexia.

Other symptoms and special features: Most common in middle age (30–50 years) but may occur in children. Both sexes are affected equally. Later stages are marked by paroxysmal spasms and pseudoanginal chest pain.

Causes: Neuromuscular disorder marked by failure of relaxation of the lower esophageal sphincter (presumably based on degeneration of the Auerbach plexus).

Diagnosis:

● Typical history and symptomatology.

● Radiography: Barium swallow (aperistalsis; megaesophagus; elongated, funnel-shaped to thread-like gastroesophageal segment; "wine glass" figure).

● Esophagoscopy.

● Esophageal manometry.

Differentiation is required from esophageal carcinoma, benign tumor, scleroderma, and peptic ulcer.

Special Form:

Hypermotile Achalasia

Powerful esophageal contractions accompanied by cramping retrosternal pain. *"Nutcracker dysphagia"* is based on a greatly elevated lower esophageal sphincter pressure (up to 180 mmHg or more!).

High Achalasia (Cricopharyngeal Achalasia)

Main symptoms: Dysphagia, occasionally with aspiration of the bolus into the larynx and trachea. Failure of glottic closure leads to vigor-

Table 8.**10**   Causes of cricopharyngeal achalasia (after F. H. Ellis)

Central nervous system:	— Cerebrovascular insult — Bulbar poliomyelitis — Multiple sclerosis — Parkinsonism
Muscular diseases:	— Muscular dystrophy — Dermatomyositis — Myasthenia gravis — Thyrotoxic myopathy
Miscellaneous:	— Postoperative dysphagia — Recurrent nerve paralysis — Gastroesophageal reflux
Primary coordination defects:	— Pharynoesophageal diverticula

ous but ineffectual coughing when deglutition is attempted.

Causes: Paralysis of cranial nerves IX–XI and occasionally of nerve XII. See also Table 8.**10**.

Extrinsic Compresssion and Displacement

Dysphagia may be caused by external compression of the healthy esophagus by extraesophageal mediastinal tumors, benign and malignant thyroid tumors, mediastinal lymphomas, cysts, blood vessels (dysphagia lusoria, see p. 380), cervical spine lesions (especially the fifth to seventh vertebrae), kyphoscoliosis, or by a widened aortic arch and enlarged left atrium (mitral stenosis). Thoracic surgical procedures can affect the esophagus by leaving postoperative contractures or causing nerve lesions that alter tonus and motility.

Presbyesophagus

Prolonged bolus transit due to faulty coordination of esophageal movements with increased tertiary contractions and atonic phases. *Diagnosis* of this *age-related* conditions is made by radiography and manometry.

Globus Hystericus (Globus "Nervosus")

Main symptoms: Paroxysmal and sometimes painful foreign-body sensation in the troath, usually most pronounced at the level of the cricoid cartilage. Independent of eating, al-

though the sensation is sometimes perceived as hampering food ingestion, thus mimicking true dysphagia. Peak occurrence is over age 40, with a 3:1 female preponderance. Symptoms generally are exacerbated by physical and emotional stress, and episodes become more frequent. Prolonged asymptomatic intervals can occur, however.

Causes: Multifactorial. Disturbance of cricopharyngeal muscle innervation due to autonomic, endocrine, pharmacologic, or mechanical influences (larynx including dysphonia, vertebral column, esophagus, great cervical vessels, etc.). Also depression and carcinophobia.

Diagnosis:
● Typical clinical presentation. There is almost always a sensation of pressure or tightness behind the cricoid arch: usually digital pressure at that point will briefly reproduce the globus sensation. Organic lesions cannot be demonstrated.
● Barium swallow studies do not demonstrate functional or organic esophageal stenoses. Radiographs can be useful for excluding a mass lesion in the neck or mediastinum and spinal pathology.
● Endoscopy may be performed as far as the gastroesophageal junction if desired to exclude demonstrable disease.
● Phoniatric examination can exclude hyperfunctional or hypofunctional autonomic laryngeal dystonia.
● A trial course of a psychoactive drug such as chlordiazepoxide (Librium) may be adminis-

Table 8.**11**   The most common esophageal tumors

Benign	
Epithelial	– Papillomas
	– Adenomas
Mesenchymal	– Leiomyomas
	– Fibromas ("polyps")
	– Hemangiomas
	– Lipomas
	– Neurofibromas
	– Neuromas
	– Myoxomas
Malignant	
Epithelial	– Squamous cell carcinomas (90%)
	– Adenocarcinomas (usually by upward extension from the cardia)
Mesenchymal (very rare)	– Various sarcomas
	– Carcinosarcomas
	– Melanomas

tered in low dosage to assist differential diagnosis.

Differentiation is required from true dysphagia due to functional or organic causes (see Tables 4.**25** and 8.**8**).

Benign Neoplasms

The principal benign tumors of the esophagus are listed in Table 8.**11**. These neoplasms have a very *low* overall incidence. The most common are myomas, which usually occur in the lower half of the esophagus, affect males more than females, and are most prevalent in middle age.

Symptoms: Long, nonspecific history. Increasing dysphagia, regurgitation, and retrosternal pressure that may progress to back pain during eating. Heartburn.

Diagnosis:
● Radiography.
● Esophagoscopy and biopsy. A number of benign esophageal tumors are *pedunculated*.

Differentiation is required from an aneurysm or malignant tumor.

Malignant Neoplasms

The most common esophageal malignancy (>90%) is *squamous cell carcinoma*, many of which are histologically undifferentiated. Other forms are *adenocarcinoma* (which usually involves the distal esophagus as a proximal extension of gastric carcinoma) and the rare *sarcomas*, which present a variety of histologic compositions.

Main symptoms: Retrosternal or interscapular pain is not unusual in the early stage. Progressive dysphagia is first experienced only with solid foods. Other symptoms are retrosternal pressure or burning, hiccups, regurgitation, vomiting (which may be blood-tinged), cough, weight loss, and oral fetor. Later there is hoarseness (recurrent nerve paralysis) and occasional Horner syndrome (cervical sympathetic trunk lesion). Cachexia, severe dysphagia or aphagia, and severe pain usually develop by about 4–5 months. Paraesophageal, mediastinal, abdominal, and cervical tissues are involved by lymphogenous spread. Hematogenous metastasis is to the liver, lungs, bone, and brain.

Other symptoms and special features: Esophageal malignancies most commonly affect males (3:1) over 60 years of age, most of whom have a history of heavy alcohol use and smoking. Other *predisposing factors* are previous caustic injury. Plummer–Vinson syndrome, diverticula, hiatal hernia, peptic ulcer, achalasia, Barrett esophagus, and reflux esophagitis. Many esophageal carcinomas arise by extension from adjacent structures (thyroid, larynx, bronchi, stomach). Esophageal involvement by distant metastases is uncommon. Mesenchymal malignancies and melanomas are *very* rare.

Diagnosis:
● Contrast radiography shows an asymmetric stenosis with irregular margins. Tomography and CT.
● Esophagoscopy and biopsy.

Symptom   **Hematemesis**

The vomitus is usually dark or black with a "coffee ground" appearance. Vomitus originating from the stomach has an acrid odor.

The most common causes of hematemesis are listed in Table 8.**12**.

Table 8.**12** Causes of hematemesis

Synopsis	
Cause	Typical associated features
Esophageal varices	Jaundice, epistaxis, alcoholism, vascular "spiders," hepatic cirrhosis
Gastric ulcer, duodenal ulcer, erosive gastritis	History of "stomach problems"
Esophagitis (reflux, ulcerating)	Heartburn, retrosternal pain
Mallory–Weiss syndrome	Frequent, severe vomiting; vomiting immediately preceding copious bleeding
Anastomotic ulcers	History of anastomotic surgery
Malignant tumor of the esophagus or stomach	Poor general health, weight loss; regurgitation; retrosternal or epigastric pain
Hemorrhagic diathesis	History or symptoms consistent with bleeding tendency
Hereditary hemorrhagic telangiectasis	Typical vascular markings in the mouth, face, and sometimes on the extremities
Caustic injury (acid, lye)	Typical history; traces of caustic injury in the mouth and pharynx
Barrett esophagus	Acquired brachyesophagus; symptoms resemble those of hiatal hernia
Boerhaave syndrome	Complete spontaneous rupture of the esophagus with severe retrosternal pain, prostration, and rapid downhill course. Shock. "Acute abdomen"

9. Mediastinum

Pathologic processes of the neck, esophagus, or tracheobronchial tree can lead to diseases of the pleura, while diseases of the mediastinum can spread to involve the foregoing structures and systems. Thus, the *upper anterior mediastinum* in particular is apt to figure in the differential diagnosis of otorhinolaryngologic disorders. Corresponding symptoms may be produced by inflammatory conditions, *injuries and their sequelae*, or by *benign* and *malignant mass lesions*.

Diagnostic Options

Diagnosis is based on the history, *palpation* of the cervical soft tissues, *percussion, auscultation*, and especially *radiologic* procedures: chest radiographs and fluoroscopy, biplane films, conventional tomograms and/or CT scans, and contrast esophagography. A recent addition is *magnetic resonance imaging (MRI)*, which offers new capabilities of localization and tissue discrimination. Symptoms may warrant the use of *esophagoscopy, tracheobronchoscopy*, and/or *mediastinoscopy* (Table 9.1), which may be combined with *biopsy* or the collection of material for microbiologic analysis. Consultation with a thoracic surgeon or internist is urgently indicated in patients whose history and symptoms are suggestive of mediastinal disease.

The following mediastinal diseases are of primary interest to the ENT physician:
○ Acute and chronic mediastinitis
○ Expansile or space-occupying lesions
  − Malformations
    (cysts, dermoid cysts, teratomas)
  − Vascular lesions (aneurysms)
  − Benign and malignant neoplasms
    (intrathoracic goiter, thymoma, lipoma, fibroma, neuroma, angioma, lymphoma, parathyroid adenoma, etc.)

Acute Mediastinitis

Main symptoms: Severe, rapidly progressive systemic signs with severe pain behind the sternum or between the scapulae and occasionally in the neck. High fever with chills, greatly elevated ESR, and a marked left shift in the white differential blood count. Dysphagia and odynophagia. Tachycardia, shortness of breath, and usually severe unrest. Frequent singultus or vomiting. Historical evidence of a primary disease.

Other symptoms and special features: Mediastinal emphysema (which may spread to the lower cervical soft tissues) is especially common after an instrumental perforation (endoscopy) or with a perforating foreign body. Less common are signs of inflow stasis from obstruction of the superior vena cava.

Causes: Frequently traumatic, such as perforation by esophagoscopy, tracheobronchoscopy, or a perforating foreign body. Closed or open injury between the neck and diaphragm. Spontaneous perforation caused, for example, by an esophageal ulcer or a malignant tumor of the esophagus, tracheobronchial tree, or neck. Hematogenous and lymphogenous mediastinal infections can also occur.

Diagnosis:
● History (trauma is frequently present).
● Radiographic studies (chest film: widening of the mediastinal band, "chimney sign"; decreased mobility of the diaphragm; tomograms and/or CT scans; esophagogram).
● Esophagoscopy and/or tracheobronchoscopy, as indicated.

Table 9.**1** Principal indications for mediastinoscopy and scalene node biopsy

	Mediastinoscopy	Scalene node biopsy
Substrate	Paratracheal, tracheobronchial, bronchopulmonary lymph nodes	Lymph nodes in front of the anterior scalene muscle in the omoclavicular trigone; "sentinal node" at the junction of the thoracic duct with the lower left "great" venous angle (Fig. 10.**2**)
Goal	Extend the intrathoracic and mediastinal lymph node evaluation	Investigate the diagnostically important collecting site for lymphatic drainage from the chest and abdomen
Frequently detectable diseases	Hodgkin lymphoma Non-Hodgkin lymphoma Tuberculosis Sarcoidosis Lymphogenous metastatic carcinoma	Sarcoidosis Hodgkin lymphoma Non-Hodgkin lymphoma Mediastinal tumors Bronchial carcinoma Gastrointestinal carcinoma Pancreatic malignancies Gynecologic cancers

● Laboratory values are consistent with a severe, acute inflammation.

Differentiation is required from myocardial infarction, pleuritis, pericarditis, pancreatitis, and gastric perforation.

Chronic Mediastinitis

Main symptoms: Similar to those of acute mediastinitis, but less dramatic and pursuing a milder course.

Causes: May progress from acute mediastinitis. Otherwise may result from tuberculosis, Boeck disease, syphilis, histoplasmosis, (blasto)mycosis, or a foreign body.

Diagnosis is like that for acute mediastinitis and may additionally require mediastinoscopy or thoracotomy.

Expansile or Space-occupying Lesions

These lesions tend to produce *different symptoms* from inflammatory processes. Typically there is a long history of gradually progressive symptoms such as dyspnea, intrathoracic pressure, cough, and possibly stridor. Retrosternal pain and back pain *may* be present. The same applies to cardiac and circulatory abnormalities. Later stages are marked by increasing dysphagia (esophageal displacement) and occasional odynophagia. Even a benign mass can cause a compression of the superior vena cava leading to edematous swelling about the head, neck, and upper arm and visible venous congestion (upper inflow stasis). Recurrent nerve paralysis (hoarseness), the Horner syndrome (miosis, ptosis, enophthalmos), and elevation of the diaphragm are more characteristic of malignant neoplasms. Some mediastinal masses remain clinically silent for some time, however, and may be discovered incidentally on radiographs.

Besides the above procedures, other special studies available for the *diagnosis* of mediastinal masses include mediastinal venography, radionuclide scanning (thyroid), pneumomediastinography, and *endoscopic procedures* (esophagoscopy, tracheobronchoscopy, mediastinoscopy) that may include *incisional biopsy, direct transtracheal or transbronchial needle aspiration, or scalene node biopsy* (see Table 9.**1**).

The *differential diagnosis* of this disease group should include the various types of autochthonous benign neoplasms and malformations as well as pleural malignancies and tumors that involve the mediastinum by direct extension or distant metastasis. It should also include systemic diseases (see below), diaphragmatic hernias, distended diverticula, and aortic aneurysm.

Mediastinal (secondary) *lymph node involvement* is most common in patients with lymphogranulomatosis, tuberculosis, sarcoidosis, immunoblastic lymphoma (see p. 408), leukemia, and especially bronchial carcinoma (see Table 9.**1**).

10. Neck

The Symptoms

○ Pain, p. 390

○ Neuralgia and neuralgiform complaints, p. 392

○ Blood flow abnormalities in the great cervical vessels, p. 395

○ Morphologic change (swelling, tumor, malformation), p. 397

○ Morphologic change in the thyroid gland, p. 408

○ Important syndromes, p. 412

Although "the neck" represents a topographic region with well-defined subregions, it is difficult to define it precisely in clinical terms. As the connecting link between the head and trunk, the neck contains numerous vitally important organs and structures that perform bridging functions between the head and thorax without distinct anatomic boundaries. Accordingly, a number of disciplines are concerned with the clinical aspects of the neck.

While the present chapter is oriented toward the requirements of otorhinolaryngologic differential diagnosis in the neck region, attention is also given to essential differential diagnostic aspects of neighboring specialties.

Principal Diagnostic Methods

○ *Inspection* and *palpation*, combined with the *history*, often play a *decisive* role in differential diagnosis! Important *criteria for palpation* are *size, shape, consistency, mobility, pulsation, tenderness*, and overlying *skin changes*. Complete relaxation of the cervical soft tissues is necessary for reliable palpation with an optimum yield. This in turn requires that the patient be placed in a sitting position with the head tilted forward, and that the examiner palpate the neck bimanually from both the anterior and posterior sides.

○ *Diagnostic imaging procedures:* The principal radiographic studies are *soft-tissue films* (emphysema, foreign bodies), *cervical spine films* (in various functional positions!), and especially *tomography and CT. Contrast medium* may be used in these studies if desired. Various arterial and venous *angiographic methods* are available for demonstrating the cervical vessels (digital subtraction angiography of the carotid or vertebral artery system, superselective angiography, venography, etc.).

Increasingly, radiographic procedures are being supplemented or replaced by *magnetic resonance imaging (MRI)*, which is particularly rewarding in the neck owing to its capacity for soft-tissue discrimination.

○ An equally rewarding modality in the neck region is *sonography* (ultrasound), especially using the B-mode technique (high-contrast images of various tissues and tissue planes, identification of lymph nodes). The A scan is still used for the diagnosis of cysts and other cavitary structures. Doppler ultrasound permits the determination of flow rates in the cervical vessels.

○ *Endoscopic procedures* (tracheobronchoscopy, esophagoscopy, and mediastinoscopy) are indispensable in the differential diagnosis of many neck diseases and for establishing a tissue diagnosis by *biopsy*.

Symptom   Pain

The most important causes of neck pain, including the submental and nuchal regions, are listed in Table 10.**1**.

Superficial Painful Inflammatory Conditions in the Neck Region

Furuncles and *carbuncles* of the neck tend to occur posteriorly. They are most common in adolescents and young adults and in patients with diabetes mellitus, endocrine changes, or weakened host defenses. Pain is also a feature of *infected atheromas* and *dermoids* and various forms of *acute* or *chronic pyoderma*.

Causes: The principal causative organisms are staphylococci and streptococci.

The **diagnosis** is based on typical local findings. If desired, the organism can be isolated, identified, and its antibiotic sensitivity determined. A diabetic metabolic status should be excluded whenever a furuncle or carbuncle is found.

Deep (Acute) Inflammatory Conditions

These can have diverse clinical presentations:

Compartmental Abscess

Main symptoms: Constant, severe pain, odynophagia, swelling of the oral floor and/or one side of the neck with exquisite tenderness and possible circumscribed redness and tension of the overlying skin. Severe systemic signs with high fever. Elevated ESR and a pronounced left shift in the white blood count.

Other symptoms and special features: The head and neck are held in a guarded position, and trismus may occur. In later stages there may be chills, septic fever, and rapid deterioration reflecting thrombophlebitis or generalizing sepsis. Antibiotic therapy can mask the classic symptoms!

Causes: Abscess formation in one of the fascial compartments of the neck, usually originating in the mouth or pharynx (glossitis, lingual abscess, dental focus, osteomyelitis of the mandible, tonsillitis or peritonsillitis, injury of pharyngeal mucosa). May also result from lymphadenitis. Spread of inflammation tends to follow a descending path. Abscess formation may also originate from the thyroid gland or may follow surgery of the mouth or neck.

Diagnosis:
- Typical history and clinical picture.
- Endoscopic search for the primary focus (teeth, tonsils, pharynx, etc.).
- Diagnostic imaging: CT, possibly MRI.
- Sonography is useful for locating sites of liquefaction.
- Needle aspiration with diagnostic (including microbiology and sensitivity testing!) and therapeutic intent.

Ludwig Angina

This is a cellulitic process involving the oral floor *above* the hyoid bone (see also p. 234). The submental area is hard, bulging, and extremely tender with tense, reddened skin. The condition may progress at any time to a deep compartmental abscess or descending cervical cellulitis! The diagnosis is like that for a compartmental abscess (see above).

Cervical Cellulitis

Main symptoms: "Bull neck." Severe systemic illness with high, occasionally septic temperatures, dysphagia, and possibly dyspnea and stridor. Rapid downhill course. Rapidly spreading inflammation with exquisite tenderness of affected areas. Possible symptoms of thrombophlebitis of the internal jugular vein (see below) or mediastinitis (see p. 386).

Causes: Diffuse, usually fulminating bacterial soft-tissue infection of the neck dissecting along the planes of the cervical fascia and great blood vessels and spreading chiefly toward the jugular fossa, with potential for mediastinal involvement. The infection often originates in the tonsils and occasionally in the major salivary glands (parotid, submandibular, sublingual). Some infections are dentogenic. See pp. 233, 234, 263, and Figure 4.**2**.

Diagnosis is like that for compartmental abscess (see above).

Thrombophlebitis of the Internal Jugular Vein

Main symptoms: Tenderness and protective resistance along the anterior border of the sternocleidomastoid muscle, i.e., over the vascular sheath. Antibiotics can mask this characteristic tenderness and reduce the protective defense. Chills with septic temperatures. Soft, rapid pulse. Generally there is coexisting inflammatory disease of the tonsils, ear, or mandible and dentition with regional cervical lymphadenopathy. Severe malaise. Greatly elevated ESR, left shift in white blood count. Occasional splenomegaly and/or hematogenous seeding of purulent metastases (lung, liver).

Causes: Extension of a hematogenous, lymphogenous, or contiguous bacterial infection of the mouth, pharynx, or ear into the regional venous system (see also pp. 41, 214, 262).

Diagnosis:
● Complete ENT examination to identify and eradicate the primary focus.
● Noninvasive evaluation of the internal jugular vein (by ultrasound or MRI).
● Identification of the causative organism in the blood may be attempted.
● Referral to an internist is indicated to evaluate for septic metastasis.

Nonspecific Lymphadenitis

Main symptoms: Tender, enlarged lymph nodes at the mandibular angle, in the submental area, along the internal jugular vein (especially at the "jugulofacial angle"), and less commonly in the supraclavicular fossa or nuchal area (see Fig. 10.**4**). In long-standing cases the lymph nodes become indurated and less painful. Occasional liquefaction (fluctuation) is followed by spontaneous eruption through the skin with the formation of a fistula. Peak occurrence is form 1 to 10 and 50 to 70 years of age.

Causes: Bacterial and/or viral infection of the regional lymph nodes arising from a primary head and neck focus. Cervical lymph node involvement is a feature of many inflammatory

Table 10.**1**   *Symptom*   Pain

Synopsis
Inflammatory conditions
Superficial
– Furuncle
– Carbuncle
– Infected atheroma or dermoid
– Pyoderma
Deep
– Compartmental abscess
– Ludwig angina
– Cervical cellulitis
– Thrombophlebitis of the internal jugular vein
– Nonspecific lymphadenitis
– Mononucleosis, see p. 231
– Specific lymphadenitis, see Table 10.**9**
– Chronic lymphadenitis, see p. 399
Injuries
Neuralgias and neuralgiform complaints
– Posterior neck pain, see p. 392 and Table 10.**2**
– Myoarthropathies, see p. 17
– Whiplash injury
– Vertebragenic headache
– Cervical syndromes (upper, middle, lower)
– Pain in dysphonias, see p. 339 ff.
– Cervical rib syndrome (costoclavicular compression syndrome)
– Scalenus syndrome
– Glossopharyngeal neuralgia, see p. 162
– Neuralgia of the vagus nerve and/or its superior laryngeal branch, see pp. 163, 350
– Odynophagia, see pp. 279, 380
Neoplasms

processes of diverse etiologies affecting this region. These secondary lymphadenopathies are clinically indistinguishable from one another, so their presence is not suggestive of a special underlying disease. At the same time, all cases of acute cervical lymphadenitis warrant a very thorough search for a cause in the head and neck region!

Diagnosis:
● Complete ENT examination to identify the primary focus. If a focus is not found, referral to an internist or pediatrician is indicated.
● In suspicious cases a lymph node biopsy should be taken for histologic analysis.

Differentiation is required from systemic disease of the lymphatic system, AIDS (HIV, see p. 245), infected neck cyst, and metastatic malignancy. See also Table 10.**6**.

Injuries

Main symptoms: Most patients have an obvious history and corresponding local findings. With *sharp* injuries, there is significant risk of involvement of nerves, blood vessels, and the respiratory and digestive tracts. *Blunt* trauma is characterized by pain and rapid swelling of cervical soft tissues (hematoma, emphysema). Trauma that breaches the jugular vein system carries a risk of air embolism (cyanosis, dyspnea, unconsciousness, convulsions, cardiac arrest). Involvement of the carotid sinus (contusion) leads reflexly to an acute fall of blood pressure and/or asystole. With hematoma formation and "internal" trauma, an initial asymptomatic interval may be followed by dyspnea and dysphagia, and cervical cellulitis and/or mediastinitis may ensue! Laryngeal and tracheal involvement are discussed on pp. 316, 324, and 363. Late sequelae of injury to the cervical vessels include arteriovenous fistulae and aneurysms, which most commonly involve the great vessels.

Diagnosis:
● A detailed evaluation of traumatized neck structures is generally undertaken *during* the operative treatment that follows primary emergency care measures.
● In milder cases without open injury, palpation, endoscopy, and tomography may provide and adequate workup.

Special Form:

Fracture of the Hyoid bone and/or the Superior Horn of the Thyroid Cartilage

Main symptoms: Odynophagia, swelling of adjacent cervical soft tissues; possible transient dysphonia. With malunion or nonunion, odynophagia may become permanent.

Diagnosis: Palpation to locate site of tenderness. Radiographic demonstration of the fracture may be tried.

Symptom   **Neuralgia and Neuralgiform Complaints**

Posterior Neck Pain

The principal causes are summarized in Table 10.**2**.

Whiplash Trauma and Other Cervical Spine Injuries

Main symptoms: History of trauma (or rear-end collision) capable of causing a transient subluxation of the cervical spine. Symptoms and course may resemble classic cervical spondylosis, with symptoms developing gradually (after an asymptomatic interval) or appearing immediately after the trauma. Differential diagnosis can be quite difficult, because the effects of the trauma often are *not* demonstrated by radiographs. Posttraumatic complaints tend to subside in 2–6 months, however.

Diagnosis:
● An accurate history and thorough clinical evaluation are important for forensic and other reasons.
● Radiographic studies are frequently unrewarding!
● Neurologic and orthopedic consultation may be indicated.

Differential diagnosis:
See Tables 2.**11** and 2.**12**.

Vertebragenic (Spondylogenic) Headache

Main symptoms: Pain on movement of the head and neck, radiating to the nuchal area and occasionally to the forehead ("helmet" pain). Pain is predominantly *unilateral* and may project to the shoulder region (brachialgia). The head is held in a guarded position. Pain is often provoked by a sustained, unfavorable body posture or position, by loading of the cervical spine, by an extreme head position, by prolonged work with the neck flexed or extended, etc.

Other symptoms and special features: Restriction of cervical spine motion (with crepitation), radicular sensory disturbances and/or loss of reflexes in the neck, shoulder, and arm. Acute pain is precipitated by excessive head movements, sneezing, coughing, straining, etc. Vertebrobasilar vertigo may occur (see pp. 102, 106, 113). Tenderness is noted along the cervical spine and in the paravertebral neck muscles. Hyperesthesia of the scalp, sensation of scalp tension. See also Table 10.3.

Causes: Osteoarthritic changes or skeletal anomalies of the cervical spine, especially involving C0 and C1 or less commonly C2.

Diagnosis:
- Assessment of cervical spine mobility, tenderness of the paravertebral neck muscles and about the uncinate process; pain on axial compression of the cervical spine.
- Radiographs show typical osteoarthritic vertebral changes (marginal osteophytes, narrowing of the foramina and intervertebral spaces, impingements, displacements, posttraumatic deformities and contour defects). *But:* There is often a marked discrepancy between the clinical presentation and radiographic findings!
- Diagnosis is aided by trial manipulations and physiotherapeutic measures and by evaluating the "dynamics" of the intervertebral joints and uncovertebral connections.

Differential diagnosis:
See Tables 10.2 and 2.11.

Table 10.2   Causes of nuchal pain

Subtentorial organic diseases
Congenital anomalies at the craniocervical junction – Platybasia – Basilar impression
Osteolytic processes involving the occipital bone and atlas – Rust syndrome
Functional and/or organic disturbances of the cervical spine – Atlantoaxial dislocation – Subaxial dislocation – Spondylosis and spinal osteoarthritis (at C0–C1 to C2–C3) – Joint "restriction" or segmental dysfunction (e. g., at C2–C3) – Upper cervical syndrome
Herniated intervertebral disk
Anomaly ⎫ Inflammation ⎬ Involving the cervical spine or adjacent structures Neoplasia ⎭
Previous cervical spine injury
Musculotendinous irritation (e. g., due to unphysiologic loading of the deep neck muscles)
Ante- or retroflexion headache
Tension headache, see p. 164
Neuralgia of the occipital nerves, see p. 163
Vertebral artery insufficiency, see p. 396
See also Tables 2.11 and 10.3

Cervical Syndromes

Main symptoms:

a) *Upper* cervical syndrome: See previous section on Vertebragenic Headache.

b) *Middle* cervical syndrome: Dull, diffuse, often bilateral pain radiating to the dermatomes of C3, C4 (phrenic muscles), and C5 (deltoid and biceps muscles). *No* sensory or motor deficits. There may be accompanying autonomic symptoms such as palpitations, cardiac arrhythmias, and phrenic dysfunction.

c) *Lower* cervical syndrome: Analogous symptoms involving the dermatomes for C6, C7, C8, and/or T1 ("shoulder–arm syndrome").

Examination of the cervical spine often demonstrates abnormal motion of the interverte-

Table 10.**3** Criteria for the diagnosis of spondylogenic headache (from M. Mumenthaler, F. Regli: Der Kopfschmerz. Thieme, Stuttgart 1990)

---

1. Located in the nuchal or occipital region
2. Frequently radiates to the forehead (helmet pattern)
3. Sometimes as in (1) and (2), but confined to one side
4. Usually occurs in prolonged episodes that recur with some frequency
5. Episode may be precipitated by stress on the cervical spine (e. g., prolonged maintenance of the same head position)
6. Associated with, or previous history of:
   - Evidence of cervical spine pathology
     - Torticollis
     - Cervicobrachialgia
   - Evidence of cervical spine lesion
     - Direct trauma
     - Whiplash injury
7. On examination:
   - Restricted mobility of the cervical spine
   - Paravertebral tenderness, often unilateral
     - Nuchal muscles
     - Occipital attachments of the nuchal muscles
   - Radiologic changes
     - Anomalies
     - Degenerative bone changes
     - Posttraumatic changes
     - Functional changes
8. Exclusion of other (occipital) causes of headache (see Tables 2.**10** and 2.**11**)
9. Positive response to specific therapy

See also Tables 2.**11** and 10.**2**

---

bral joints and/or tenderness at the insertions of the short back muscles.

Causes: "Pseudoradicular" symptoms arise as a protective response to functional disturbances or organic lesions involving single or multiple joints in the cervical spine.

Diagnosis:
● Exclusion of ENT pathology.
● Radiographic examination of the cervical spine in the lateral and AP projections, possibly supplemented by "functional" views.
● Consultation with a neurologist, orthopedist, and perhaps a physical therapist.

Differentiation is required from true radicular syndrome (boring, gnawing pain in the affected dermatomes with sensory and/or motor deficits, sometimes involving multiple roots). Referred pain from a focus in the abdominal organs or shoulder and arm joints. Inflammatory or degenerative arthritis of the cervical spine. Soft-tissue rheumatoid manifestations in the neck and cervical spine. Another possibility is psychosomatic pain. See also Table 10.**3**.

Cervical Rib Syndrome (Costoclavicular Compression Syndrome)

Main symptoms: Circulatory impairment in the forearm and hand, brachialgia, occasional pain radiating to the neck. Brachial plexus paralysis. Occipital headache, possible intermittent cerebral ischemia. The typical symptoms can be provoked by extreme head rotation to the affected side (scalenus syndrome, see below), by raising the arm (costoclavicular syndrome), or by carrying a heavy load.

Causes: Supernumerary cervical rib belonging to the seventh or sixth cervical vertebra; anomalous insertion of the scalenus anterior muscle. Compression of the brachial plexus and/or the subclavian artery and vein. Fully developed symptoms usually appear between 40 and 50 years of age, with a 3:1 preponderance of females. Overt clinical symptoms develop in only about 10–15% of radiographically demonstrable cases.

Diagnosis:
● The supernumerary rib may be palpable. Stenotic bruit is occasionally audible over the subclavian artery in the supraclavicular fossa.
● The Adson test: Head rotation to the affected side and deep inspiration abolish the radial artery pulse.
● Radiographic studies: Cervicothoracic skeletal survey view may be supplemented by functional angiography of the subclavian artery.

Differentiation is required from osteochondrosis of the cervical spine, inflammatory or neoplastic spinal disease, and shoulder–arm syndrome.

Scalenus syndrome (caused by an anomalous insertion of the scalenus anterior muscle) presents practically the same symptoms but is not associated with skeletal anomalies.

Neuralgia of the Glossopharyngeal Nerve

See p. 162.

Neuralgia of the Vagus Nerve

See p. 163.

Odynophagia

See pp. 279, 380.

Neoplasms

Benign and even malignant neoplasms of the cervical region generally do not cause pain in their early stage, and other symptoms suggest the diagnosis (morphologic changes, functional deficits). Pain may, however, be the *first* warning sign of a benign or malignant tumor that is irritating cervical nerve tissue, such as a sympathetic neuroma (schwannoma) or sympathicoblastoma. Pain may also signal a paravertebral chordoma, a chondroma or chondrosarcoma (radicular symptoms), or a pharyngeal or laryngeal carcinoma (see p. 326). The *Pancoast tumor* (pulmonary sulcus carcinoma) and *malignant goiter* can cause pain radiating to the neck and shoulder and can also incite the Horner syndrome.

Symptom	**Blood Flow Abnormalities in the Great Cervical Vessels**

Disturbances of blood flow in the great cervical vessels are reviewed in Table 10.4.

Carotid Insufficiency

Main symptoms: The *sudden* occlusion of a *common carotid artery, internal carotid artery,* or *brachiocephalic trunk* (by trauma, embolism, etc.) causes permanent central nervous deficits (ranging to complete hemiplegia) in at least 50% of patients. A *slowly progressive* unilateral occlusion of these vessels (by tumor compression or obliteration, arteriosclerosis, etc.) may cause no central neurologic deficits if an adequate collateral circulation is established via the circle of Willis.

Carotid stenoses not caused by trauma or neoplasia (e.g., due to atherosclerosis) may be asymptomatic. The symptoms depend on the degree of the stenosis (see Table 10.5).

A unilateral occlusion of one *external carotid artery*, even when sudden, is generally tolerated without functional deficits. When the vessel is ligated, however, there is a risk of retrograde thrombosis with embolism distant from the ligature. A sudden bilateral occlusion of the external carotid artery can lead to severe

Table 10.**4** *Symptom* Abnormal blood flow in the great cervical vessels

Synopsis
Carotid insufficiency
– Common carotid artery
– Internal carotid artery
– External carotid artery
– Brachiocephalic trunk
– Acute complete occlusion
– Gradual complete occlusion
– Carotid stenosis
Vertebral artery insufficiency
– Basilar insufficiency
– Subclavian steal syndrome
Internal jugular vein insufficiency
Posttraumatic arteriovenous fistula

necrosis at various sites in the head and neck (e.g., the tongue).

Causes: Obstruction or occlusion of the vessel lumen by atherosclerotic wall thickening, embolism, extrinsic compression, ligation, or by abnormal kinking, looping, or coiling of the

Table 10.5   Stages of carotid insufficiency

Stage I:	No neurologic deficits, but angiographically demonstrable stenosis or occlusion of the internal carotid artery
Stage II:	Intermittent but still reversible symptoms of several minutes' duration such as hemiplegia, speech and gait disturbance, and lapse of consciousness
Stage III:	Stroke with gradually progressive, irreversible focal deficits and loss of consciousness, caused by complete occlusion of the internal carotid artey
Stage IV:	Permanent damage with neurologic deficits; end stage

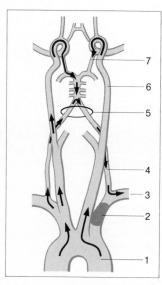

Fig. 10.1   Collateral circulation in subclavian steal syndrome (after Hollinshead)

1 Aortic arch
2 Occlusion of the subclavian artery
3 Subclavian artery
4 Vertebral artery
5 Foramen magnum
6 Internal carotid artery
7 Circle of Willis

vessel. Insufficiency of the *internal* carotid artery can also result from *blunt trauma* (e.g., thrombus formation following a closed neck injury).

Diagnosis:
● If a stenosis is suspected: Auscultation of the carotid bifurcation (a marked stenotic bruit is heard when luminal reduction exceeds 40%).
● B-mode sonography.
● Doppler sonography.
● Diagnosis may be aided by DSA (digital subtraction angiography) or CT.

Vertebral(−Basilar) Insufficiency (Vertebrobasilar Insufficiency)

Main symptoms: Episodic or persistent ataxia, unsteady and/or rotatory vertigo, spontaneous nystagmus (central vestibular, see pp. 106, 113). Cochlear hearing impairment (see p. 81). Visual disturbances. Transient impairment of consciousness and drop attacks. Sensory and motor deficits may ensue. The Wallenberg (oblongata) syndrome may also develop. Incidence is highest in the 6th decade or later.

Causes: Stenosis of the vertebral artery (occasionally bilateral) or basilar artery due, for example, to atherosclerosis, embolism, or extrinsic compression (cervical spondylosis). Predisposing factors are diabetes, hypertension, and general vascular diseases. See also p. 113.

Special Situation:

Subclavian Steal Syndrome:

A stenosing lesion in the proximal subclavian artery or brachiocephalic trunk can cause a reversal of flow in the ipsilateral vertebral artery, which "steals" blood from the vertebrobasilar system (Fig. 10.1). The *cardinal symptoms* of obtundation, vertigo, visual disturbance, dysarthria, etc., are most pronounced during exercise of the ipsilateral arm (cause: reversible ischemic foci in the brain stem).

Diagnosis:
● Doppler sonography of the vertebrobasilar system (transcranial Doppler flowmetry of the vertebral and basilar arteries). DSA may be used as an adjunct.
● Provocative test for suspected subclavian steal syndrome: fist clenching or exercise of the ipsilateral arm.

- Pulse and blood-pressure measurements *in both arms* (when the syndrome is present, the right–left discrepancy exceeds 20 mmHg).
- Stenotic sounds may be audible over the subclavian artery.

Differentiation is required from aortic arch syndrome and a dissecting aneurysm.

Obstruction of the Internal Jugular Vein

A *unilateral* interruption of blood flow is not associated with clinically apparent deficits. A *concomitant bilateral* obstruction usually leads to very severe congestive phenomena with impending edema formation in the head and neck region that may become acutely life-threatening! The symptoms gradually regress over a period of weeks.

Carotidynia
See p. 167.

Symptom   **Morphologic Change (Swelling, Tumor, Malformation)**

The most common relevant diseases are listed in Table 10.**6**.

Important *lymph node groups draining the head and neck* are reviewed in Table 10.**7** (see also Fig. 10.**4**). The differential diagnosis of *enlarged lymph nodes* is reviewed in Table 10.**8**, and the principal *causes of head and neck lymphomas* are listed in Table 10.**9**.

Drug-induced Lymphadenopathy

A number of drugs can, with prolonged use, incite a bilateral lymph node swelling that shows little or no tenderness and regresses when the drug is withdrawn. This type of lymphadenopathy can affect the cervical, axillary, inguinal, mediastinal, or abdominal nodes. Often the blood count initially shows leukocytosis, which is succeeded by eosinophilia with leukopenia. Presumably based on an allergic or pseudoallergic response. Drugs known to incite lymphadenopathy are listed in Table 10.**10** (see p. 401).

Chronic Soft-tissue Inflammatory Conditions

Chronic Cellulitis

An acute cellulitic process in the neck (see pp. 233, 234) may progress to a subacute and chronic stage depending on the type of infect-ing organism, its virulence, and individual host defenses. The cardinal symptom of pain is succeeded by other *main symptoms*: hard swelling ("wooden phlegmon"), livid skin discoloration, and the possible formation of one or more fistulae. Systemic signs are only moderate. The *causative organisms* are generally antibiotic-resistant "problem organisms" such as *Pseudomonas, Proteus, E. coli*, anaerobes, or less commonly encountered organisms such as *Actinomyces, Blastomyces, Brucella*, etc. Foreign bodies and bony suppuration (mandible) can likewise sustain a chronic phlegmonous process. The *diagnosis* is based on otorhinolaryngologic findings, identification of the causative organism, and possibly the demonstration of a sequestrum, foreign body, or even a malignant tumor!

Actinomycosis

Main symptoms: Hard, "board-like" soft-tissue infiltration (neck, oral floor, cheek, etc.), usually with the formation of multiple abscesses and fistulae. Livid discoloration of the overlying skin. Pus from the abscesses is usually yellow and frequently contains greenish granules (agglomerations of filaments and spores). Actinomycosis has become a very rare infection.

Causes: Infection with the anaerobic gram-positive species *Actinomyces israeli* and accompanying bacteria (staphylococci and streptococci). Small eptihelial defects in the mouth or

Table 10.**6**   *Symptom*   Morphologic change (swelling, tumor, malformation, etc.)

Synopsis

Inflammatory swellings

Acute

- Acute superficial soft-tissue inflammatory conditions, see p. 390
- Acute deep soft-tissue inflammatory conditions, see p. 390
- Ludwig angina, see p. 390
- Acute nonspecific lymphadenitis, see p. 391
- Mononucleosis, see p. 231
- Drug-induced lymphadenopathy

Chronic

- Chronic soft-tissue inflammatory conditions
  - Chronic cellulitis
  - Actinomycosis
- Chronic nonspecific lymphadenitis
- Lymph node involvement in
  - Tuberculosis
  - Sarcoidosis (Besnier–Boeck–Schaumann disease)
  - Syphilis
  - AIDS, see p. 245
  - Toxoplasmosis, see pp. 66, 290
  - Cat scratch fever, see p. 286
  - Tularemia, see p. 290
  - Other infections, see Table 4.**28**
  - Local and generalized lymph node enlargements, see Table 10.**8**
- Inflammatory swellings of the salivary glands, see p. 299 ff.
- Inflammatory swellings of the thyroid gland, see p. 411

Malformations

- Cervical cysts and fistulae
  - Lateral cervical cyst and fistula
  - Aural–cervical cyst or fistula, see pp. 32, 402
  - Midline cervical cyst or fistula

- Laryngocele, see p. 328
- Teratoma
- Torticollis (may be acquired!)
- Klippel–Feil syndrome
- Goldenhar syndrome

Tumors

Benign tumors

- Madelung neck
- Fibroma
- Lipoma
- Cystic hygroma
- Cervical hematocele
- Hemangioma simplex
- Carotid body tumor
- Neoplastic lymphadenopathy
- Neuroma
- Neurinoma
- Ameloblastoma

Malignant tumors

- Lymph node metastases
- Lymphogranulomatosis (Hodgkin disease)
- Non-Hodgkin lymphoma (malignant lymphoma)
- All advanced, outward-projecting carcinomas and sarcomas of the cervical organs and major salivary glands

Morphologic changes in the thyroid gland

Goiter

- Dystrophy
- Euthyroid goiter
- Hypothyroid goiter
- Hyperthyroid goiter (Basedow disease)
- Strumitis
- Malignant goiter

pharynx, carious teeth, and fracture sites form portals of infection.

Diagnosis:

● Identification of the causative organism in pus or tissue samples (needle biopsy) and in culture.

● Serologic tests (agglutination, complement binding, precipitation) and intradermal tests are not considered sufficiently reliable.

Differentiation is required from other infectious agents (problem organisms, tuberculosis, etc.), suppuration about a sequestrum (osteomyelitis following trauma, irradiation, ect.), and malignancy.

Table 10.**7** Lymphatic drainage of the head and neck (see also Fig. 10.**2**)

Important lymph node groups in the head and neck region	Areas drained
Mandibular angle	Mouth, tonsils, teeth, tongue (posterior portion and base). Submental and submandibular region. Pharynx
Retroauricular	External auditory canal, auricle, temporal scalp
Preauricular	Anterior scalp, external ear, lateral eyelids, upper face, parotid gland
Submaxillary, submandibular, submental	Lower half of facial skin, lips, teeth, tongue (anterior part and borders), nose, salivary glands
Nuchal	Skin of the head and occiput
Superior (deep) cervical group	Receives drainage from the entire head and upper neck region
Inferior (deep) cervical group	Lower neck, axilla, arm, chest

Chronic Lymphadenitis

Main symptoms: Common childhood sequel (see p. 391) to an infectious disease or minor injury (scratch wound, etc.). May also result from a specific infection (see below). Affected nodes are firm, usually nonpainful, and enlarged (mandibular angle, submental, deep jugular chain, etc.). Mobility of the nodes may be normal or moderately decreased. Possible liquefaction, abscess and fistula formation. Peak occurrence is from 1–10 and 50–70 years of age. Spontaneous regression follows elimination or resolution of the cause.

Causes: Infection with a variety of pathogenic organisms (see below).

Table 10.**8** Diagnostic evaluation of enlarged lymph nodes (slightly modified from U. Bucher. In: W. Hadorn, N. Zöllner: Vom Symptom zur Diagnose. Karger, Basel 1979)

History

Age

Acute onset:
- Viral and bacterial infections
- Acute hemoblastoses

Pain:
- Inflammatory conditions
- Acute hemoblastoses

Fever:
- Especially common with infectious lymphadenopathies, also occurs with proliferative forms (Hodgkin disease)
- Acute hemoblastoses

Environment, occupation:
- Contact with animals: brucellosis, toxoplasmosis, tularemia, cat scratch fever, etc.
- Farmers: actinomycosis
- Schools, military bases, etc.: mononucleosis

Anorexia, weight loss, night sweats:
- Consumptive lymph node diseases (malignant lymphomas, hemoblastoses, metastasizing tumors, tuberculosis, etc.)

Pruritis (with or without cutaneous lesions):
- Lymphogranulomatosis, chronic lymphatic leukemia, malignant lymphoma

Alcoholic pain (lymph node pain induced by alcohol consumption)
- Sarcoidosis (Besnier–Boeck–Schaumann disease)
- Lymphogranulomatosis (Hodgkin disease)

Drugs (see Table 10.**10**)

Anemic complaints, hemorrhagic diathesis:
- Consumptive disease, bone marrow involvement (e. g., hemoblastoses)

Diagnostic findings

Palpation of the lymph nodes:
- Isolated or generalized lymph node involvement
- Moveability
- Consistency
- Collateral edema
- Fistula formation

Complete ENT examination including tonsils, salivary glands, teeth, and thyroid. Basic laboratory workup and possibly serologic tests

B-mode sonography

Radiography (lung, etc.)

Other general signs of disease: spleen, liver, joints, skin changes, etc.

Excisional or percutaneous biopsy

Table 10.**9**   Lymph node enlargement in the head and neck region

Disease group	Disease	Additional information in text
Localized (isolated) lymphomas Inflammatory		
Acute lymphadenitis (site depends on area drained)	Usually an accompanying bacterial infection, less commonly virogenic	See p. 311
	Syphilis (primary focus in the head region)	See pp. 247, 401
	HIV	See p. 245
	Diphtheria	See p. 233
	Plaut–Vincent tonsillitis	See p. 260
Chronic lymphadenitis (site depends on portal of entry)	Tuberculosis (lymphogenous)	See p. 401
	Toxoplasmosis (may also be generalized)	See Table 4.**28**
	Listeriosis	See Table 4.**28**
	Cat scratch fever	See Table 4.**28**
	Leishmaniasis	See Table 4.**28**
	Tularemia (may also be generalized)	See Table 4.**28**
	Brucellosis	See Table 4.**28**
	Actinomycosis	See p. 397
Neoplastic	Lymphogenous tumor metastasis (regional metastasis)	See p. 406
	Lymphogranulomatosis	See p. 407
Generalized lymphomas Inflammatory		
Sepsis Viral infection	Infectious mononucleosis (EBV)	See p. 231
	Measles	See pp. 11, 66
	Rubella	See p. 91
	Mumps	See pp. 65, 300
	Cytomegalovirus (infants)	See p. 302
Chronic lymphadenitis	Tuberculosis (hematogenous)	See p. 401
	Secondary syphilis	See pp. 247, 401
	Leprosy	See Table 4.**28**
	HIV (AIDS)	See p. 245
	Brucellosis	See Table 4.**28**
	Listeriosis	See Table 4.**28**
	Toxoplasmosis	See Table 4.**28**
	Generalized fungal infections	See Table 4.**28**
Various reactive diseases	Drug-induced lymphadenopathy	See p. 397
	Serum disease	
	Sarcoidosis	See pp. 255, 401
	Chronic rheumatoid arthritis	
	Disseminated lupus erythematosus	See p. 210
	Chronic dermatoses and collagen diseases	
	Immunodeficiency diseases	
Storage diseases	Gaucher disease	
	Hand–Schüller–Christian disease	
	Niemann–Pick disease	
Neoplastic	Acute leukosis	
	Lymphogranulomatosis (Hodgkin disease), advanced stages	See p. 407
	CLL (chronic lymphatic leukemia)	See p. 408
	Non-Hodgkin lymphomas	See p. 408
	Hematogenous (distant) metastases	

Diagnosis: These steps are generally followed in the evaluation of chronic cervical lymphadenitis:
- History with attention to potential sources of infection.
- Complete ENT examination.
- Differentiation from simple acute lymphadenitis and from tuberculous or syphilitic lymphadenitis, including routine laboratory studies.
- Serologic search (CBR, agglutination, precipitation, etc.) for possible causative organisms (see Tables 10.6 and 4.28).
- Biopsy for histologic *and* microbiologic evaluation. Biopsy in *children* is generally deferred until lymph node enlargement has proven unresponsive to broad-spectrum antibiotics or persists for 6−8 weeks following elimination of the putative cause.

Differentiation is required from systemic diseases (lymphoma), cervical cyst, salivary gland diseases, AIDS (HIV infection, and malignant metastases.

The following *forms of lymphadenitis* (especially when *chronic*) should be considered in the differential diagnosis:

○ **Tuberculous Lymphadenopathy**

Main symptoms: Painless swelling of various groups of cervical lymph nodes, sometimes bilateral. Most prevalent in children and adolescents but increasingly common in the 20−50 age range. The lesions may be solitary, multiple, small or large, firm or fluctuant, and may be associated with fistula formation.

Causes: Infection (mainly postprimary hematogenous infection with the human strain of tubercle bacilli).

Diagnosis:
- History, giving special attention to contact with infected persons and trips abroad (Africa, Asia).
- Radiographic examination: Cervical soft tissues (calcium shadows) and chest.
- Intradermal tuberculin test.
- Consultation with a pediatrician or internist.

Differential diagnosis: See above.

Table 10.**10** Drugs that can cause lymphadenopathy

Hydantoin
Penicillin
Streptomycin
Sulfonamides
Isoniazid (INH)
Diaminodiphenylsulfone
Thiouracil
Viomycin
Heparin
Phenylbutazone
Salicylates
Phenacetin
Meprobamate
Iron dextran
Typhus antigen
Antitoxins
Follicular hormone, etc.
The swollen lymph nodes are usually symmetrical and nonpainful
Cervical manifestations may be accompanied by axillary, inguinal, mediastinal, and abdominal lymphadenopathies
Blood count: Initial leukocytosis is often succeeded by eosinophilia and leukopenia
Symptoms regress after withdrawal of the offending drug

○ **Sarcoidosis**
   (Besnier−Boeck−Schaumann Disease)

Main symptoms: See p. 391. The supraclavicular lymph nodes are the most commonly affected *cervical* nodes (approximately 70%). Concomitant mediastinal lymph node involvement is very common.

○ **Syphilis**

Cervical lymph node involvement is generally present in *secondary* and *tertiary* syphilis. Given a suitable portal of infection, these nodes become symptomatic (firm and painful) about 1−2 weeks following the primary infection. In *generalized stage II* infec-

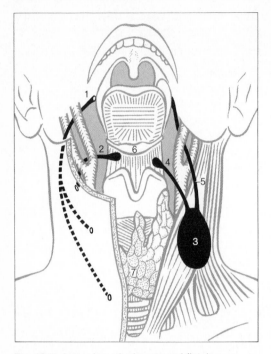

Fig. 10.**2**   Lateral cervical cysts and fistulae

1 Lateral cervical fistula (remnant of the second branchial apparatus). Fistulous tract passes through the carotid bifurcation, with openings in the tonsillar fossa and at the anterior border of the sternocleidomastoid muscle
2 Blindly terminating tract of a short lateral cervical fistula (e.g., derived from the third branchial apparatus)
3 Lateral cervical cyst with a tract that terminates blindly at the level of the hyothyroid membrane (4) or with a cleft remnant ascending to the level of the tonsillar fossa (5)
6 Body of the hyoid bone
7 Thyroid

tions, cervical lymphadenopathy is usually evident *before* the outbreak of mucocutaneous eruptions, even with a distant portal of infection, and is generally ubiquitous. *Congenital and tertiary syphilis* are usually not associated with overt lymphadenopathy. See p. 247 for further details.

○ **AIDS.** See p. 245

○ **Toxoplasmosis**
See p. 66 and Table 4.**28**

○ Many other infections by various pathogens are likewise associated with enlargement of the cervical lymph noses. See Tables 10.**9** and 4.**28**.

Differential diagnosis: See Table 10.**9**.

Malformations

Cervical Cysts and Fistulae

Figures 10.**2** and 10.**3** illustrate the typical manifestations of cystic and fistulous anomalies in the neck region that are of primary interest in terms of differential diagnosis.

Lateral Cervical Cysts and Fistulae (Remnants of the Second or Third Branchial Apparatus) (Fig. 10.2)

Main symptoms: Development of a tense, slowly enlarging cystic mass on the side of the neck (at the anterior border of the sternocleidomastoid muscle). These anomalies become clinically apparent at varying times from infancy to early adulthood (2nd–4th decades). An open fistula may be present at birth, or a fistula may develop later from an initially intact cyst (especially after attempted subtotal surgical removal). Pain occurs only if the cyst and its contents become inflamed. Most branchial cysts are unilateral, fluctuant, and relatively fixed with respect to underlying tissues.

Other symptoms and special features: Fistuale may terminate blindly in the cervical soft tissues or may establish a direct communication between the oropharynx and cervical skin. Fistulae and cysts can arise from various pharyngeal pouches.
○ Typical configuration of cervical fistulae derived from the *second branchial apparatus* (Fig. 10.**2**,1): The fistulous opening is usually in the middle or lower third of the neck, anterior to the sternocleidomastoid muscle. The fistulous tract ascends below platysma in front of the vascular sheath, turns medially *between the external and internal carotid arteries*, and passes to the lateral oropha-

rynx above the glossopharyngeal nerve and below the stylohyoid ligament, where it terminates blindly or opens near the tonsillar fossa. Cysts related to this apparatus are usually at the level of the carotid bifurcation, lateral to the internal jugular vein.

○ Typical configuration of cervical fistulae derived from the *third branchial apparatus* (Fig. 10.**2**, 2): The lower skin opening and course are similar to those of fistulae related to the second branchial cleft. The tract runs to the hyothyroid membrane and piriform sinus, passing above and anterior to the hypoglossal nerve and superior laryngeal nerve, below the glossopharyngeal nerve, and *posterior to the internal carotid artery.* This type of fistula is rare.

Causes: Remnants of the embryonic branchial apparatus (see above).

Diagnosis:

● Typical local findings (tense cystic mass) at the anterior border of the sternocleidomastoid muscle and occasionally in the "carotid triangle."

● In doubtful cases, aspiration of the cyst yields a viscous, greenish-yellow fluid. When a fistula is present, a probe can always be inserted into the external opening and can sometimes be passed along the full length of the tract. Free communication between the external and internal openings can be demonstrated by instilling methylene blue into the lower orifice (appearance of dye near the ipsilateral tonsil).

● Usually the entire tract can be demonstrated radiographically by injecting contrast material into the opening.

● Sonography (A-mode, B-mode) is also informative.

Differentiation is required from dentocutaneous fistula, postoperative fistula (e.g., following tumor resection), cold abscess, cystic hygroma (see p. 405), laryngocele, and lymphangioma.

Acquired Fistulae

These can result from trauma to various structures including the lymphatic system ("chyle fistulae") or salivary glands and may present as a draining lymphadenitis or strumitis, a dento-

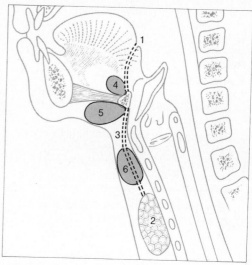

Fig. 10.**3**   Midline cervical cysts

1   Foramen cecum at the base of the tongue
2   Thyroid
3   Embryonic thyroglossal duct
4   Suprahyoid midline cyst
5   Subhyoid midline cyst
6   Low midline cyst

cutaneous fistula, a postoperative or posttraumatic fistula, or a cold abscess with fistulous drainage.

Midline Cervical Cysts and Fistulae (Thyroglossal Duct Remnants)
(Fig. 10.**3**)

Main symptoms: Tense, painless cystic mass with smooth contours, usually poorly displaceable on underlying tissues. These cysts tend to develop between 5 years of age and early adulthood. Most are located in the midline at the hyoid level, but they may occur as low as the jugular fossa. If a fistulous opening is present, it too is located on the midline, although fistulae recurring after inadequate surgery may open farther laterally.

Causes: Persistence of remnants of the embryonic thyroglossal duct (see Fig. 10.**3**).

Diagnosis:

● Typical local findings: A midline cyst or fistula follows the movements of the hyoid bone when the patient swallows.

Table 10.**11** Torticollis (causes) (from W. Becker, H. H. Naumann, C. R. Pfaltz: Ear, Nose, and Throat Diseases)

Muscular

– Spastic disorders
– Inflammatory lesions, as in tuberculosis, or neoplastic infiltration of the sternocleidomastoid muscle and overlying skin
– Removal of the sternocleidomastoid muscle (e. g., as part of a neck dissection)
– Paralysis of the accessory nerve (can also result from mechanical irritation by the vertrebral artery)
– Rheumatoid torticollis, myogelosis
– Progressive ossifying myositis
– Neuralgic–neurovascular symptom complex in scalenus syndrome, see p. 394

Osseous

– Atlantoaxial torticollis sencondary to inflammation, irradiation, or nasopharyngeal surgery (= Grisel disease)
– Klippel–Feil syndrome (in some cases), see Table 4.**26**
– Goeminne syndrome, see Table 4.**26**
– Goldenhar syndrome (in some cases), see Table 2.**13**
– Traumatic dislocation of a cervical vertebra

Symptomatic

– Ocular reflex torticollis to compensate for unilateral visual or oculomotor disturbances
– Guarded neck position due to a peritonsillar, retrotonsillar, or parapharyngeal abscess, see pp. 233, 262
– Acute or subacute lateral cervical lymphadenitis, see Tables 10.**6**, 10.**9**
– Congenital: unilateral contracture of the sternocleidomastoid muscle due to fibrous transformation (cause unknown, hereditary factors involved) (see also Osseous Causes)
– Scarring (e. g., postoperative or postirradiation)
– Congenital cystic hygroma, see p. 405
– Bezold mastoiditis, see p. 12
– Unilateral labyrinthine dysfunction, see pp. 73, 104 ff.

Psychogenic, neurotic

● A probe introduced into a midline fistula generally encounters the hyoid. The tract may occasionally extend behind the body of the hyoid to the foramen cecum at the base of the tongue!

● If necessary, the fistulous tract can be delineated by sonography or contrast radiography.

Differentiation is required from dermoid cyst, (submental) lymphadenitis or lymphoma, lymphangioma, cystic hygroma, an enlarged thyroid pyramidal lobe, ectopic thyroid tissue, and laryngocele.

Torticollis (Wryneck)

The most common forms of torticollis are reviewed in Table 10.**11**. Only a few are classified as malformations.

Klippel–Feil Syndrome

See Table 4.**26**.

Goldenhar Syndrome

See Table 2.**13**.

Tumors

Benign and malignant neoplasms of the neck that are not derived from the skin or mucosa (such as advanced or invading laryngeal or pharyngeal carcinoma, tracheal tumors, etc., also skin cancers, melanomas, etc.) have a mesenchymal, neuroectodermal, or vascular matrix. Except for lymphomas (see p. 408), these nonepithelial neoplasms occur rarely in the neck. This group includes *fibromas, lipomas, hemangiomas, lymphangiomas, histiocytomas, neurofibromas, schwannomas* (neurilemomas), and *rhabdomyomas*. Rarer still are the corresponding malignant forms. A *Kaposi sarcoma*, a common lesion of AIDS (see p. 246), also occurs in the neck. Differential diagnosis ultimately rests on biopsy, so a detailed discussion is unnecessary in this context.

Benign Neoplasms

Characteristic benign neck masses, aside from the rare true benign lymphomas, are:

○ *Madelung neck* (multiple lipomas, typical notched contour in the nuchal midline).

○ *Cystic hygroma* (congenital cystic lymphangioma) and congenital *cervical hematocele* (analogous derivative of the vascular system). Both anomalies tend to enlarge and can cause significant mechanical aerodigestive obstruction (see below).

○ *Carotid body tumor* (chemodectoma; see below).

○ *Goiter*, which can also occur in a malignant form (see p. 412).

Cystic Hygroma (Congenital Cystic Lymphangioma of the Neck)

Main symptoms: Soft, boggy, compressible, diffuse subcutaneous mass, usually most prominent on one or both sides of the neck. Associated internal mass effects can displace tissues toward the oropharynx and hypopharynx, larynx, trachea, and esophagus, causing potentially life-threatening dyspnea, stridor, and/or dysphagia. A mechanical wryneck position ("pseudotorticollis") can also occur. Many hygromas enlarge during the first years of life, causing speech impairment.

Causes: Congenital cavernous and cystic multilocular *lymphangiomas.*

Diagnosis:
● Typical clinical presentation from birth.
● Needle aspiration may be considered in doubtful cases.
● Delineation of tumor margins by radiography, sonography, and endoscopy.

Differentiation is required from hemangioma (see below), cervical cyst, teratoma, and other congenital anomalies.

Rare Forms

○ *Cervical hematocele:* An analogous congenital anomaly derived from the *vascular system.* This entity requires *differentiation* from:

○ *Hemangioma simplex*, which, while common in the facial, oral, and parotid regions, may also affect the back or sides of the neck in a capillary or cavernous form. Though usually present at birth, many of these vascular tumors do not become clinically

apparent for several years. They may occur symmetrically as nevus flammeus; they may form soft, diffuse, subcutaneous, asymmetrical swellings; or they may extend more deeply into the soft tissues of the neck (e.g., the muscles of the oral floor and tongue, parapharyngeal, etc.). See also pp. 146, 308.

Main symptoms: Soft, compressible swelling, sometimes with marked redness of the overlying skin or mucosa. Superficial lesions are occasionally subject to recurrent bleeding, and sufficiently large hemangiomas can hamper speech and deglutition. Hemangiomas are relatively common in complex malformation syndromes (e.g., the Sturge–Weber syndrome, see Table 2.**13**).

Diagnosis: See previous section (Cystic Hygroma).

Carotid Body Tumor (Chemodectoma, Glomus Tumor)

Main symptoms: Firm, spherical or slightly nodular swelling located below the mandibular angle at the level of the carotid bifurcation, anterior to and below the sternocleidomastoid muscle. This very slow-growing tumor is movable laterally but cannot be displaced up and down. Tumors attaining sufficient size can cause globus sensation and dysphagia. Marked transmitted pulsations are usually palpable, and auscultation often discloses a pulsatile sound.

Other symptoms and special features: Compression of the tumor by turning the head or other manipulations *may* provoke dizziness, a fall in blood pressure, faintness, or occasionally tinnitus (carotid sinus symptoms). The tumor is bilateral in 2–5% of patients. Peak occurrence is in the 3–5th decades. Five percent (to 10%) of tumors project into the oropharyngeal lumen. There is an estimated 5–10% incidence of malignant transformation.

Cause: Tumor arising from the carotid body at the carotid bifurcation (= nonchromaffin paraganglioma).

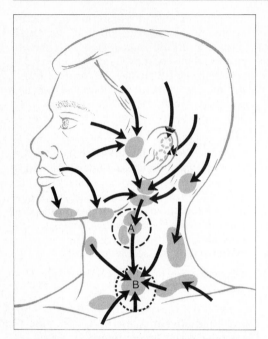

Fig. 10.**4**   Lymphatic drainage of the head and neck (highly schematic) Drainage from peripheral tributaries to the various regional lymph node groups

A   Lymph node group at the "superior" venous angle (chiefly drains the head region)
B   Drainage center at the jugulosubclavian "inferior" venous angle (drains the ipsilateral head and neck; also receives drainage from sites throughout the body [thoracic duct, etc.] with varying distribution on each side)

Diagnosis:
● Long asymptomatic history. Typical site of occurrence, typical palpable and often audible findings.
● Imaging studies: Carotid angiography (DSA) (egg-shaped widening of the carotid bifurcation, spongy vascular pattern within the tumor boundaries). MRI and sonography also may be used.

Differentiation is required from aneurysms of the cervical vessels, lateral cervical cyst, external laryngocele, cervical lymphoma (see below), neurogenic neck tumors, and lymph node metastases.

Neoplastic Lymphadenopathy

True benign lymph node tumors are rare in the neck. The slow-growing *localized benign lymphoma* requires differentiation from inflammatory lymph node swelling (see Table 10.**9** and pp. 391, 397, 399 ff.) and from *reactive lymph node hyperplasia*, which is most common in children and adolescents.

Malignant Neoplasms

Malignant Lymph Node Tumors

These have major significance in both children and adults, particularly since cervical lymphadenopathy is often the *first clinical sign* of generalized malignant disease.

Differential diagnosis: Malignant lymph node tumors are classified into three broad groups:

○ Lymph node metastases (carcinomas, less commonly melanomas, sarcomas, etc.)
○ Hodgkin disease (lymphogranulomatosis)
○ Non-Hodgkin lymphomas ("malignant lymphomas" in the older nomenclature)

Lymph Node Metastases

Main symptoms: Metastatic lymphadenopathy is rare in juveniles and becomes more common with advancing age. It is characterized by single or multiple, hard, nodular lymph nodes, initially mobile but gradually becoming fixed, in one of the cervical chains (Fig. 10.**4**).

Metastases from head and neck tumors most commonly involve the deep jugular chain, especially at the *superior* venous angle (Fig. 10.**4**). Lymph node metastases are frequently bilateral, depending on the type and location of the primary tumor. Initially the nodes are nontender until inflammation supervenes. In later stages involvement of the cervical plexus, vagus nerve, or sympathetic trunk can lead to sensory and motor dysfunction (e.g., neck−shoulder−arm syndrome, the Horner syndrome, diaphragmatic paralysis, etc.). The frequency of cervical lymph node metastases for various primary tumor sites is shown in Table 10.**12**.

Figure 10.**4** shows a highly schematic representation of the interdependence between tumor site and the anticipated sites of lymph node metastasis.

Causes: Most lymph node metastases result from the lymphogenous dissemination of malignant cells from head and neck tumors (including the thyroid) or from tumors of the bronchial region, esophagus, or even the breast and gastrointestinal tract ("sentinal node").

Diagnosis:
● Bilateral palpation of the cervical lymph nodes (Fig. 10.**4**).
● History, endoscopic findings, and radiologic findings for localization of the primary tumor. Incisional biopsy or fine-needle aspiration biopsy.
● Tomographic, CT, or sonographic evaluation of the cervical soft tissues, cervical lymph node system, and adjacent extranodal structures (large vessels, fascial compartments, cervical organs).
● Special inquiries (metastasis from the abdominal or thoracic cavity) may necessitate scalene node biopsy and mediastinoscopy (see Table 9.**1**).

Differentiation is required from malignant lymphoma, Hodgkin disease, tuberculosis, and chronic adenopathies (see Table 10.**9**).

Hodgkin and Non-Hodgkin Lymphoma

Hodgkin disease (lymphogranulomatosis) and *non-Hodgkin lymphoma* are *generalized* lymphatic diseases that can have primary and ongoing manifestations in the neck region. Thus, the otolaryngologist is often concerned with their differential diagnosis, which requires close communication with the oncologist, pathologist, and radiologist. We therefore limit our remarks to a brief summary of the symptoms and nomenclature(s) that are most significant to the ENT physician. Further evaluation and staging are handled by the attending oncologist.

Hodgkin Disease (Lymphogranulomatosis)

Main symptoms (with cervical involvement): The initial sign is very often a firm, painless, unilateral swelling of cervical lymph nodes, which initially remain mobile. Nonspecific sys-

Table 10.**12** Incidence of clinical lymph node involvement by head and neck carcinoma at the time of diagnosis (from W. Becker, H.H. Naumann, C.R. Pfaltz. Ear, Nose, and Throat Diseases. Thieme, Stuttgart 1989)

Organ	% (approximate)
Hypopharynx	65
Oropharynx	60
Nasopharynx	60
Oral cavity	40
Salivary glands	25
Larynx (depending on site)	0–60
Skin	15
Internal nose and paranasal sinuses	10

temic signs include fatigue, an undulant fever that rises slowly to moderate levels with afebrile intervals, night sweats, weight loss, and pruritus. Later there is usually significant subjective malaise. Incidence is bimodal, with the first peak between ages 10 and 35 and the second after age 50.

Other symptoms and special features: Hematologic values are initially normal but later demonstrate anemia, lymphopenia, an elevated ESR, and possibly eosinophilia. Splenomegaly and sometimes hepatomegaly subsequently develop. There is about a 10% incidence of primary extranodal involvement (e.g., nasopharynx, oropharynx, digestive tract, skin, bones, etc.).

Causes: Unknown: *Four histologic types* are recognized (characterized by lymphocyte predominance, nodular sclerosis, lymphocyte depletion, and mixed cellularity).

Diagnosis:
● Laboratory status.
● Chest radiographs (in two planes), sonography (neck and upper abdomen), thoracic and abdominal CT.
● Excisional biopsy of a cervical lymph node, perhaps supplemented by mediastinoscopy and/or scalene node biopsy.
● Positive findings warrant consultation with a (pediatric) internist. Radiologic consultation may also be advised.

Table 10.**13** Nomenclature of non-Hodgkin lymphomas

Kiel classification (Lennert)	Former designation
Low grade of malignancy	
Lymphocytic	
– Chronic lymphatic leukemia	Chronic lymphatic leukemia
– Hairy-cell leukemia	Lymphoid reticulosis
– Mycosis fungoides	Mycosis fungoides
– T-zone lymphoma	Atypical lymphogranulomatosis
Lymphoplasmacytic	Waldenström macroglobulinemia
Plasmacytic	Plasmocytoma
Centrocytic	Lymphocytic lymphosarcoma
Centroblastic-centrocytic	Follicular lymphoma, Brill–Symmers lymphoma
High grade of malignancy	
Centroblastic	Included with lymphoblastic sarcoma
Lymphoblastic	Included with lymphoblastic sarcoma
Immunoblastic	Reticulosarcoma (retothelial sarcoma)

Other classifications in current use:
○ I.W.F. = International Working Formula
○ Classification of Rappaport
○ Classification of Lukes and Collins

Non-Hodgkin Lymphoma (Old Name: Malignant Lymphoma)

Main symptoms (with cervical involvement): Early stage is marked by solitary or multiple swollen cervical lymph nodes, initially nontender, which generally are softer than in Hodgkin disease. No subjective malaise. In contrast to lymphogranulomatosis, whose initial manifestation is usually confined to the cervical nodes, non-Hodgkin lymphomas can be readily demonstrated in regions outside the neck. Later stages are marked by fever, lethargy, and weight loss. The disease can occur at any age, but the peak incidence is about 15–20 years higher than in Hodgkin disease patients.

Other symptoms and findings: In later stages the lymph nodes become matted and fixed or less mobile. The blood count shows early anemia and occasionally "lymphosarcoma–cell" leukemia. There is early enlargement of the liver and spleen. Extranodal manifestations in the nose, oropharynx, and paranasal sinuses are relatively common! These manifestations, as well as orbital and thyroid involvement, should be excluded by careful endoscopic (and possibly radiologic) examination.

Cause: Unknown. There is no standard international *nomenclature* for non-Hodgkin lymphomas. The *Kiel classification* is perhaps the most widely used nomenclature in Germany at present (Table 10.**13**). Older designations applied to malignant lymphomas are contrasted with the current nomenclature in Table 10.**13**.

Diagnosis: Same as for Hodgkin disease.

Differentiation is required from toxoplasmosis, tuberculosis, drug-induced and/or allergic lymphadenopathy, and metastatic carcinoma.

Symptom   Morphologic Change in the Thyroid Gland

(See synopsis in Table 10.**6**).

Thyroid function testing is the task of the endocrinologist or internist. But because the thyroid gland is located in the neck and can play a primary or secondary, active or passive role in diseases involving the neck, it falls within the scope of otorhinolaryngologic differential diagnosis, which often aids in treatment selection for cervical disorders that involve the thyroid (e.g., malignant tumors, tracheal stenosis, trauma, etc.).

Table 10.**14**   Diagnostic evaluation of thyroid disease

History: Duration of the thyroid change, increase in neck circumference (collar size), thyroid nodules, pain, hoarseness, dyspnea or dysphagia, nervousness or lethargy, cardiac complaints, excess sweating, sleeplessness, weight loss, finger tremor, hair loss, malaise, etc.	*Radionuclide scanning* (^{99}Tc or ^{131}I, detection of ectopic thyroid tissue, function test of iodine uptake by the glandular parechyma) – Cold nodule: Hypofunctioning area produced by simple goiter, cyst, hemorrhage, or rarely by a thyroid malignancy – Warm nodule: Slightly hyperfunctioning area produced by a compensated autonomous adenoma – Hot nodule: Markedly hyperfunctioning area produced by a decompensated autonomous adenoma
Inspection: Neck contours, size of the thyroid gland, symmetry, ectopic thyroid tissue, laryngeal displacement	
Palpation: Bimanual palpation from the front and back with the patient in a sitting position; assessment of gland consistency (soft, hard, homogeneous, nodular, symmetric, asymmetric); tenderness to pressure; mobility of the gland in its bed and movement of the gland during swallowing	*Tracheobronchoscopy and/or esophagoscopy* is indicated when there are symptoms of compression or displacement of the trachea, bronchi, or esophagus
	In vitro function tests:
Auscultation for vascular thrill or bruit	T_3 Triiodothyronine
Laryngoscopy: Vocal cord function	T_4 Thyroxine; normal range: 5–13 µg iodine/ 100 mL serum. T_4 radioimmunoassay (RIA) and T_4 enzyme immunoassay (EIA)
Radiography: Standard chest films (2 planes) Spot films of trachea (2 planes), as indicated Barium swallow, as indicated Tomograms and/or CT scans (for special inquiries)	TBI Thyroxine binding index; normal range: 0.9–1.1 µg iodine/100 mL serum
	TRH Thyrotropin-releasing hormone
	TSH Tyhroid-stimulating hormone
Sonography: The thyroid gland is readily accessible to diagnostic ultrasound	ETR Effective thyroxine ratio = combination of T_4 test and TBI test
	Histologic *(biopsy)* and/or cytodiagnostic *(fine-needle aspiration)* examination. (The latter study has a false-negative rate of approximately 10%)

The size and shape of the thyroid gland are not meaningful indicators of thyroid function. Nevertheless, changes in the shape and consistency of the gland provide the most immediate differential diagnostic criteria from the *otolaryngologic perspective.* The present discussion is therefore limited to a table that reviews the principal diagnostic options for thyroid diseases and to a survey of the most common thyroid disorders that are associated with conspicuous enlargement of the gland (goiter).

Methods for the Diagnosis of Thyroid Disordes (Table 10.**14**)

Goiter

Goiter (struma) denotes a visible and/or palpable enlargement of the thyroid, *independent of the functional state* of the gland.

Three *size classes* of goiter are recognized:
1. The thyroid is *palpably* enlarged. *Visible* enlargement is apparent only when the head is dorsiflexed
2. The thyroid is visibly enlarged in *all* head positions
3. The thyroid is so greatly enlarged that it projects into the retrosternal space and may cause regional complications

The following *types of goiter* are distinguished:

o Dystopic "goiter"
o simple euthyroid goiter
o Hypothyroid goiter
o Hyperthyroid goiter
o Thyroiditis (strumitis)
o Malignant goiter

It should be recalled that hormonal disturbances can also occur in a thyroid of normal size. However, functional disturbances that are associated with thyroid enlargement are of particular interest within the context of otorhinolaryngologic differential diagnosis.

Dystopic Goiter

Forms include *lingual goiter, intratracheal goiter, multiple foci* of dystopic thyroid tissue occurring throughout the neck (chiefly involving the lateral cervical area or the area of the former thyroglossal duct), and *thoracic (mediastinal) goiter.* A normal thyroid gland may coexist at the usual site, or part or all of the normal gland may be absent. This must be determined before any potentially troublesome ectopic thyroid tissue is removed (radionuclide scanning).

Simple Euthyroid Goiter

Main symptoms: Visible thyroid enlargement, either with diffuse parenchymal proliferation (as in juvenile goiter) or with the formation of single or multiple nodules (as in nodular goiter or colloid goiter of middle age). Females are predominantly affected. Occurrence may be endemic or sporadic. The lesion is painless, but large goiters can interfere with movement, respiration, eating, etc.

Other symptoms and special features: Large goiters can cause threatening regional complications (trachea, esophagus, larynx [see p. 371], recurrent nerve paralysis [p. 350], retrosternal space). There is *no* disturbance of thyroid function!

Causes: Proliferative intraglandular processes caused by a deficient iodine supply, impaired iodine utilization, and/or a disturbance of endocrine regulation. As the condition progresses, degenerative changes occur in the form of colloid cysts, organized hemorrhagic foci, adenomatous nodules, calcium, deposits, nodule formation, etc.

Diagnosis:
● Simple goiter is mobile, nontender, has a smooth or nodular surface and a variable consistency.
● Radiography and radionuclide scanning (see Table 10.**14**).
● Function tests demonstrate *euthyroid* values.

Hypothyroid Goiter

Main symptoms: Endemic or sporadic thyroid enlargement. Findings are analogous to simple goiter but are accompanied by signs of diminished mental activity (apathy, lethargy, increased sleep requirement). Skin is dry, scaling, and thickened. Menstrual disturbances and sexual dysfunction are common. Myxedema or hypothyroid cretinism may occur.

Other findings and special features: Frequently the voice is deep and harsh, and speech may be slowed. Inner ear symptoms (hearing loss, vertigo) also occur.

The Pendred syndrome: Sensorineural hearing loss, disturbance of iodine metabolism, and goiter (see p. 87, Tables 1.**43** and 4.**26**).

Causes: Deficient peripheral supply of thyroid hormones despite compensatory parenchymal hyperplasia. Deficient iodine utilization. Endemic goitrogens. Exogenous insult by drug side effects or inadequate hormone therapy.

Diagnosis: Besides characteristic local findings (see above), diagnosis relies mainly on function tests: elevated TSH levels, decreased T_4 and/or T_3 levels.

Cold Nodule

Nonfunctioning area of thyroid parenchyma on radionuclide scan. The causes of this phenomenon can be very diverse: Degenerative changes, colloid cysts, inactive adenomas, calcific foci, and even carcinomas (in about 10% of cases!). For safety, therefore, a cold nodule should be removed for histologic analysis.

Hyperthyroid Goiter

Main symptoms: The Merseburg triad (nodular or diffuse goiter, tachycardia, and exophthalmos) is not always complete! Weight loss, restlessness, sweating, hair loss, sleeplessness, fatigue, increased appetite. Typical ocular signs: glossy eye, eyelid flutter with infrequent blinking. Fine tremor of the fingers. Psychomotor unrest, occasional psychopathologic reactions.

Other symptoms and special features: Emaciation and temperature elevation. The skin is often moist. Women over age 30 are predominantly affected. A special complication is unilateral or bilateral endocrine orbitopathy: Exophthalmos with ocular protrusion, conjunctivitis, eyelid swelling, chemosis, and periocular edema.

Progression to *thyrotoxic crisis* can occur. Suggestive signs: Aggravation of hyperthyroid symptoms (see above), high fever, sleeplessness, severe weight loss, and extreme physical and mental excitation to the point of delirium.

Causes: Unknown. The most common clinical forms are: a) diffuse hyperthyroidism (Basedow disease), b) localized hyperthyroidism (toxic adenoma), and c) thyrotoxicosis factitia caused by excessive administration of thyroid hormone. May relate to aberrant central regulation of hormone production and/or (auto)immune mechanisms.

Diagnosis:
- Typical history and clinical presentation.
- Palpable findings; a solitary nodule is suggestive of autonomous (toxic) adenoma.
- Low serum cholesterol.
- Radionuclide scan can differentiate between toxic adenoma ("warm" [compensated] or "hot" [decompensated] nodule) and diffuse hyperthyroidism.
- Function tests: T_3 and T_4 are generally increased, TRH test is usually negative.

Thyroiditis (Strumitis)

Acute, Purulent Inflammation

Painful swelling of the thyroid gland, local tenderness, fever, redness of the overlying skin. The patient favors a sitting posture with the head tilted forward (to relieve discomfort). Severe odynophagia, sometimes radiating to the ear. Severe swelling can cause dyspnea. Abscess formation may occur.

Causes: Bacterial inflammation, trauma, radiotherapy.

Diagnosis: Typical clinical signs of inflammation and corresponding laboratory findings.

Differentiation is required from malignant goiter and lymphadenitis.

Granulomatous (de Quervain) Thyroiditis (Subacute, Nonpurulent Inflammation)

Firm, moderately tender thyroid swelling, often following several weeks after a systemic *viral infection* (influenza, mumps, coxsackievirus, etc.). Odynophagia with pain radiating to the ear is not uncommon. General weakness and malaise. Often only portions of the gland are inflamed (induration). Regional lymph nodes may be involved.

Diagnosis:
- Laboratory findings: Elevated ESR. Leukocytosis is absent or moderate.
- Possible demonstration of thyroid antibodies.
- Fine-needle biopsy or incisional biopsy.

Lymphocytic (Hashimoto) Thyroiditis (Subacute, Nonpurulent Inflammation)

Insidious, oligosymptomatic course with little or no pain. The thyroid has a soft, elastic feel on palpation and may or may not be enlarged. Most patients are women over 40 years of age. There is *no* regional lymphadenopathy.

Causes: Unclear. Probably an autoimmune basis.

Diagnosis:
- Laboratory findings: Elevated ESR, greatly increased gamma globulin and thyroglobulin antibody levels (suggestive of autoimmune disease).
- Function tests: Euthyroid or increasingly hypothyroid.
- Fine-needle biopsy or incisional biopsy.

Table 10.**15** Malignant thyroid tumors (after 1974 WHO classification)

Epithelial malignancies
- Follicular carcinoma
- Papillary carcinoma
- Squamous cell carcinoma
- Undifferentiated (anaplastic) carcinoma (spindle-cell type, giant-cell type, small-cell type)
- Medullary carcinoma

Nonepithelial malignancies
- Fibrosarcoma
- Other sarcomas, etc.

Miscellaneous malignancies
- Carcinosarcoma
- Malignant lymphoma

Metastases
- From breast, kidney, bronchus, etc.

Malignant Goiter

Malignancies with an epithelial or mesenchymal matrix may be autochthonus thyroid tumors or may be metastatic to the thyroid gland from the breast, kidney, or bronchi (Table 10.**15**). Usually there are no initial warning signals except for *rapid* growth! Later the gland becomes painful and increasingly immobile. Regional lymph node involvement is relatively swift. A very hard, palpable mass in the thyroid or regional lymph nodes, combined with pronounced weight loss, should always lead one to suspect malignancy. Females predominate by about 2:1. Isotope scans usually demonstrate a nonfunctioning area (cold nodule) in the gland. Malignant involvement of adjacent structures is manifested by hoarseness (recurrent nerve), dysphagia, the Horner syndrome (sympathetic trunk), venous congestion, prominent fixed lymph nodes, and bone metastases ("rheumatoid" symptoms!).

Diagnosis:
- Palpable findings.
- Radionuclide scan (cold nodule).
- Incisional biopsy or, if necessary, fine-needle biopsy.

Important Syndromes Involving the Neck

Selected syndromes that involve the neck are reviewed in Table 10.**16**.

Table 10.**16** Syndroms that commonly produce symptoms in the neck region

Designation	Classification	Typical ENT deficits	Other symptoms
Fibrositis syndrome	Extra-articular rheumatism. Soft-tissue symptoms, myogeloses, tendon and/or fascial involvement, myositis. Variable course and substrates	Isolated painful cervical muscle groups. Tendon and fascial pain in the neck region; foci of periostosis and insertional tendinopathy	Occurs in all body regions
Kawasaki syndrome	Acute, febrile mucocutaneous lymphadenopathy	Cervical lymphadenitis. Red, fissured lips; enanthema with involvement of the tongue	High fever, disease of childhood, may also include involvement the abdominal organs
Cervical rib syndrome	See p. 394		
Klippel–Feil syndrome	See Table 4.**26**		
Löfgren syndrome	Acute form of sarcoidosis	See p. 255	
Pendred syndrome	See p. 87		
Rust syndrome (malum suboccipitale)	Bone destruction involving the atlas and axis	Nuchal pain. Stiff carriage of the head. Possible posterior cranial nerve dysfunction	A malignant tumor in the suboccipital region usually has causal significance
Subclavian steal syndrome	See p. 396 and Fig. 10.**1**		
Tangier syndrome	Congenital lipoprotein deficiency (hypochloesterolemia, high triglyceride level, indirect hyperbilirubinemia)	Enlarged, yellow-orange tonsils. Enlargement of cervical lymph nodes	Generalized lymph node enlargement. Hepatosplenomegaly. Typical laboratory blood findigs
Wallenberg syndrome (oblongata syndrome)	Disease of lateral medulla oblongata due to occlusion of the vertebral artery and posterior inferior cerebellar artery (atherosclerosis, syphilis, embolism)	Vertigo, nystagmus, vomiting, tendency to fall toward the affected side. Severe facial pain. Dysphagia. Crossed sensory disturbances. Possible ipsilateral abducens paralysis. Ipsilateral recurrent nerve palsy	Possible contralateral hemiparesis. Corneal reflex may be absent, and multiple other neurologic deficits may involve the trunk and extremities
Cervical syndrome (several subgroups)	See p. 393		

Further Reading
(Overviews and Selected Monographs)

Arnold, W. J., J. A. Laissue, I. Friedman, H. H. Naumann: Diseases of the Head and Neck. Thieme, Stuttgart 1987

Ballenger, J. J.: Diseases of the Nose, Throat, Ear, Head and Neck. 14th edition. Lea & Febiger, Philadelphia, 1991

Batsakis, J. G.: Tumors of the Head and Neck, 2nd ed. Williams & Wilkins, Baltimore 1979

Beck, C.: Otogene Sinusthrombosen. In: Berendes, J., R. Link, F. Zöllner: Hals-Nasen-Ohren-Heilkunde in Praxis und Klinik, 2. Aufl., Bd. VI. Thieme, Stuttgart 1980

Becker, W., J. Haubrich, G. Seifert: Krankheiten der Kopfspeicheldrüsen. In: Berendes, J., R. Link, F. Zöllner: Hals-Nasen-Ohren-Heilkunde in Praxis und Klinik, 2. Aufl., Bd. III. Thieme, Stuttgart 1978

Becker, W., H. H. Naumann, C. R. Pfaltz: Ear, Nose and Throat Diseases. A Pocket Reference. 2nd edition. Thieme, Stuttgart 1994

Beckmann, G.: Akute und chronische Entzündungen des Kehlkopfes. In: Berendes, J., R. Link, F. Zöllner: Hals-Nasen-Ohren-Heilkunde in Praxis und Klinik, 2. Aufl., Bd. IV/1. Thieme, Stuttgart 1982

Belenky, W. M., J. E. Medina: First branchial cleft anomalies. Laryngoscope 90 (1980) 28

Berendes, J.: Leitsymptom Kopfschmerz. In: Berendes, J., R. Link, F. Zöllner: Hals-Nasen-Ohren-Heilkunde in Praxis und Klinik, 2. Aufl., Bd. I. Thieme, Stuttgart 1977

Boenninghaus, H. G.: Ohrverletzungen. In: Berendes, J., R. Link, F. Zöllner: Hals-Nasen-Ohren-Heilkunde in Praxis und Klinik, 2. Aufl., Bd. V. Thieme, Stuttgart 1979

Bohnstedt, M.: Krankheitssymptome an der Haut, 2. Aufl. Thieme, Stuttgart 1965

Bordley, J. E. et al.: Ear, Nose and Throat Disorders in Children. Raven Press, New York 1986

Bork, K., N. Hoede, G. W. Korting: Symptome und Krankheiten der Mundschleimhaut und der Perioralregion. Schattauer, Stuttgart 1984

Brandt, R. H.: Endoskopie der Luft- und Speisewege. Springer, Berlin 1985

Braun-Falco, O., G. Plewig, H. H. Wolff: Dermatologie und Venerologie, 3. Aufl. Springer, Berlin 1984

Burgener, F. A., M. Kormano: Röntgenologische Differentialdiagnose, 6. Aufl. Thieme, Stuttgart 1988

Burkhardt, A.: Oral cavity and oropharynx. In: Arnold, W.-J., J. A. Laissue, I. Friedman, H. H. Naumann: Diseases of the Head and Neck. Thieme, Stuttgart 1987

Caldarelli, D. D.: Craniofacial anomalies. Otolaryngol. Clin. N. Amer. 14 (1981) 763

Cembirek, H., F. Frühwald, N. Gritzmann: Kopf-Hals-Sonographie. Springer, Wien 1988

Chandler, J. R., B. Mitchell: Branchial cleft cysts, sinuses and fistulas. Otolaryngol. Clin. N. Amer. 14 (1981) 175

Conley, J.: Salivary Glands and the Facial Nerve. Thieme, Stuttgart 1975

Cooper, B. C.: Nasorespiratory functions and orofacial development, Otolaryngol. Clin. N. Amer. 22 (1989) 413

Dalessio, D. J.: Wolff's Headache and other Head Pain, 4. ed. Oxford University Press, New York 1980

Deck, K. A.: Endokrinologie. Thieme, Stuttgart 1976

Eder, M., P. Gedigk: Lehrbuch der Allgemeinen Pathologie und der Pathologischen Anatomie, 31. Aufl. Springer, Berlin 1984

Eeckhout, van den J., F. Estienne: Diagnostics différentiels. Office International de Librairie, Brüssel 1977

Eichmann, F., U. W. Schnyder: Das Basaliom. Springer, Berlin 1981

Ellis, F. H.: Upper Esophageal Sphincter in Health and Disease. Surg Clin North Am 51 (1971) 553

English, G. M.: Otolaryngology. Harper & Row, Hagerstown 1976

Ewerbeck, H.: Differentialdiagnose von Krankheiten im Kindesalter, 2. Aufl. Springer, Berlin 1984

Feldmann, H.: HNO-Notfälle, 2. Aufl. Springer, Berlin 1981

Ferlinz, R.: Internistische Differentialdiagnostik, 2. Aufl. Thieme, Stuttgart 1989

Fleury, P., Y. Lacomme, F. Legant, J. Marchand, M. Wayoff: Les affections dermatologiques en O. R. L. Librairie Arnette, Paris 1977

Frey, K. W., K. Mees, Th. Vogl: Radiologische Unfalldiagnostik in der HNO-Heilkunde. Aktuelle Oto-Rhino-Laryngologie, H. 10. Thieme, Stuttgart 1988

Germer, W. D., H. Loebe, H. Stickl: Infektions- und Tropenkrankheiten, AIDS, Schutzimpfungen, 3. Aufl., Springer, Berlin 1987

Graf, K., U. Fisch: Geschwülste des Ohres und des Felsenbeins. In: Berendes, J., R. Link, F. Zöllner: Hals-Nasen-Ohren-Heilkunde in Praxis und Klinik, 2. Aufl., Bd. V. Thieme, Stuttgart 1979

Gross, D., R. Frey: Kopfschmerz. Fischer, Stuttgart 1981

Grossmann, W.: Spannungskopfschmerz 1982. IMP Verlagsgesellschaft, Neu-Isenburg 1982

Hanafee, W. N., P. H. Ward: The Larynx. Thieme Medical Publ., New York 1990

Hansen, W. E.: Gastrointestinale Symptome. Springer, Berlin 1984

Hadorn, W., N. Zöllner: Vom Symptom zur Diagnose, 7. Aufl. Karger, Basel 1979

Headache Classification Committee of the International Headache Society: Classification and diagnostic criteria for headache disorders, cranial neuralgias and facial pain. Cephalalgia 8 (1988) Suppl. 7

Heberer, G., W. Köle, H. Tscherne: Chirurgie, 3. Aufl. Springer, Berlin 1980

Heyck, H.: Der Kopfschmerz, 5. Aufl. Thieme, Stuttgart 1982

Hollwich, F.: Augenheilkunde, 11. Aufl. Thieme, Stuttgart 1988

Holt, G. R., D. E. Mattox, G. A. Gates: Decision Making in Otolaryngology. Decker, Philadelphia; Mosby, St. Louis 1984

Hommerich, K. W.: Gutartige Geschwülste der Nase und Nasennebenhöhlen. In: Berendes. J., R. Link, F. Zöllner: Hals-Nasen-Ohren-Heilkunde in Praxis und Klinik, 2. Aufl., Bd. II. Thieme, Stuttgart 1977

Hopf, H. C., G. Haferkamp: Schmerzen im Kopfbereich. In: Ferlinz, R.: Internistische Differentialdiagnostik. Thieme, Stuttgart 1989

Hornstein, O. P.: Entzündliche und systemische Erkrankungen der Mundschleimhaut. Thieme, Stuttgart 1974

Hornstein, O. P.: Klinik und Diagnose des malignen Melanoms. In: Weidner, F., J. Tonak: Das maligne Melanom der Haut. Perimed, Erlangen 1981

Jacoby, H.: Veränderungen der Zunge in der Diagnostik des praktischen Arztes, 2. Aufl., Schattauer, Stuttgart 1960

Jaffé, L.: Hals-Nasen-Ohren-Heilkunde in den Tropen und Subtropen. In: Berendes, J., R. Link, F. Zöllner: Hals-Nasen-Ohren-Heilkunde in Praxis und Klinik, 2. Aufl., Bd. III. Thieme, Stuttgart 1978

Janzen, R., H. A. Kühn: Neurologische Leit- und Warnsymptome bei inneren Erkrankungen. Thieme, Stuttgart 1982

Jawetz, E., J. L. Melnick, E. A. Adelberg: Medizinische Mikrobiologie, 5. Aufl., Springer, Berlin 1980

Kaboth, W., E. Heilmann: Erkrankungen des Blutes. In: Losse, H., E. Wetzels: Rationelle Diagnostik in der inneren Medizin, 3. Aufl., Thieme, Stuttgart 1982

Kecht, B.: Parasitosen. In: Berendes, J., R. Link, F. Zöllner: Hals-Nasen-Ohren-Heilkunde in Praxis und Klinik, 2. Aufl., Bd. III. Thieme, Stuttgart 1978

Keller, W., A. Wiskott: Lehrbuch der Kinderheilkunde, 5. Aufl., hrsg. von K. Betke, W. Künzer. Thieme, Stuttgart 1984

Kirstein, R.: Krankheiten der Lippen und der Mundschleimhaut. In: Berendes, J., R. Link, F. Zöllner: Hals-Nasen-Ohren-Heilkunde in Praxis und Klinik, 2. Aufl., Bd. III. Thieme, Stuttgart 1978

Kleinsasser, O.: Pathologie der Geschwülste des Hirnschädels. In: Handbuch der Neurochirurgie, Bd. IV/1. Springer, Berlin 1960

Kleinsasser, O.: Bösartige Geschwülste des Kehlkopfs und des Hypopharynx. In: Berendes, J., R. Link, F. Zöllner: Hals-Nasen-Ohren-Heilkunde in Praxis und Klinik, 2. Aufl., Bd. IV. Thieme, Stuttgart 1983

Kleinsasser, O.: Tumoren des Larynx und des Hypopharynx, Thieme, Stuttgart 1987

Köhn, K.: Nase und Nasennebenhöhlen, Kehlkopf und Luftröhre. In: Doerr, W., G. Seifert, E. Uehlinger: Spezielle pathologische Anatomie, Bd. IV, Springer, Berlin 1969

Komisar, A.: Nasal obstruction due to benign and malignant neoplasms. Otolaryngol. Clin. N. Amer. 22 (1989) 413

Kuemmerle, H. P., N. Goossens: Klinik und Therapie der Nebenwirkungen, 3. Aufl., Thieme, Stuttgart 1984

Kuriloff, D. B.: Nasal septal perforations and nasal obstruction. Otolaryngol. Clin. N. Amer. 22 (1989) 333

Lee, K. J.: Essential Otolaryngology, 2nd ed. Huber, Bern 1977

Lee, K. F.: Differential Diagnosis in Otolaryngology. Arco, New York 1978

Leiber, B., G. Olbrich: Die klinischen Syndrome, Bd. I u. II. 6. Aufl., Urban & Schwarzenberg, München 1981

Lucente, F. E., S. M. Sobol: Essentials of Otolaryngology. Raven Press, New York 1983

McAuliffe, G. W., H. Goodell, H. G. Wolff: zit. in: Ballantyne, J., J. Groves: Diseases of the Ear, Nose and Throat. 4th ed. Vol. I. Butterworths, London 1979

Male, O.: Medizinische Mykologie für die Praxis. Thieme, Stuttgart 1981

Manz, A.: Gewerbliche Schäden der oberen Luftwege. In: Berendes, J., R. Link, F. Zöllner: Hals-Nasen-Ohren-Heilkunde in Praxis und Klinik, 2. Aufl., Bd. I. Thieme, Stuttgart 1977

Marx, H.: Kurzes Handbuch der Ohrenheilkunde, 2. Aufl., Fischer, Jena 1947

Marx, H.: Nasenheilkunde, Lieferung 1−6. Fischer, Jena 1949−1953

Matthys, H.: Akute Atemnot und ihre pathophysiologischen Grundlagen. In: Ungeheuer, E., H. Walcha: Akute Atemnot. Perimed, Erlangen 1985

Maurer, H.: Entzündungen des Rachens. In: Berendes, J., R. Link, F. Zöllner: Hals-Nasen-Ohren-Heilkunde in Praxis und Klinik, 2. Aufl., Bd. III. Thieme, Stuttgart 1978

May, M.: The Facial Nerve. Thieme, Stuttgart 1986

McConnel, F. M. S., D. Erenko, M. S. Mendelsohn: Manofluorographic analysis of swallowing. Otolaryngol. Clin. N. Amer. 21 (1988) 625

Metzel, E.: Pathologische Prozesse der Schädelbasis. In: Berendes, J., R. Link, F. Zöllner: Hals-Nasen-Ohren-Heilkunde in Praxis und Klinik, 2. Aufl., Bd. VI. Thieme, Stuttgart 1980

Miehlke, A.: Fazialislähmungen. In: Berendes, J., R. Link, F. Zöllner: Hals-Nasen-Ohren-Heilkunde in Praxis und Klinik, 2. Aufl., Bd. V, Thieme, Stuttgart 1979

Miehlke, A., E. Stennert, R. Arold, R. Chilla, H. Penzholz, A. Kühner, V. Sturm, J. Haubrich: Chirurgie der Nerven im HNO-Bereich. Arch. Oto-Rhino-Laryngol. 231 (1981) 89

Moser, F.: Oto-Rhino-Laryngologie, Bd. I u. II. VEB Fischer, Jena 1986

Müller, E.: Narben und Defektbildungen im Mittelohr und begleitende Entzündungen. In: Berendes, J., R. Link, F. Zöllner: Hals-Nasen-Ohren-Heilkunde in Praxis und Klinik, 2. Aufl., Bd. V. Thieme, Stuttgart 1979

Müller, F., O. Seifert: Taschenbuch der medizinisch-klinischen Diagnostik, 71. Aufl., hrsg. von G. A. Neuhaus. Bergmann, München 1985

Mumenthaler, M.: Neurologie, 8. Aufl., Thieme, Stuttgart 1986

Mumenthaler, M.: Neurologische Differentialdiagnostik, 2. Aufl., Thieme, Stuttgart 1983

Mumenthaler, M., F. Regli: Der Kopfschmerz. Thieme, Stuttgart 1990

Mündnich, K., K. Terrahe: Mißbildungen des Ohres. In: Berendes, J., R. Link, F. Zöllner: Hals-Nasen-Ohren-Heilkunde in Praxis und Klinik, 2. Aufl., Bd. V. Thieme, Stuttgart 1979

Nager, G. T., D. W. Kennedy, E. Kopstein: Fibrous dysplasia. Ann. Otol., Suppl. 92 (1982)

Nasemann, Th.: Viruskrankheiten der Haut, der Schleimhäute und des Genitales. Thieme, Stuttgart 1974

Naumann, H. H.: Kurze Pathophysiologie der Nase und ihrer Nebenhöhlen. Banale Entzündungen der Nase und ihrer Nebenhöhlen. In: Berendes, J., R. Link, F. Zöllner: Hals-Nasen-Ohren-Heilkunde, Bd. I. Thieme, Stuttgart 1964

Naumann, H. H., W. H. Naumann: Kurze Pathophysiologie der Nase und ihrer Nebenhöhlen. In: Berendes, J., R. Link, F. Zöllner: Hals-Nasen-Ohren-Heilkunde in Praxis und Klinik, 2. Aufl., Bd. I. Thieme, Stuttgart 1977

Neumann, O. G.: Gutartige Tumoren und Pseudotumoren des Larynx. In: Berendes, J., R. Link, F. Zöllner: Hals-Nasen-Ohren-Heilkunde in Praxis und Klinik, 2. Aufl., Bd. IV. Thieme, Stuttgart 1983

Nolting, S., K. Fegeler: Medizinische Mykologie, 3. Aufl., Springer, Berlin 1986

Noyek, A. M., A. J. Maniglia: Congenital disordes in otolaryngology. Otolaryngol. Clin. N. Amer. 14 (1981) H. 4

Paparella, M. M., D. A. Shumrick: Otolaryngology, Vol. 1–4. 3rd ed. Saunders, Philadelphia 1990

Patten, J. P.: Neurologische Differentialdiagnose. Springer, Berlin 1982

Pauser, G., F. Gerstenbrand, D. Gross: Gesichtsschmerz. Fischer, Stuttgart 1979

Pfaffenrath, V., A. Schrader, I. S. Neu: Primäre Kopfschmerzen. MMV Medizin Verlag, München 1984

Rankow, R. M., I. M. Polayes: Diseases of the Salivary Glands. Saunders, Philadelphia 1976

Reifferscheid, M., S. Weller: Chirurgie, 7. Aufl., Thieme, Stuttgart 1986

Rosemann, G. E., K. H. Vosteen: Spezifische Infektionen der Nase und der Nasennebenhöhlen. In: Berendes, J., R. Link, F. Zöllner: Hals-Nasen-Ohren-Heilkunde in Praxis und Klinik, 2. Aufl., Bd. I. Thieme, Stuttgart 1977

Rosenthal, W., W. Bethmann, A. Bienengräber: Spezielle Zahn-, Mund- und Kieferchirurgie, 3. Aufl. Barth, Leipzig 1971

Rudert, H.: Tumoren der Oropharynx. In: Berendes, J., R. Link, F. Zöllner: Hals-Nasen-Ohren-Heilkunde in Praxis und Klinik, 2. Aufl., Bd. IV/2. Thieme, Stuttgart 1983

Samii, M., P. J. Jannette: The Cranial Nerves. Springer, Berlin 1981

Savary, M., G. Miller: Der Ösophagus. Gassmann, Solothurn 1976

Schmidt, D., J.-P. Malin: Erkrankungen der Hirnnerven. Thieme, Stuttgart 1986

Schuermann, H., A. Greither, O. Hornstein: Krankheiten der Mundschleimhaut und der Lippen, 3. Aufl. Urban & Schwarzenberg, München 1966

Seifert, G.: Mundhöhle, Mundspeicheldrüsen, Tonsillen und Rachen. In: Doerr, W., E. Uehlinger: Spezielle pathologische Anatomie, Bd. I, Springer, Berlin 1966

Seifert, G.: Salivary glands. In: Arnold, W. J., J. A. Laissue, I. Friedman, H. H. Naumann: Diseases of the Head and Neck. Thieme, Stuttgart 1987

Seifert, G., A. Miehlke, J. Haubrich, R. Chilla: Speicheldrüsenkrankheiten. Thieme, Stuttgart 1984

Seiferth, L. B., F. Wustrow: Verletzungen im Bereich der Nase, des Mittelgesichts und seiner Nebenhöhlen sowie frontobasale Verletzungen. In: Berendes, J., R. Link, F. Zöllner: Hals-Nasen-Ohren-Heilkunde in Praxis und Klinik, 2. Aufl., Bd. I. Thieme, Stuttgart 1977

Siebert, K.: Gewerbeerkrankungen der Luftwege. In: Berendes, J., R. Link, F. Zöllner: Hals-Nasen-Ohren-Heilkunde, Bd. I. Thieme, Stuttgart 1964

Siegenthaler, W.: Differentialdiagnose innerer Krankheiten, 16. Aufl., Thieme, Stuttgart 1988

Siewert, R., A. L. Blum, F. Waldeck: Funktionsstörungen der Speiseröhre. Springer, Berlin 1976

Silver, C. E.: Laryngeal Cancer. Thieme Medical Publ., New York 1991

Soyka, D.: Der Gesichtsschmerz. Schattauer, Stuttgart 1973

Soyka, D.: Kopfschmerz. Edition Medizin, Weinheim 1984

Stevenson, D. D.: Allergy, atopy, nasal disease and headache. In: Dalessio, D. J.: Wolff's Headache and other Head Pain, 4. ed. Oxford University Press, New York 1980

Suen, C. E., E. N. Myers: Cancer of the Head and Neck. Churchill Livingstone, New York 1981

Theissing, G., J. Theissing: Spezifische Krankheiten in Mund und Rachen. In: Berendes, J., R. Link, F. Zöllner: Hals-Nasen-Ohren-Heilkunde in Praxis und Klinik, 2. Aufl., Bd. III. Thieme, Stuttgart 1978

Tiedemann, R.: Seröse und seromuköse Entzündungen des Mittelohres. In: Berendes, J., R. Link, F. Zöllner: Hals-Nasen-Ohren-Heilkunde in Praxis und Klinik, 2. Aufl., Bd. V. Thieme, Stuttgart 1979

Ungerecht, K.: Ösophagus. In: Berendes, J., R. Link, F. Zöllner: Hals-Nasen-Ohren-Heilkunde in Praxis und Klinik, 2. Aufl., Bd. III. Thieme, Stuttgart 1978

Vogl, H.: Differentialdiagnose der medizinisch-klinischen Symptome I und II. UTB E. Reinhardt, München 1978

Vosschulte, K., H. G. Lasch, F. Heinrich: Innere Medizin und Chirurgie, 2. Aufl., Thieme, Stuttgart 1981

Walthard, B.: Die Schilddrüse. In: Doerr, W., G. Seifert, E. Uehlinger: Spezielle pathologische Anatomie, Bd. IV. Springer, Berlin 1969

Wey, W.: Schilddrüsenkrankheiten. In: Berendes, J., R. Link, F. Zöllner: Hals-Nasen-Ohren-Heilkunde in Praxis und Klinik, 2. Aufl., Bd. II. Thieme, Stuttgart 1977

Wustrow, F.: Die Tumoren des Gesichtsschädels. Urban & Schwarzenberg, München 1965

Wustrow, F.: Bösartige Tumoren der Nase und ihrer Nebenhöhlen. In: Berendes, J., R. Link, F. Zöllner: Hals-Nasen-Ohren-Heilkunde in Praxis und Klinik, 2. Aufl., Bd. II. Thieme, Stuttgart 1977

Zehm, S.: Geschwülste des Nasenrachens. In: Berendes, J., R. Link, F. Zöllner: Hals-Nasen-Ohren-Heilkunde in Praxis und Klinik, 2. Aufl., Bd. II. Thieme, Stuttgart 1977

Zenner, H. P.: Allergologie in der Hals-Nasen-Ohren-Heilkunde. Springer, Berlin 1987

Differential Diagnosis of Hearing Disorders (K. Schorn)

Biesalski, P., F. Frank: Phoniatrie, Pädaudiologie. Thieme, Stuttgart 1982

Bluestone, C. D., S. E. Stool: Pediatric Otolaryngology. Saunders, Philadelphia 1983

Federspil, P.: Nebenwirkungen in der HNO-Heilkunde. In: Kuemmerle, H. P., N. Goossens: Klinik und Therapie der Nebenwirkungen, 3. Aufl. Thieme, Stuttgart 1984

Gervin, K. S., A. Glorig: Detection of Hearing Loss and Ear Disease in Children. C. C. Thomas, Springfield, IL 1974

Greiner, G.F., C. Conraux, P. Felblot: Zentrale und psychogene Hörstörungen. In: Berendes, J., R. Link, F. Zöllner: Hals-Nasen-Ohren-Heilkunde in Praxis und Klinik, 2. Aufl., Bd. VI/2. Thieme, Stuttgart 1980

Huizing, E.H.: Hereditäre Innenohrschwerhörigkeit. In: Berendes, J., R. Link, F. Zöllner: Hals-Nasen-Ohren-Heilkunde in Praxis und Klinik, 2. Aufl., Bd. VI/2. Thieme, Stuttgart 1980

Ilberg, C. von: Toxische Schäden des Hörorgans. In: Berendes, J., R. Link, F. Zöllner: Hals-Nasen-Ohren-Heilkunde in Praxis und Klinik, 2. Aufl., Bd. VI/2. Thieme, Stuttgart 1980

Koniksmark, B.B., R.J. Gorlin: Genetic and Metabolic Deafness. Saunders, Philadelphia 1976

Lehnhardt, E.: Clinical Aspects of Inner Ear Deafness. Springer Verlag, New York 1984

Shulman, A., J.-M. Aran, J. Tonndorf, H. Feldmann, J.A. Vernon: Tinnitus: Diagnosis, Treatment. Lea & Febiger, Philadelphia 1991

Stange, G., R. Neveling, E.H. Huizing: Hörsturz. In: Berendes, J., R. Link, F. Zöllner: Hals-Nasen-Ohren-Heilkunde in Praxis und Klinik, 2. Aufl., Bd. VI/2. Thieme, Stuttgart 1980

Stephens, S.D.G., L. Luxon, R. Hinchcliffe: Immunological disorders and auditory lesions. Audiology 21 (1982) 128

Differential Diagnosis of Vestibular Disorders (H. Scherer)

Baloh, R.W., V. Honrubia: Clinical Neurophysiology of the Vestibular System. 2nd ed. Davis, Philadelphia 1989

Barber, H.O., J.A. Sharpe: Vestibular Disorders. Yearbook, Chicago 1987

Brandt, Th., W. Büchele: Augenbewegungsstörungen. Fischer, Stuttgart 1983

Brandt, Th., M. Dieterich: Phobischer Attacken-Schwank-Schwindel. Münch. med. Wschr. 128 (1986) 247

Brandt, T.: Vertigo: its multisensory Syndromes. Springer, Berlin 1991

Clark, A.H., W. Tennis, K. Waltmans, H. Scherer: Threedimensional aspects of caloric, nystagmus. Part II: Caloric induced tonic torsional deviation. Acta Otolar (in press)

Dix, M.R., J.D. Hood (Eds.): Vertigo. Wiley, Chichester 1984

Gay, A., N.M. Newman, J.C. Keltner, M.H. Strond: Eye Movement Disorders. Mosby, St. Louis 1974

Graham, M.D., J.L. Kemink (Eds.): The Vestibular System: Neurophysiologie and Clinical Research. Raven Press, New York 1987

Häusler, R., J. Pampurik: Die chirurgische und physiotherapeutische Behandlung des benignen, paroxysmalen Lagerungsschwindels. Z. Laryng. Rhinol. 68 (1989) 349

Honrubia, V., M. Brazien (Eds.): Nystagmus and Vertigo: Clinical Approach to the Patient with Dizziness. Academic Press, San Diego 1982

Kornhuber, H.H.: Vestibular system. In: Handbook of Sensory Physiology, Vol. VI/1 + 2. Springer, Berlin 1974

Leigh, R.I., J.S. Lee: The Neurology of Eye Movements. F.A. Davis, Philadelphia 1991

Marx, P.: Augenbewegungsstörungen in Neurologie und Ophthalmologie. Springer, Berlin 1984

Megighian, D., C.L. Schmidt: Diagnostik der peripheren Vestibularisstörungen. In: Berendes, J., R. Link, F. Zöllner: Hals-Nasen-Ohren-Heilkunde in Praxis und Klinik, 2. Aufl., Bd. VI. Thieme, Stuttgart 1980

Moser, M., G. Ranacher: Die Gleichgewichtsuntersuchung. Maudrich, Wien 1984

Mumenthaler, M.: Neurologische Differentialdiagnostik, 3. Aufl. Thieme, Stuttgart 1988

Mumenthaler, M.: Neurologie, 8. Aufl. Thieme, Stuttgart 1986

Oosterveld, W.J. (Ed.): Otoneurology. Wiley, New York 1984

Pfaltz, C.R., F. Ildiz: The optokinetic Test: Interaction of the Vestibular and Optokinetic System in Normal Subjects and Patients with Vestibular Disorders. Arch. Oto-Rhino-Laryngol. 234 (1982) 21

Poeck, K.: Neurologie. Springer, Berlin 1984

Rudge, P.: Clinical Neuro-Otology. Churchill Livingstone, New York 1983

Sano, K., H. Sekino, Y. Tsukamoto: Stimulation and destruction of the region of the interstitial nucleus in cases of torticollis and see-saw nystagmus. Confin. neurol. 34 (1972) 331

Scherer, H.: Das Gleichgewicht, Teil I. Springer, Berlin 1984

Scherer, H.: Das Gleichgewicht Teil II. Springer, Berlin 1992

Scherer, H.: Nebenwirkungen von Medikamenten auf das Gleichgewicht. Z. Laryng. Rhinol. 65 (1986) 467

Stoll, W., D.R. Matz, E. Most: Schwindel und Gleichgewichtsstörungen. Thieme, Stuttgart 1986

Index

"Vs. (versus)" indicates a specific differential diagnosis.